BLOOD, PURE AND ELOQUENT

BLOOD, PURE AND ELOQUENT

A Story of Discovery, of People, and of Ideas

Maxwell M. Wintrobe
M.D., Ph.D., M.A.C.P., hon. D.Sc.

Member, National Academy of Sciences, U.S.A.
Distinguished Professor of Internal Medicine
College of Medicine
University of Utah

McGraw-Hill Book Company

New York St. Louis San Francisco Auckland Bogotá Hamburg Johannesburg London Madrid
Mexico Montreal New Delhi Panama Paris São Paulo Singapore Sydney Tokyo Toronto

BOWLING GREEN UNIV. LIBRARY

This book was set in Palatino by York Graphic Services, Inc.
The editors were J. Dereck Jeffers and Moira Lerner;
the designer was Joan E. O'Connor;
the production supervisor was Robert A. Pirrung.
R. R. Donnelley & Sons Company was printer and binder.

BLOOD, PURE AND ELOQUENT

1 2 3 4 5 6 7 8 9 0   DODO   8 9 8 7 6 5 4 3 2 1 0

Library of Congress Cataloging in Publication Data

Main entry under title:

Blood, pure and eloquent.

    Includes index.
    1. Blood. I. Wintrobe, Maxwell Myer, date
[DNLM: 1. Blood. WH100.3 B655]
QP91.B656   612'.11   79-21157
ISBN 0-07-071135-6

TO BECKY

CONTENTS

vii

7 Iron and Heme: Crucial Carriers and Catalysts

Irving M. London

8 The Life Span of the Red Blood Cell and Circumstances of Its Premature Death

John V. Dacie

9 Blood and Mountains

Allan J. Erslev

LIST OF CONTRIBUTORS

ERNEST BEUTLER, M.D.
Member, National Academy of Sciences, U.S.A.; Chairman, Department of Clinical
Research, Scripps Clinic and Research Foundation, La Jolla, California

WILLIAM B. CASTLE, M.D., M.A.C.P., hon. F.R.C.P., M.D., D.Sc.
Member, National Academy of Sciences, U.S.A.; Francis Weld Peabody Faculty
Professor of Medicine, Emeritus, Harvard Medical School, Cambridge; Former
Distinguished Physician, U.S. Veterans Administration

C. LOCKARD CONLEY, M.D., F.A.C.P., F.R.C.P.
Distinguished Service Professor of Medicine and Head of the Hematology
Division, Department of Medicine, The Johns Hopkins University School of
Medicine, Baltimore

CHARLES G. CRADDOCK, M.D., F.A.C.P.
Clinical Professor of Medicine, University of California, Los Angeles

WILLIAM H. CROSBY, M.D., F.A.C.P.

Colonel (Ret.), Medical Corps, United States Army; Head, Division of Hematology-Oncology, Scripps Clinic and Research Foundation; Adjunct Professor of Medicine, University of California, San Diego

SIR JOHN V. DACIE, M.D., F.R.S., hon. M.D.

Emeritus Professor of Haematology, University of London; Formerly Head, Department of Haematology, Royal Postgraduate Medical School, London, England

LOUIS K. DIAMOND, M.D., F.A.A.P.

Adjunct Professor of Pediatrics, Research Associate, Cancer Research Institute, University of California, San Francisco; Professor of Pediatrics Emeritus, Harvard Medical School; Former Director, Blood Grouping Laboratory; Former Director, Blood Bank and Transfusion Service, Children's Hospital Blood Center, Boston

ALLAN J. ERSLEV, M.D., F.A.C.P.

Cardeza Research Professor of Medicine; Director, Cardeza Foundation for Hematologic Research, Jefferson Medical College of Thomas Jefferson University, Philadelphia

WILLIAM L. FORD, M.A., D.Phil., M.R.C.P.

Professor of Experimental Pathology, Department of Experimental Pathology, University of Manchester, England

FREDERICK W. GUNZ, M.D., Ph.D., F.R.C.P., F.R.A.C.P., F.R.C.P.A.

Director of Medical Research, Kanematsu Memorial Institute, Sydney Hospital, Australia

GERALD D. HART, M.D., F.R.C.P.(C), F.A.C.P., F.R.A.I., F.R.N.S.

Associate Professor, Department of Medicine, University of Toronto; Physician-in-Chief and Director, Department of Haematology, Toronto East General Hospital, Canada

CHARLES A. JANEWAY, M.D., hon. M.A., M.D.

Professor of Pediatrics, Harvard Medical School; Physician-in-Chief, Emeritus, Senior Associate in Medicine and Immunology, Children's Hospital Medical Center, Boston

LASLO G. LAJTHA, M.D., D. Phil.
Professor of Experimental Oncology, University of Manchester; Director, Paterson Laboratories, Christie Hospital and Holt Radium Institute, Manchester, England

IRVING M. LONDON, M.D., hon. Sc.D.
Member, National Academy of Sciences, U.S.A.; Professor of Medicine, Harvard Medical School; Grover M. Hermann Professor of Health Sciences and Technology and Professor of Biology, Massachusetts Institute of Technology; Director, Harvard-MIT, Division of Health Sciences and Technology; Director, Whitaker College of Health Sciences Technology and Management-MIT, Cambridge, Massachusetts

OSCAR D. RATNOFF, M.D.
Member, National Academy of Sciences, U.S.A.; Professor of Medicine, Case-Western Reserve University, Cleveland; Career Investigator of the American Heart Association

THEODORE H. SPAET, M.D.
Head, Hematology Department, Montefiore Hospital; Professor of Medicine, Albert Einstein College of Medicine, New York

MEHDI TAVASSOLI, M.D.
Associate in Hematology, Scripps Clinic and Research Foundation, La Jolla, California

DAVID J. WEATHERALL, M.D., F.R.C.P., F.R.S.
Nuffield Professor of Clinical Medicine, University of Oxford, England

MAXWELL M. WINTROBE, M.D., Ph.D., M.A.C.P., hon. D.Sc.
Member, National Academy of Sciences, U.S.A.; Distinguished Professor of Internal Medicine, College of Medicine, University of Utah, Salt Lake City

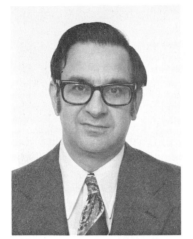

Ernest Beutler

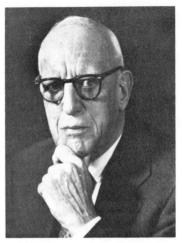

William B. Castle

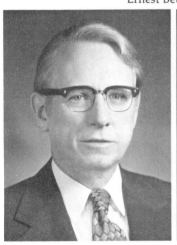

C. Lockard Conley

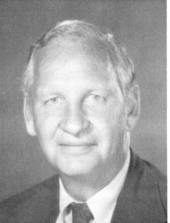

Charles G. Craddock

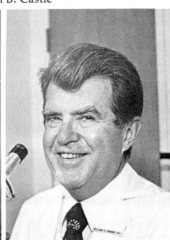

William H. Crosby

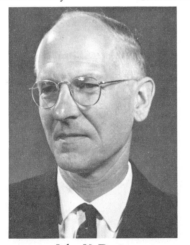

John V. Dacie

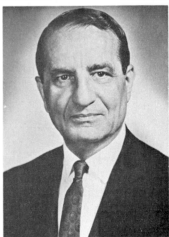

Louis K. Diamond

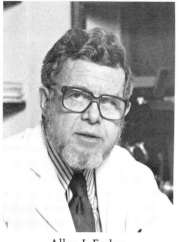

Allan J. Erslev

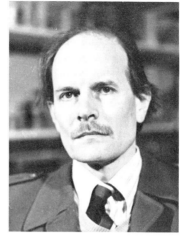

William L. Ford

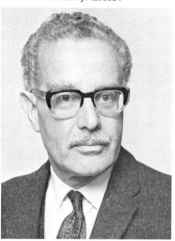

Frederick W. Gunz

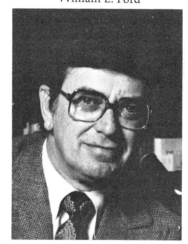

Gerald D. Hart

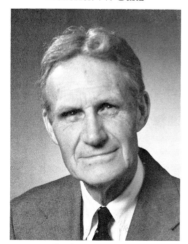

Charles A. Janeway

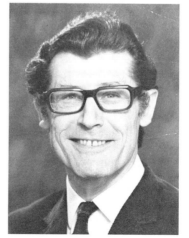

Laslo G. Lajtha

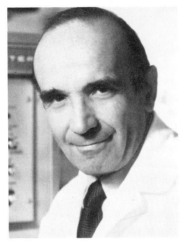

Irving M. London

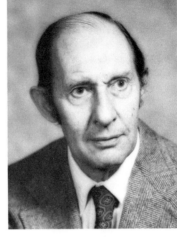

Oscar D. Ratnoff

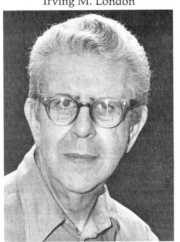

Theodore H. Spaet

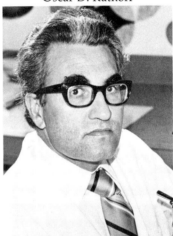

Mehdi Tavassoli

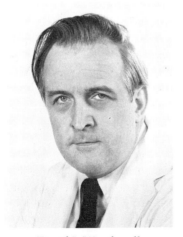

David J. Weatherall

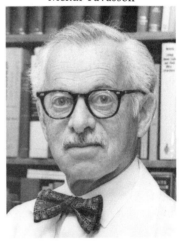

Maxwell M. Wintrobe

PREFACE

Interest in discovery and in its practical consequences has grown tremendously, and the results of research have been widely publicized. What has received less attention is the story of how our knowledge has been gained, the kinds of people who provided the ideas and carried them to fruition, and the circuitous but often exciting path that has been followed to attain what we know today. The story is worth telling.

The present monograph is designed to tell how the study of the blood began, how understanding developed, and what degree of comprehension we have today. Circulating as it does throughout the body and being at the same time that part of ourselves that can be most easily sampled and analyzed, the blood has yielded to research facts of profound significance concerning its components, the blood-forming organs, and the so-called blood diseases, and also about the human organism as a whole.

And what have we learned? Far more than we had ever dreamed of. But in addition we have discovered that everything is vastly more complicated—and more wondrous—than we had imagined. Moreover, each solution has opened the door to still more areas for exploration, more questions to answer. And this has made it all that much more exciting.

The reader, whether layman or scientist, should find the story instructive as well as interesting: the kinds of people who made the significant observations and how they came to do so; how these observations were regarded; what stood in the way of the exploitation of findings; and the totally unpredictable consequences of their development. These, as well as the benefits reaped by mankind, are facts that, if they were not true, would have to be classified as science fiction. At first the growth of knowledge was very slow, but it has accelerated at an ever more rapid pace. The achievements of the past 50 years have been tremendous, and in the last 30 years in particular they have multiplied even more rapidly.

There are now more than the usual reasons for making available this fascinating story. Not only are more and more people becoming interested in information concerning various aspects of science and matters affecting health, but also, more than ever before, the body public is becoming involved in the support of scientific research. This makes it especially desirable—in fact, essential—that people not only learn about the results of research but also understand how that knowledge has been gained.

What few appreciate is that the activities included under the name *research* are very diverse. There is research that truly explores the unknown, asks questions to which there are as yet no answers and requires delving into areas that are obscure and uncharted. At the other extreme is the collection of data that are available for the asking, although they are not yet gathered together in appropriate juxtaposition. The latter calls for effort and funds but not the imagination, the determination, and the stubbornness in the face of opposition and failure which the first may require.

When one questions the unknown, the answer is rarely found quickly. An observation is made, but its meaning and ultimate value are usually not obvious; the analysis of a new observation or a new set of phenomena may be complex, and to a certain extent success may be fortuitous. In pursuing an idea the scientist may start off in one direction, but an unforeseen finding or accidental observation may point the way along a different path. Those who are lost in a dark forest, must use all their senses and all their ingenuity in seeking the clues that may lead them to the light.

Our story is told in a way that intelligent readers, even those with a limited background in science, will in large measure, even though not always in detail, be able to understand. We have sought to explain technical terms in the text as they have been used. In addition, a small glossary is provided. The various chapters have been prepared with the same care as any scientific document, and this has been done by world-renowned experts on the various aspects of hematology. The authors of each of the chapters have themselves participated in and contributed to the advances that have been made in the past 20 to 30 years; some have even been involved as many as 50 years. They are therefore in a position to present a first-hand account. This, significantly, is the period of time during which more has been learned about the blood and blood diseases than in all the preceding centuries for which history is recorded. And yet, as will be seen, it is on that earlier background that the present body of knowledge has been built.

In a book of this kind, photographs of some of the persons who have contributed to the field in an important way add considerable interest. The choice as to which ones should be included, however, is difficult and is one that may not always meet with universal agreement. As a general rule, it has seemed best to exclude photographs of living persons, but in this respect one could not be rigid. In the end, the final choice has been left to the authors of each of the chapters.

When I presented the idea of a collection such as the present one to an old friend, Dr. John Bowers, president of the Macy Foundation, I found not only wholehearted encouragement and enthusiastic support but also many very useful suggestions. Moreover, in a short time the Macy Foundation provided generous financial support, for which I express sincere thanks.

This volume is the outgrowth of discussions initiated originally with Lockard Conley, Clement Finch, Ernest Simon, and Wolf Zuelzer and subsequently with other colleagues, especially William B. Castle. I am deeply indebted to all of these friends and to many others. I wish also to express my appreciation for help and advice in regard to the early historical material in Chapter 1 to Professor Owsei Temkin, Professor Emeritus of the History of Medicine, Johns Hopkins University. I am especially grateful to Elena (Mrs. Carlos) Eyzaguirre, librarian at the Spencer Eccles Library of the University of Utah College of Medicine, without whose unflagging and always willing and efficient assistance my task would have been immensely more difficult. I am happy also to acknowledge the help of my secretary, Judy Staples, and to thank Ruth Henson for some editorial assistance. Still others whose help I should mention include the staff of the National Library of Medicine in Bethesda, Maryland, and Dr. Peter Reizenstein of Stockholm, Sweden. With great pleasure, I acknowledge the wholehearted cooperation of the publishers, the McGraw-Hill Book Company, and the McGraw-Hill Book Company staff.

Finally, I cannot begin to thank sufficiently the authors of the various chapters in this book for their hard work. Fortunately, as they have said themselves, they found their efforts extremely enjoyable and rewarding. In particular, I thank them for their patience with the editor, whose demands must have seemed interminable. Obviously, without their skillful explorations and lucid accounts, the book would not have been written.

Maxwell M. Wintrobe, M.D.

BLOOD, PURE AND ELOQUENT

CHAPTER 1

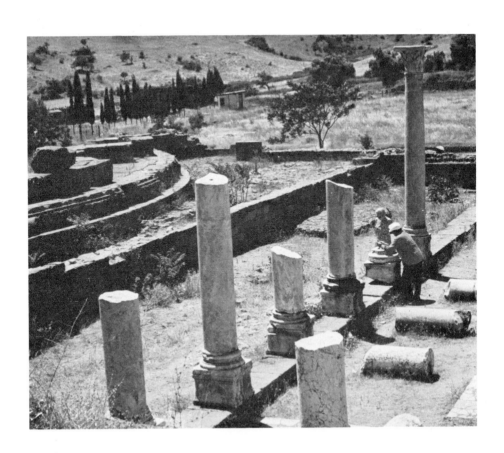

MILESTONES ON THE PATH OF PROGRESS

Maxwell M. Wintrobe

The blood has always fascinated humanity. Blood has been regarded as a living substance, the very essence of life. Poets have written of thick blood and thin, pale blood, red blood and blue blood, royal blood, and pure and eloquent blood. Goethe[1] regarded blood to be "ein ganz besondrer Saft."

It was John Donne,[2] poet of seventeenth-century England, who spoke of pure and eloquent blood:

. . . her pure and eloquent blood,
Spoke in her cheekes, and so distincktly wrought,
That one might almost say, her bodie thought.

But it is for the scientist that the blood has been especially eloquent. As the series of essays that follows will show, the study of the blood and of disorders usually regarded as "blood diseases" has led to discoveries of great practical importance, discoveries that have had such seminal consequences that whole new fields of science have been opened or their development has been immeasurably enhanced. Molecular biology is just one example of the latter.

This should come as no surprise. Irvine Page[3] called the blood "the

Chapter Opening Photo   The Aesculapium at Pergamum in 1968.

circulatory computer tape" that carries coded messages, cellular and humoral, to integrate and to serve the intricate demands of the various organs and tissues of the body. Easily obtained by sterile puncture of a vein with a hollow needle or from fingertip with a lancet, the blood is readily accessible for study.

Ancient Concepts

It is reasonable to assume that even millennia before anything was known about its circulation or its functions, blood was regarded as essential for life. In addition to food and air, which primitive peoples no doubt recognized as necessary for survival, they must have noted that there is a substance within the body that is a vital fluid. They must have recognized that when enough blood was lost, life ceased. Quite early also, the blood seems to have been thought to be related to the heart, that mysterious organ whose motion ceased as life ended. This association is suggested by a drawing of a mammoth by an Aurignacian man in a cave of Paleolithic times in northern Spain.[4]

Most of what has been transmitted to us regarding ancient beliefs about blood dates back only a few millennia. That the Sumerians (third millennium B.C.) paid attention to it is indicated by their pictograph for blood, $\wedge$ (a branching blood vessel?).[5] According to ancient Hebrew thought, blood was the vital principle, identical with the soul, and the drinking of blood was prohibited.[6] The Bible uses the term *to shed blood* in the sense of "to kill." As judged by the Papyrus Ebers from Thebes (about 1550 B.C.),[7] the Egyptians thought that food in the stomach is turned into blood by the heart. Opinions about the content of the blood vessels differed, but a widely held belief was that expressed by Erasistratus (ca. 310–250 B.C.). He held that the arteries contained air (pneuma), this being sublimated as the "vital spirit" after leaving the lung; the veins carried the blood.[8]

Underlying the various speculations regarding biology was the pervading concept of matter. This was founded on the interrelationship of the four elements, fire, earth, water, and air. As Sigerist[9] pointed out, these elements surely must have played an important part in the thinking of many peoples. However, it is Empedocles of Agrigentum (504–443 B.C.) who, possibly influenced by Egyptian and Babylonian philosophies as well as by the earlier pre-Socratic philosophers such as Thales, is credited with having put forward clearly a concept of the Creation that was based on the interrelationship of fire, earth, water, and air.[10]

This theory was accepted as a very workable concept for interpreting the cosmos, the world as a whole. Compatible with, and perhaps arising from, this concept of matter was the doctrine of the four humors which were thought to constitute the human body. This doctrine is set out clearly in one of the Hippocratic writings (about 400 B.C.), and was systematized into a complex pattern by Galen (ca. A.D. 130–200).[11] In this form, the doctrine of the four humors reigned for about 1400 years, dominating medical thinking even to the time of Sydenham (1624–1689). It was believed that the body is made up of four humors, blood, phlegm, black bile, and yellow bile; health and disease were seen as the consequence of the proper equilibrium or imbalance, respectively, of these four components. Like the four elements, the four humors were regarded as possessing the four basic qualities, namely, hot, cold, moist, and dry.[12] Remnants of the humoral theory of antiquity still survive in the words *sanguine, phlegmatic, melancholic,* and *bilious.*

Fahraeus[13] (no ancient despite his name but the twentieth-century Swedish physician who devised the erythrocyte sedimentation test) made the interesting suggestion that the theory of the four humors was based on clinical observation rather than solely on speculation. He pointed out that when blood is allowed to flow into a tall transparent container, it first seems to be a homogeneous red fluid but that after clotting and clot retraction, a clear yellow fluid appears. At the bottom of the vessel, a deep red, almost black, jellylike material collects. Above this is a thinner layer of red blood. Still nearer the top of the clot, a pale green or whitish layer may be discerned, especially if the subject of the venesection has been ill (Figure 1-1).

Here we can see the separation of the blood into the "four humors" as it loses its "innate heat and dies," to quote the ancient philosophers. From the bottom to the top, we now know that the four layers consist of deoxygenated red cells; red cells possessing more oxygen and therefore red; other cellular elements and fibrin; and, finally, blood serum. It is easy to see how they could have been named black bile, sanguis or blood, phlegm, and yellow bile.

Because the phlegm or pale greenish layer, the *crusta phlogistica* (as it later

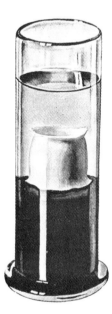

Figure 1-1 The appearance of blood after clotting in a large vessel, showing the dark red cells at the bottom, somewhat lighter-colored red cells above, the layer of white cells and fibrin above these, and the blood serum. (*From Fahraeus, R.: The suspension stability of blood, Acta Med Scand 55:1–228, 1921.*)

came to be called), consists mainly of white blood cells and fibrin, it was more readily seen in sick people. The assumption that this was the *cause* of illness, rather than a manifestation of disease, is easy to understand. It would not be the last time that cause and effect would be confused.

Such concepts quite naturally harmonized with the idea of bloodletting as a means of ridding the body of its fouled fluids. Phlebotomy (bloodletting) can be traced back to the earliest days of medicine;[14] it was actively practiced by the Hippocratic school (Figure 2-2). It was a practice that continued even into the nineteenth century. The drawing of the "bloodletting man" in the calendar of Regiomontanus (1475) showed the points of election for bloodletting as related to the signs of the zodiac.[15] Strongly advocated by the renowned American physician and signer of the Declaration of Independence Benjamin Rush (1745–1813), venesection, together with copious purging, was almost universally practiced in the treatment of the victims of yellow fever during the 1793 epidemic in Philadelphia; it likely played a significant role in the high mortality. As a result of such well-intentioned therapy,[16] many victims were literally bled to death.[17]

As described in the next chapter, the earliest anticipation of the good to be gained by the opposite, blood transfusion, was suggested, according to one view, by the myth which gave Asclepius, the Greek god of medicine, credit for reviving the dead by means of the Gorgon's blood.[18] How Harvey's account of the circulation of the blood (1628) led to the transfusion of blood in humans is fully described in a most interesting fashion by Dr. Diamond in Chapter 19. The ultimate death in Paris of a deranged man who had been transfused in December 1667 by Jean-Baptiste Denys with the blood of a calf,[19] and the furor which this raised, slowed that form of therapy for a hundred years.

Clinical descriptions of conditions now considered to be blood disorders can be found in the writings of the ancients. Thus, the interdiction in the Babylonian Talmud[20] of circumcision if it had been fatal in two successive sons indicates an awareness of a familial bleeding disorder, now termed hemophilia. Paleopathologists have found among ancient remains manifestations of disorders which are now considered as affecting the blood-forming system. In the next chapter, Hart describes some of the objects of art and coins, medals, and votives as well as paintings that provide clues about the illnesses from which our ancestors suffered.

HIPPOCRATES, GALEN, AND THE LATER AGES

Among the ancients, the supernatural and the magical dominated their concepts of disease. The introduction of a new approach has been attributed to Hippocrates (460–375 B.C.).[21] The origins of this famous teacher are uncertain; we do know he was born on the island of Cos and was one of the physicians who considered Asclepius (Asklepios, Aesculapius), the mythical god of healing,[22] their patron. The Asclepiads claimed descent, at least spiritual descent, from him.

Hippocrates' reputation is based on the Hippocratic writings,[23] but whether any were written by him is a moot question. His "Works" nevertheless represent the best of medicine at that time. Observation and reasoning, rather than mysticism, were emphasized; no doubt in the course of time the Asclepiads accumulated a large body of observations, for some of the physicians of Hippocrates' time were keen observers. They made careful and systematic examinations of their patients' conditions, and some of their descriptions of disease have hardly been improved to this day. A critical attitude of mind began to emerge, and failures were described as well as successes.

The greatest scientific name after Hippocrates is that of Aristotle (384–322 B.C.), another Asclepiad, but Aristotle was at his weakest in physics and physiology, contributing more in embryology insofar as medicine was concerned.[21] Thus it was that, after the time of Hippocrates and of Aristotle, the center of Greek medicine moved to Alexandria, where attention was given to anatomical studies. Then, well into the second century A.D., a number of great practitioners of Greco-Roman medicine became renowned, such as Rufus of Ephesus, who lived during the reign of Trajan (A.D. 98–117),[24] and Soranus.[25]

After Hippocrates, however, the most distinguished medical figure was Galen[11] (ca. A.D. 130–200). He was born in the Greek city of Pergamum in Asia Minor (Chapter Opening Photo) and was schooled there as well as in Smyrna and in Alexandria, and his renown spread throughout the Europe of the day. His main contribution lay in his anatomical studies; in his experiments, such as the effects of transection of the spinal cord at different levels; and in his insistence that medicine must be based on theory *and* experience. He was a brilliant observer and a wise physician; he introduced an elaborate system of polypharmacy founded on the knowledge of his predecessors and on his own acquaintance with the therapeutic effects of plants and herbs, accumulated as the result of his travels. He also developed a system of pathologic physiology, which he based on his own observations and upon the doctrine of the four humors, as well as on Platonic and Aristotelian principles. Many of his observations were astute; however, as would be expected, his philosophical system was not free from contradictions and, unfortunately, much was in error. Nevertheless, Galen's system preserved the idea of medicine as a unit.

So great was Galen's reputation that his views held sway for more than 14 centuries. Physicians in later times rarely questioned his authority. Consequently, the practice of founding one's medical judgments on observation and reason and of profiting from experience gradually died out; for many succeeding centuries the advance of medical knowledge practically came to a standstill. Even Rhazes (850–932),[26] Avicenna (Ibn Sina, 980–1037)[27,28] and Maimonides (1135–1204),[29] all outstanding physicians of their day, mainly codified the medical knowledge of their times, generally attempting to fit it with the observations of Hippocrates and the system of Galen. The intellectual liberation from scholasticism, which Roger Bacon (1214–1294) attempted to initiate in the thirteenth century, was a very slow process. It took Paracelsus (1493–1541) to dare to discard Galenism and the four humors.[30]

As mentioned earlier, the contents of the veins and arteries were not regarded as identical by the Ancients. According to Galen, the veins contained blood, a blend of blood in the strict sense and of more or less of the other humors, together with some smoky "pneuma" (spirit).[31] The veins carried the food for most of the organs. On the other hand, the arteries contained a refined vaporous blood together with a finer pneuma and maintained the vital activities and body heat. It took William Harvey (1578–1657) to convincingly describe the circulation of the blood from the heart through the lungs and back to the heart and then into the arteries and back through the veins;[32] he emphasized that the "pneuma" did not exist independently of the blood and that both the arteries and veins contained only one substance, namely the blood.

Harvey, however, did not know how the arteries and veins are connected; it was only later that Marcello Malpighi described the capillaries (Chapter 17). Furthermore, Harvey was not able to explain satisfactorily the difference in the color of venous and arterial blood. Even the speculations made later in the seventeenth century on the various chemical particles and the revelations of microscopy did not essentially alter the old idea of the blood as a "living substance." Harvey believed that ". . . life . . . resides in the blood (as we are also informed in our sacred writings). . . . blood is the generative part, the fountain of life, the first to live, the last to die, and the primary seat of the soul."[33] In a similar way, John Hunter, the leading surgeon and medical scientist of the eighteenth century, believed that the blood was connected with the principle of life. Only with the discovery of the process of oxidation in 1775 and, years later, after the recognition of hemoglobin and of its unique property with respect to oxygen, as will be described below, was insight gained regarding the primary function of the red corpuscles in the transport of oxygen. It is, therefore, not difficult to understand that even in the early nineteenth century, the ancient beliefs still persisted, and many and varied human ailments were attributed to disorders of the blood. Even today the concept that "the blood is bad" as an explanation for troubling symptoms is not unusual.

The Dawning of Microscopy

For the field of hematology, the invention of the microscope was of unique significance. With it, a world was disclosed that even the most imaginative students of nature had not conceived. In a sense, that farseeing monk of the thirteenth century, Roger Bacon, might be considered the inventor of the simple microscope, for he described the use of single convex lenses.[34] However, he was imprisoned, and his writings remained hidden. Consequently, beyond the use of such lenses as spectacles and hand magnifiers, little was accomplished in microscopy until Zacharias Janssen, a spectacle maker of Middleburg, Holland, together with Hans Lippershey in 1590 invented a means for combining glass lenses in a tube to make an instrument for magnifying minute objects. In 1665, Robert Hooke, the Curator of the Royal Society of London, described a greatly improved compound microscope. However, these early compound microscopes had limited usefulness.[35] Magnifications were usually of the order of 30 diameters, the field was far from flat, and objects appeared to be surrounded by fringes of color *(chromatic aberration)*. Other faults were those caused by *spherical aberration,* arising from the fact that a lens brings axial rays to a different focus than marginal ones, thereby causing poor image quality, and *coma,* which refers to the appearance of a smear of light resembling a comet where there should be a small circle. These microscopes served well enough for the examination of insects and plants, and these became objects for the attention of many amateur naturalists, whose reports were beautifully illustrated. Swammerdam's *Book of Nature* contains many fine examples of this work.[36] Elegantly designed instruments, like those of Madame de Pompadour[37] and of George III,[38] also were produced, and it became fashionable to marvel at the design of a bee's wing or the body of a louse.

For these reasons, until 1830,[39] when Joseph Jackson Lister, a wine merchant and the father of the famous Lord Lister, showed how one could combine lenses of different light dispersion in a way that avoided the faults described above, the single-lens simple microscope proved to be the more useful instrument. Although the field of view was much smaller than that seen through the compound microscope, the image was not distorted and magnifications of 300 to 400 diameters could be achieved. However, the effectiveness of a simple microscope (Figure 1-2) depended on the skill with which the lens was ground and on the manner of illumination.

ANTONJ VAN LEEUWENHOEK

Especially skillful and indefatigable in the grinding of lenses was Antonj van Leeuwenhoek (1632–1723) (Figure 1-3), chamberlain (janitor) of the Council Chamber of the Worshipful Sheriffs of Delft, Holland, and otherwise employed in a linen drapery shop.[40] The Dutchman Jan Swammerdam (1637–1680) and the Italian Marcello Malpighi (1628–1694) are often credited with describing the red blood corpuscles before Leeuwenhoek, but Swammerdam only referred to the presence of ''ruddy globules'' in the blood and doubted that blood in its vessels contains such globules,[36] while Malpighi's interest seems to have been only casual. It is Leeuwenhoek, therefore, who

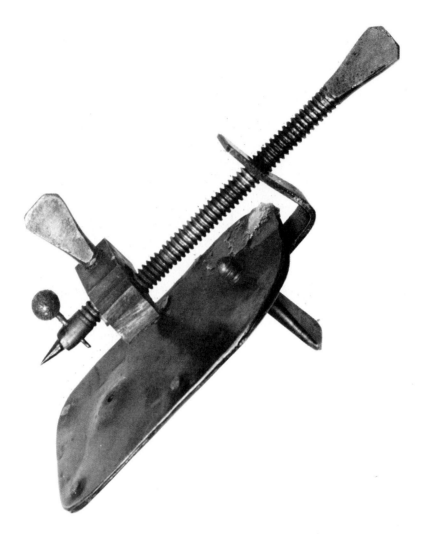

Figure 1-2 Leeuwenhoek's microscope consisted of two plates $1\frac{3}{16}$ x $\frac{3}{4}$ inch, rivetted together, between which a $\frac{1}{16}$ inch biconvex lens was fixed. To these plates an L-shaped brace was fixed. From the top of the L a $1\frac{3}{4}$ inch screw extended to a block in the center of the plate. Through the block, a $\frac{1}{2}$ inch-long pointed screw was inserted and on this the object to be examined was fixed. (*Courtesy of the Smithsonian Institution, Washington, D.C.*)

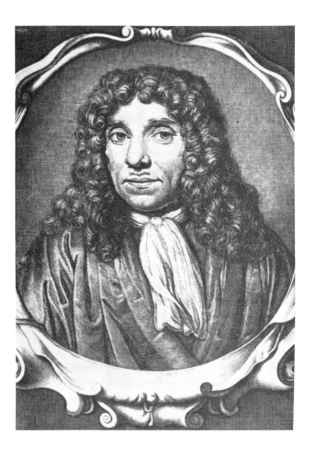

Figure 1-3 Antonj van Leeuwenhoek (1632–1723). *(Courtesy of Dr. Marcus Jacobson.)*

deserves the credit for having provided the first real description of the red
blood cells.*[41] He was untutored and had had little formal education, but he
was a person of infinite curiosity and patience.[40,42] He examined his own
blood, described the red corpuscles, and even measured their diameters, doing
this with remarkable accuracy. How he accomplished this is unclear, for
Leeuwenhoek kept the details of his method secret.[40] His microscopes consisted of a minute biconvex lens mounted between two thin oblong plates of
brass or other metal. To this, mechanical accessories for focusing the object to
be viewed were fixed. In his first report,[41] he described how he drew blood
into a glass "pipe" (pipette) "not thicker than a man's hair" and how he
attached this to the pin of his microscope with the aid of his "spittle." One
marvels how he managed so successfully to display before his magnifying lens
the objects he chose to study. How he illuminated them he never divulged.

* "The Blood is composed of exceeding small particles, named globules, which, in most animals
are of a red color, swimming in a liquor, called by physicians, the serum. . . . These particles or
globules are so minute that 100 of them, placed side by side, would not equal the diameter of a
common grain of sand; consequently, a grain of sand is above a million times the size of one such
globule."

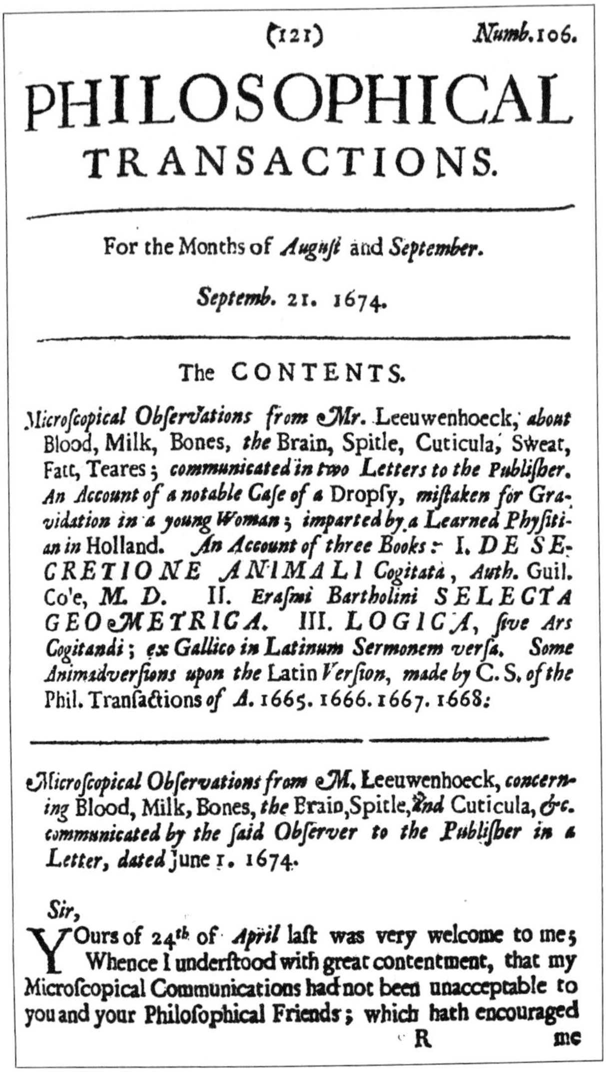

(121)   *Numb.* 106.

PHILOSOPHICAL
TRANSACTIONS.

For the Months of *August* and *September.*

Septemb. 21. 1674.

The CONTENTS.

Microfcopical Obfervations from &Mr. Leeuwenhoeck; *about* Blood, Milk, Bones, *the* Brain, Spitle, Cuticula; Sweat, Fatt, Teares; *communicated in two Letters to the Publifher. An Account of a notable Cafe of a* Dropfy, *miftaken for Gravidation in a young Woman; imparted by a Learned Phyfitian in* Holland. *An Account of three Books:* I. *DE SE-CRETIONE ANIMALI Cogitatâ, Auth.* Guil. Co'e, *M. D.* II. *Erafmi Bartholini SELECTA GEOMETRICA.* III. *LOGICA, five Ars Cogitandi; ex Gallico in Latinum Sermonem verfa. Some Animadverfions upon the* Latin *Verfion, made by* C. S. *of the* Phil. Tranfactions *of A.* 1665. 1666. 1667. 1668:

Microfcopical Obfervations from &M. Leeuwenhoeck, *concerning* Blood, Milk, Bones, *the* Brain, Spitle, *and* Cuticula, &c. *communicated by the faid Obferver to the Publifher in a Letter, dated* June 1. 1674.

Sir,

YOurs of 24ᵗʰ of *April* laft was very welcome to me; Whence I underftood with great contentment, that my Microfcopical Communications had not been unacceptable to you and your Philofophical Friends; which hath encouraged
                                                     · R   me

Figure 1-4 Leeuwenhoek's first report of his microscopical observations. (*Courtesy National Library of Medicine, Bethesda, Md.*)

Perhaps he employed some form of dark-field illumination.[43] He did not seem to find useful the globules of molten glass which Father de la Torré presented to the Royal Society, and neither did Hewson.[44]

That the observations of this self-made scientist became known is a tribute to the remarkable open-mindedness of the Fellows of the Royal Society of London, to whose secretary Leeuwenhoek's friend, the physician Reinier de Graaf, submitted Leeuwenhoek's letter describing his observations (Figure 1-4). This was the first of no less than 375 communications from Leeuwenhoek which were published in the society's *Transactions* in the succeeding 50 years.

Thus it was that the tiny constituents of the blood, the so-called red corpuscles (the erythrocytes), which carry oxygen about the body, were first seen; and it was with similar rudimentary equipment that the cells concerned with the defenses of the body, discussed in Chapter 13, the "white" or colorless corpuscles (the leukocytes) may have been observed, perhaps first by Malpighi and by Leeuwenhoek, but certainly by William Hewson. Platelets, the tiny translucent objects which participate in stemming the flow of blood from its natural paths, to be discussed in Chapter 16, were discovered only after Lister devised a means for greatly improving the compound microscope.[38]

MICROSCOPY AFTER 300 YEARS

It is unnecessary to discuss here all the improvements and modifications that have come about in the field of microscopy. These have made it possible to achieve magnifications of 50,000 diameters and greater and to visualize the three-dimensional configurations of the blood cells as well as intimate details of their structure. These tiny globules, whose very existence was once questioned, and whose significance was long doubted, later, with the development of staining methods, became the main focus of attention during the morphologic era of hematology.

For microscopic examination, the blood usually was spread in a thin film on glass slides (the *blood smear* of routine blood examination), allowed to dry, and then was stained with various dyes. Much was learned from the study of these "flattened, brilliantly colored cadavers," as Bessis[45] called them. With the introduction of phase contrast and electron microscopy, however, still another world was opened up. It became possible to visualize the intricate inner structure of the cells: the nucleus that contains, through its content of deoxyribonucleic acid (DNA), the "blueprint" of the cell and controls the synthetic activities specific for that cell; the mitochondria, which supply the necessary energy; the ribosomes and Golgi complex, which manufacture proteins; the microfilaments and vacuoles, which are concerned with the cell's movement as well as with the entry and exit of various materials into and out of the cell; the lysosomes, which serve as organs of digestion; and the plasma membrane of the cell (Figure 1-5). The discovery of the extraordinarily complex inner structure of these cells, coordinated with information derived by other means, like the initial discovery of the microscope, has opened new vistas and has provided a degree of insight about the role of the cells of the blood in biology that has proved to be of unparalleled importance.

WILLIAM HEWSON

Of several persons who have come to be called the "father of hematology," William Hewson (1739–1774) was the first (Figure 1-6). The son of an apothecary and surgeon in Northumberland, he came to London at the age of 20 and

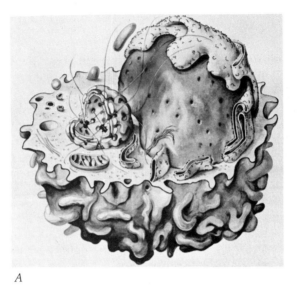

A

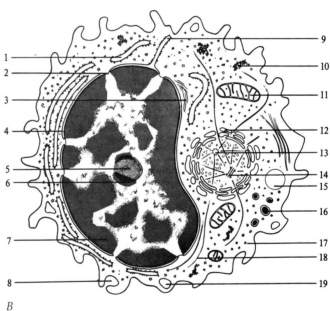

B

Figure 1-5 (*A*) Three-dimensional model of a lymphocyte. (*B*) Diagram of a section of a lymphocyte, based on electron microscopic examinations: (1) rough endoplasmic reticulum (RER), (2) nuclear pore, (3) microfilaments, (4) nuclear envelope, (5) nucleolus, (6) perinuclear chromatin, (7) chromocenter, (8) beginning of pinocytosis, (9) RER communicating with nuclear envelope, (10) aggregate of glycogen, (11) mitochondrion, (12) Golgi complex, (13) centriole (cut transversely), (14) centriole (cut longitudinally), (15) contractile vacuole, (16) lysosome, (17) polyribosome, (18) microtubule, and (19) end stage of pinocytosis. (*Reproduced by permission from Bessis, M: Blood Smears Reinterpreted. Springer International, 1977.*)

became associated with the famous Hunters, John and then William, participating with them in dissection, in teaching, and in research.[46] He discovered
the lacteal and lymphatic vessels in birds, reptiles, and fishes; he examined the
red blood corpuscles with improved lenses,[44] noting that in serum they were
flat rather than globular; and he described the leukocytes. Because leukocytes
are few in number as compared with the red corpuscles, and are colorless, they
are easily overlooked. He contrived to observe them by diluting blood with
serum rather than water, as others had done. His most important contribution,
however, was his demonstration of the essential features of blood coagulation,[47,48] thus proving that it is due to the clotting of the plasma rather than
because of changes in the cellular constituents, as will be explained in Chapter
18. In addition, as described in Chapter 14, his observations on the anatomy
and the functions of the lymphatic system were remarkably accurate, and his
ideas regarding the thymus were prophetic of concepts that only began to take
hold almost 200 years after his death. Hewson, whose treatise on the lymphatic system was dedicated to Benjamin Franklin, married the daughter of the
lady in whose home the American representative resided during his 15 years
in London. Unfortunately, Hewson died at the age of 35, at the peak of his
career, from an infection sustained during dissection.

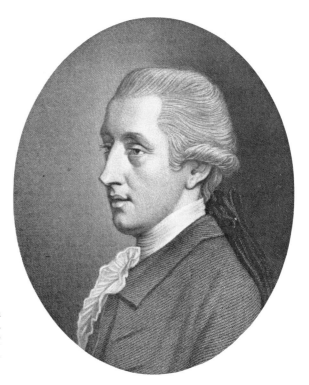

Figure 1-6 William Hewson
(1739–1774), "father of hematology." *(Courtesy National
Library of Medicine, Be-
thesda, Md.)*

EARLY REACTIONS TO MICROSCOPY

In spite of the observations of Leeuwenhoek, Hewson, and others, progress was extremely slow. Not only were technological advances very gradual, but, for more than 2 centuries after the red blood corpuscles were first described, disclosures about the world of the infinitely small, like the earlier revelations of the telescope, strained even great minds to an unacceptable degree. Hewson wrote: "Some have gone so far as to assert that no credit could be given to microscopes, that they deceive us by representing objects different from what they really are."[44] Even in 1829 Goethe wrote:[49] "Microscope and telescope confuse in reality the pure human judgment." * Although Hippocrates, as long before as the Golden Age of Greece, stressed the importance of observation, few trusted what they could see for themselves and, instead, put their faith in dogma and hypothesis. Those who thought for themselves and observed nature, rather than accepting the concepts of the past, often suffered ignominy and were soon forgotten.

Of course, a few voices made themselves heard. Thus, Hewson insisted that the "small round globules" which Malpighi, Swammerdam, and Leeuwenhoek had observed in the blood must be "of great use" because they were found "so generously" among all species of animals.[44] An early clue to that function was provided by Richard Lower (1631–1691), who, in 1669,[50] noted that exposure of venous blood to air in the lungs or in the bleeding basin restored its arterial crimson. This was a century before Lavoisier[51] demonstrated in 1775 that animal life is a process of oxidation. Recognition of the presence of iron in the blood has been attributed to Nicolas Lémery (1645–1715);[52] and Otto Funke[53] in 1851 discovered hemoglobin, the main constituent of the red corpuscles. However, it was the investigations of Felix Hoppe-Seyler (1825–1895)[54] that were epochal in the sense that they demonstrated the significance of these findings. He showed that hemoglobin has the property of readily taking up and discharging oxygen. This made understandable the ancient concept that the arteries contain *air* ("pneuma") and the veins, *blood*. Ultimately, the red blood corpuscles came to be recognized as uniquely designed vehicles for the transport of oxygen throughout the body. The manner in which they carry this vital substance and yet consume essentially none of it themselves, as well as other aspects of the continuing growth of understanding about the functions of these structures, will be found in Chapters 6 and 7.

Introduction of Quantification

These early observers laid the first milestones along the path of progress. The introduction of quantification as a supplement to observation was the next important step in the study of the blood. As we have seen, study of the

---

* "Mikroskope und Fernrohre verwirren eigentlich den reinen Menschensinn."

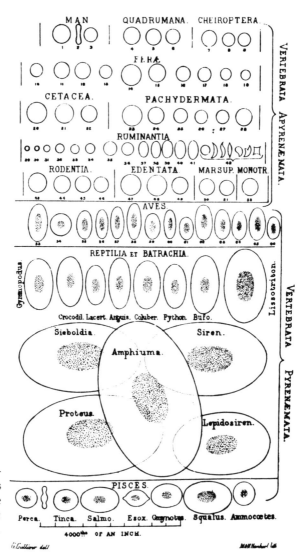

Figure 1-7 Gulliver's observations on the sizes and shapes of the red corpuscles of the blood of vertebrates. *(From Gulliver, G: Proc Zoological Soc, London, 1875, p. 474.)*

invisible world was made possible by the single-lens microscope. But it was only after 1830 that the principles were determined whereby an achromatic objective could be produced; then, as Robb-Smith has pointed out,[38] "The optical instrument makers lost no time in providing scientists with microscopes which would further their enquiries. . . ." Then it became possible for William Addison[55,56] (Chapter 13) and George Gulliver[57,58] to describe their observations on the "rough or granulated, colourless corpuscule"[56] (the

COURS

DE

MICROSCOPIE

COMPLÉMENTAIRE DES ÉTUDES MÉDICALES

ANATOMIE MICROSCOPIQUE ET PHYSIOLOGIE

DES

FLUIDES DE L'ÉCONOMIE

PAR

AL. DONNÉ

DOCTEUR EN MÉDECINE, EX-CHEF DE CLINIQUE DE LA FACULTÉ DE PARIS,
PROFESSEUR PARTICULIER DE MICROSCOPIE, ETC.

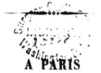

A PARIS

CHEZ J.-B. BAILLIÈRE

LIBRAIRE DE L'ACADÉMIE ROYALE DE MÉDECINE.
RUE DE L'ÉCOLE-DE-MÉDECINE. 17

LONDRES, CHEZ H. BAILLIÈRE, 219, REGENT-STREET

1844

Figure 1-8 Title page of Donné's syllabus for his course on microscopy. (*Courtesy National Library of Medicine, Bethesda, Md.*)

modern granulocyte) and on the 8 or 10 times smaller "loose or independent molecules"[56] (the platelets). Gulliver[58] also published detailed measurements of the sizes of the red corpuscles in various species of animals[59] (Figure 1-7).

It was in Europe that the earliest steps were taken to enumerate the constituents of the blood. Thus, in 1851, Karl Vierordt[60] published the first blood cell counts, and a few years later Welcker[61] reported blood counts and hemoglobin estimations in many different diseases. At first the methods employed were ingenious but time-consuming and quite tedious. Vierordt's procedure required 3 hours or more to complete. He used a capillary pipette calibrated in diameter but not in length; the latter had to be laboriously determined by placing it beside a micrometer on the microscope stage. The contents of the pipette were expelled onto a flat slide where they were mixed with diluting and preserving fluid, and the entire spread was then counted with the aid of a finely squared micrometer in the eyepiece of the microscope.

In the course of the next 60 years, a multitude of modifications of this basic procedure were introduced; they are described in great detail by Gray.[62] For measuring, or for measuring and mixing blood, pipettes were designed which held a fixed volume. For counting the blood, a great variety of ruled chambers of a uniform, known depth were devised, and various diluting solutions were introduced. For the measurement of hemoglobin, devices were designed that attempted to match against arbitrary standards the intensity of its color when released from the red cells. Among the contributors to these technological developments were Cramer, Potain, Malassez, Hayem and Nachet, Gowers, Thomas Bürker, and Neubauer.

Even before improved methods for enumerating cells became available, however, there were a few men of imagination who foresaw the usefulness of microscopy for the study of disease and the potential utility of qualitative and quantitative examinations of the blood. Thus, Alfred Donné (1801–1878) organized classes in clinical microscopy and put together a syllabus[63] (Figure 1-8), while Gabriel Andral (1797–1876) (Figure 1-9) published a monograph on hematology[64] (Figure 1-10). In the latter, anemia in pregnancy, in lead poisoning, and in other conditions was discussed, and, among other topics, he noted the remarkably small size of the red corpuscles in chlorosis, the "green sickness," which was such a popular subject of the artists of the sixteenth and

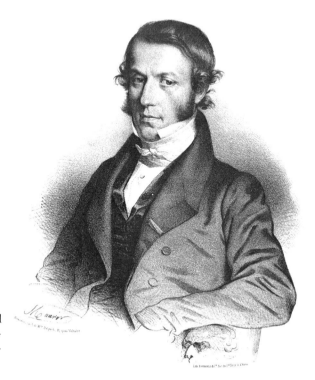

Figure 1-9 Gabriel Andral (1797–1876). (*Courtesy National Library of Medicine, Bethesda, Md.*)

seventeenth centuries, especially those of the Flemish school.[65] Even the possibility that anemia results from excessive destruction of red cells was considered by Andral.

The ideas of Andral and Donné represented an important and revolutionary departure in clinical medicine. Although by the nineteenth century, the constituents of the blood had begun to interest the natural scientist, many of the leading physicians were still suspicious and mocked those who saw the potential value of the microscope.[66] For the most part, it was regarded as an amusing plaything rather than a scientific instrument. Andral remarked that his elders rejected the microscope as useless and feared it as a source of error,[64] while Donné stated in regard to his teaching of microscopy that he "founded this teaching at my cost, my risks and perils."* Nevertheless, he wrote, he

* "J'ai fondé cet enseignement à mes frais, à mes risques et périls;"

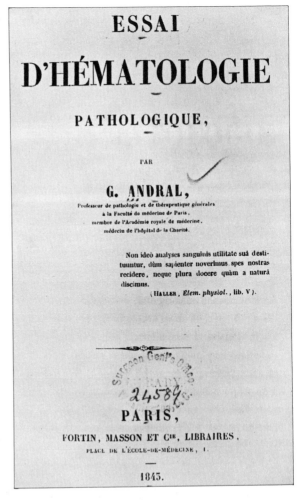

ESSAI

D'HÉMATOLOGIE

PATHOLOGIQUE,

PAR

G. ANDRAL,

Professeur de pathologie et de thérapeutique générales
à la Faculté de médecine de Paris,
membre de l'Académie royale de médecine,
médecin de l'hôpital de la Charité.

Non ideò analyses sanguinis utilitate suâ destituuntur, dùm sapienter noverimus spes nostras recidere, neque plura docere quàm a naturâ discimus.
(HALLER , Elem. physiol., lib. V).

24589

PARIS,

FORTIN, MASSON ET Cⁱᵉ, LIBRAIRES,
PLACE DE L'ÉCOLE-DE-MÉDECINE, 1.

1843.

Figure 1-10 Title page of the first monograph on hematology. *(Courtesy National Library of Medicine, Bethesda, Md.)*

drew great satisfaction from his efforts despite the indifference and obstacles with which he was met.[63] It is true, of course, that the technology employed was crude. It would be another 90 years before something approaching accuracy came into general use and before normal values for red cells, hemoglobin, leukocytes, and platelets, based on the examination of statistically significant numbers of healthy individuals of different ages and sexes, began to be established. However, it was people like Donné, Andral, and Piorry,[67] as well as Vierordt, Welcker, and others, who foresaw the potential of the new approach and labored to demonstrate its value.

The Era of Morphologic Hematology

Notwithstanding the atmosphere of skepticism and the general unwillingness of many of the physicians of the time to entertain new ideas, by the middle of the nineteenth century investigations were begun by a number of scientists that would profoundly influence the future course of medicine. This was especially apparent in Germany. It was a time of political unrest, and the ferment affected scientific thought as well. The contributions of Henle, the anatomist; Helmholtz and Ludwig, the physiologists; Liebig, the chemist; Virchow, the pathologist; and Frerichs, Traube, and Wunderlich, the clinicians, are respected today, as they came to be then.[68] Of these great people, Rudolph Virchow[69] (1821–1902) was a particularly prominent figure. He was noted not only for his emphasis on the essential role of alterations in cells, the basic components of tissues and organs, in the development of disease but also for his encouragement of those who wished to test hypotheses, including his own. His willingness to alter his views when shown to be in error was unusual. His interests were universal and included such diverse areas as politics and archaeology. He even dug for a time with Schliemann in Troy. His name will appear repeatedly in the chapters that follow, for example, in relation to the investigations of Metchnikov (Chapter 13) and in connection with the description of leukemia (Chapter 15).

PAUL EHRLICH

It was into such an atmosphere that Paul Ehrlich (1854–1915) was born.[68] A young man of great intelligence and exceptional dedication, he was a model of Virchow's principle, as expressed in Virchow's graduation thesis: "A Life Filled with Toil and Work Is Not a Burden but a Blessing."[69] As a student in Breslau, Ehrlich came under the influence of Ferdinand Cohn, often regarded as the greatest botanist of all time after Linnaeus; here he also was associated with Rudolf Heidenhain, successor to Purkinje, the teacher of Pavlov, and Julius Cohnheim, one of the greatest of all experimental pathologists and a pupil of Virchow.[70,71] This was a period in which research was venerated, and the system of medical education encouraged good students to find their own way, free from spoon-feeding.

It was at this time that an important technological advance was made. By furnishing a means for the differential staining of the cells in tissue specimens, thereby illuminating their study, the newly developing German chemical industry, which had just discovered the aniline dyes, provided a boon to microscopy.[72] Ehrlich's cousin Carl Weigert, 9 years his senior and an assistant of Julius Cohnheim, already was one of the masters in developing methods for staining tissues and was one of Ehrlich's mentors. Thus it was that in 1877, while he was still a medical student, Ehrlich developed a triacid stain that permitted the clear definition of the nucleus, the cytoplasm, and the other details of cells in thin dried films of blood.[73] With the aid of the greatly improved compound microscopes by then available, this technique permitted him to discover features in the blood that had hitherto been unseen and unsuspected. He differentiated various types of white cells in the blood (Chapter 13)[74] and described the cells of the blood in health and disease, including the nucleated red cells characteristic of the bone marrow in pernicious anemia *(megaloblasts);*[75] he was the first to distinguish aplastic from the other forms of anemia and made many other contributions to clinical hematology.[76] His name will appear repeatedly in these pages.

In their day these contributions marked the beginning of a new era in hematology. And yet they represented only a small part of Ehrlich's contributions to medical science. For example, his concept of molecular structure and his studies of the oxygen consumption of specific tissues[77] anticipated the dawning of a new science, *cytochemistry;* his genius in formulating scientific hypotheses laid the foundations for the disciplines of *immunology* and of *chemotherapy.* It is said that he approached research like a detective on a trail, and it is not surprising that his favorite diversions were the novels of Conan Doyle, whose signed portrait hung on the wall of his study.

Ehrlich's longtime secretary Martha Marquardt has furnished a delightful account of this great man.[78] He was a person who, even from his student days, concentrated his efforts and worked with burning intensity at a pitch of constant excitement. So great was his early fascination and concentration on tissue staining that had he not had the support and encouragement of one of his early professors, Waldeyer, his failure to attend the lectures of his teachers might have caused him great difficulties in medical school. So focused was his drive and so unconcerned was he about his surroundings that he not only always had stains on his hands and his clothing from the dyes with which he was experimenting, but, in his unheeding concentration on his goal, even the table in Waldeyer's laboratory became covered with spots of all colors, as did the towels in the room of the inn where he later lived in Leipzig and the billiard table on which, for lack of any other place to work, he conducted some of his experiments. His laboratory was always stacked with bottles and papers; there was scarcely an empty chair on which to sit (Figure 1-11). Yet, although his laboratory appeared crowded, disorganized, and confused, he knew where to find whatever he wanted. It is not surprising that a servant attempting to clean

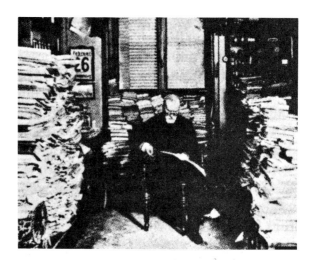

Figure 1-11 Paul Ehrlich (1854–1915) in his study. (*Reproduced from Marquardt, M. Paul Ehrlich. New York, Henry Schuman, 1951.*)

his laboratory inadvertently lit the small iron stove on which he happened to have left some slides to dry, for lack of a suitable stand. He had been attempting unsuccessfully to stain a sputum specimen from a patient with tuberculosis and proposed to examine it the next morning. Imagine his consternation, soon turned to amazement, when he looked at his dried, and now heated, slides and found the bacilli stained with the acidic dye. As a result of this accident, the method for staining tubercle bacilli was discovered, which medical students for many subsequent decades were taught to employ in the study of their patients.

Ehrlich's path through life was not a smooth and easy one, but, fortunately, there were people of understanding and influence who recognized his unusual attributes so that means continued to be found which permitted him to pursue his investigations. Fortunately he required little equipment, and he was satisfied with simple facilities. Visitors frequently expressed their astonishment at the simplicity of his laboratory. Although during his lifetime Ehrlich was acclaimed and received many honors, including the Nobel Prize in medicine and physiology, his last years were unhappy ones. Because his concepts were novel and imaginative, it was natural that they were attacked. His treatment for syphilis ("606," "914"), which was only replaced several decades ago by the discovery of penicillin, supplied ammunition to his critics, for it was not free from serious adverse side effects.

Ehrlich has been called the father of hematology, of immunology, and of chemotherapy. Few men have contributed so much to the health of humanity. The introduction of Ehrlich's staining techniques was quickly appreciated and facilitated the work of such giants as Aschoff, Maximow, Pappenheim, and others, whose contributions will be discussed in these pages. These techniques initiated what has been called the morphologic era of hematology.[79] In the last quarter of the nineteenth century and for several decades of the present one, hematologists became absorbed in viewing and interpreting the colorful and fascinating panorama of cells which can be seen in the blood, both in health and in disease. As an aid in discovering the presence and nature of various types of infection, as well as an indication of the response of the body to such infections and to other disorders, and even as measures of prognosis, the differential leukocyte counts, which Ehrlich's procedures made possible, have proved to be of immense value.[80]

The half-century that followed the introduction of staining procedures, including the staining of living tissues *(vital staining)*, was one of considerable progress to which many contributed, for example, Georges Hayem (1841–1935)[81] (Figure 1-12), Florence Sabin (1871–1953),[82] Hal Downey (1877–1959),[83] and many others. Nevertheless, it is astonishing to realize how relatively little

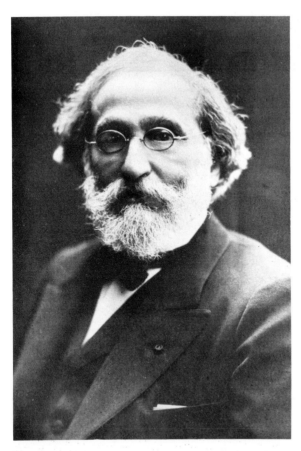

Figure 1-12 Georges Hayem (1841–1935). Another "father of hematology."

additional *understanding* about most disorders of the blood had been achieved even in the 50 years after Ehrlich's important contributions. The relevant sections of Osler's *Principles and Practice of Medicine*, published in 1928, differ little from those pages in the first edition, published in 1892.[84] The morphologic alterations of the blood in disease had been beautifully described, but the causes of the changes observed still were obscure. Fifty years ago, clinical examinations provided superb illustrations of the incisive perceptions of which the trained human being is capable; the outstanding clinicians were amazingly astute. Nevertheless, beyond painstaking microscopic observations of the patient's blood, little else of a laboratory nature was done. Physiologic measurements at the clinical level were primitive or nonexistent, not only in the field of hematology but also in most of the other branches of medicine. Furthermore, the techniques for making quantitative blood examinations were still crude and even the so-called normal values for red blood cell counts and hemoglobin levels were mainly guesses, based on a half-dozen measurements made 75 years earlier.[85] Hemoglobin values determined by very crude methods were expressed in percent of normal, even though no adequately founded standard of normal had been established. Anemias were classified as *primary* or *secondary*, but this served only to distinguish the more severe cases of pernicious anemia from other forms of anemia and fostered confusion rather than providing illumination. Understanding of the leukemias, lymphomas, and bleeding disorders was no better.

The Modern Era

Insofar as it is possible to set a date, the modern era of hematology may be said to have begun in 1926 with the announcement of an important discovery. Some years before, George Whipple (1878–1976) had begun a quantitative study of foods that favor hemoglobin production; he had found liver to be particularly effective. The subsequent application of his observations to the treatment of pernicious anemia by George Minot (1885–1950) and his associates, together with the ingenious experiments of William Castle (1897–   ), which were designed to gain an understanding of the pathogenesis of this disease, excited everyone's imagination and virtually revolutionized the field of hematology. These achievements set the stage for a new era. It is of relatively little moment today that liver was effective in pernicious anemia for a very different reason than that which caused hemoglobin production in Whipple's dogs. What mattered was the fact that *investigation*, based on painstaking observation and measurement, would be the rule of the future. The story is told in Chapter 10.

Starting in the 1920s, from the descriptive discipline dominated by the study of blood cell morphology that it had been, hematology began to be transformed into a science founded on quantitative measurement that employs physiologic and biochemical methods with all their refinements. Improved methods of blood examination were introduced; especially useful in this respect was the hematocrit devised by Wintrobe.[86] This provided a simple and accurate method for determining the relative quantities of red cells and plasma in a specimen of blood. The hematocrit also served as the basis for calculating the average size and hemoglobin content of the red cells and led to his introduction of the indexes MCV (mean corpuscular volume), MCH (mean corpuscular hemoglobin), and MCHC (mean corpuscular hemoglobin concentration) that now are used universally. A logical consequence was the development of a system for classifying the various anemias according to both morphologic and etiologic criteria[87] and the establishment for the first time of statistically valid standards of normality of the blood in men, women, and children of different ages. In this way the study of anemia was given a rational basis. Armed with these more accurate quantitative assessments, and aided by a growing understanding of the physiology of the blood and the hematopoietic system, physicians began to think about disorders of the blood in physiologic and quantitative terms.

As will be related in the chapters that follow, beginning in the 1930s new knowledge concerning the physiology of the blood, the blood-forming organs, and the diseases affecting them, developed at an ever accelerating pace. The vacuum, however, at first was enormous and much had to be learned. So great was our ignorance that, in the light of what is understood today, even in mid-century the deficiencies were profound. Thus, as recently as 1951[88] the manner in which hemoglobin is held within the red blood corpuscle was in doubt. Whether the erythrocyte possesses a definite membrane was debated. The uniqueness of the mammalian red corpuscle as a carrier of oxygen that consumes essentially no oxygen itself was appreciated; yet it was not realized that its efficiency in the transport of a cargo with a potential for its own oxidative destruction is related in large measure to the nonoxidative metabolism of glucose. As discussed in Chapter 6, we now know that instead of being an inert particle, the red corpuscle possesses a sequence of enzymes on which its active metabolism is based. In addition, we now know that anemias caused by increased red cell destruction may result from a variety of inherited deficiencies of one of these enzymes. Also, several disorders of the red cell membrane, hereditary in nature or acquired, have been postulated, and the fascinating structure of hemoglobin itself has been elucidated. The various abnormal hemoglobin disorders (see Chapter 11) and thalassemia ("Mediterranean" anemia, Cooley's anemia, in Chapter 12) represent a wholly new or greatly broadened area of knowledge. Similarly, in striking contrast to the period before 1926 and even in comparison with what was known at the time the third edition of my textbook of hematology was published in 1951,[88] in our understanding of the process of coagulation, related in Chapter 18, the function of the platelets (in Chapter 16), and the defense mechanisms of the body and the role the leukocytes play in this respect (Chapters 13 and 14), as well as in many other areas, the field of hematology today is in a greatly accelerated and most exciting phase of growth.

Practical benefits have also accrued. With the discovery of liver extract and, later, of folic acid, effective treatment of pernicious anemia and of nutritional anemias became possible; and with the isolation of vitamin B_{12}, the beneficial effects of liver were explained, and therapy became simplified and convenient. Furthermore, observations concerning the effect of folic acid on tumor growth[89] led to the development and production of *folic acid antagonists*,[90] substances which interfere with cell growth, as discussed in Chapter 15.

The study of agents capable of interrupting the growth of cells had actually begun after World War I as a result of the investigations of the biologic effects of poison gases. During World War II the destructive effects of the so-called nitrogen mustards on lymphoid tumors were observed,[91,92] and out of these investigations modern chemotherapy and the burgeoning field of oncology arose.

Beginning with the study of a white blood cell, the lymphocyte, whose nature and functions long were enigmatic, the field of immunology, both humoral and cellular, was born and continues to flourish (Chapter 14). The discovery of the blood groups, including the Rh and other factors, has made possible advances in the technology of blood transfusion and also has provided a means for the treatment of hemolytic disease of the newborn and even the prevention of this frightening threat (Chapters 19 and 20). The new insights regarding immunology, advances in the technology of blood transfusion, and greater understanding of the process of coagulation have made possible the extraordinary contributions of modern surgery and the development of organ transplantation techniques. In Table 1-1, some of these developments are outlined.

The course of discovery in various areas of hematology has often been circuitous but always fascinating. Entirely unforeseen vistas of understanding have resulted from the quests to answer seemingly uncomplicated questions. Investigations begun at the bedside have led to completely unexpected additions to our knowledge, and research directed towards the blood diseases has led to important developments in other disciplines, such as those of nutrition and human genetics. Thus, investigations of the sickling phenomenon, begun at the bedside, eventually led to the discovery that a specific alteration in a normal molecule can produce such ill effects as to result in serious disease; so Linus Pauling's term *molecular disease* was coined (Chapter 11). This and many other ramifications of the new approaches to the study of disease that saw their first use in the field of hematology will be described in the various chapters that follow.

Table 1-1 *Some ramifications of research on blood*

ORIGINAL RESEARCH	PROGRESSIVE PHASES OF INVESTIGATION		APPLICATION
Blood clotting and bleeding disorders →	Recognition of multiple clotting factors	Better understanding of bleeding disorders (e.g., hemophilia)	Purification of clotting factors; Improved diagnosis	Specific and simplified treatment of hemophilia, etc.; Genetic counseling
	Study of factors interfering with coagulation of blood	Study of means of preventing thrombosis	Application in therapy	Coronary occlusion; Pulmonary embolism; Thrombophlebitis; Strokes; Open heart surgery
Blood transfusion →	Discovery of blood groups A, B, AB, O; Rh factors; others	Improved collection and preservation of blood; Blood banks	Component therapy (red cells, platelets, white cells, albumin, globulin, etc.); Understanding of hemolytic disease of newborn (HDNB)	Facilitation of cancer therapy, transplantation, surgical procedures; Forensic medicine; Prevention of HDNB
Role of foods in production of hemoglobin (Hgb) →	Liver therapy of pernicious anemia (PA)	Discovery of folic acid, vitamin B$_{12}$	Simplified treatment of ....; Development of folic acid antagonists of cell growth	Nutritional anemias, pernicious anemia; Chemotherapy of leukemia and other malignancies

Nature of:
sickle-cell anemia
thalassemia → Recognition of molecular diseases → Growth of science of molecular biology
Study of hereditary mechanisms for globin synthesis → Flourishing of human genetics research → Antenatal diagnosis
Genetic counseling

Mode of action of:
mustard gas
nuclear energy → Understanding of their effects on cell growth → Development of various alkylating agents → Treatment of malignant tumors (leukemias, Hodgkin's disease, breast, colon, etc.)
Development of radioisotopes → Use of radioisotopes in diagnosis and treatment

Search for antimalarial compounds → Discovery of glucose-6-phosphate dehydrogenase (G6PD) deficiency → Understanding of red cell anaerobic metabolism → Discovery of nature of: hereditary hemolytic anemias and, by use as cell "marker," other diseases

References

1   Goethe JW von: *Faust* (1808). Hrsg, und erläutert von Erich Trunz, Hamburg, C. Wegner, 1949, part I, line 1740.
2   Donne J: The second anniversary, line 244, in Manley F (ed): *The Anniversaries (1611–1612)*. Baltimore, The Johns Hopkins Press, 1963, 209 pp.
3   Page IH: Blood—the circulatory computer tape. *Perspect Biol Med* 15:219–220, 1972.
4   Breuil H, Obermaier H: *The Cave of Altamira at Santillana del Mar, Spain*. Madrid, Tip. de Archivos, 1935, plate XIX.
5   Majno G: *The Healing Hand*. Cambridge, Harvard University Press, 1975, 571 pp, p 59.
6   Leviticus 17:14.
7   Ebbell B (trans): *The Papyrus Ebers*. Copenhagen, Levin and Munksgaard, Ejnar Munksgaard, 1937, 135 pp.
8   Garrison FH: *An Introduction to the History of Medicine*, 4th ed. Philadelphia, Saunders, 1929, 996 pp, p 103.
9   Sigerist HE: *A History of Medicine*. New York, Oxford University Press, 1961, vol II, 352 pp, p 200.
10 Sigerist, ibid., p 104.
11 Siegel RE: *Galen's System of Physiology and Medicine*. Basel and New York, S. Karger, 1968, 419 pp.
12 Sigerist, op. cit., pp 317–335.
13 Fahraeus R: The suspension stability of the blood. *Acta Med Scand* 55:1–228, 1921.
14 Sigerist, op. cit., vol I, 564 pp, p 116.
15 Garrison, op. cit., p 200 (illustration).
16 Holmes C: Benjamin Rush and the yellow fever. *Bull Hist Med* 40:246–263, 1966.
17 Powell JH: *Bring Out Your Dead*. Philadelphia, University of Pennsylvania Press, 1949, 326 pp.
18 Sigerist, op. cit., vol II, p 44.
19 Denys J: Lettre Écrite à Monsieur de Montmor, touchant deux expériences de la transfusion faites sur les hommes, Paris, 1668; lettre touchant une folie inveterée qui a eté guérie depuis peu par la transfusion du sang. Paris, Jean Cusson, 12 Janvier, 1668.
20 Garrison, op. cit., p 70.
21 Garrison, op. cit., pp 92–101.
22 Sigerist HE: *The Great Doctors*. New York, WW Norton, 1933, 422 pp, pp 22–28.
23 Adams F: *The Genuine Works of Hippocrates*, trans from the Greek, with a preliminary discourse and annotations. New York, W. Wood, 1891, 2 vols, 390 pp, 366 pp.
24 Talbott, JH: *A Biographical History of Medicine. Excerpts and Essays on the Men and Their Work*. New York, Grune and Stratton, 1970, 1211 pp, p 10.
25 Sigerist, *The Great Doctors*, pp 61–67.
26 Talbott, op. cit., p 18.
27 Talbott, ibid., p 20.
28 Sigerist, *The Great Doctors*, pp 78–87.
29 Rosner F, Muntner S: *The Medical Aphorisms of Moses Maimonides*. New York, Yeshiva University Press, 1970, vol 1, 265 pp and vol 2, 244 pp.
30 Garrison, op. cit., pp 204–207.

31 Temkin O: On Galen's pneumatology. *Gesnerus* 8:180–189, 1951.

32 Garrison, op. cit., pp 246–248.

33 *The Works of William Harvey, M.D.*, Willis R (trans). London, Sydenham Society, 1847, pp 376–377.

34 Haden RL: The origin of the microscope. *Ann Med Hist*, Ser. 3, 1:30–44, 1939.

35 Bracegirdle B: The performance of seventeenth- and eighteenth-century microscopes. *Med Hist* 22:187–195, 1978.

36 Swammerdam J: *The Book of Nature; or, The History of Insects*, Floyd T (trans). London, CG Seyffert, 1758, pp xx, 236, 153, lxii, p 31.

37 Dreyfus C: *Some Milestones in the History of Hematology*. New York, Grune and Stratton, 1957, 87 pp, p 28.

38 Robb-Smith AHT: Why the platelets were discovered. *Br J Haematol* 13:618–637, 1967.

39 Bracegirdle B: JJ Lister and the establishment of histology. *Med Hist* 21:187–191, 1977.

40 Dobell C: *Antony van Leeuwenhoek and his "Little Animals."* New York, Dover, 1960, 435 pp, pp 313–338.

41 Leeuwenhoek A van: Microscopical observations. *Philos Trans R Soc Lond* 9:121–128, 1674; Hoole S (trans): *The Select Works of Antonj van Leeuwenhoek Containing his Miscroscopical* [sic] *Discoveries in Many of the Works of Nature*, London, published by the author, in 2 vol, vol I 1798, vol II 1807, vol I, p 89.

42 Bender GA, Thom RA: *Great Moments in Medicine*. Detroit, Northwood Institute Press, 1966, 421 pp, pp 108–114.

43 Casida LE Jr: Leeuwenhoek's observation of bacteria. *Science* 192:1348–1349, 1970.

44 Hewson W: On the figure and composition of the red particles of the blood, commonly called the red globules. *Phil Trans 63* (part II):303–323, 1773.

45 Bessis M: *Blood Smears Reinterpreted*, Brecher G (trans). Berlin, Heidelberg, New York, Springer International, 1977, 270 pp.

46 Talbott, op. cit., pp 311–314.

47 Hewson W: *Experimental Inquiries*. Part 1, 2d ed. London, T Cadell, 1772, 223 pp. Part 2, *Containing a Description of the Lymphatic System*. London, J Johnson, 1774, 239 pp. Part 3, *Description of the Red Particles of the Blood* [*posthumous*, F Magnus (ed)]. London, T Longman, 1777, 144 pp.

48 Gulliver G: *The Works of William Hewson, F.R.S.* London, The Sydenham Society, 1846, part III, lvi, 360 pp, p 214.

49 Goethe JW: *Werke, Maximen und Reflexionen.* Hamburg, Wegner Verlag, 1963, vol XII, p. 418.

50 Lower R: Tractatus de corde (Latin). London, J. Allestry, 1669, 220 pp, pp 170 et seq.

51 Lavoisier AL: Sur la nature du principe qui se combine avec les métaux pendant leur calcination, et qui en augmente le poids (a). *Histoire de l'academie royale des Sciences, 1775*, Paris, 1778, pp 520–526.

52 Garrison, op. cit., p 284.

53 Funke O: Über das Milzvenenblut. *Z Rat Med* 1:172–218, 1851.

54 Hoppe-Seyler F: Über die Oxydation in lebendem Blute. *Med-chem Untersuch Lab* 1:133–140, 1866–1871.

55 Addison W: Colourless globules in the buffy coat of the blood. *Lond Med Gaz NS* 27:477–479, 1840–1841.

56 Addison W: On the colourless corpuscles and on the molecules and cytoblasts in the blood. *Lond Med Gaz NS* 30:144–148, 1841–1842.

57 Gerber F: *Elements of General and Minute Anatomy of Man and the Mammalia*, With notes and an appendix comprising observations on the blood, chyle, lymph &c, &c, by Gulliver G. London, H Baillière, 1842, vi 71 pp, xvi 390 pp, app 106 pp.

58 Gulliver G: *Gulliveriana: An Autobiography*. Canterbury, 1881. Quoted in Robb-Smith, Why the platelets were discovered.

59 Gulliver G: Observations on the sizes and shapes of the red corpuscles of the blood of vertebrates, with drawings of them to a uniform scale, and extended and revised tables of measurements. London, *Proc Zool Soc*, 474, 1875.

60 Vierordt K: Zählungen der Blutkörperchen des Menschen. *Arch Physiol Heilk* 11:327–331, 1852.

61 Welcker H: Blutkörperchenzählung und farbeprüfende Methode. *Vrtljschr Prakt Heilk* 44:11–80, 1854.

62 Gray H: Cell-counting technic: a study of priority. *Am J Med Sci* 162:526–557, 1921.

63 Donné A: *Cours de Microscopie complémentaire des Études medicales*. Paris, Baillière, 1844, 550 pp.

64 Andral G: *Essai d'Hématologie pathologique*. Paris, Fortin, Masson et Cie Lib, 1843, 186 pp.

65 Fowler MM: Chlorosis—an obituary. *Ann Med Hist* 8:168–177, 1936.

66 Dreyfus, op. cit., p 21.

67 Piorry PA: *Traité de Médecine pratique et de Pathologie iatrique ou medicale*, Cours professé a la faculté de médecine de Paris. Paris, Pourchet & J-B. Baillière, 1841–1851, 8 v., 8° Atlas, 42 pl.

68 Temkin O: The era of Paul Ehrlich. *Bull NY Acad Med* 30:958–967, 1954.

69 Talbott, op. cit., pp 681–684.

70 Talbott, ibid., pp 709–711.

71 Jokl E: Paul Ehrlich—man and scientist. *Bull NY Acad Med* 30:968–975, 1954.

72 Rhoads CP: Paul Ehrlich in contemporary science. *Bull NY Acad Med* 30:976–987, 1954.

73 Ehrlich P: Beitrag zur Kenntnis der Anilinfärbungen und ihrer Verwendung in der mikroskopischen Technik. *Arch Mikr Anat* 13:263–277, 1877.

74 Ehrlich P: Methodologische Beiträge zur Physiologie und Pathologie der verschiedenen Formen der Leukocyten. *Z Klin Med* 1:553–560, 1879–1880.

75 Ehrlich P: *Farbenanalytische Untersuchungen zur Histologie und Klinik des Blutes*. Berlin, A Hirschwald, 1891, 137 pp.

76 Himmelweit F (ed): *The Collected Papers of Paul Ehrlich*. London, Pergamon Press, 1956, vol I, pp 1–286.

77 Ehrlich P: *Das Sauerstoff-Bedürfniss des Organismus. Eine farbenanalytische Studie*. Berlin, A Hirschwald, 1885, 167 pp.

78 Marquardt M: *Paul Ehrlich, With an Introduction by Sir Henry Dale*. New York, Henry Schuman, 1951, 255 pp.

79 Sabine JC: A history of the classification of human blood corpuscles. *Bull Hist Med* 8:696–720, 785–805, 1940.

80 Wintrobe MM: Diagnostic significance of changes in leukocytes. *Bull NY Acad Med* 15:223–240, 1939.

81 Dreyfus C: Georges Hayem (1841–1935). *J Lab Clin Med* 27:855–865, 1942.
82 Sabin FR: On the origin of the cells of the blood. *Physiol Rev* 2:38–69, 1922.
83 Wells, LJ, McKinlay CA: Hal Downey, Ph.D. *Journal-Lancet,* 80:445–448, 1960.
84 Osler W: *Principles and Practice of Medicine,* 1st ed. New York, Appleton, 1892, 1079 pp, pp 684–711.
85 Wintrobe MM: Erythrocyte in man. *Medicine* (Baltimore) 9:195–255, 1930.
86 Wintrobe MM: A simple and accurate hematocrit. *J Lab Clin Med* 15:287–289, 1929; and Wintrobe, MM: Macroscopic examination of the blood. *Am J Med Sci* 185:58–73, 1933.
87 Wintrobe MM: Anemia. Classification and treatment on the basis of differences in the average volume and hemoglobin content of the red corpuscles. *Arch Intern Med* 54:256–280, 1934.
88 Wintrobe MM: *Clinical Hematology,* 3d ed. Philadelphia, Lea and Febiger, 1951, 1048 pp
89 Heinle RW, Welch AD: Experiments with pteroylglutamic acid and pteroylglutamic acid deficiency in human leukemia. *Proc Am Soc Clin Invest,* May 1948. *J Clin Invest* 27:539, 1948 (abst).
90 Farber S, Diamond LK et al: Temporary remissions in acute leukemia in children produced by folic acid antagonist, 4-aminopteroyl-glutamic acid (Aminopterin). *N Engl J Med* 238:787–793, 1948.
91 Gilman A, Phillips FS: The biological actions and therapeutic applications of the β-chloroethyl amines and sulfides. *Science* 103:409–415, 1946.
92 Goodman LS, Wintrobe MM, Dameshek W, Goodman MJ, Gilman A, McLennan MT: Nitrogen mustard therapy. *JAMA* 132:263–271, 1946.

CHAPTER 2

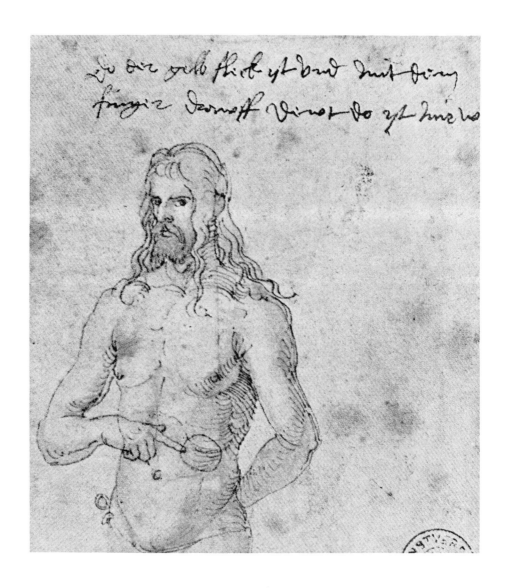

ANCIENT DISEASES OF THE BLOOD
Gerald D. Hart

D isease is as ancient as life itself. The bones and fossilized remains of prehistoric animals and ancient humans show evidence of trauma, infection, arthritis, tumors, and endocrine and other abnormalities.

Paleopathological Sources

Information about life and death in ancient times is recorded in the bones, bodies, and art of the people. Many diseases affect the skeleton. Through the collaboration of archaeologists, anthropologists, and paleopathologists, an accurate diagnosis of certain diseases can be reached from the study of ancient bones. The archaeologist assigns a date to a skeleton after considering burial depth, accompanying artifacts and structures, and the method of burial. Meticulous excavation techniques are necessary, however, in order to obtain material suitable for study.

At a recent dig of an Iron Age site in England, an archaeologist discovered a thin eggshell-like object within the thoracic cage of a skeleton. An inexperienced excavator might have damaged, destroyed, or ignored this object, but it

Chapter Opening Photo Self-portrait by Albrecht Dürer, indicating left upper quadrant abdominal pain probably due to a splenic infarct.

33

was recognized as having probable major paleopathologic significance and was referred to an expert for further study.[1] Dr. Calvin Wells thought that the object was a calcified hydatid cyst. This results from a parasitic disease caused by exposure to sheep and dogs; it is still common in agricultural areas of the world. The parasite lodges in the lungs, spleen, liver, bones, and brain. The cells of the body attempt to isolate the organism by producing a wall of tissue around the invader. Dr. Wells' cyst is the earliest example of the disease yet found and demonstrates that over the span of many hundreds of years the human race has not improved its ability to adapt to this parasite.

The anthropologist routinely deduces from bones the owner's age, sex, and parity (if female) and may see evidence of congenital, inflammatory, traumatic, degenerative, or neoplastic disease.

The paleopathologist applies modern investigative techniques to ancient materials. Bones and bodies may be x-rayed, studied under the microscope, and analyzed chemically. These findings are then correlated with archaeologic and anthropologic information to establish a clinical diagnosis. In the recent past, because of inadequate consultation and collaboration among these three disciplines, some erroneous diagnoses of disease in ancient humans were made. For example, multiple myeloma, a malignant disorder of the bone marrow, causes extensive destruction of the skeleton; it occurs in middle age or later and, in its advanced form, produces punched-out holes in the skull (Figure 2-1A). However, such skeletal lesions are not unique to myeloma. Many anthropologists have ignored the differential diagnosis of punched-out skull lesions and have overdiagnosed myeloma;[2] destructive bone lesions may be caused by other more common tumors, such as metastatic carcinoma of the breast (Figure 2-1B). By correlating the potentialities of anthropology, archaeology, and laboratory and clinical medicine, the modern paleopathologist has made some remarkable and interesting diagnoses about the diseases suffered by ancient peoples.[3]

Ancient desiccated bodies (mummies) have been found in many areas of the world. Bodies may be preserved by dehydration, freezing, or tanning. Careful dissections with microscopic examination and biochemical analysis of tissues have led to a better understanding of the lives led by these peoples and their deaths. On many occasions these bodies may contain evidence of a particular blood cell type or a parasite which can provide enough information on which to base a diagnosis.

Since ancient times, portraits and sculptures have depicted disease; sometimes this detail was accidental but often it was part of the artist's accurate depiction of the subject. In other instances, these ancient medical illustrations were intended to depict disease; for example, the votives of Greece and Rome and the clay forms of ancient Mexico. The fifteenth century German painter Albrecht Dürer even sent his physician a self-portrait indi-

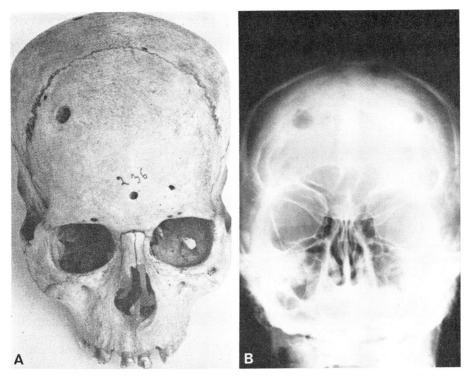

Figure 2-1 *(A)* Ancient Egyptian skull showing multiple punched-out lesions in bone. This may result from invasion of the bone marrow by a variety of malignancies. *(Courtesy of Calvin Wells. Reproduced with permission of the Journal of Laryngology and Otology.)* *(B)* Skull x-ray of a 38-year-old woman with metastatic carcinoma of the breast.

cating that he suffered pain in the region of his spleen (Chapter Opening Photo).

Our historic past was violent and included many traumatic causes of blood loss. Skeletons may show sword cuts and may have imbedded in them arrowheads, bullets, and other artifacts of war. These may be mute testimony to a violent hemorrhagic death. A 2000-year-old peat-bog mummy from Denmark has been found with an ear-to-ear slash across the throat.[3]

Bloodletting as a form of medical treatment has been practiced since the doctrine of the four humors (Chapter 1) was formulated. The instruments used included scalpels, cupping vases, and bleeding bowls. In the Louvre, there is a fifth-century B.C. Athenian vase which depicts a bleeding bowl with a physician about to make an incision over the cubital vein of a patient (Figure 2-2). The coins of the ancient Greek city of Epidaurus advertised the medical facilities of their Asclepian temple complex by depicting a cupping

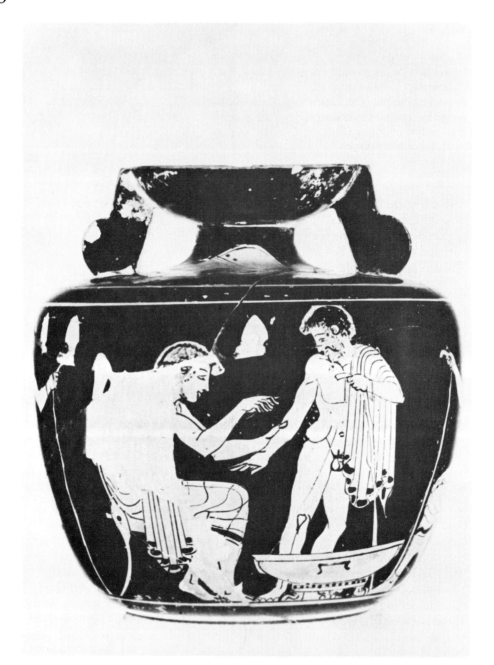

Figure 2-2 Athenian vase (fifth century B.C.). Depicts a physician about to bleed a patient. Below the patient is an ancient bleeding bowl. (*Courtesy of Maurice Chazeville, Paris, and reproduced with the permission of the Secretary General of the Louvre Museum, Paris.*)

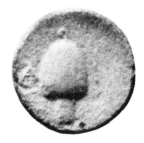

Figure 2-3 Ancient coin from Epidaurus depicting a cupping vessel used in the treatment of disease at the famous Asclepian Temple of Epidaurus. Many ancient coins portrayed local products, gods, or legends as identification for their source of origin. *(Reproduced by permission of the trustees of the British Museum.)*

vessel (Figure 2-3). Repeated bloodletting, however, would have resulted in iron-deficiency anemia. It is hard to understand why the numerous nonphysiologic indications for venesection were accepted for so many centuries. Perhaps the answer lies in the fact that both patient and physician saw the practice as a tangible attack on disease, and both were reassured by this.

BONE MARROW OVERGROWTH AND ITS EFFECTS ON THE SKELETON

Changes in the bone marrow may be reflected in the skeleton. In children, these changes are expressed in the skull and the long bones, but in adults they are usually seen only in the skull. In 1888, the German anthropologist H. Welcker described a corallike porosity in the parietal and frontal bones of the skull in some excavated Egyptian skeletons (Figure 2-4).[5] He called these changes *porotic hyperostosis*, a term that is still used but has been modified by some authorities to *symmetrical hyperostosis*. Such skeletal changes are the sequelae of prolonged marrow overgrowth (hyperplasia) and are the hallmark of severe anemia of long standing.

The skull is formed of an inner and an outer layer of hard protective (cortical) bone. These layers make up 25 percent of the skull. Sandwiched between these protective layers is the spongy (diploic) bone which makes up the remaining 75 percent and contains the blood-producing marrow cells. The overall thickness of the three layers at fixed anatomical points is consistent in normal persons.[6] However, with marrow proliferation, these measurements vary. Marked multiplication of red cells (erythroid hyperplasia) results in expansion of the diploë and ultimately may produce pressure atrophy of the outer table of the skull. Continued hyperplasia may even cause the outer table of the cortex to disappear with the result that the periosteum (the outer lining of the bone) may bulge outwards. In this situation, the periosteal bone-forming cells (the osteoblasts) are stimulated to lay down new bone around the blood vessels that occupy the expanding marrow. Anatomically, the end result of this process is symmetrical hyperostosis. In lateral radiographs of the skull the expanded diploë is surrounded by bone which has replaced the outer

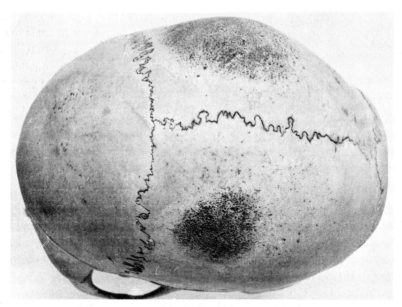

Figure 2-4 Symmetrical hyperostosis of skull showing coral- or sievelike perforations of the parietal bones. *(Roman skull courtesy of Calvin Wells.)* This finding was first described by Welcker in 1888. *(Photographed by Mary Kipper.)*

cortex (Figure 2-5). Roentgenographically such skulls have a "hair-on-end" appearance.[7]

These changes are nonspecific and may be the result of any long-standing severe anemia in infancy or childhood. In 1930, Vogt, a radiologist at the Children's Hospital of Boston, called attention to the similarity of the symmetrical hyperporosis of skulls discovered by anthropologists and archaeologists and the "hair-on-end" changes seen in the skulls of patients with thalassemia major (Chapter 12) and in other congenital hemolytic anemias.[8] Failure to demonstrate radiologic changes in the skulls of adults with severe anemia has been explained by Dr. Philip Lanzkowsky on the grounds that symmetrical hyperostosis (the hair-on-end appearance) does not develop unless the anemia that is causing erythroid hyperplasia develops in association with premature birth, protein malnutrition, or nutritional rickets, all of which cause the bone to be more pliable than normally.[9]

A less dramatic but more common skeletal manifestation of anemia is the appearance of multiple perforations in the bone above the eye socket. This condition, known as *cribra orbitalia,* has fascinated anthropologists since its original description by Welcker.[5] Some have regarded this as a manifestation of iron deficiency, but, in reality, it represents the aftermath of intense, prolonged marrow stimulation from any cause. The supraorbital area of bone is thin and is susceptible to erosion by the proliferating marrow.

Symmetrical hyperostosis and cribra orbitalia illustrate the purposeful functional design of the body. Marrow proliferation never erodes internally, for if it did the increased number of cells would result in increased pressure on the brain with profound upset in cerebral function. Marrow grows outwards under the scalp or into the sinuses. This may result in changes in facial features (thalassemia facies) or in the forehead outline (Bahima disease).

Symmetrical hyperostosis has been found in skeletons from around the world; e.g., in Greece, Turkey, Peru, Mexico, the United States, and Canada. Professor J. Lawrence Angel, Director of Anthropology at the Smithsonian Institute, has assembled impressive archaeological data from Greece and Turkey suggesting that in these areas this lesion is due to thalassemia (Chapter 12).[10] Dr. Mahumid Y El-Najjar at Case Western Reserve University has impressive data which indicate that iron deficiency is the factor underlying

Figure 2-5 "Hair-on-end" radiographic appearance of symmetrical hyperostosis. This change is common in the skulls of patients with thalassemia major, sickle-cell anemia, and other severe congenital anemias.

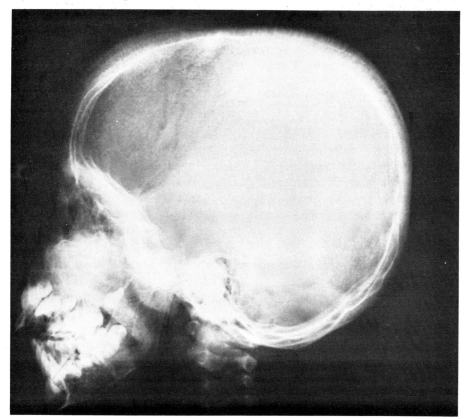

Table 2-1 *Social influence on incidence of symmetrical*
hyperostosis (east Mediterranean)

LIFESTYLE	PERIOD	INCIDENCE, %
Advanced hunters	15,000–8000 B.C.	2
Early farmers	6500–2000 B.C.	50
Proto-city dwellers	2000–1200 B.C.	12
City-state dwellers	650–300 B.C.	2

Source: From Angel JL, 1966,[10] 1967.[6]

symmetrical hyperostosis among the Indians from New Mexico and Arizona.[11,12]

Table 2-1 summarizes Angel's anthropologic findings in the Eastern Mediterranean. In the period 15,000 to 8000 B.C., symmetrical hyperostosis was rare (2 percent), but in the period 6500 to 2000 B.C., the incidence increased to 50 percent. He believes that symmetrical hyperostosis increased after the eighth millennium B.C., when ancient peoples switched from hunting to farming; coincident with this social change, falciparum malaria appeared. It is thought that patients with thalassemia, sickle-cell disease (Chapter 11), and G6PD enzyme deficiency (Chapter 6) have a greater resistance to falciparum malaria than do normal individuals. Dr. Angel has proposed that the increase in symmetrical hyperostosis after the eighth millenium B.C. in Greece and Turkey reflects the selective survival of people with thalassemia in a malarial community. This hypothesis is further supported by the relative rarity of symmetrical hyperostosis among those farming in the high, dry, and, consequently, low-risk malarial communities as compared with those farming in the low-lying, high-risk malarial communities (Table 2-2). Generally, better drainage of farmland, lower water levels, and a lower mosquito population may explain the decreasing incidence of symmetrical hyperostosis after the second century B.C. (Table 2-1).

Table 2-2 *Geographical influence on the incidence of*
symmetrical hyperostosis in early farmers (8000 B.C.)

Inland drainage areas with marshy soft soil	
Catal Hügük (Turkey)	41%
Macedonia	60%
Dry rocky areas	
Khirokitia (Cyprus)	9%
Kephalia	11%

Source: From Angel JL, 1966,[10] 1967.[6]

Table 2-3 *Symmetrical hyperostosis in southwestern American Indians*

	270 CANYON DWELLERS OF NORTHERN ARIZONA AND NEW MEXICO	269 PLAINS DWELLERS OF SOUTHERN ARIZONA AND NEW MEXICO
Total series	54.1%	14.5%
Children	76.6%	17.3%
Females	49.0%	11.9%
Males	36.9%	13.3%

Source: From El-Najjar y M, et al., 1975,[11] 1976.[12]

Symmetrical hyperostosis among the Indians of the southwestern United States (Table 2-3) was, according to Dr. El-Najjar, due to long-standing iron deficiency.[11,12] The incidence of symmetrical hyperostosis in Indians living in the canyons of northern Arizona and northern New Mexico was 54 percent as compared to 14.5 percent among those living on the plains of southern Arizona and southern New Mexico. He concluded that the differences in diet explained these differences. Archaeological studies have shown that the canyon dwellers ate little meat and their diet consisted mainly of maize. Maize is low in iron, and the presence of phytate in its outer husk impairs absorption of dietary iron. On the other hand, the plains Indians had ready access to a variety of animal foods in addition to maize. This more balanced diet would give them considerable protection against iron-deficiency anemia. The incidence of symmetrical hyperostosis was higher in children than in women and lowest in men, corresponding to the well-known tendency of children and women to develop iron deficiency and its relative absence in men. Recent clinical studies have shown the "hair-on-end" x-ray changes in the skulls of children with severe iron deficiency.[13] The absence of historical or archaeological evidence of malaria or hemoglobinopathies in the New World before contact with Europeans further supports the contention that iron deficiency produced the symmetrical hyperostosis in the canyon dwellers of northern Arizona and New Mexico.

OTHER SKELETAL EVIDENCE OF BLOOD DISEASE

In addition to symmetrical hyperostosis, the skull may show other evidence of blood disease. Multiple myeloma, a malignant disorder of the plasma cells in the bone marrow, was mentioned earlier. The archaeologist may see not only "punched-out" areas of bone destruction due to tumors but also bone infarcts, such as occur with sickle-cell disease. The marrow hypertrophy which accompanies the anemia of thalassemia major often is so marked that it obliterates the sinuses and pushes forward the incisor teeth. Chronic infections such as tuberculosis, syphilis, and leprosy may also produce destructive changes in the skeleton. Traumatic hemorrhage of soft tissues may heal and leave as a sign of its former presence metastatic ossification at the site of muscle insertions.

COPROLITES

Studies of coprolites (fossilized excrement) from the bowels of mummies, from ancient cesspits, or from sites of human and animal habitation yield valuable information about diets and about parasitic infestation in ancient times. Before they are studied, the coprolites are rehydrated with trisodium phosphate and concentrated with formalin-ether. Numerous parasite ova have been found. Jansen, who studied materials of human origin from a site in northwest Germany that was occupied between 100 B.C. and A.D. 500, identified the ova of *Ascaris lumbricoides*, *Trichuris trichiura*, *Taenia ovis* or *T. globosa*, *T. solium* or *T. saginata*, and *Diphyllobothrium latum*.[14]

Many intestinal parasites may induce blood loss and iron-deficiency anemia. The Commonwealth Institute of Helminthology at St. Albans, Herts., England, maintains a catalogue and bibliography of paleopathologic discoveries in this field. The presence of the parasite *Diphyllobothrium latum* indicates ingestion of uncooked fish and thus of tapeworms that have an avid appetite for the host's dietary vitamin B_{12}. Infestation with fish tapeworm, which is common in the Baltic States, produces megaloblastic anemia. Eggs resembling those of the fish tapeworm have also been found in mummies from Moorland in East Prussia[15] and from the Chicama Valley in Peru.[16]

Egyptian Mummies

During the mummification process, the brain was removed via the nasal cavity, and the cranial cavity was sealed with pitch. (The ancient Egyptians believed that the brain had no function.) The heart was thought to be the seat of the mind and in it was recorded the owner's good and evil. This organ was left in the body so that the gods could weigh it to determine if the deceased was worthy of heaven. The stomach, liver, intestines, and lungs were removed and mummified separately. They were returned to the body in the form of organ packages or were placed outside the body in separate jars. These *Canopic jars* carried on their lids the portrait of a god for which that organ was sacred.

Unfortunately, the Egyptian process destroyed a great deal of tissue that would have been of value to the paleopathologist. Sir Marc-Armand Ruffer, who in 1910 performed some of the earliest medical studies on Egyptian mummies, was able to rehydrate the tissues and then embed them in paraffin and process them in a routine histological fashion.[17] His rehydrating techniques used a mixture of absolute alcohol, calcium carbonate, and formaldehyde, which is still in use as *Ruffer's solution*. He was the first to discover the fluke *Bilharzia haematobia* (*Schistosoma haematobium*) in mummies.

In 1974, an international team at the University of Toronto performed an autopsy on a naturally dehydrated mummy of a 16-year-old Egyptian weaver named Nakht from the Twentieth Dynasty (1150 B.C.). The body showed remarkable preservation of detail and demonstrated presumptive evidence of anemia. The examiners found intact red cells and were able to determine the youth's blood group.[18]

X-ray studies made prior to unwrapping the body showed this to be a naturally dehydrated mummy.[19] This method of body preservation had been practiced by the ancestors of dynastic Egypt (prior to 3200 B.C.). The bodies were buried in shallow sand graves, where the drying and desiccation occurred naturally. As the Egyptians became more prosperous, they placed their dead in elaborate tombs. Unfortunately, the body, which was so important for the spirit's afterlife, was not well preserved in this setting. The Egyptian mummification process was developed to preserve the body artificially—humans imitating nature. The key to the ancient Egyptian mummification process was the removal of the organs and dehydration. The latter was accomplished chemically by the use of *natron*. This naturally occurring substance was called *netjery* by the ancient Egyptians, from which comes the modern chemical symbol Na for sodium. Netjery or natron is made up of sodium bicarbonate, sodium chloride, and sodium sulfate.[20]

Nakht was a working man, and his family could not afford this elaborate process; they settled for an inscribed casket.[21] His preservation by natural means offered an ideal subject for study. The organs had been left intact and were preserved remarkably well.

The inscription on the outside of the coffin clearly identified the occupant as Nakht, a weaver from the funeral temple of King Setnakht. *ROM I* is the scientific descriptive name identifying the first mummy from the Royal Ontario Museum collection to undergo a detailed medical and scientific study.

When the abdominal cavity was opened, the bowel was readily visible as paper-thin material. The liver was shrunken but had retained its shape. The spleen seemed enlarged, relatively speaking, and the splenic bed contained dark pigment, which probably represented antemortem or postmortem splenic rupture. The bladder was shrunken, but the kidneys could not be identified.[22] Histologic preparations of the organs demonstrated remarkable preservation of structural detail. The proportion of fibrous tissue in the liver was greater than normal, and it contained *Schistosoma* ova. These ova had a lateral spine which identified them as being of the species *haematobium*. The increased fibrous tissue in the liver suggested additional infestation by *Schistosoma* of the *mansoni* type. Similar ova were found in the bowel and bladder; the latter contained intact red cells, suggesting the typical picture of bilharziasis, which is seen in Egypt today.[23]

The bowel contained numerous ova characteristic of *Taenia*, a tapeworm. These have a double radiate shell containing a larva with three pairs of hooklets. When the eggs were concentrated, electron microscopic studies showed a remarkable preservation of the details (Figure 2-6).[24] The bowel also contained red cells, and these (Figure 2-7) are the oldest known human red cells (3200 years).

Nakht was the victim of a common cause for anemia, bilharzia infestation of the kidney, bowel, bladder, and liver.

Intact red cells and white cells (Figure 2-8) were isolated from a blood clot in the sigmoid sinus of the skull. Testing of the antigens of these cells revealed that Nakht's blood belonged to group B.

ANCIENT BLOOD GROUPS

Blood group antigens A, B, and H are complex carbohydrates, which may be preserved and hence can be detected after disintegration of the red cell. These antigens are also detectable in the tissue fluids of the 75 percent of the population who, because they possess the dominant secretor gene, are called *secretors*.

The two tests used to detect the presence of blood group antigens in tissue

Figure 2-6 Egg of *Taenia* species from the Egyptian mummy Nakht. Arrows indicate hooklets. Magnification 18,800X. *(Courtesy of Horne and Lewin. Reproduced with permission of the Canadian Medical Association Journal.)*

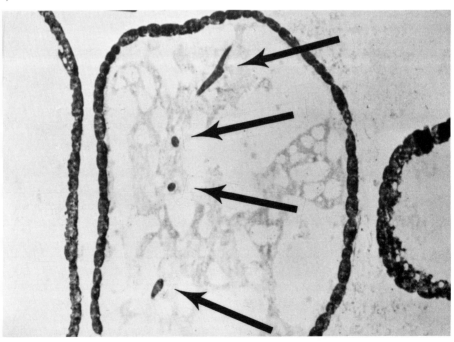

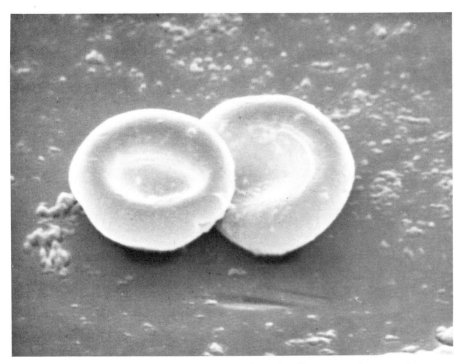

Figure 2-7 Red cells from intestinal contents of Nakht. (Scanning electron microscope photograph. Magnification 6500X.) Note the preservation of the concave disc shape. *(Courtesy of Horne and Lewin and reproduced with permission of the Canadian Medical Association Journal.)*

stains or after disintegration of the red cells are the serologic micromethod and the agglutination inhibition test. The presence of blood group O is signaled by the absence of a reaction with anti-A or anti-B serum or by the production of agglutination with anti-H sera (group O cells contain a high concentration of H substance). This technique has been used by forensic laboratories for many years. In the mid-1930s, it was applied to archaeological material.[25,26] In one study of 11 ancient Egyptian skeletons, Candela demonstrated blood group B in six, blood group AB in three, and blood group O in two.[27] With it, Connolly and Harrison affirmed the kinship of the ancient Egyptian kings Smenkhkare and Tutankhamen by demonstrating the presence of blood group A_2.[28] Hart, Kvas, and Soots enhanced the sensitivity of this technique by adding an antihuman serum (Coombs' serum) to the test system.[29,30]

The agglutination inhibition test strengthens and confirms the results of the serologic micromethod. Here, antiserum (anti-A, anti-B, anti-H) of known potency is tested with the unknown substance; if the specific antigen is present, the measured potency of the serum will decrease when retested with

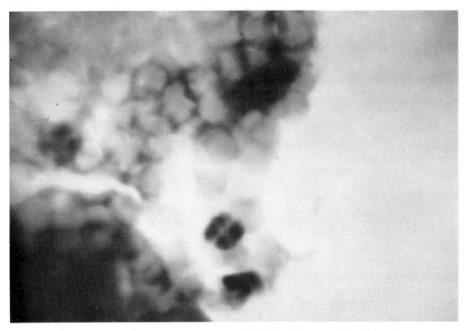

Figure 2-8 Blood clot from sigmoid sinus of Nakht showing the oldest known preserved white cells and red cells. (Magnification 1000X.) *(Courtesy of Peter Lewin, The Hospital for Sick Children, Toronto.)*

the specific cells; e.g., anti-B serum known to produce agglutination of B cells at a dilution of 1:1024 is mixed with an unknown. If the unknown contains B substance, some of the anti-B serum will be absorbed by the antigen, and the potency of the serum will be decreased. A drop in titre from 1:1024 to 1:64, for example, would indicate the presence of B antigen in the unknown material.

Unfortunately, the blood group antigens A and B are not specific for human red cells; that is, many bacterial, animal, and vegetable substances contain A or B antigen. Pigs have blood group A and oxen and rabbits have blood group B; some plants have blood group A; the bacteria *E. coli* have blood group B. This lack of specificity impairs the value of blood group testing on ancient human remains.

HOW LONG CAN BLOOD GROUP ANTIGENS BE PRESERVED?

The mummy Nakht (ROM I) provided striking evidence that blood group antigens could be preserved for over 3200 years. Testing of the splenic material was positive with the agglutination inhibition test, but all tests with the serologic micromethod resulted in hemolysis (breakdown) of the test cells. The sigmoid sinus material, on the other hand, was positive for blood group B with both methods. The discrepancy was explained after an examination of the histologic sections of the splenic material; they contained no red blood cells but did contain numerous bacteria and fungal spores, which caused the breakdown of group O cells. The sigmoid sinus material, however, did contain intact red cells and was not contaminated by hemolytic spores.

Gods, Philosophers, and Anemia

According to Greek mythology, Asclepius, the god of medicine, was the illegitimate son of Apollo and was delivered from the womb of his dead mother by cesarean section. The boy Asclepius was raised by Chiron the centaur, who taught him the art of herbal medicine. Early in his medical career, Asclepius gained favor with Athena, the goddess of wisdom, who gave him some of the Gorgon's blood. By using this blood, Asclepius was able to raise the dead. (Ancient mythology does not specify the route of administration or the anticoagulant used.) This myth suggests that the ancient Greeks recognized the role of blood in sustaining life, and it anticipates the technique of blood transfusion, especially that of cadaver blood. It also contains the first historical reference to the resuscitating powers of transfusion.[31,32]

From the fifth century B.C. to the fourth century A.D., the temples of Asclepius played an important part in medical care, and the Asclepian priest-physicians practiced a form of mystical medicine. Part of their ritual required that cured patients give the temple an offering depicting the diseased part. Today most museums have in their collections votive hands, feet, ears, uteri, breasts, and penises. A votive indicating iron-deficiency anemia would depict a hand bearing spoon-shaped nails (koilonychia).

G6PD ENZYME DEFICIENCY

Demeter, the Greek goddess of harvest, forbade the members of her cult to eat beans, perhaps because the ancients had recognized favism, an explosive hemolytic anemia that develops after the eating of fava beans by individuals with a deficiency of the enzyme *glucose-6-phosphate dehydrogenase* (G6PD, Chapter 6). Modern science recognizes different types of G6PD enzyme deficiency. One type is distributed around the Mediterranean basin and extends east into northern India; the present genetic distribution of this enzyme defect follows the outline of the empire established by Alexander the Great.

Pythagoras, a mathematician, philosopher, and physician, lived in the fifth century B.C. and had a great following among the Greek colonists at the southern end of Italy. He forbade his followers to eat beans, which suggests

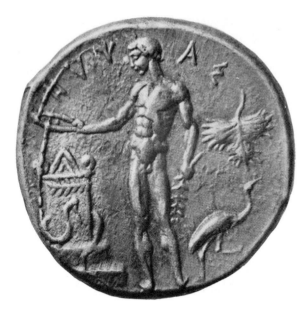

Figure 2-9 Coin of Selinus commemorating the drainage of the surrounding swamps. The river-god Selinus is shown sacrificing at the altar of Asclepius (symbolized by the serpent). The leaf is a parsley leaf symbolic of Selinus and one of its major products. The bird is a swamp bird stalking away in disgust. *(Reproduced with the permission of Hirmer Fotoarchiv München.)*

that he also recognized the condition now known as favism.[33] Even today, the highest incidence of G6PD enzyme deficiency is found in southern Italy, the location of the ancient Pythagorian school.

MALARIA

Numismatic evidence shows that the ancient Greeks and Romans recognized the role of swamps in producing disease. The ancient city of Selinus in western Sicily was surrounded by marshes, and its people reputedly suffered from malaria. Empedocles, a disciple of Pythagoras, is credited with organizing the engineering work which drained the marshes and relieved the people of local epidemics. He eliminated the stagnant water (a breeding ground for malaria-carrying mosquitoes) by joining the rivers surrounding the city—the Hypsas and the Selinus—thereby creating a fast-flowing stream, which drained the marshes. This event was commemorated on several contemporary coins (Figure 2-9). Tetradrachmas from the period 467 to 145 B.C. depict the river-god Selinus sacrificing at the altar of Asclepius. Another series beginning in 417 B.C. and continuing until the destruction of Selinus by Carthage in 409 B.C. continued to commemorate the event.[34–36]

   Credit for understanding the natural cause of malaria has been attributed to the Roman scholar Marcus Terentius Varro (ca. 100 B.C.), who postulated that tiny animals inhabiting the marshes entered the body and caused the disease.[37] There were many marshes and landlocked lakes around Rome, and, over the years, attempts were made to drain them to make the land more habitable and healthy. A coin of Hadrian celebrates one of the early efforts to drain Lake Fucinus and depicts a farm laborer standing upon a pump. A coin of Trajan also commemorates the draining of a portion of the Pontine Marshes.

The existence of splenomegaly in the ancient world is suggested by a bas-relief sculpture showing a physician palpating a mass in the left upper quadrant of a young patient (Figure 2-10). Here the patient is standing, whereas modern practice requires the patient to lie on the back or the right side in order to bring forward a slightly enlarged spleen from under the rib cage.

LEAD POISONING

Lead is a potent toxin that may give rise to anemia and other complications. In the past century, the frequency of lead intoxication has decreased markedly as a result of public health regulations which prevent casual exposure. In ancient Rome and throughout the Roman Empire, water was conducted by lead pipes and stored in lead cisterns. Pottery, especially wine jars, was lead-glazed, and

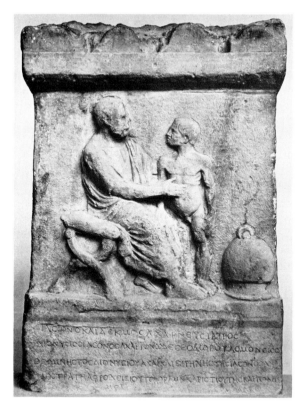

Figure 2-10 Roman physician examining the abdomen of a child. He is probably palpating an enlarged spleen. A marble relief, second century A.D. *(Photograph courtesy of the Department of Greek and Roman Antiquities, the British Museum, and reproduced courtesy of the trustees of the British Museum.)*

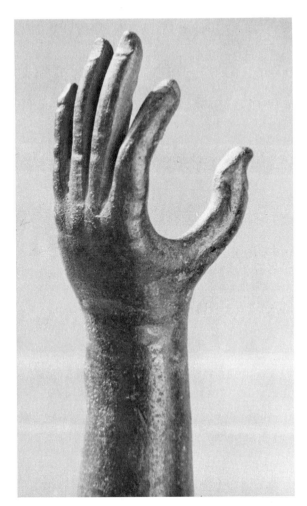

Figure 2-11 Votive hand from Lydney, England, showing spoon-shaped deformity of the nails (koilonychia). *(Courtesy of Viscount Bledisloe and reproduced with permission of the Bulletin of the History of Medicine.)*

copper cooking utensils were lead-lined. In addition to those who mined and smelted the lead, therefore, the average citizen was continuously exposed to lead intoxication; indeed one author has gone so far as to blame lead poisoning for the decline and fall of the Roman Empire.[38]

Ninety percent of the lead absorbed into the body is deposited in the bones in an inert state; before it reaches the bones, however, the lead may impair a variety of body functions and produce anemia. Bone lead can be measured chemically; currently, H. A. Waldron and Calvin Wells are studying Roman bones using atomic absorption spectroscopy.[39] These studies show a high lead concentration in bones recovered from the Roman city of York as compared to contemporary rib samples. The levels are not believed to be high enough to produce endemic lead poisoning; however, other studies on bones from Roman Cirencester show much higher lead levels, which Dr. Waldron believes could be detected by histochemical techniques.

Future studies will include controls to determine the possibility that lead may be lost from the bones into the soil or that bones can take up lead from the soil. In any case, these studies will give new information concerning lead intoxication in the ancient world.

IRON-DEFICIENCY ANEMIA AT LYDNEY,
GLOUCESTERSHIRE: FOURTH CENTURY

At Lydney, in Gloucestershire, England, there are the remains of the Celtic Temple of Nodens, which was built along the lines of an Asclepian temple complex.[40] In addition to the temple, the site contained guest houses, a bath house, and a long building of unknown use. Of the votive objects found at the site, the most important object is a bronze upper extremity. The arm is crude, but the hand is quite detailed and the nails show koilonychia (Figure 2-11). The hematologic significance of this votive can only be appreciated after considering the geographical setting of the temple. The complex is built on ancient iron workings, and behind the guest house is the only intact Roman iron mine in Britain today. The therapy of Asclepian temple medicine included taking the local waters, a practice that continues today a few miles from Lydney at the ancient Roman city of Bath. The waters of Lydney would still be helpful in treating iron deficiency, and even today no better votive could be chosen to depict severe iron deficiency than a hand with spoon-shaped nails.

Pallor and Palettes

Pallor, especially of the face, lips, and nails, is the hallmark of anemia. Extreme iron-deficiency anemia may result in a marked pallor that has a greenish cast. Persons with such an appearance were said to have chlorosis (iron-deficiency anemia) centuries before physicians could measure the hemoglobin level or examine red cells under the microscope. The term *chlorosis* comes from the Latin for green. Constantius I, father of Constantine the Great, was called Constantius Chlorus because of his pale complexion. Today when a hematologist sees an adult with a lifelong history of pallor, he or she thinks of congenital hemolytic anemia. If the person is from the Mediterranean basin, the hematologist would think about thalassemia. Constantius was of Dardanian ancestry, i.e., from a part of modern Turkey in an area that is still known for thalassemia. Patients with thalassemia minor exhibit varying degrees of pallor, and Constantius' nickname Chlorus may have been derived from this.

Today, mild iron deficiency is very common. It is estimated that 10 percent of North American women are iron deficient, and it is probable that iron deficiency was more severe and more frequent in less affluent times. It is also probable that over the centuries artists depicted the pallors and hues of anemia in their subjects.

However, the reader who wishes to examine the portraits in the art galleries of the world for evidence of anemia should be warned about the perils of pseudopathology.[41] Alterations in bone, bodies, or art due to the effects of time or environmental factors may lead to a false diagnosis. When viewing paintings, we must remember that ancient skin tone pigments may have faded or changed. For example, the skin tones in portraits by Joshua Reynolds have whitened over the years, so that most of his subjects now have a ghostly white complexion. In addition to chemical pseudopathology, we must be aware of errors based on artistic license. In this circumstance the artist might portray the subject with unnatural pallor to achieve a contrast with the surroundings or to imply the quality of purity or godliness.

To be certain of a diagnosis of "artistic" anemia, we must have a standard control; just as our hemoglobinometers are standardized against known quantities of hemoglobin, portraits must be compared with apparent contemporary normal features painted with the same pigments. In Velázquez's Bacchus, which is displayed at the Prado in Madrid, a flabby, pale Bacchus is surrounded by seven revellers. One of the habitues has marked pallor, in contrast to the robust, somewhat plethoric countenance of his colleagues. This man is probably the eighteenth century counterpart of today's alcoholic who presents with a hemoglobin of 4 to 5 g per 100 ml of blood (normal range is 15 to 16), which is caused by megaloblastic anemia induced by a diet high in alcohol and low in folic acid.

Contemporary portraits of the six wives of Henry VIII offer a hematologic challenge.[42] Jane Seymour is pale, and Catherine Parr shows marked pallor. The latter portrait, which is attributed to W. Scrotts (1545), also depicts auburn hair and a beautiful crimson dress. Have skin pigments and other colors remained true? The nails, which are clearly visible, do not show koilonychia; however, many patients with iron deficiency do not show this change. Catherine Parr remarried after Henry's death, and she died following childbirth. Did severe anemia contribute to some of the maternal deaths among the aristocracy of sixteenth century Britain?

The world has preserved a rich heritage of art from Roman and Greek times. Many of the Roman wall paintings and Greek vases depict women with varying degrees of pallor, all the more marked when compared to the suntanned skin of their male companions. In seventeenth-century Europe, pallor became symbolic of purity and feminity. Women with chlorosis were said to have the "virgin's disease." Lange, an authority of the time, recommended pregnancy as a treatment for chlorosis, but this would only aggravate iron-deficiency anemia.[43] However, the other changes accompanying pregnancy, namely marriage and perhaps a better diet or a larger share of the available food, might replenish essential vitamins and deficient iron stores.

Summary

A study of the bones, bodies, and art of earlier days thus shows that disease of the blood is as old as the human race. The physicians of ancient Thebes and Babylon did not understand the suffering of Nakht and Alexander. The ancient Macedonians and the canyon dwellers of New Mexico did not know they had marrow hyperplasia. It is doubtful that Dürer's physician understood the pain so well portrayed in the artist's self-portrait. The votive of Lydney represents a therapeutic fluke. In the chapters that follow, the steps taken by researchers to understand diseases which have afflicted the human race for thousands of years will be described.

References

1 Wells C, Dallas C: *Romano-British Pathology.* Antiquity 50, 53–55, Cambridge, England, Antiquity Publications Ltd., 1976.
2 Brooks S, Melbye J: *Skeletal Lesions Suggestive of Pre-Columbian Multiple Myeloma. Miscellaneous Papers of Paleopathology.* Museum of Northern Arizona, Technical series 7, 23–29, William Wade Edition.
3 Wells C: *Bones, Bodies and Disease.* London, Thames and Hudson, 1964, 282 pp.
4 Abel AL: Bleeding Through the Ages, Hunterian Society Annual Meeting, Address at the Talbot, London Wall, London E.C. 2 on Monday May 5, 1969. London, Metropolitan Press Ltd.
5 Welcker H: Cribra Orbitalia. Ein ethnologisch-diagnostiches Merkmal am Schädel mehrerer Menschenrassen. *Arch Anthropol* 17:1–12, 1888.
6 Angel JL: Porotic hyperostosis or osteoporosis symmetrica, in Brothwell and Sandison (eds): *Diseases in Antiquity.* Springfield, Ill, Charles C Thomas, 1967, chapter 29.
7 Mosley J: The paleopathologic riddle of osteoporosis. *Am J Roentgenol* 95:135–142, 1965.
8 Vogt EC, Diamond LK: Congenital anemias, roentgenologically considered. *Am J Roentgenol* 23:625–627, 1930.
9 Lanzkowsky P: *Osseous Changes in Iron Deficiency Anemia–Implications for Paleopathology; Porotic Hyperostosis: An Enquiry,* Paleopathology Association Monograph No 2. Detroit, The Paleopathology Association, 1977.
10 Angel JL: Porotic hyperostosis, anemias, malarias and marshes in the prehistoric eastern Mediterranean. *Science* 153:760–763, 1966.
11 El-Najjar MY, Lozoff B, Ryan DJ: The paleoepidemiology of porotic hyperostosis in the American southwest, radiological and ecological considerations. *Am J Roentgenol* 125:918–924, 1975.
12 El-Najjar MY, Robertson AL: Spongy bones in prehistoric America. *Science* 193:141–143, 1976.

13 Lie-Injo LE: Chronic iron deficiency with bone changes resembling Cooley's anemia. *Acta Haematol (Basel)* 19:263–268, 1958.

14 Jansen J, Over HJ: Het voorkomen van parasieten in terp materiaal uit Noordwest, Duitsland. *Tijdschr, Diergeneeskd* 87:1377–9, 1962.

15 Szidat L: Uber die Erhaltungsfähigkeit von Helmintheneiren in vor-und früh-geschichtlichen Moorleichen. *Z Parasitenkd* 13:265–74, 1944.

16 Callen EO, Cameron TWN: A prehistoric diet revealed by coprolites. *New Scientist* 8:35–7, 39–40, 1960.

17 Ruffer MA: Note on the presence of *Bilharzia haematobia* in Egyptian mummies of the twentieth dynasty. *Br Med J* 1:16, 1910.

18 Hart GD, Cockburn C, Millet NB, Scott JW: Lessons learned from the autopsy of an Egyptian mummy. *Can Med Assoc J* 117:415–418, 1977.

19 Rideout DF: Radiological examination (Nakht). *Can Med Assoc J* 117:463, 1977.

20 Harris JE, Weeks KR: *X-raying the Pharaohs*. New York, Scribners, 1973, 195 pp, pp 81–82.

21 Millet NB: Archaeological background (Nakht). *Can Med Assoc J* 117:461–462, 1977.

22 Scott JW, Horne PD, Hart GD, Savage H: Gross anatomic and miscellaneous studies, (Nakht). *Can Med Assoc J* 117:464–465, 1977.

23 Reyman TA, Zimmerman MR, Lewin PK: Histopathologic investigation, (Nakht). *Can Med Assoc J* 117:470–472, 1977.

24 Horne PD, Lewin PK: Electronmicroscopy of mummified tissue, (Nakht). *Can Med Assoc J* 117:472–473, 1977.

25 Boyd WC, Boyd LG: An attempt to determine the blood groups of mummies. *Proc Soc Exp Biol Med* 31:671, 1934.

26 Boyd WC, Boyd LG: Blood group tests on 300 mummies. *J Immunol* 32:307, 1937.

27 Candela PB: Blood group reaction in ancient human skeletons. *Am J Phys Anthropol* 21, 429–432, 1936.

28 Connolly RC, Harrison RD: Kinship of Smenkhare and Tutankhamen affirmed by serological micromethod. *Nature* 224:325, 1969.

29 Hart GD, Soots ML, Kvas I: Blood group testing, (Nakht). *Can Med Assoc J* 117:476, 1977.

30 Hart GD, Kvas I, Soots ML: Blood group testing of ancient material with particular reference to the mummy Nakht. *Transfusion* 18:4, 78–82, 1978.

31 Edelstein L: *Asclepius*. Baltimore, The Johns Hopkins Press, 1945, vol I, 470 pp, vol II, 277 pp.

32 Hart GD: Asclepius, god of medicine. *Can Med Assoc J* 92:232–236, 1965.

33 Russel B: *History of Western Philosophy*, 2d ed. London, Allen and Unwin, 1965, 842 pp, p 50.

34 Storer HR: *Medicina in Nummis*. Boston, Wright and Potter Printing Co, 1931, 1146 pp, pp 27–38.

35 Holzmair E: *Katalog der Sammlung*. Dr. Joseph Brettauer, 384, Wien 1937 im Selbstverlaag, 101.

36 Kraay CM, Hirmer M: *Greek Coins*. London, Thames and Hudson, 1966, 396 pp, pp 297–298.

37 Thorwald J: *Science and Secrets of Early Medicine*. London, Thames and Hudson, 1962, 92 pp.

38 Gilfillan SC: Lead poisoning and the fall of Rome. *J Occup Med* 7:53–60, 1965.

39 Mackie A, Townshend A, Waldron HA: Lead concentrations in bones from Roman York. *J Archaeol Sci* 2:235–237, 1975.

40 Wheeler REM, Wheeler TV: *Reports of the Research Committee of the Society of Antiquaries,* no. 9. Oxford, University Press, 1932, 132 pp.

41 Wells C: The study of ancient disease. Surgo; *Glasgow U Med J* 1(32):3–7, 1964.

42 Woodward GWO: *The Six Wives of Henry VIII.* London, Pitkin Pictorials Ltd., 1972, 24 pp.

43 Major RH: *Classical Descriptions of Disease,* 3d ed. Springfield, Ill, Charles C Thomas, 1945, 711 pp, pp 488–489.

CHAPTER 3

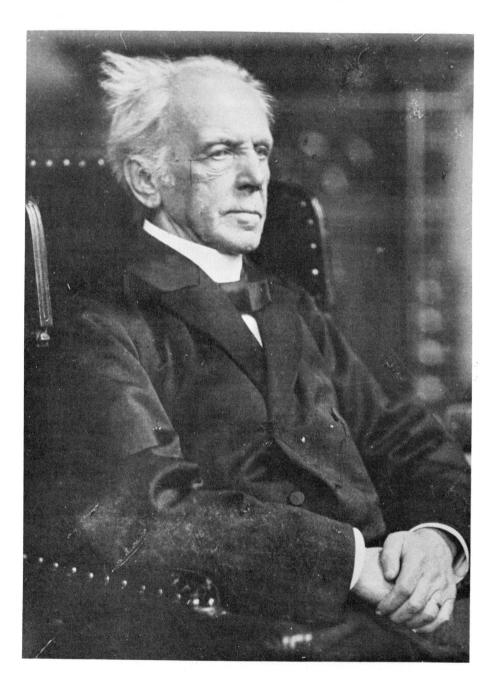

BONE MARROW: THE SEEDBED OF BLOOD

Mehdi Tavassoli

Ne cherche pas l'eau, cherche la soif
                                    Paul Claudel

Cette soif qui te fit géant
Jusqu'à l'Être exalte l'étrange
Toute-puissance du Néant!
                                    Paul Valéry

The marrow of our bones is the seedbed of our blood. Like blood, it is essential to life. It is, after the blood itself, the largest and most widely dispersed organ in our body. We harbor more than 1 trillion cells in our marrow at any one time. Every day more than 200 billion red cells, 10 billion white cells, and 400 billion platelets are produced in the marrow. Here is where all lymphocytes (our defense agents) and scavenger monocytes originate. A variety of other functions are attributed to the marrow. Birds carry air in their marrow not only to aid in levitation but apparently to serve a respiratory function as well.[1] There is an interesting cyclic change in pigeons—before ovulation, the marrow cavity is almost entirely obliterated by bone, which is then resorbed during ovulation and the bone minerals are used to form the egg shell.[2]

As one might surmise, a production center of this magnitude is highly vulnerable to malfunction or to the deleterious effects of various factors such as anticancer drugs. In fact, the marrow is currently the single most important limiting factor in cancer treatment. The reason that the treatment of cancer is often not definitive is because the marrow cannot tolerate it. On the other hand, the marrow is endowed with considerable potential for self-renewal;

Chapter Opening Photo   Ernst Neumann (1834–1918). *(Courtesy of Prof. H. Lullies.)*

57

this mitigates the impact of its exquisite sensitivity. In this regard its wide dispersion is a distinct advantage.

We have not known all this for very long. For centuries, poets, healers, and philosophers saw and described the close link between blood and life. Not so the marrow. Its role as the seedbed of blood lay hidden, like a seed in the soil. It began to sprout hardly more than a hundred years ago when Ernst Neumann (Chapter Opening Photo) and Giulio Bizzozero (Figure 3-1) established the link between blood and marrow. Ever since, marrow research has been a fertile field, fruitful not only to medicine but to the fundamental understanding of life itself. Scientists have used the marrow as a model for the elucidation of basic questions in biology. In some instances, new fields of biomedical research have emerged from studies of the marrow, e.g., radiobiology, cell kinetics, and transplantation.

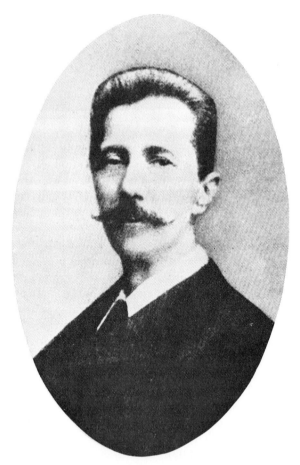

Figure 3-1 Giulio Bizzozero (1846–1901). *(From Castiglioni A: Storia della medicina [Mondadori, ed.], Milano, 1936.)*

This essay is a historical perspective to underscore how scientific ideas concerning the marrow evolved. It is not a review of current concepts, nor is it merely a chronology of events. It deals with the dynamics of the evolution of knowledge. In the words of Claudel quoted above, "It seeks not the water but the thirst."

A Trace in the Realm of Ideas

In most languages, *marrow* denotes the inmost of the central part. Metaphorically, it connotes the essence, the substance, the vital part, or the "goodness." Thus, in the prologue of *Gargantua*, Rabelais invites us to "break the bone and to suck the substantive marrow." And in *Hamlet*, we are told:

It takes
From our achievements though perform'd a height
The pith and marrow of our attribute.

From the ancient days, the marrow of animals was used for food and was considered to be rich and nutritious. During the twelfth century, marrow was considered a "dainty," and cookbooks gave recipes for preparing it. In 1539, Sir Thomas Elyot thought, "Marrowe is more dilectable than the brayne."

In modern times, as everything came to have a scientific aroma, the nutritious effect of marrow was tested by physicians. In the 1890s, first Brown-Séquard[3,4] and then others fed marrow to patients with blood dyscrasias, but to no avail. The matter was then laid to rest only to be revived in the 1920s. Whipple's study of the effects of different foods on hemoglobin production stimulated further interest (Chapter 10). Isolated, anecdotal case reports claimed that patients recovered from blood dyscrasias after eating marrow. By 1929, however, it was clear that the only nutritious effect of marrow was due to its iron content. These experiments were the forerunners of marrow transplantation, as some physicians naively hoped that they could transfer living cells by feeding the marrow.[5]

During the sixteenth and seventeenth centuries, the marrow was considered a source of warmth, energy, and inner heat: "Thy bone is marrowless, thy blood is cold," said Shakespeare. "Love" was said to burn or to "melt the marrow." Perhaps in this connotation, the marrow was also considered the seat of vitality and strength: "Marrowy and vigorous manhood," said Oliver Wendell Holmes. "Spending his manlie marrow in her armes," said Shakespeare. Prior to the discovery of its blood-forming function, the marrow was believed to be the source of bone nutrition. Identification of large bones with physical strength and manhood might have led to the designation of the marrow as a source of strength. In 1926, Mechanik,[6] who was measuring the volume of the marrow, found that "under comparable conditions, man has more marrow than woman, a highly noteworthy characteristic of the normal sex differences in man until now unknown." The major product of the marrow, red cell mass, also is known to be lower in the female sex than the male.

The Path of a Discovery

Historical events do not take place in a vacuum. The course of history is a continuum wherein every event relates to a preceding one and leads to the next. Neumann's revelation that the marrow is the seedbed of blood was the culmination of a search for the origin of red cells that had begun much earlier.

Red cells were first described in the seventeenth century (Chapter 1), but it was not until the nineteenth century that a search for their origin could begin. The intervening period, the entire eighteenth century, was spent in a seemingly endless squabble, which achieved little more than establishing the identity of the red cell. In fact, for biology as a whole, this was a century of indolence, torpor, and inaction. Nothing positive could be achieved without the synthesis of a conceptual frame that could serve as a *point de départ* for future work; and this came in 1838 with the formulation of the cell theory.

The formulation of a cell theory, the conceptualization of the cell (the "little room") as the fundamental unit of life, was the dawn of a new era in biology. It was conceived in 1838 by Mathias Schleiden[7] and Theodor Schwann.[8] From then on, biology moved rapidly. The rest of the nineteenth century was the *aurea aetas*, when the foundations of many disciplines were laid—bacteriology and immunology, pathology and histochemistry, modern biochemistry and genetics, and antisepsis and modern surgery. This was the century that provided great workers in biology. The essence of this period is well reflected in two quotations from Claude Bernard.[9] In 1855, when he was appointed professor of experimental medicine, the opening sentence of his inauguration lecture was: "Experimental medicine which I am supposed to teach you, does not exist." Some 15 years later, as the president of the Paris Academy of Sciences, he amended this statement: "The dawn of experimental medicine is now visible on the scientific horizon."

It was within this scientific ambiance that the search for the origin of red cells began and for several decades was focused on embryonic life. This was only natural—scholars of this period did not know that blood formation is a continuous process, and takes place throughout life. The finite life span of red cells, and therefore the necessity for their continuous replenishment, was not recognized. As late as 1923, as quoted elsewhere (Chapter 8), Peyton Rous wrote: "So subtly is normal blood destruction conducted and the remains of the cells disposed of, that were it not for indirect evidence one might suppose the life of most red corpuscles to endure with that of the body."[10] As late as

1905, Jolly found remnants of the nucleus in some red cells and none in others. He postulated two cell lineages and wrote: "In search of their origin, I have naturally searched the blood of mammalian embryos."[11] Evidently, the assumption was that blood cells, once formed in the embryo, remain in the body throughout life.

Neumann is rightly credited with the recognition of the marrow as the seat of blood formation. However, it is generally unrecognized that, conceptually, his most fundamental contribution was his recognition that blood formation is a continuous process, occurring during postnatal life. It was this concept that formed the frame of reference for much of the work that followed. His first brief communication[12] of 1868 does not reflect this, suggesting that he attained this conceptual view gradually. But, the opening paragraph of his 1869 note[13] reads:

> The present work intends to demonstrate the physiologic importance of the bone marrow and that it is an important organ for blood formation which has not been recognized. It operates continually in a *de novo* formation of red blood cells.

To reach this conclusion, Neumann used deductive logic based on a premise that later proved incorrect. For a different reason, however, the conclusion remains valid—Neumann thought that proliferation of marrow cells occurred inside the blood vessels of the bone marrow and reasoned that these continuously proliferating cells must also continuously move out into the general circulation, for otherwise the blood circulation in the marrow would stop. We now know that red cell proliferation does not take place inside the blood vessels; but Neumann's conclusion remains valid because all blood formation takes place within a fixed volume inside a rigid frame of bone, where for every cell that is born, within or outside the blood vessels, one must leave to maintain the fixed volume.

Here, a corrective note is necessary. Most historical introductions on the marrow suggest that a substantive contribution was made by Claude Bernard.[14,15] These all refer to volume 68 of *Comptes Rendues* of the Paris Academy of Sciences. Examination of the original document[13] indicates that in this particular year, Claude Bernard, in his capacity as a member of the Academy, introduced a paper by Neumann, who was not a member. The title reads: "The Function of Bone Marrow in the Formation of Blood. Note by *Mr. Neumann*, presented by *Mr. Claude Bernard*."

Opposition to Neumann's discovery was most intense in Paris, where almost every eminent histologist had a theory on red cell production (vide infra). Bernard recognized Neumann's depth of vision and strongly supported his views. But there is nowhere, in this or other volumes of *Comptes Rendues*, an indication that Claude Bernard himself made a substantive contribution to this subject.

A Visionary Duo

Neumann's discovery was announced in the form of a preliminary report, which appeared as the lead article in the issue of 10 October 1868 of the *Centralblatt für die medizinischen Wissenshaften.* [12] Here is a translation of *About the Significance of Bone Marrow for Blood Formation*, preliminary communication by Prof. E. Neumann.

> In the so-called red bone marrow of man as well as the rabbit, one can regularly find, in addition to the well-known marrow cell, certain other elements which have not been mentioned until now; namely nucleated red blood cells, in every respect corresponding to embryonic stages of the red blood cells.
>
> Also in the marrow rich in fat, the same cells are present but in lower quantity and their number decreases parallel to the decrease in the number of *marrow cells* and the increase in the number of fat cells.
>
> It is possible to trace the origin of these elements to the marrow cells. The high content of colorless elements in the blood of the marrow makes it likely that there is a migration of contractile marrow cells into the vessels.
>
> A thorough description of my observations will be published.

The promised thorough description appeared the next year in an extensive article in *Archiv der Heilkunde.* [16] In the interim, however, two communications appeared in Italian and were soon translated in the *Centralblatt.* [17,18] They were both by Bizzozero, confirming the observation that nonnucleated red blood cells are formed from nucleated red cells in the marrow. Bizzozero extended the blood-forming function of the marrow to include the formation of white cells.

A careful reading of these interesting communications leaves one with the impression that perhaps Bizzozero might have come to this conclusion even before Neumann, but he was unsure of the reception he might receive if his findings were announced. The rapidity with which Bizzozero's announcement appeared following publication of Neumann's announcement supports this speculation.

It is worth mentioning that Neumann was a well-established professor in the European tradition, [19] whereas Bizzozero was but a 22-year-old recent graduate facing considerable opposition in his hometown of Pavia. His appointment to the faculty of medicine was pushed through, thanks to the recommendation of his mentor, Mantegazza, in the face of opposition by other faculty members, who cited his youth. [20] It should also be noted that in some areas, the views of Neumann and Bizzozero were not exactly identical. Retrospectively, in all these instances, Bizzozero proved to be correct.

Of the two, however, Neumann was a more persistent student of the subject. He continued his work on the marrow, and toward the end of the century produced other classic contributions. Among his "firsts" were the identification of leukemia[21] and of pernicious anemia[22] as diseases of the marrow. He coined the term *myelogenous leukemia*.[23]

Like Immanuel Kant, Neumann preferred to remain a lifelong citizen of Königsberg, where he taught and worked almost all his life on blood production and blood pigments. His superb literary taste, reflected in his masterful German writings, provides the profile of a German scholar in the classical sense. Bizzozero, by contrast, led a very unsettled life. Born in Varese, he studied in Milan and completed his medical studies in Pavia. He subsequently trained with Virchow in Berlin and, for a brief period, settled in Torino. He then moved to Rome where he was assigned an honorary senate seat. The scope of his scientific interest was also varied. His early interest in the vascular system was soon replaced by interest in the marrow; but after a decade, he focused on the coagulation mechanism and recognized and coined the term *platelet*. Toward the end of his life, he developed choroiditis, which interfered with the microscopic work. His interest then turned to issues affecting public health. He died at the turn of the century, rather prematurely, at the age of 55.

Even before Neumann and Bizzozero, the transition of the nucleated to nonnucleated red cell had been seen in the liver by Kölliker,[24] a German scholar. The French anatomist Charles Robin[25] had also come close to this discovery, but he did not recognize the kinship of red cells to marrow cells. He coined the term *marrow cells (médullocelles)*, which apparently is what Neumann referred to as "bekannten Markzellen"[12]—the well-known marrow cells.

This frontier of knowledge, thus, was being explored intensively. Had not Neumann made his discovery known, it would surely have been made by others. It is the curious nature of science that, in Bergsonian terms, it has its own *élan vital*, its own momentum. With some exceptions, humanity is but an instrument of this momentum to expand the boundary of knowledge: "It is not the men that make science; it is science that makes the men."[26]*

The Maze of Theories

The findings of Neumann and Bizzozero had two components. One related to the *cellular origin* of the red cell; it stated that nonnucleated red cells in the blood are derived from nucleated precursors. The second related to the *tissue origin* and stated that this process takes place in the marrow.

---

* Variations on this theme also appear in Paul Valéry's *Mauvaises pensées ou autres* (1941, Paris, Corti), wherein he concludes: "Ce qui fait un ouvrage n'est pas celui qui y met son nom. Ce qui fait un ouvrage n'a pas de nom." (The one who does a piece of work is not the one who puts his name on it. The one who does the work has no name.) Bertold Brecht's *Galileo* is even more emphatic on this note: "There is no scientific work that one man alone can write." (*Collected Plays*, 1972, N.Y., Vintage.)

The first component stood in contrast to a great number of divergent theories of that time,[14,27,28] perhaps reflecting the intensity of search for the origin of the red cell. A number of investigators supported the nuclear origin of the red cell. Erb[29] maintained that red cells are products of disintegration of white cell nuclei. Wharton Jones[30] believed that the nuclei of precursor cells swelled by acquiring hemoglobin and became red cells. Pouchet[31] maintained that red cells might be derived from white cells by *hemoglobinic degeneration,* similar to fatty degeneration. Weber,[32] on the other hand, thought that red cells were made from fat globules in the liver. Several scholars played different notes on the tune that red cells are protoplasmic offsprings of a precursor cell which is in a state of continuous expansion and budding. To this group belonged Rindfleisch,[33] Rollet,[34] and Malassez.[28] Generation of hemoglobin in the cytoplasm of *vasoformative cells* (scavenger cells) was the theory of Ranvier,[35] who maintained that from these cells, red cells are released, plasmid-like, into the circulation. Hayem[36] thought red cells were made by platelets. Arndt[37] believed that any protoplasmic fragment could absorb hemoglobin and turn into a red cell. Apparently, in drawing a parallel with nucleated red cells in birds, several investigators, including Boettcher,[38] Löwit,[39] and Stricker,[40] were of the opinion that mammalian red cells also had a nucleus *(Innenkörper),* albeit not as well defined as that of their avian counterparts.

Some of these theories may now appear strange and even naive, but it should be remembered that during this period, the viable nature of red cells had not yet been established. More than a quarter of a century later, Jolly[27] observed that "these theories diverted the researchers in a direction completely inconsistent with the viable nature of the red cell." It was against this background that the observations of Neumann and Bizzozero appeared. To see straight through this cloud of confusion, vision was needed; that is what Neumann and Bizzozero offered. They belonged to a generation of scientists who could expand the range of possibilities and of whom Ehrlich (Chapter 1) was a superior example.

Despite the intensity of the search, Neumann's observations did not catch on easily. His ideas were received with the same skepticism with which Immanuel Kant's *Critique of Pure Reason* had been greeted almost a century before. Neumann was supported by Bizzozero and by Claude Bernard, but there were also Pouchet and Hayem to repudiate him and Robin to accuse him of adding to the confusion by postulating yet another theory. Georges Hayem wrote an entire book in repudiation of Bizzozero! The preface of this book,[36] despite a haughty tone, is but a *lamentoso* for plausible theories that were about to sink. Later, in reference to Hayem, Jolly[27] deplored the "unfortunate" influence that did not permit Neumann's theory to be accepted universally for about 20 years.

To understand this skepticism, we may remember that during this period, all students of the subject had their pet theories, which they defended vehemently. Moreover, in their initial presentations, Neumann and Bizzozero could not provide compelling evidence to override the maze of theories. They saw nucleated red cells in the marrow and concluded that they are the source of nonnucleated red cells. Naturally, this was received as "yet another theory." At any rate, "compelling evidence" in those days consisted of demonstrating the transition forms between the two cells: *post hoc ergo propter hoc.*

The confusion may not have been all that unjustified. During this period, histologists were working at the limits of their methodological potential. Without further developments in fixation and staining techniques, little substantive information could be gained. Charles Robin is an example. He studied the marrow in 1849 using acetic acid in his preparations. Consequently, the hemoglobin was leached out of nucleated red cells, and he was unable to recognize their kinship to their nonnucleated products.[25] Apparently, with reference to Robin and mindful of his mistake, both Neumann and Bizzozero repeatedly emphasized the necessity of using a neutral fixative or no fixative at all.

Despite all the opposition, however, within two decades, Neumann's discovery was a scientific axiom! The brilliance of truth may first be blinding, but ultimately it supersedes all artificial illuminators.

Pitting of the Cell

Science is a never-ending inquiry. Answers inevitably lead to new questions. The concept of the derivation of red cells from nucleated precursors inevitably led to the question of how the nucleus is lost.[27,28] One school of thought maintained that the nucleus was not lost, but simply changed its character so that in routine preparations it was no longer visible. Attempts were then made to visualize the invisible nucleus with the aid of various chemicals.[38,40]

Among those who believed in elimination of the nucleus, two mechanisms were invoked. The first, and at that time the dominant, theory maintained that the nucleus was resorbed. Neumann was a proponent of this. The second theory maintained that the nucleus was extruded; this view was advanced by Rindfleisch[33] and held by Bizzozero.[41] Transitional stages between nucleated and nonnucleated cells should have provided an answer; but few of them were to be seen, and Neumann was forced to conclude that nuclear resorption occurred very rapidly.

If most histologists were in search of transitional stages for an answer, Malassez[28] was different. This French histologist invoked a logical argument. He maintained that if the nucleus is resorbed, the volume of the red cell should be equal to that of its nucleated precursor; while if the nucleus is extruded, the volume of the red cell should be less than that of its nucleated precursor. Thus, he made a series of measurements, remarkable for the time, and concluded that the nucleus could not have been resorbed.

The ingenious argument, alas, did not come upon a *tabula rasa,* an open mind. Like most of his contemporaries, Malassez had his own pet theory. He maintained that red cells bud off continuously from a nucleated precursor whose cytoplasm is in a state of continuous growth. Thus, he also denied the extrusion of the nucleus in favor of his *"théorie de bourgeonnement protoplasmique"*: like Daedalus, a prisoner of his own intellectual labyrinth!

At the turn of the century, after the introduction of newer staining methods, Pappenheim[42] tried to bring the two theories together. He suggested a sequence of nuclear degeneration, fragmentation, and then extrusion. During the next half-century, this question was buried amid other more fashionable questions. Enucleation of red cells was somehow *demodé*. The lack of suitable techniques perhaps was responsible, for it was not until the advent of microcinematography in the 1950s that Bessis and others[43] recorded expulsion of the nucleus. With the advent of electron microscopy, the controversy now seems to have subsided in favor of nuclear extrusion.[44]

A related question that was not faced earlier concerns the role of the marrow in the enucleation of the red cell—the concept of a marrow-blood barrier.[44] The synthesis of this concept needed three elements. First, the comparative studies of the nineteenth century established that avian red cells are nucleated whereas those of mammals are not. This curious fact did not attract much attention. Not much was known of the function of the nucleus in those days, and, because birds were considered lower in the evolutionary scale, the presence of a nucleus in the red cell was considered a "sign of inferiority."[27] In the early twentieth century, a second difference became apparent—in birds, red cells are formed inside the blood vessels; in mammals, this process takes place outside the vessels. A third element arose from the concept of "pitting" that takes place in the spleen. Cells that contain inclusions lose them in passing through the spleen (Chapter 5). A comparable "pitting" occurs in the marrow much as stones are pitted from fruits. When a nucleated red cell migrates through the vascular wall to enter the circulation, it loses its nucleus. The cytoplasm is malleable and squeezes through, but the nucleus is rigid and remains behind.[45]

These three elements form the basis of a synthesis. There exists a screening barrier, the vascular wall, between the marrow and the blood. It controls what can enter the circulation, or at least what cannot. In mammals, the red cells must pass through this barrier, which retains their nuclei; thus, mammalian red cells are nonnucleated. In birds, the cells develop beyond this barrier, and to enter the circulation they need not pass through it. Thus, circulating red cells in birds are nucleated.

The Life of an Unfortunate Concept

In his second paper,[18] Bizzozero reported on the presence in the marrow of large cells containing pigmented granules similar to red cells. He drew a parallel to similar cells observed by Virchow in bleeding foci and by Kölliker in the spleen. Clearly, the description is that of scavenger cells containing red cell debris. Bizzozero concluded that the marrow, in addition to being the seat of blood formation, is also the site of blood destruction. One can be impressed by Bizzozero's interpretation because Ranvier[35] saw similar granules and thought these cells generated hemoglobin, which was then condensed to form red cells.

At this point, history replays an instructive note. Science is a search for truth, but the truth may not necessarily be plausible. Human beings, however, are wont to take plausibility for truth, and misinterpretations of facts that are based on plausibility often last long and may resist replacement by correct interpretation.

When in 1838, Schleiden, a lawyer-turned-botanist, enunciated his cell theory, one of its main components related to the mechanism of cell formation.[46,47] He maintained that new cells are formed by the aggregation and confluence of granules of various sorts by a process similar to that of crystal formation. Being basically a physical process, according to Schleiden, living cells are not necessary for the formation of a new cell.[7] Although shortly thereafter, Virchow[48] placed the cell theory in proper context by indicating that new cells are formed by division of preexisting living cells, *omnis cellula e cellula*, Schleiden's fallacious theory was to live on for about a century, dictating the conceptual frame for many minds in biology. It was not accidental that during this same period, Pasteur's germ theory met with resistance by those who clung to the belief in the spontaneous generation of microbes.[49] The formation of red cells, which were not really considered "true" cells, was particularly susceptible to the influence of this concept.

It was against this background that many students of embryology developed the opinion that red cells originate inside larger cells (*blutkörperchenhaltige Zellen*) by the aggregation and confluence of pigmented granules and through a process similar to crystal formation. The unlikely member of this group was Ernst Neumann. The essence of this thinking is evident in his communication of April 1869, where he takes issue with Bizzozero's interpretation of pigment-containing cells.[16] Later, he saw nucleated red cells within the cytoplasm of scavenger cells and concluded that the nucleated red cells are formed within, and extruded from, the cytoplasm of these parent cells.[50] Nearly a decade passed before Neumann abandoned this viewpoint[51] and agreed with Bizzozero that the cells containing pigmented granules must be regarded as scavenger cells.

Schleiden's concept concerning cell origin, however, was not yet to be abandoned. Its undue influence on concepts of red cell formation lasted well into our century, when Harvey Jordan revived it, modified it, and maintained that red cells originate inside megakaryocytes.[52] He found Wright's theory of platelet formation (Chapter 16) not incompatible with his own theory of red cell formation from megakaryocytes. This, fortunately, was the swan song of that unfortunate concept; for after Jordan, Schleiden's specter was finally removed from the conceptual frame of red cell formation.

Beyond the Marrow

The observations of Neumann and Bizzozero related not only to the *cellular origin* but also to the *tissue origin* of the red cell. They stated that the marrow is the major production center of red cells. On this issue, the scientific ambiance was less opinionated and this concept should have fared better. Actually, it did not. Scholars of that period, being deeply entangled in the theories of the *cellular origin* of the red cell, were oblivious to the tissue in which the search should be made. Most searched in the blood; few found it necessary to look in other tissues. The epitome of this attitude is shown by the work of Georges Pouchet.[53] In 1878, he reported on the regeneration of red cells in a dog who was bled. He examined the blood but not the marrow. He found no nucleated red cells and concluded that nucleated cells could not be the origin of red cells; for were it so, "it would be difficult to admit that none of these elements could find their way into the circulation." He then observed an increased number of platelets, now a well-recognized occurrence after blood loss, and concluded that platelets were the source of red cells. "In the field of experimentation, chance favors only the prepared mind," said Louis Pasteur,[54] who, during the same period, was engaged in a battle with another Pouchet, Félix. The latter, believing in the spontaneous generation of microbes, repudiated Pasteur's germ theory.[49]

We may remember, however, that during this time, researchers were studying various species from frog to bat to human. Nucleated red cells had been seen in many other tissues, and even after the function of the marrow in blood formation had been generally accepted, there was no reason that this site should exclude other sites. Thus, in defense of their view, Neumann and Bizzozero began a systematic study of various tissues in a variety of species. Their studies lasted nearly two decades and showed that in adult humans, red cell production is limited to the marrow.[55,56] The only dissent came from Harvey Jordan, who, some 30 years later, maintained that lymph nodes also could produce red cells.[57] He argued that plasma cells were but aborted red cells. This is the more interesting because during this period, Jordan[58] raised another dissenting voice, this time against, to quote Florence Sabin,[59] the "majority opinion" that red cells originate from the vascular wall. The minority of one, Jordan, proved to be correct in his dissent and proved once again that truth is not achieved by consensus. Indeed, science is not a democratic domain.

The Favorable Environment

The "majority opinion" to which Sabin refers had evolved as a corollary to Neumann's discovery. Once the marrow was established as the site of blood cell formation, it was natural to search in the marrow not only for the immediate parent cells but also for their ancestors. This led to the assumption that the ancestor cells of blood cells *originate* in the marrow. Again, assumption was based on plausibility, not logic. The bone marrow is certainly a production center for blood cells, but no logical dictum requires that the ancestor cells originate there. Simply because a product comes out of a factory, we do not assume that its basic constituents also originate there.

Yet, this assumption provided the frame of reference for students of the marrow during the first quarter of our century and formed the basis for the "majority opinion" that the ancestor cell of the red cell is derived from the vascular wall.[60] Again, it was the advent of more appropriate methodology, radiobiologic methods and the transplantation technique (Chapter 4), that placed the question in perspective—the marrow is a production center whose environment is favorable to the proliferation and growth of blood cells. The ancestor of these cells, the common stem cell, however, might circulate. In its course, it may pass through many organs, but, upon arrival in the marrow, it "homes" and begins to proliferate and produce blood cells like a seed in a fertile soil.[61] In our age of acronyms, this concept has become known as *HIM*, for hematopoietic inductive microenvironment.[62]

The foundation for this thinking was evident as early as the first decade of this century in the writings of such scholars as Max Askanazy,[63] a pupil of Neumann. Danchakoff,[64] who subscribed to the "majority opinion," remarked that in birds, red cells were produced inside the blood vessels; not so the white cells. They arose on the outside and wandered in. She was of the opinion that the vascular wall gave rise to both red and white cells, and, thus, concluded that the environment on the two sides of the wall must be different and must determine which cell type is produced. A few years later, in 1916, in a lecture before the College of Physicians and Surgeons of Columbia University, she was arguing the case for the existence of a common stem cell.[65] She drew an analogy to a heap of tree seeds. In a moderate climate the seeds will grow into tall trees, but in arctic lands they will develop into trees no higher than our moss:

> How would it be possible to know if there were differences in the seeds? The only possibility of solving this problem would consist of sowing the seeds of arctic trees in our climate and vice versa. If the seeds of our tall trees again produce dwarf trees in the arctic lands, the seeds of the different products of development will have been shown to have been identical.
>
> Similar experiments may be carried out with the haematopoietic tissue.

Her prophecy was realized some 50 years later, thanks to the advent of transplantation techniques, which proves that in the absence of appropriate methods, the most brilliant concepts may lead nowhere but to oblivion or stagnation.

Morphologic Era and a Dichotomy

There is a repeating sequence in the history of science that is almost axiomatic—controversies arise when scientists are working on the boundary of the potential of their methods and may be overstepping the circle of permissible conclusions. New methods must be developed to expand the boundary of possibilities by a quantum and to permit new exploitations and expansion of knowledge. When the new boundary is reached, new controversies arise. The two elements, methods and permissible conclusions, are in a continuous state of interaction and cross-fertilization—the movement is *legato*.

Toward the end of the nineteenth century, a series of rapid advances in morphologic methods took place, the pinnacle of which was Paul Ehrlich's introduction of the use of aniline dyes and of heat-fixed films of blood and marrow in hematology. Recognition of marrow as the site of blood production must have been a stimulus for these advances because they were immediately applied to the study of the blood and the marrow, expanding our knowledge of blood production.

Ehrlich's methods were soon replaced by the simpler Romanowsky methods for staining of air-dried smears; this gave the cytology of blood and marrow a new dimension. The new method was exploited by many scholars, foremost among them, Pappenheim, Ferrata, and Naegeli. Their studies form the basis for our present knowledge of blood and marrow cytology, in technique as well as interpretation, in health as well as in disease. This was the golden age of hematologic morphology.

Parallel with these developments, a number of anatomists focused on blood production in the embryo; foremost among them were two Russians, Alexander Maximow and Vera Danchakoff. Maximow worked primarily on mammals; Danchakoff on birds. Their studies form the basis of our current knowledge of embryonic blood production.

Whereas Pappenheim, Ferrata, and their followers worked with dry smears, Maximow and Danchakoff used sectioned tissues. The two methods offer different potentials and, expectedly, limitations. The smear technique permits the detailed study of single cells but not their relation in the tissues. The opposite is true of the section technique.

As long as the two groups worked well within the boundaries of their methodologic potentials, their findings were mutually helpful, but this period did not last long. Soon, both groups exhausted the possibilities of their respective methods and were working on the boundaries again. At this point, Pappenheim and Ferrata were engaged in giving their field an artistic dimension by providing atlases and color plates; the proponents of tissue section, on the other hand, began a series of conceptualizations and wide-ranging speculations. The findings of the two groups no longer coincided but were in sharp opposition. A dichotomy appeared.

The literature of this period is rather amusing in that the two camps, basically identified by their methodologic orientations, criticized each other precisely on that score—technique. Each group recognized the methodologic limits of the other but not their own. Downey, a proponent of the smear technique, believed that the section did not "bring out the finer details of structure, especially of the nuclei, seen in dry smear."[66] Similar criticisms were directed at Maximow by many others who felt that "his persistent unilateral slant on the all-sufficiency of sectioned material prevented him often from properly evaluating the importance of nuclear morphological changes as specific expressions of cell ancestry and maturation."[14]

By contrast, from the other camp we hear Maximow announcing that the dry smear method is "inadequate for solving the general problems of the origin of blood cells."[60] He then makes a somewhat caustic remark about clinicians:

> Among clinicians, however, the dualistic theory is more popular. Operating with minute differences in the nuclear and protoplasmic structures of normal and pathological blood cells, it supplies them with a convenient, detailed, though somewhat artificial classification of these elements.

Danchakoff, the very eloquent and somewhat argumentative proponent, also turns the edge of the sword on the "pathologist-clinician":

> Facing the various highly differentiated products, the pathologist-clinicians could not but admit a polyphyletic origin for various blood cells. The red cells possessed their own stem cells, as also the different leukocytes and lymphocytes.[65]*

One might think the choice of method determines a researcher's particular interpretive leaning; but the preconception also dictates the interpretation irrespective of the method. Thus, in 1909, during a blood symposium in Berlin, when Ferrata studied some of Maximow's tissue preparations, he came to an entirely different conclusion from that of Maximow himself, supporting the concept of multiple ancestral cells.[67]

Red and Yellow Marrow

In the course of evolution, the bone marrow is a latecomer in the task of blood production; but it probably has achieved a high plateau of efficiency. Nature tried a few other tissues for the task before settling on the marrow—the spleen, the liver, the kidney, and even the wall of the gut. Because the marrow is within the bone, only those species with a backbone have marrow. In the evolutionary scale, the frog is the first to have blood-producing marrow, but

---

* This topic is discussed more fully in Chapter 4.

then only transiently during the summer; however, when the frog's spleen is removed, the marrow assumes all the blood-producing function. In the reptile, the marrow and the spleen bear the burden equally. In birds and mammals, the marrow is the major site, but other sites retain minor roles. It is only in primates that the task of blood production is limited to the marrow. Similarly, only during the last part of primate fetal life does marrow supersede the other organs and take its unique place in blood production.

There are two types of marrow: blood-producing marrow, which is red because of its hemoglobin content, and yellow marrow, containing mostly fat, which imparts a yellowish color. It was Xavier Bichat[68] who first, at the end of the eighteenth century, recognized the two types of marrow and coined the terms "red" and "fatty" marrow. He thought that the red marrow was seen in the fetus and the yellow or "true" marrow, in the adult. He recognized that the marrow fat is distinct from the usual variety of fat. Bichat could not yet know of the link between the blood and the marrow; nor could he discuss the change from red to fatty marrow. The presence of red marrow in the adult was to be recognized later, including even the transitory state between the two, the gelatinous marrow.[69]

Again, it was Neumann who provided us with the classic statement. In 1882, he enunciated the rule governing the development of yellow marrow. In effect, he recognized a phenomenon that is sometimes referred to as *Neumann's law*.[70] It states that at birth, all bones that contain marrow contain red marrow. With age, the blood-producing activity contracts toward the center of the body, leaving the more peripheral bones with only fatty marrow.

For about 50 years, students of the marrow did not know what to make of this phenomenon. During the morphologic era, a favorite preoccupation of researchers was to make the marrow inactive and then to stimulate it at will. This was done to overcome the crowding of the marrow by the blood-forming cells and, so, to appreciate better the underlying organization. Hence, the literature of this period is full of such jargon as "simplified marrow" or "unmasked blood formation."[59]

The mechanism underlying the development of yellow marrow after birth was not studied until 1936, when Charles Huggins and his coworkers[71] observed a parallel phenomenon—at birth, the temperature of the marrow is comparable in all bones, but, soon after birth, cooling takes place in the bones of the extremities. This observation immediately suggested a relationship—the thermal environment in the bones of the extremities after birth is not optimal for blood production; consequently, the sites for blood production contract and are confined to the warmer bones in the central parts of the body. To test this hypothesis, they looped the rat tail, which contains yellow marrow, and placed it within the warmer environment of the abdomen. Soon, the part located inside the abdomen became red.[71] Here again, one is faced with two separate elements—the contraction of red marrow and the concomitant cooling of the bones; their discoveries were separated by a period of 50 years. Both discoveries, however, were necessary before a logical synthesis could be formulated and tested.

Huggins' explanation has now proved to be an oversimplification. Genetic, functional, and developmental influences may be even more important for the development of yellow marrow.[72]

Of the Bone and its Marrow

The most ancient views about the function of the marrow are related to its strange case, the bone. Hippocrates maintained that the marrow is the source of the nutrient supply to the bone, an opinion also held by Galen. Aristotle took the opposite view, viz., the marrow is a waste product of the bone (excrementum ossium).[73]

Impressed by the extensive vascularity of the marrow, anatomists of the eighteenth century expounded on the Hippocratic view and maintained that the marrow is but the vascular component of the bone and is located in the inner part for protection. Considerable interest centered around an ill-defined membrane, the "medullary membrane," which was believed to be an elaborate barrier controlling the nutrition of bone.[73] In 1700, the French anatomist Duverney[74] argued that many bones, like those of the middle ear, do not have marrow; thus, the marrow could not be all that essential to the nutrition of bone. In the nineteenth century, Charles Robin[73] noted that in the course of development, the marrow is formed after the bone and, therefore, it cannot be the source of bone nutrition any more than it can be the origin of its development.

This was an era in science when mechanomorphic views were beginning to become popular. Robin postulated a purely mechanical function for the marrow in relation to the bone. He argued that of two cylinders of similar weights and substance, the one with an empty core, i.e., with a larger diameter, is stronger. Thus, the presence of a marrow cavity in the long bones strengthens them without adding to their weight and, in addition, creates more surface area for the insertion of muscles and ligaments than otherwise would be possible, a postulate hardly testable or contestable.

Experimental medicine, which was then beginning to thrive, provided an opportunity for exploring the relation between the bone and its marrow. Several researchers separated the two tissues by removing bits of the marrow out of the bone and grafting them elsewhere, usually in the abdomen. Some of the first such experiments were done by the French experimentalist Goujon[75,76] and later, by Bailkow,[77] who noted a somewhat surprising phenomenon; the grafted marrow may disappear entirely, but if it survives, it transforms into a piece of bone which has neither the volume nor the shape of the grafted tissue.

These were the first observations made on the bone-forming potential of the marrow. No marrow could be obtained from the grafted marrow in these experiments. Indeed, it was not until the present century that marrow was obtained after implantation of the marrow, and this marrow was still within a shell of bone.[78] Thus, the Hippocractic postulate was reversed—the bone must somehow be essential for the function of the marrow. This was the frame of reference for the marrow researchers of the 1920s. Sabin[59] sets the tone by pointing out that bone provides a nonexpansile frame for the marrow and "when there is any increase of cells in marrow, something has to pass out to make room." For lack of suitable methods, the question remains unresolved.

Marrow Vessels

In a general way, one may say that marrow blood vessels, more than any of its components, have intrigued researchers. They also exemplify how the advance of knowledge depends on appropriate methods.

In ancient times, when the marrow was believed to be a source of nutrient supply to the bone, it was perceived as a mass of vessels interspersed with fat. During the eighteenth century, when the medullary membrane theory was fashionable, Duverney,[74] and, later, Bichat,[68] thought of it essentially as a vascular membrane. Duverney drew an analogy with the spinal cord. Both the marrow and the spinal cord are protected within a rigid frame of bone, and both are very soft tissues with a high fat content. Since the spinal cord has a vascular membrane, the arachnoid, so must the marrow. During the nineteenth century, Miescher exaggerated these views and considered the entire marrow cavity as a single, enormously enlarged vascular channel.[73]

By the mid-nineteenth century, however, methodologic developments permitted a more realistic view of the marrow vasculature, and by the turn of the century, the problem had been reduced to two related questions. One question concerned the nature of the circulation in the marrow and asked whether it is a closed system or open to the extravascular space. This question involved enigmatic vascular structures for which the term *sinusoids* was soon to be coined by Minot.[79] The second question related to the site of blood production and whether it is inside or outside the vessels. Thus, the lines were drawn for a battle which was to last for about half a century.

In 1892, Van der Stricht[80] recognized that the sites of red cell formation differ in birds and mammals. In birds, he maintained that the circulation is a closed system and red cell formation takes place within the vessels, an opinion that was later confirmed. In mammals, however, he thought the circulation is wide open with maturing red cells wandering about and entering the circulation only when fully mature (Figure 3-2). During the 1920s, a concerted effort by many students of the marrow led to the formulation of a coherent view, if not a complete answer.[58] It was only after the advent of new microscopic techniques that a picture began to emerge, according to which, in mammals,

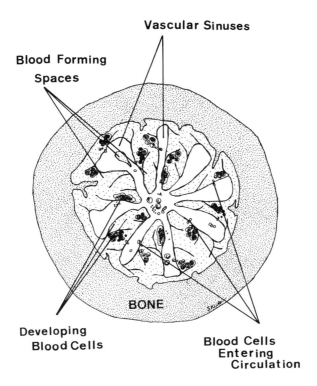

Vascular Sinuses

Blood Forming Spaces

BONE

Developing Blood Cells

Blood Cells Entering Circulation

Figure 3-2 A diagrammatic cross section of a long bone in mammals. The bone surrounding the marrow cavity may send small branches into the marrow cavity. The marrow cavity basically consists of two elements—vascular spaces and blood-forming spaces. Blood cells are developed outside the vessels in blood-forming spaces. Normally, these spaces are crowded with blood-forming cells. In this diagram, the blood-forming spaces have been intentionally drawn with fewer cells to make the phenomenon better appreciated. In the scale of this diagram, developing blood cells are purposely magnified to make their appreciation easier. In several areas mature blood cells are squeezing through the vascular barrier to enter the vascular sinuses and from there into the central vein and general circulation.

red cells are formed outside the vessels and delivered to the circulation through the "sinusoid" barrier. Now other questions puzzle us—the nature of the sinusoid wall, the mode of cellular migration across the wall, and the regulation of this phenomenon.

There is no final answer for a scientific question, only metamorphosis.

Acknowledgments

Among many, I am particularly indebted to Professor Emanuele Salvidio of Genova, who not only compensated for my inadequacies in German and

Italian languages but also located and provided me with the photograph of Giulio Bizzozero (Figure 3-1). For the photograph of Ernst Neumann (Chapter Opening Photo), I am indebted to Professor H. Lullies.

References

1 Meyer AL, Meltzer SJ: On continuous insufflation through the humerus in fowls. *Am J Physiol* 40:126–127, 1916.

2 Bloom W, Bloom MA, McLean FC: Calcification and ossification. Medullary bone changes in the reproductive cycle of female pigeon. *Anat Rec* 81:443–475, 1941.

3 Brown-Séquard CE, d'Arsonval A: Recherches sur les extraits liquides retirés des glandes et d'autres parties de l'organisme et sur leur emploi en injections, sous-cutanées, comme méthode thérapeutique. *Arch Physiol* 3(series 5):491–506, 1891.

4 Brown-Séquard CE, d'Arsonval A: Des injections sous-cutanées ou intra-veineuses d'extraits liquides de nombre d'organes comme méthode thérapeutique. *C R Acad Sci (Paris)* 114:1399–1405, 1892.

5 Pegg DR: *Bone Marrow Transplantation.* Chicago, Year Book Medical Publishers, 1966, 192 pp, p 11.

6 Mechanik N: Untersuchungen über das Gewicht des Knochenmarkes des Menschen. *Anat Entwickl* 79:58–99, 1926.

7 Schleiden MJ: Beiträg zur Phytogenesis. *Müller's Arch Anat Physiol Wissensch Med* 5:137–176, 1838, pp 231–263. (An English translation of Schleiden's monograph with some additional notes has appeared as an appendix to the English translation of Schwann's "Mikroskopische Untersuchangen.")

8 Schwann T: *Microscopical Researches into the Accordance in the Structure and Growth of Animals and Plants,* Smith H (trans). London, Sydenham Society, 1847, 268 pp.

9 Bernard C: in Greene JE (ed): *100 Great Scientists.* New York, Washington Square Press, 1964, 489 pp, p 259.

10 Rous P: Destruction of red blood corpuscles in health and disease. *Physiol Rev* 3:75–105, 1923.

11 Jolly MJ: Sur l'évolution des globules rouges dans le sang des embryons de mammifères. *C R Soc Biol* (Paris) 58:593–594, 1905.

12 Neumann E: Ueber die Bedeutung des Knochenmarkes für die Blutbildung. *Zentralbl Med Wissensch* 6:689, 1868.

13 Neumann E: Du rôle de la moelle des os dans la formation du sang. *C R Acad Sci (Paris)* 68:1112–1113, 1869.

14 Michels NA: Erythropoiesis. A critical review of the literature. *Folia Haematol* (Leipz) 45:75–128, 1931.

15 Ness PM, Stengle JM: Historical introduction, in Surgenor DM (ed): *The Red Blood Cell.* New York, Academic Press, 1974, 612 pp, p 10.

16 Neumann E: Ueber die Bedeutung des Knochenmarkes für die Blutbildung. Ein Beitrag zur Entwicklungsgeschichte der Blutkörperchen. *Arch Heilk* 10:68–102, 1869.

17 Bizzozero G: Sulla funzione ematopoetica del midollo delle ossa. *Zentralbl Med Wissensch* 6:885, 1868.

18 Bizzozero G: Sulla funzione ematopoetica del midollo delle ossa. Seconda communicazione preventia. *Zentralbl Med Wissensch* 10:149–150, 1869.

19 Askanazy M: Ernst Neumann. *Zentralbl Allg Pathol Pathol Anat* 29:409–421, 1918.

20 Dizienarie Biog degli Italiani. Alberto M Ghisalberti (ed). Instituto della Enciclopedia Italiana, Rome, 1960, vol I, Article: Bizzozero, Giulio, pp 747–751.

21 Neumann E: Ein Fall von Leukämie mit Erkankung des Knochenmarkes. *Arch Heilk* 10:1–15, 1870.

22 Neumann E: Ueber das Verhalten des Knochenmarkes bei progressiver perniziöser anaemie. *Berl Klin Wochenschr* 14:865–866, 1877.

23 Neumann E: Ueber myelogene Leukämie. *Berl Klin Wochenschr* 15:69, 1878.

24 Kölliker A: Ueber die Blutkörperchen eines menschlichen Embryo und die Entwicklung der Blutkörperchen bei Sängethieren. *Z Rat Med (Zürich)* 4:112–159, 1846.

25 Robin C: Sur l'existence de deux espèces nouvelles d'éléments anatomique qui se trouvent dans le canal médullaire. *C R Soc Biol (Paris)* 1:149–150, 1849.

26 Chargaff E: A quick climb up Mount Olympus. *Science* 159:1448–1449, 1968.

27 Jolly MJ: Recherches sur la formation des globules rouges des mammifères. *Arch Anat Microsc Morphol Exp* 9:133–314, 1907.

28 Malassez L: Sur l'origine et la formation des globules rouges dans la moelle des os. *Arch Physiol* 9(series 2):1–47, 1882.

29 Erb W: Zur Entwickelungsgeschichte der rothen Blutkörperchen. *Virchows Arch* 34:138–193, 1865.

30 Jones TWharton: The blood corpuscle considered in its different phases of development in the animal series. I. Vertebrata. *Philos Trans R Soc Lond (Biol)* 136:63–88, 1846.

31 Pouchet G: De l'origine des hématies. *C R Soc Biol* (Paris) 30:77–79, 1878.

32 Weber EH: Ueber die Bedeutung der Leber für die Bildung der Blutkörperchen der Embryonen. *Z Rat Med (Zürich)* 4:160–167, 1846.

33 Rindfleisch GE: Ueber Knochenmark und Blutbildung. *Arch Mikr Anat* 17:21–42, 1880.

34 Rollet A: Ueber Zersetzungsbilder der rothen Blutkörperchen. *Untersuch Inst Physiol Histol Graz Leipz* 1:1–31, 1870.

35 Ranvier LA: De development et de l'accroissement des vaisseaux sanguins. *Arch Physiol* 11(series 2):429–445, 1874.

36 Hayem G: *Du sang et de ses altérations anatomiques.* Paris, G Masson, 1889, 1035 pp.

37 Arndt R: Untersuchungen an den rothen Blutkörperchen der Wirbelthiere. *Virchows Arch* 83:15–41, 1881.

38 Boettcher A: Untersuchungen über die rothen Blutkörperchen der Wirbelthiere. *Virchows Arch* 36:342–434, 1866.

39 Löwit M: Die Anordnung und Neubildung von Leukoblasten und Erythroblasten in den Blutzellenbildenden. *Arch Mikr Anat* 38:524–612, 1891.

40 Stricker S: Mikrochemische Untersuchungen der rothen Blutkörperchen. *Arch Ges Physiol* 1:590–600, 1868.

41 Bizzozero G: Ueber die Bildung der rothen Blutkörperchen. *Virchows Arch* 95:26–45, 1884.

42 Pappenheim A: Ueber Entwickelung und Ausbildung der Erythroblasten *Virchows Arch* 145:587–643, 1896.

43 Bessis M, Bricka M: Aspect dynamique des cellules du sang. Son études par la microcinématographie en contraste de phase. *Rev Hematol* 7:407–435, 1952.

44 Tavassoli M: Red cell delivery and the function of the marrow-blood barrier: A review. *Exp Hematol* 6:257–269, 1978.

45 Tavassoli M, Crosby WH: Fate of nucleus of marrow erythroblast. *Science*

173:912–913, 1973.

46   Karling JS: Schleiden's contribution to the cell theory. *Biol Symp* 1:37–57, 1940.

47   Conklin EG: Predecessors of Schleiden and Schwann. *Biol Symp* 1:58–66, 1940.

48   Virchow RLK: *Cellular Pathology as Based upon Physiological and Pathological Histology.* Collection of lectures delivered in Pathological Institute of Berlin during 1858 and published in 1859 as "Die Cellularpathologie." Translated from second edition of the original by Frank Chance. Philadelphia, Lippincott, 1863, 554 pp.

49   Dubos RJ: *Louis Pasteur: Freelance of Science.* Boston, Little Brown, 1950, 418 pp, pp 159–187.

50   Neumann E: Neue Beiträge zur Kenntnis der Blutbildung. *Arch Heilk* 15:441–476, 1874.

51   Neumann E: Ueber Blutregeneration und Blutbildung. II. Lymphdrüsen und Milz als Blutbildungsorgane. *Z Klin Med* 3:417–425, 1881.

52   Jordan HE: A contribution to the problems concerning the origin, structure, genetic relationship and function of the giant cells of hemopoietic and osteolytic foci. *Am J Anat* 24:225–269, 1918.

53   Pouchet G: Sur la régénération des hématies mammifères. *C R Soc Biol (Paris)* 30:37–38, 1878.

54   Pasteur L: in Greene JE (ed): *100 Great Scientists.* New York, Washington Square Press, 1964, 489 pp, p 284.

55   Bizzozero G, Torre A: Ueber die Entstehung der rothen Blutkörperchen bei den verschiedenen Wirbeltierklassen. *Virchows Archiv* 95:1–25, 1884.

56   Neumann E: Ueber die Entwicklung roter Blutkörperchen in neugebildetem Knockenmark. *Virchows Arch* 119:835–398, 1890.

57   Jordan HE: The erythrocytogenic capacity of mammalian lymph nodes. *Am J Anat* 38:255–297, 1926.

58   Jordan HE, Baker JP: The character of the wall of the smaller blood vessels in the bone marrow of the frog with special reference to the question of erythrocyte origin. *Anat Rec* 35:161–174, 1927.

59   Sabin FR: Bone marrow. *Physiol Rev* 8:191–244, 1928.

60   Maximow AA: Relation of blood cells to connective tissues and endothelium. *Physiol Rev* 4:533–563, 1924.

61   Tavassoli M: Studies on hemopoietic microenvironments. *Exp Hematol* 3:213–226, 1975.

62   Trentin JJ: Influence of hematopoietic organ stroma (hematopoietic inductive microenvironments) on stem cell differentiation, in Gordon AS (ed): *Regulation of Hematopoiesis.* New York, Appleton-Century-Crofts, 1970, 765 pp, pp 161–186.

63   Askanazy M: Über die physiologische und pathologische Blutregeneration in der Leber. *Virchows Arch* 205:346–371, 1911.

64   Danchakoff V: Über die Entwicklung des Knochenmarks bei den Vögeln und über dessen Veränderungen bei Blutentziehungen und Ernährungsstorungen. *Arch Mikr Anat* 47:855–926, 1909.

65   Danchakoff V: Origin of blood cells. *Anat Rec* 10:397–414, 1916.

66   Downey H: The myeloblast, in Downey H (ed): *Handbook of Hematology III.* New York, Paul B Hoeber, 1936, 3136 pp, p 2021.

67   Ferrata A: in Berliner Hämatologische Gesellschaft. *Folia Haematol (Leipz)* 8:392–398, 1909.

68 Bichat X: Auszug aus Bichat's Abhandlung über die Membranen. *Arch Physiol* 5:169–275, 1802 (Excerpts from Xavier Bichat's monograph entitled *Traité des membranes en general et de diverses membranes en particular.*)

69 Gosselin L, Regnauld J: Recherches sur la substance médullaire des os. *Arch Gen Med* 10:257–275, 1849.

70 Neumann E: Das Gesetz der Verbreitung des gelben und roten Knochenmaarkes. *Zentralbl Med Wissensch* 20:321–323, 1882.

71 Huggins C, Blocksom BH: Changes in outlying bone marrow accompanying a local increase of temperature within physiological limits. *J Exp Med* 64:253–274, 1936.

72 Tavassoli M, Crosby WH: Bone marrow histogenesis: A comparison of fatty and red marrow. *Science* 169:291–293, 1970.

73 Robin C: La moelle des os. *Dictionnaire encyclopédique des sciences médicales*, 1875, 796 pp, pp 1–33.

74 Duverney M: De la structure et du sentiment de la moelle. *Histoire de l'academie royale des sciences, 1700*, pp 202–205.

75 Goujon E: Greffe de la moelle des os, productions osseuses. *C R Soc Biol (Paris)* 18:42–44, 1866.

76 Goujon E: Recherches expérimentales sur les propriétés physiologiques de la moelle. *J Anat Physiol* 11:399–412, 1869.

77 Bailkow A: Ueber Transplantation von Knochenmark. *Zentralbl Med Wissensch* 24:371–373, 1870.

78 Tavassoli M, Crosby WH: Transplantation of marrow to extramedullary sites. *Science* 161:54–56, 1968.

79 Minot CS: On a hitherto unrecognized form of blood circulation without capillaries in the organs of vertebrata. *Proc Bost Soc Nat Hist* 29:185, 1901.

80 Van der Stricht O: Nouvelles recherches sur la genèse des globules rouges et des globules blancs du sang. *Arch Biol* 12:199–344, 1892.

CHAPTER 4

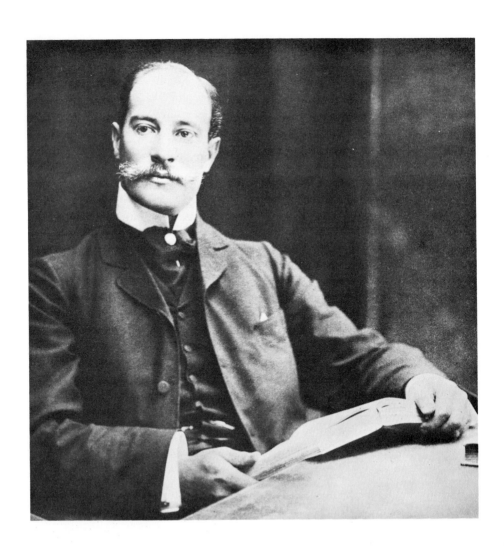

THE COMMON ANCESTRAL CELL
Lazlo G. Lajtha

B ecause the search for the ancestral cell inevitably has involved the whole process of the origin and development of the blood cells, an alternative title to this chapter could be: "Search for the early cellular events during blood cell formation." This question emerged as soon as it was discovered that the blood is not merely a solution of chemicals (salts and proteins) but also a suspension of cells. The first question posed was simple: Where in the body, and by what type of cells, are the blood cells produced?

The history of this question, looking back with the hindsight of today, is almost an illustration of the rather curious statement (made, probably not for the first time, in 1704, by Richard Mead):[1] "At vero cum temporis decursu philosophorum decretis accommodari coepisset medicina. . . ."* It is indeed an illustration of how statements, made originally on quite inadequate evidence, may be verified later by appropriate experimentation when suitable analytical techniques become available.

Almost 100 years after Leeuwenhoek measured the size of red blood cells,

---

* Indeed, with the passage of time, medicine begins to accommodate the statements of philosophers.

as mentioned in Chapter 1, William Hewson, in many respects the true "father of hematology," remeasured them and described them as "flat as a guinea"; he also described the comparatively much less numerous "coulourless" blood cells as well. He had already raised a question about their origin and, based on his observations on lymph nodes and the thoracic duct, proposed the theory that the site of origin is the lymphatic tissue, which feeds the cells into the blood circulation through the thoracic duct. Although he did not—at that time could not—try to do more than indicate the *site* (not the cell, or cells) of origin of blood cells, his theory dominated the field for some 100 years. And when it was revived in the 1900s, it formed one aspect of the great debate on the cell (or cells) of origin of the blood cells, a debate that lasted well into the middle of the present century.

Site of Origin

With the improvement of microscopic techniques, the question of the *site of origin* was tackled at two levels during the middle of the nineteenth century—the site of origin during embryonic development and during adult life. There is, of course, no a priori reason why either the same or different sites should operate in these two instances—however, one might expect that embryonic development, employing as it does initial or "temporary" solutions during the growth of the various organs, might differ from the steady state situation operating in the fully mature organism. Nevertheless, with the still limited histologic techniques available, it was easier and not entirely unreasonable to look at the de novo situation in the embryo, where hematopoiesis first begins. In 1846, Weber and Kölliker[2] had already extended their observations to state that in a stage of fetal life, the liver is the main site of hematopoiesis. Later work, however, demonstrated that hepatic blood cell formation is not the first, but already a "later," transient phase in embryonic development and that the first blood cells are formed in the "blood islands" of the early extraembryonic tissues, the area opaca and the yolk sac. The embryologic studies, by looking at the early development in the embryo as opposed to the cell lineages occurring in the adult, inadvertently contributed to some of the later controversies by trying to extrapolate from the embryonic to the adult situation.

By 1868, Neumann[3] (see Chapter 3) and also, independently, Bizzozero[4] demonstrated that in the adult organism, the main site of blood cell formation is the bone marrow. This was, of course, contrary to what Hewson had said 100 years earlier, and also contrary to what the highly respected embryologists were saying. It was predictable that Neumann's statement would not be easily accepted. Indeed, no less an authority than the great French physician Hayem accused Neumann of "encumbering science" by ill-founded statements. Later work by histologists, however, amply confirmed Neumann's findings, and by the end of the century, the question of the site of hematopoiesis had been settled and accepted—hematopoiesis shifts from the yolk sac to the liver during fetal development, "homing" and eventually locating in the bone marrow in early postnatal life.

The question about the cell (or cells) of origin had hardly been raised until then. That the blood contains more than one kind of cell was known, but the real diversity of blood cells and, even more so, their complicated development from earlier forms of "precursor cells" could not be appreciated until the introduction of better analytical methods for the morphologic identification of different cells in the bone marrow. Quite early, however, the question of origin and its importance in the understanding of blood formation occupied many minds, and in 1892 Van der Stricht[5] summarized the scientific sentiments: "La formation des globules rouges et blancs est une des questions les plus épineuses et les plus controversées de l'embryologie et de l'histogenese."*

Speculations on the Basis of Morphology

The first important analytical technique for recognizing the different cell types was made available with the discovery by Paul Ehrlich[6,7] that, with appropriate staining methods, it is possible to classify (and subclassify) the various blood and bone marrow cells. Ehrlich used smears of bone marrow. His method involved heating the slides on which the cells were spread to fix them, and he used a triacid mixture of stain. This enabled him to describe (among various other cell types) a "primitive" large basophilic mononuclear cell with a vesicular nucleus and few or no granules. He called this the *Myelozyt* (marrow cell) and considered it to be the specific precursor of granulocytes. He classified the lymphocytes as having an entirely different line of development, being derived from lymphatic tissue, thus proposing a dualistic concept of blood formation. This was perhaps the first attempt to describe the "ancestral" cell or, to be more precise, *an* ancestral cell in the hematopoietic series. It was also the beginning of the concept of the *stem cell*—a cell type that can maintain its own numbers by cell division and yet can provide descendants which eventually "mature" into the various blood cells.

Ehrlich's work was followed by Pappenheim's (Chapter Opening Photo), who, from 1898 onwards, used the improved staining method of Romanowsky (a combination of eosin and methylene blue azure), which permitted the viewer to make a finer distinction between the different characteristics of the cells than the original triacid method of Ehrlich.[8,9] Perhaps because of the greater range of detail he was able to observe, he noted that the various transitional forms of cells could be systematized into a scheme that could be

---

* The formation of red cells and white cells is one of the most prickly and controversial questions of embryology and histogenesis.

traced backward to a relatively featureless "primitive" type of mononuclear cell—a cell which he called *Lymphoidozyt*. He advanced the proposal that this cell was so primitive (on morphologic grounds) that it could be considered to be the common ancestor of *all* blood cells; i.e., it was *the* totipotential undifferentiated hematopoietic stem cell. Although the idea of a common ancestor cell was new, it was, in a sense, a revival of the earlier Hewsonian principle of the lymphoid origin of all blood cells. With this, the great debate—between the dualistic concept of Ehrlich and the monophyletic theory of Pappenheim—began, to last for over 3 decades. The techniques available did not allow a precise functional correlation of the different features of the cells; the purpose of the investigations was to pinpoint the *most primitive* cell (or cells) that might be fulfilling the role of the stem cell.

This was the era of truly great morphologists, who studied cellular hematology with the microscope, an era of sometimes bitter arguments, and an era of dogmatic statements strongly felt but weakly founded. It was an authoritarian era, when great hematologists each had to have their stem cells; the lesser ranks became aligned with one or the other school of thought. (My first teacher in hematology had been a pupil of the great Naegeli; when he taught me the difference between myeloblasts and lymphoblasts I happened to ask: "And why is this cell called *lymphoblast?*" His answer was characteristic: "Because Naegeli said so!") The truth of the matter was (and it is perhaps surprising that this was not more appreciated by the participants) that—as in every case when a great scientific debate goes on—there was insufficient evidence to enable anyone to draw a scientifically tenable or valid conclusion. Painstakingly careful descriptions were made, but the protagonists used different staining methods or even different hematological material—embryonic tissues, normal adult bone marrow, or leukemic cells. There were almost no efforts to organize "workshops" to compare the same material and use the different analytical methods, apart from a meeting in early 1909.[10] As late as 1938, William Bloom[11] rightly complained: "Many hematologists trace cell lineages on a series of transition forms in their own material, yet protest vigorously against other investigations reaching different conclusions on the basis of transition forms in their preparations."

The embryologists—perhaps understandably, in view of their material—tended to favor a monophyletic view; after all, every tissue must originate from *a* cell at some time during embryonic development. Thus, van der Stricht[5] in 1892 described the intravascular origin of red cells (i.e., cells arising from the inner lining of the blood vessels in embryologic hematopoietic sites), a view confirmed by both Dantschakoff[12,13] and Maximow[14,15] between 1907 and 1910. They described an undifferentiated (i.e., relatively featureless) cell that was presumed to originate from embryonic mesenchyme and that they held to be the stem cell. Because "featureless" mononuclear cells and some lymphocytes can be almost indistinguishable, Maximow accepted the monophyletic view of Pappenheim and his "lymphoidocyte" stem cell.

In 1900, Naegeli,[16] the great Swiss authoritarian, who was opposed to this monophyletic view, took up his mighty cudgel of supercritical analysis in favor of Ehrlich's dualistic theory. He claimed a recognizable distinction between his *myeloblast,* which he regarded as the ancestor of the granulocytic cells, and the *lymphoblast,* which was responsible for the lymphoid lines of cells. Based on his morphologic studies, and emphasizing the clinical differences between myeloid and lymphatic leukemias, he wrote in 1931: "Ich habe in 1900 die Myeloblasten als die Vorstufe aller weissen Knochenmarkszellen beschrieben und damit die damals erschütterte Lehre des Erhlichschen Dualismus auf festen Boden gestellt. . . ."[17]* A bold statement, indeed, but typical of the man.

The debate was on, from 1900 to almost 4 decades later—Pappenheim and Maximow as monophyleticists, followed by their pupils Ferrata and Bloom, respectively, as well as Weidenreich, Jordan, and Downey, versus the dualists (or pluralists) Naegeli, Türk, Schilling, Sabin, and Doan, to name only a few of the great protagonists. The debate, frequently sharp and sometimes quite bitter, is very well illustrated in the hematologic literature, particularly between 1910 and 1930. It was well reviewed by both sides in great detail, albeit by that time in a somewhat mellowed style, in the multiauthored *Handbook of Hematology,* which was edited in 1938 by Downey.[18]

The illuminating aspect in a reading of the contemporary papers is that the differences between the competing views were more apparent than real, however strongly felt. By the late 1930s, there is evidence of this realization, even by the main participants, although not verbalized. It was realized that it was futile to argue about fine morphologic differences when the methods of producing cell preparations were as different as supravital stains of living cells versus fixed cells, and materials as different as embryonic tissues versus adult marrow or leukemic blood. Moreover, even the fundamental arguments were "fuzzy" in the sense that, for example, Naegeli's dualism (myeloblast for granulopoiesis and lymphoblast for lymphopoiesis) did not really include the erythropoietic precursors in any clear fashion; in fact, Pappenheim,[10] Maximow, and Bloom later modified their monophyletic concepts to say that the "lymphoidocyte/hemocytoblast" is *capable* of providing all cell types, if need arises, but in normal steady state conditions, the separate sublines can maintain their own numbers.

By the 1940s, the heterogeneity of even the lymphocyte population began to be appreciated, and so did the impossibility of any clear-cut solution to the question with the methods then available. By then it became clear that even the term *lymphocyte* may hide a number of functionally different cell types, and that there were no clear-cut experimental methods with which to pin functional differences onto the fine variations among the early cell types. It was possible to characterize the biochemical and functional properties of the late,

---

* In 1900, I described the myeloblast as the precursor of all the white cells in the bone marrow, and, thereby, I established the then shaken dualistic view of Ehrlich on firm grounds.

mature forms of, for example, normoblasts during their hemoglobinization, but not the early "undifferentiated" cells. The noise of the debate died down—the question, however, kept on smoldering.

How Does a Stem Cell Function?

With today's hindsight, it might be considered surprising that in spite of the strong convictions on ancestry, no one asked the question *how* any stem cell population would function or how its proliferation or differentiation could be controlled—all the arguments were essentially morphologic. To be sure, it was probably realized that the difficult question of *how* could not be answered until new scientific tools became available, but this did not deter the more dynamically thinking Edwin E. Osgood[19] from tackling the problem, even if only in a theoretical fashion. His concepts of asymmetric division of the stem cell (i.e., providing an immature daughter cell that forms another stem cell as well as one that will mature into one of the specialized blood cells) were formulated well before the arrival of the experimental tools necessary for their testing. Osgood (Figure 4-1) was a man who was, in many respects, ahead of his time throughout his life. His mathematical modeling of cell growth and differentiation is only now being verified by experimentalists. He had a feel for mathematics as a tool for biological understanding, in contrast to many who try to fit biology into mathematical strait jackets.

Essentially, the great debate was among morphologists, who, by the late 1930s, realized the limitations of their arguments. Perhaps because cellular hematology was mainly concerned with morphology and cytochemistry, when new tools became available, from the mid-1940s onward, they did not come from hematology, but mainly from a new scientific discipline to which many hematologists then turned—radiation biology. They involved the use of radioactive isotopes, tissue grafting, chromosome cytogenetics, and later, with the development of the new discipline of immunology, the use of immunogenetic markers.

By the 1950s, it had been demonstrated that animals can be protected against otherwise lethal doses of whole-body irradiation either by partial shielding of hematopoietic tissue, e.g., the spleen,[20] or by grafting hematopoietic cells into irradiated recipients.[21] At first thought to be due to a humoral factor, within the next 5 years this radioprotective effect was clearly shown to be cellular, i.e., some cells in the shielded area or in the graft were responsible for the restoration of the hematopoietic tissues;[22,23] this was convincingly demonstrated in 1956 by Ford and his colleagues at Harwell by using chromosomally "marked" bone marrow as the graft.[24]

The fact that cellular growth was responsible for hematologic restitution—i.e., that recolonization occurs from the grafted cell or cells—did not *prove* either that stem cells are involved or that a monophyletic stem cell is

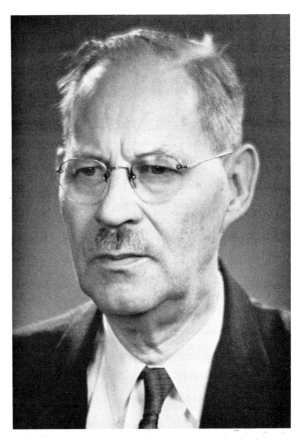

Figure 4-1 Edwin E. Osgood (1899–1969). *(Courtesy of Dr. Robert E. Koler, University of Oregon Medical School.)*

responsible. Both the monophyletic and dualistic (or pluralistic) schools had recognized the proliferative potential of myelocytes and other "recognized" marrow elements, the only cell types in the marrow in which high mitotic indices could be observed. They talked about the "homoplastic" growth of these cells under normal conditions and thus did not even need to "draw" on a stem cell (or cells). The question then was: is the regeneration from the shielded or grafted cells due to stem cell proliferation or merely an expansion of the growth potential of more mature cells? To answer this, one had to learn which cell type can proliferate in the marrow and to discover to what extent it can proliferate. This information was provided by radioactive *tagging* of bone marrow cells. Precursors of deoxyribonucleic acid (DNA) were synthesized which contained radioactive labels (radiophosphorus, radiocarbon, or tritium). Such labeled precursors could then be taken up and incorporated into cells that were proliferating (i.e., synthesizing new DNA), and the labeled cells could then be identified in stained preparations covered with a thin layer of photographic emulsion. Such *autoradiographic* studies, carried out at Oxford, England, and Brookhaven, New York, in particular, by measuring the proportion of labeled cells in a cell population, provided the information necessary to determine the proliferation rates and capacities of the various types of bone marrow cells. As a result of such cell cycle measurements of the duration of the various phases of the proliferation cycle in "recognizable" bone marrow cells, by 1960 it became clear that all the morphologically recognizable and classifiable erythroid and granulocytic cells are only "transit" populations. Their proliferation potential is limited to only a few cell divisions.[25] Hence, not only in any case of regeneration or repopulation of the bone marrow, but also in steady state maintenance of hematopoiesis, some "earlier" (e.g., stem) cell populations must be actively involved. Once again, the stem cells became important, for it was on them, on their growth potential, that hematologic regeneration—either after radiation or following drug-induced toxic damage—really depended. It was clear that a merely morphologic search for the stem cell was unrewarding, and with the 1960s, the era described by McCulloch as "hematology without the microscope" began.

Hematology without the Microscope

It was the time for multidisciplinary research. By the teaming up of a physicist-radiobiologist and a physician-hematologist, Till and McCulloch in Toronto[26] in 1961, using the spleen-colony method, proved the existence of a single stem cell with pluripotential capacity. This was accomplished by showing that if hematopoietic cells were injected into lethally irradiated mice, their spleens would develop macroscopic nodules.

Each such nodule (or colony) was found to consist eventually of more than one million cells. Such colonies were shown to originate from single cells (*the colony-forming stem cells*), which possessed the full developmental capacity to form large colonies of erythroid or granulocytic type cells. Using cells from donor animals with chromosome markers or, even better, cell suspensions containing cells with unique chromosomal abnormalities (e.g., induced by radiation), it could be shown that the same *single* stem cell (*colony-forming cell*, CFC or *colony-forming unit in spleen*, CFU-S) could give rise to granulocytes, monocytes, and erythrocytes.[27] Pluripotent yet monoclonal hematopoiesis was also shown to occur in chronic myelocytic leukemia (CML) by using chromosome or isoenzyme markers in patients who had inherited two forms of a particular enzyme, one form of which appeared in any one cell. All cells in the CML patients showed the same chromosomal abnormality and one form of the enzyme only, thus indicating that the abnormal stem cell population in this disease probably originates from a single pluripotent stem cell.[28,29]

By the mid-1960s, the monophyletic view of the totipotential (in respect to hematopoiesis) stem cell, first postulated by Pappenheim some 60 years before, was operationally vindicated. Indeed, the time had come for the proper definition of the term *stem cell.* The early search was for the ultimate ancestral cell, from which the hemic cells originate in adult life. It became clear that there is *a* pluripotential cell type which can serve this purpose, but it also was evident that this cell type had great growth potential—it can recover and restore its numbers if damaged.

With the extension of colony-type (clonogenic) assays to the study of a variety of tumor cells and normal tissues (e.g., skin, intestinal epithelium, cartilage), the concept of "stemness" has undergone a subtle change. The essential criterion of stemness becomes its extensive self-replicating capacity— the tumor stemline maintains the tumor growth, the skin (or gut) stem cells maintain skin-cell proliferation to compensate for the continuous desquamation of skin (or gut) cells, and the hematopoietic stem cell maintains the production of more than 200 billion (2×10^{11}) blood cells per day. The fact that hematopoietic stem cells happen to have the capacity of differentiation, i.e., that they can "turn into" a number of different ephemeral sublines, is an additional feature, namely self-maintenance. It is, of course, this additional feature which makes them pluripotential stem cells.

However, the link between the pluripotential stem cell and the various hemic cell lines still remained to be elucidated. This was provided by the development of other methods during the early and mid-1960s. In vitro culture techniques were designed in which specific blood cell development could be studied. The first of these, simultaneously but independently developed in Australia[30] and in Israel[31] in 1966, enabled granulocytic colonies to be grown in a medium which was "stiffened" by the inclusion of agar. Agar provides a suspending framework for the cells to sit in, rather than becoming attached to the glass surface. Initially the Israeli group thought that the cells so grown were phagocytic macrophages. The Melbourne workers showed that the type of colonies grown depends on the culture conditions; they can appear as macrophages or as classical granulocytes. Granulocytes were grown on the addition of "conditioned media," obtainable from a variety of organ cultures which contained what has been termed *colony-stimulating activity* (CSA). With this method, human granulocytic colonies could be grown in a clonal fashion, i.e., each colony originated from a single colony-forming cell (*colony-forming unit in culture* or CFU-C). Later, with appropriate modification of the culture conditions and using the humoral factor which stimulates erythropoiesis in vivo (erythropoietin, see Chapter 9), Canadian workers[32] succeeded in growing erythroid colonies in a similarly clonal fashion. They called the early colony-forming cell the *erythroid "burst-forming unit"* (BFU$_E$).

Comparison of the properties of the spleen colony-forming pluripotent stem cells with those of the granulocytic CFU-C and the erythroid BFU$_E$ clearly indicated that there are three different kinds of cells; moreover, between the morphologically recognizable early erythroid or granulocytic cells and the pluripotent stem cell, there are intercalated "committed" precursor lines. Neither the CFU-C nor the BFU_E were recognizable as granulocytic or erythropoietic cells. The important corollary of these observations was that although both CFU-C and BFU_E were "committed" to later differentiation into their respective recognizable descendants, they were found to possess considerable growth capacities, i.e., they could divide several times *as* CFU-C and BFU_E, respectively. This meant that these "committed" cells were serving also as intercalated amplifying populations; each committed precursor differentiating from the stem cell was capable of producing more than 30 descendants *before* further differentiation into the morphologically classifiable erythroid or granulocytic pathway. In the latter, they undergo another greater than 30-times amplification! (See Figure 4-2.) This also implied that there are two steps of differentiation involved; one step in which a pluripotent stem cell turns into a "committed" precursor, and a second step in which the committed precursor cell, having undergone some degree of amplification and probably also maturation, turns into a "recognizable" precursor, e.g., a pronormoblast. Further amplification and maturation lead to the fully mature red cells.

Figure 4-2 Diagram of amplification in transit populations during hematopoiesis. The first transit population consists of "committed" precursor cells, which, undergoing, e.g., five cell cycles, amplify by a factor of 32X. The second transit population, the "recognizable" cells (e.g., normoblasts), may also undergo five cell cycles, with a further 32X amplification resulting in an overall number of 1024 cells from the original stem cell which had entered this differentiating transit pathway.

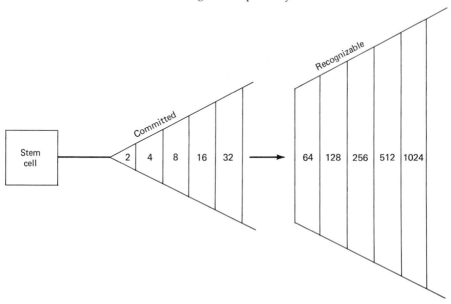

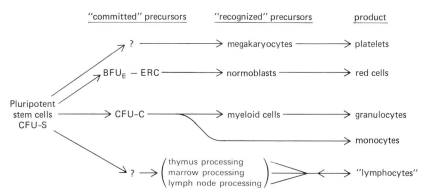

Figure 4-3 The degree of amplification during transit through the "committed" and "recognizable" precursors is such that one stem cell entering differentiation may give rise to, e.g., 2000 red cells or granulocytes. CFU-S = spleen colony-forming pluripotent stem cells. BFU_E = in vitro erythroid "burst-forming" cells (detectable in suitable in vitro bone marrow cultures). ERC = erythropoietin-responding cells (detected in vivo in animals stimulated with the erythropoiesis-inducing factor erythropoietin). CFU-C = in vitro granulocytic colony-forming cells (detectable in bone marrow cultures containing specific colony-stimulating factors). The term *lymphocytes* indicates that this morphologically simple cell population contains a variety of functionally different cells.

This, of course, means that the proportion of stem cells in the marrow can be very much smaller than would have been expected without such intercalated amplification. With such low proportions of stem cells, it is not surprising that they are difficult to locate and recognize. Even though there are now physical techniques to separate hematopoietic cells into fractions depending on their size, density, and electric charge, the stem-cell-enriched fractions rarely contain more than 30 percent stem cells, and these mainly are featureless middle-sized mononuclear cells—no good specific morphologic marker can be attached to them.

The radiobiological techniques mentioned earlier also enabled the measurement of proliferation rates in almost all the types of hematopoietic cell populations and, with the availability of good quantitative operational assays, at least for some of the various subpopulations of the hematopoietic cell hierarchy (Figure 4-3), it became possible to investigate the kinetics and mode of regulation of stem cells. Although somewhat difficult to accomplish because no one had *seen* the pluripotent stem cells (nor the in vitro CFU-C or the BFU_E cell for that matter!), the radiobiologic techniques could be adapted. If radioactive DNA precursors taken up by the cells could betray their presence in autoradiographic preparations, the task was to give even "hotter" radioactive DNA precursors, such as thymidine labeled with tritium. In this way, enough radioactivity could be incorporated into the cell nucleus for the radiation to become lethal for the cell. By means of such a radioactive thymidine "suicide" (or, more precisely, "murder"), the proportion of splenic or culture colony-forming cells in DNA synthesis could be determined as accurately (by eliminating them) as autoradiographs could indicate the proportion of labeled myelocytes or normoblasts. Indeed, this method was one of the first to show that the pluripotent CFU-S and the agar granulocytic CFU-C are different—the radioactive thymidine method in mice killed 40 to 50 percent of the CFU-C but only 5 to 10 percent of the CFU-S.[33] This surprising finding meant that in the normal mouse, the rate of stem cell proliferation is very low indeed.

Judging on the basis of the numbers cited in Figure 4-2, it appears that a very considerable amplification (probably over 1000X) is attained from a single stem cell that enters the differentiation pathway. With such amplification during maturation, the daily production of red cells and granulocytes does not need to "draw" on many stem cells. Consequently, it would appear that most of the stem cells at any one time do not need to be proliferating.

This observation has led to a wider biological concept, that of the G_0 state.[34,35] This was defined as a state in which the cell does not prepare for, or is not in the process of, DNA synthesis or mitosis; it is not in the proliferative cell cycle, but in a state from which it can be triggered to enter into the proliferative cycle. It has been suggested that a prolonged G_0 state is particularly necessary for stem cells, for it may be a time for "genetic housekeeping," i.e., for the repair and correction of the genome in a more effective fashion than would be possible if the cells were actively proliferating.

By the early 1970s, it came to be realized that proliferation control in hematopoietic cells is "local" in nature. The factor(s) responsible for this control are being unraveled at the present time.[36] The recent development of new culture methods[37] enables stem cell growth to be maintained in vitro for months and gives valuable insight into the interrelationship between stem cells and their immediate neighboring cells (Figure 4-4), as well as into the mechanisms involved in the transformation of normal stem cells into leukemic stem lines.

Thus, a stage of understanding has been attained wherein manipulation of stem cell behavior has become a realistic probability and will almost certainly become practical within the next decade. As a consequence, it may become possible to hasten hematopoietic recovery from cytotoxic damage and to protect stem cells against drugs that preferentially damage cells in a proliferative state.

The Outcome

Thus, the story of the search for the ancestral cell has followed the lines of all scientific investigations: solutions are found and further questions are raised as new techniques become available. The first meaningful approaches were made

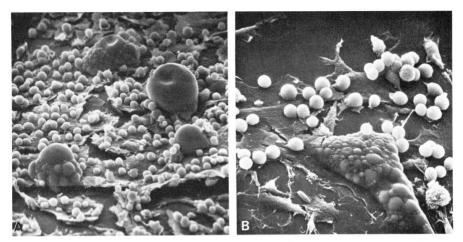

Figure 4-4 Scanning electron microscope view of hematopoietic foci in vitro.[37] Demonstration of intercell interactions and the dependence of stem cells on appropriate micromilieu. The small round cells are the hematopoietic cells, including stem cells. Their presence depends on either closeness to gigantic fat-containing cells or to large, flattened cells which prevent them from sticking and flattening on glass or plastic surfaces. The absolute number of large fat cells determines the absolute number of stem cells in these cultures. (A) 20 μm; (B) 10 μm.

possible by the improved microscopes and the staining techniques of the nineteenth century; this could result only in morphologic studies, however. These reached their limitations sooner than some of the investigators were then prepared to admit. Of the later methods, many—like microscopy itself—were not specifically forged for hematology, yet were fruitfully exploited by scientists who perceived their potential in the search for the ancestral cell.

We still cannot visualize the common stem cell in morphologic terms. It is clear, however, that this is not of prime importance. The operational and functional assays are specific and quantitative; they "tell" much more about the hematopoietic stem cell than any morphologic method can do. Furthermore, the new understanding about the nature and the properties of stem cells has given scientists a great deal of basic information concerning the behavior of cells in general, information that transcends the framework of hematology itself.

References

1 Mead R: *De Imperio Solis ac Lunae in Corpora Humana et Morbis inde Oriundis.* London, R Smith, 1704, 197 pp, p 2.
2 Weber EH, Kölliker A: Ueber die Bedeutung der Leber für die Bildung der Blutkörperchen der Embryonen. (Schreiben von Weber an Kölliker mit einem Vor- und Nachwort von dem Letzteren.) *Z Rat Med* 4:160–167, 1846.

3 Neumann E: Ueber die Bedeutung des Knochenmarkes fur die Blutbildung. *Zentralbl Med Wissensch* 6:689, 1868.

4 Bizzozero G: Sulla funzione ematopoetica del midollo delle ossa. *Zentralbl Med Wissensch* 6:885, 1868.

5 Van der Stricht O: Nouvelles recherches sur la genese des globules rouges et des globules blancs du sang. *Arch Biol (Liege)* 12:199–344, 1892.

6 Ehrlich P: Ueber die specifischen Granulationen des Blutes. *Arch Anat Physiol, Physiol Abt*, 571–579, 1879.

7 Ehrlich P, Lazarus A: Normale und Pathologische Histologie des Blutes, vol 1, *Die Anämie*, Vienna, Holder, 1898, 200 pp.

8 Pappenheim A: Abstammung und Entstehung der roten Blutzelle. *Virchows Arch (Pathol Anat)* 151:89–158, 1898.

9 Pappenheim A: Von den gegenseitigen Beziehungen der verschiedenen farblosen Blutzellen zu einander. *Virchows Arch (Pathol Anat)* 159:40–85, 1900.

10 Pappenheim A: Meeting of the German Haematologic Society. *Folia Haematol (Leipz)* 8:390–409, 1909.

11 Bloom W: Lymphocytes and monocytes: Theories of hematopoiesis, in Downey H (ed): *Handbook of Hematology.* New York, Hoeber, 1938, vol I, 698 pp, p 417.

12 Dantschakoff W: Über das erste Auftreten der Blutelemente im Hühnerembryo. *Folia Haematol* 4(Suppl):159–166, 1907.

13 Dantschakoff W: Untersuchungen über die Entwickelung des Blutes und Binde-gewebes bei den Vogeln. *Anat Hefte* 1 (abt 37):471–589, 1908.

14 Maximow A: Untersuchungen über Blut und Bindegewebe. 1. Die frühesten Entwickelungstadien der Blut- und Bindegewebszellen beim Saugetierembryo bis zum Angang der Blutbildung in der Leber. *Arch Mikr Anat* 73:444–561, 1909.

15 Maximow A: Untersuchungen über die Blut und Bindegewebe. III. Die embryonale Histogenese des Knockenmarks der Saugetiere. *Arch Mikr Anat* 76:1–113, 1910.

16 Naegeli O: Ueber rothes Knockenmark und Myeloblasten. *Dtsch Med Woechenschr* 18:287–290, 1900.

17 Naegeli O: *Blutkrankheiten und Blutdiagnostik*, 5th ed. Berlin, Springer, 1931, 704 pp, p 1.

18 Downey H: *Handbook of Hematology.* New York, Hoeber, 1938, 4 vol, 3136 pp.

19 Osgood EE: A unifying concept of the etiology of the leukaemias, lymphomas and cancers. *J Natl Cancer Inst* 18:155–166, 1957.

20 Jacobson LO, Marks EK, Gaston EO, Robinson M, Zirkle RE: The role of the spleen in radiation injury. *Proc Soc Exp Biol Med* 70:740–742, 1949.

21 Lorenz E, Uphoff D, Reid TR, Shelton E: Modification of irradiation injury in mice and guinea pigs by bone marrow injections. *J Natl Cancer Inst* 12:197–201, 1951.

22 Lindsley DL, Odell TT, Tausche FG: Implantation of functional erythropoietic elements following total body irradiation. *Proc Soc Exp Biol Med* 90:512–515, 1955.

23 Mitchison NA: The colonisation of irradiated tissue by transplanted spleen cells. *Br J Exp Pathol* 37:239–247, 1956.

24 Ford CE, Hamerton JL, Barnes DWH, Loutit JF: Cytological identification of radiation chimeras. *Nature* 177:452–454, 1956.

25 Lajtha LG, Oliver R: Studies on the kinetics of erythropoiesis: a model of the erythron. *Ciba Foundation Symposium on Haemopoiesis*, pp 289–314, 1960.

26 Till JE, McCulloch EA: Direct measurement of the radiation sensitivity of normal mouse bone marrow cells. *Radiat Res* 14:213–222, 1961.

27 Wu AM, Till JE, Siminovitch L, McCulloch EA: A cytological study of the capacity for differentiation of normal haemopoietic colony forming cells. *J Cell Physiol* 69:177–184, 1967.

28 Fialkow PJ, Gartler SM, Yoshida A: Clonal origin of CML in man. *Proc Natl Acad Sci USA* 58:1468–1472, 1967.

29 Trujillo JM, Ohno S: Chromosomal alteration of erythropoietic cells in chronic myeloid leukaemia. *Acta Haematol (Basel)* 29:311–316, 1963.

30 Bradley TR, Metcalf D: The growth of mouse bone marrow cells *in vitro*. *Aust J Exp Biol Med Sci* 44:287–300, 1966.

31 Pluznik DH, Sachs L: The induction of clones of normal mast cells by a substance from conditioned medium. *Exp Cell Res* 43:553–563, 1966.

32 Axelrad AA, McLeod DL, Shreeve MM, Heath DS: Properties of cells that produce erythrocytic colonies *in vitro*, in Robinson WA (ed): *Hemopoiesis in Culture*. DHEW Publication No (NIH) 74–205. Washington, 1974, 489 pp, pp 226–237.

33 Lajtha LG, Pozzi LV, Schofield R, Fox M: Kinetic properties of haemopoietic stem cells. *Cell Tissue Kinet* 2:39–49, 1969.

34 Lajtha LG, Oliver R, Gurney CW: Kinetic model of a bone marrow stem cell population. *Br J Haematol* 8:442–460, 1962.

35 Lajtha LG: On the concept of the cell cycle. Symposium on macromolecular aspects of the cell cycle. *J Cell Physiol* 62(suppl 1): 143–145, 1963.

36 Lord BI, Mori KJ, Wright EG, Lajtha LG: An inhibitor of stem cell proliferation in normal bone marrow. *Br J Haematol* 34:441–445, 1976.

37 Dexter TM, Allen TD, Lajtha LG: Conditions controlling the proliferation of haemopoietic stem cells *in vitro*. *J Cell Physiol* 91:335–344, 1977.

CHAPTER 5

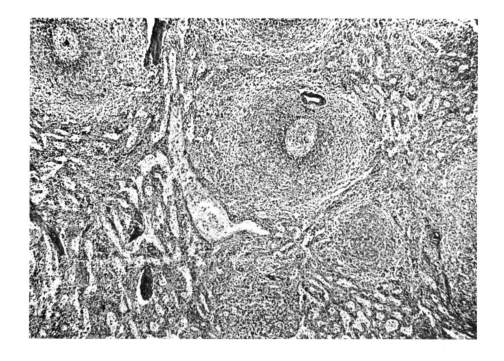

THE SPLEEN
William H. Crosby

-Et de longs corbillards, sans tambours ni musique,
Défilent lentement dans mon âme; l'Espoir,
Vaincu, pleure, et l'Angioisse atroce, despotique,
Sur mon crâne incliné plante son drapeau noir.

{—And hearses—without drums or music—roll,
In languishing procession through my soul.
While Hope destroyed lies weeping, Agony
Unfurls on my bowed skull his black drupee.}

Spleen, Charles Baudelaire

The viola is like the spleen. We have
one but no one knows why or what it's doing
there.

Harry Rumpler, violist

T he above quotations—the first, an expression of Baudelaire's morbid melancholy and the second, Harry Rumpler's teasing description of his viola—both demonstrate how the spleen, like a Shakespearean or mythological motif, has become a point of classical allusion. The title of Baudelaire's poem refers to the spleen's supposed depot of black bile and dark emotions, while Rumpler recalls the mystery that for centuries surrounded the spleen's true function.

Historically, the spleen from time to time was assigned a variety of functions—anatomical counterbalance of the liver, digestive organ, source of emotions, ductless gland. The antique mystery of splenic function has long since been solved. Structurally, it is part of the vascular system, and functionally, it is dedicated to the blood. As it has turned out, the spleen does not have one single function but a dozen, at least, if we count some pernicious activities of abnormal spleens. And there may be others we have not yet perceived. The most important functions of the normal human spleen may be grouped under two headings, those pertaining to the blood cells and those pertaining to immunity. In some animals, the spleen can modify the blood volume to increase or decrease its size "on demand."

Chapter Opening Photo Microscopic appearance of the spleen. The round structures are Malpighian follicles. The upper left and lower right areas are dominated by the irregular sinuses characteristic of the cords of Billroth. Magnification 75X.

97

Of all the parts of the hemic system, the spleen is the only one that can be totally removed. The history of splenectomy, like the history of splenic function, has been long in evolution, and we do not yet completely comprehend all of the consequences of eliminating splenic activity. The two lines of historical development have been interrelated: with better understanding of the functions of the spleen, the indications for splenectomy have been clarified, while removal of the spleen, in turn, has helped to clarify its functions.[1]

The normal human spleen is a medium-sized organ, smaller than the blood and the brain and larger than the tongue and the testes. It is nested in the dome of the diaphragm behind the left edge of the ribs and connected with the rest of the body only by blood vessels (Figure 5-1). It is a dusky, livid oblong, whose function could not be surmised from its size, location, or configuration.

The ancients assigned the spleen to the digestive system.[2,3] Fascinated by the body's symmetry, they often paired the spleen with the liver. Erasistratus, one of the first anatomists, believed that, aside from maintaining the symmetry of the abdomen, the spleen had no function at all. Plato claimed its function was to keep the liver "bright and shining." Hippocrates proposed a vital balance of four essential humors—blood, phlegm, golden bile, and black bile. The liver was the source of golden bile, the spleen, the source of black bile. Later, Galen assigned it yet another function, the withdrawal from the stomach of the watery part of food. The inability to assign other than imaginary functions to the spleen may have resulted from its lack of any aperture. The kidneys, the liver, the lungs, and the stomach all empty themselves into something. Even the brain (the supposed source of phlegm) was thought to drain through the nose. But the spleen lay isolated. Erasistratus' concept of a spleen without any function offended Galen, that giant of the second century, known to hematologists as the aphorist who coined the numbing expletive, "Plenum mysterii organon." Surely this was a Galenic sarcasm referring to the mystification of Erasistratus and his followers. Neither the spleen nor anything else held mysteries for Galen. It is impossible to describe his certitude concerning the structure and functions of every morsel of the body. Does the spleen lack an outlet? Galen asserts one into existence. "Humors unsuitable for its nutriment are discharged by the spleen through a canal into the stomach." M.T. May gently put it that Galen's devotion to theory again had led him to distort the facts.[4]*

---

* Vesalius, the great Belgian physician and anatomist of the sixteenth century, probably did more than anyone to end the darkness of the Galenic era. On this particular point, that of the spleen's excretory ducts, for example, he demonstrated by accurate examination that no channel to the stomach exists.[5] Henry Gray, the nineteenth century English anatomist, a student of the spleen and author of the still contemporary *Gray's Anatomy*, commented thus of Vesalius and the splenic-gastric channel, "It was by means of these simple anatomical observations that he overthrew an opinion advocated by one of the most celebrated physiologists, an opinion which, as we have seen, was supported by many able anatomists and taught in the ancient schools for more than a thousand years."[6]

Galen's extant writings on medicine aggregate some 2.5 million words in 119 catalogued works, and this may represent only half of them. As described in Chapter 1, this massive compendium of stultifying opinions remained the last word of medical authority for 1400 years. From his mighty presence, twentieth century hematologists have inherited a single phrase, the spleen is the *plenum mysterii organon*, the organ filled with mystery, a phrase that carries an overtone of humility, suggesting that here was a person who knew when he was stumped.

What an irony.

The doctrine of the four bodily humors not only dominated physiological concepts of life for 2000 years but left a special mark upon our language. The black bile of the spleen is second only to blood in the richness of its linguistic legacy.

Melancholy (μελαζ, *black*, + χολη, *bile*) is only the beginning. Examine the *Oxford English Dictionary* (OED), published in 1933, where one can find a

Figure 5-1 The spleen in the abdomen. The spleen (1) lies behind the stomach represented by a dashed outline (2) and beneath the diaphragm (3). It often touches the tip of the pancreas (4) and the top of the left kidney (5). Its arterial blood vessels come from the aorta (6). Venous vessels drain into the portal vein (7), which empties into the liver, also represented by a dashed outline (8). *(Adapted from Dameshek, W, Estren, S: The Spleen and Hypersplenism. New York, Grune and Stratton, 1947.)*

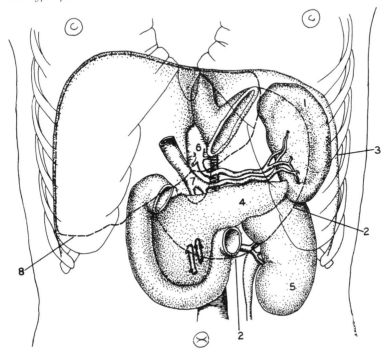

splendid list of words derived from spleen (OF. *esplen*, L. *splen*, Gr. σπλην related to Skr. *plihan*, L. *lien*). The OED's anatomical definition of spleen is "a ductless gland of irregular form which in mammals serves to produce certain changes in the blood; the milt or melt." Thereafter, other meanings are listed: (1) The seat of melancholy or morose feelings, (2) the seat of laughter or mirth,* (3) jest or play, (4) merriment, gaiety, sport, (5) a sudden impulse, whim, caprice, changeable temper, (6) hot or proud temper, high spirit, courage, (7) impetuosity, eagerness, (8) violent ill-nature, irritable or peevish temper, (9) a fit of temper, a passion, (10) a grudge, a spite, (11) amusement, delight, (12) indignation, (13) excessive dejection or depression of spirits, gloominess and irritability, melancholia.

Then come the adjectival forms, such as spleen-stone, and then the verbs: "*trans.* to regard with ill humor, to make angry. *intrans.* to feel deep anger."

Here are the words derived from spleen, almost all descriptive of passion: spleenful, spleenish, spleeny, splenalgia,† splenatic, splenative, splenectomy,† splenetic, splenicness, splenetical, splenetive, splenetize,† splenial, splenic,† splenical,† splenification,† splenify,† splenitic,† splenitis,† splenitive, splenization,† splenous. The words marked with a dagger have an anatomical or medical meaning. In some there is a double meaning, medical jargon sharing word meanings with ordinary speech, relics of a time when disordered emotions, anger, and melancholy represented a splenetic (or splenative or spleeny) disease, which might have been treated with spleen-stone or spleenwort or poultices or concoctions of spleen or milt.

Milt (or melt) is another word for spleen. The OED quotes Jehan Palsgrave's explanation (1530) of a need for two words, "The splene in man, in a beest the melte." OED suggests that "milt" comes "perhaps from the root of melt with reference to the supposed digestive function of the spleen," yet "melt" carries none of the peevish, angry, melancholy meanings that have been associated with the word *spleen*. The obsolete verb *to melt* means "to knock down; properly by a stroke in the side, where the *melt* or spleen lies," which recalls the knobbed club used by assassins in Indonesia, where, years ago, massively swollen spleens were so commonplace that a sharp blow to the left upper abdomen could often cause a fatal rupture of the splenic capsule.

Nowadays, most of the meanings of the spleen-derived words are obsolete. Angry people still vent their spleens, enamored people console their melancholy babies, but, on the whole, by improving our knowledge of the functions of the spleen, we have reduced somewhat the richness of our tongue.

Together with the black bile, we have lost some other concepts of the spleen:

---

* The Talmudists, who comment upon every aspect of God and His works, did not overlook the spleen. Contrary to the Greek tradition, the Talmudists held that the spleen is the origin of laughter.[7]

A curious discussion, persisted in since antiquity, is as to the supposed influence of the spleen on the ability of couriers. For ages runners have believed that the spleen was a hindrance to their vocation, and that its reduction was followed by greater agility on the course. With some, this opinion is perpetuated to the present day. In France there is a proverb, 'Courir comme un dérate.' [To run like a man without a spleen.] To reduce the size of the spleen, the Greek athletes used certain beverages, the composition of which was not generally known; the Romans had a similar belief and habit. Pliny speaks of a plant called *equisetum*, a decoction of which taken for three days after a fast of twenty-four hours would effect absorption of the spleen. The modern pharmacopeia does not possess any substance having a similar virtue, although quinine has been noticed to diminish the size of the spleen when engorged in malarial fevers. Strictly speaking, however, the facts are not analogous. Hippocrates advises a moxa of mushrooms applied over the spleen for melting or dissolving it. Godefroy Moebius is said to have seen in the village of Halberstadt a courier whose spleen had been cauterized after incision; and in about the same epoch (seventeenth century) some men pretended to be able to extirpate successfully the spleen for those who desired to be couriers. This operation we know to be one of the most delicate in modern surgery, and as we are progressing with our physiologic knowledge of the spleen, we see nothing to justify the old theory in regard to its relations to agility and coursing.[8]

The Story of Splenectomy

Demonstrations that the spleen is not necessary for life continued for several centuries to be a source of astonishment. The spleen had been removed many times from animals without harm.[9] Indeed, Sir Christopher Wren, England's greatest architect, around 1660, while serving as professor of astronomy at Oxford, performed such an experiment upon a dog.[10] Adelmann, from medical publications of the sixteenth, seventeenth, and eighteenth centuries, collected nine examples of human spleens removed after the organ had protruded from a wound of the belly, and in all cases the amputee survived in good health.[11] As early as 1740, Pohl described cases of congenital absence of the spleen discovered postmortem in adults.[12] Yet, despite this information that the spleen is not an essential organ, splenectomy was still being reported as newsworthy well into the nineteenth century.

The first splenectomy of record in America was performed in San Francisco, California, by E. O'Brien,[13] a surgeon of the Royal Navy:

Joseph Raphael Gamaz, aetat. 39, born in the city of Carrittano, in the province of Mexico, by trade a taylor, was wounded at Port St. Francisco, on Friday, the 24th of January, 1814, at 7 o'clock in the afternoon, while attempting to commit a rape on a female of the place. The wound was inflicted in the left side, under the last floating rib, by a *large clasp knife,* such as is generally carried by the natives in the boot; and which was snatched from the villain at the moment of the assault. It is probable, that the female still kept hold of the knife after it was plunged into the man's side, and considerably enlarged the wound; for, on the knife being with-drawn, the spleen protruded; and in this state it remained till twelve o'clock on Sunday morning following, when it first came under my cognizance.

It was now in a very advanced state of inflammation, and its organization so much destroyed, that no chance remained of its ever again being restored to vitality, or of its performing its function in the animal economy, whatever that function may be. Its removal, therefore, was determined on; and, as it was only attached to the wound by the vessels of the organ itself, and some cellular substance, a ligature was first applied round them, to prevent haemorrhage, and then the viscus was removed by the knife.

A very high symptomatic fever ensued, though every part of the most rigorous antiphlogistic treatment was rigidly enforced.

On the 13th of February, the last slough came away, leaving a clean wound, the edges of which were approximated by bandages and adhesive plaister; and on the 20th of March, the man was discharged perfectly cured.

I had an opportunity of seeing this man some months afterwards, when he appeared, and asserted himself, to be in perfect health.

Another accidental splenectomy occurred at the battle of Dettingen in 1743. A British Dragoon was grievously wounded

. . . and left all night in the field weltering in his blood, with the spleen hanging out of his body, in a mortified state. Next morning he was carried to the Surgeon, who immediately extirpated it, after tying a ligature round the large vessels, and the patient recovered to be able to do duty in the regiment.[14]

The first battlefield splenectomy of record?

Often cited as the first deliberate splenectomy was an operation per-formed in Naples in April 1549 by a stonecutter, Andriano Zaccerello, on a 24-year-old woman, the wife of a Greek centurion. Her spleen had grown to such a size as to fill the entire abdomen, and, when the old man made an incision, the organ immediately protruded. The organ itself was cut, the "membranes were separated," the wound closed, and the woman then recovered.[15] Because this belly-filling organ weighed only 2 pounds after delivery, it has been suggested that it might have been an ovarian cyst that lost its fluid during the manipulation.[16] This case was reported by Leonardo Fioravanti, who is mentioned incredulously by William Stukeley as the "first mountebank of Europe."[17]

With Lister's introduction of antiseptic surgery, invasion of the belly became practicable. Thereafter, most surgical deaths during attempted sple-nectomy resulted from bleeding, the failure of mechanical hemostasis. In 1887, on his fourth attempt, Sir Spencer Wells performed one of the first successful splenectomies in England.[18] The case is of more than ordinary hematological interest because the patient's son[19] and later her granddaughter[20] came to the attention of Lord Dawson of Penn, who demonstrated that Wells' original patient represented a familial problem, hereditary spherocytosis (see Chapter 8). Thus, Wells inadvertently produced the first surgical cure of hemolytic anemia. He had operated on his 24-year-old patient expecting to find a uterine fibroid, but instead found a 1000-g spleen, a "wandering spleen with a long attachment." Wells marveled at the disappearance of the patient's chronic jaundice after the operation. Dawson commented, "He cured the patient without knowing why."[20]

During the last quarter of the nineteenth century, many spleens were removed because they were large. The early results were dreadfully bad. A tabulation by Adelmann reveals that of the 53 splenectomies performed before June 1887, only 15 patients survived; 7 of these had "wandering spleen," that is to say, the spleen had a long pedicle, making easy the problem of mechanical hemostasis.[11] With so few patients surviving, it was difficult to perceive valid indications for splenectomy; yet surgeons continued for many years to remove large spleens from patients with leukemia and malaria. It seems that they felt vindicated when the patient survived. Perusal of the index catalog of the Library of the Surgeon General leaves an impression that every "successful" splenectomy was separately reported, some of them four and five times. Many titles are a variation upon "Enlargement of the spleen, with serious difficulties of digestion, respiration, and circulation. Intolerable pain. Splenectomy. Cure." Much less common are reports entitled, "Enlargement of the spleen. Splenectomy. Death from hemorrhage."

Toward the end of the century, the results were improving. Vanverts, for an 1898 thesis, was able to collect 274 reported cases of splenectomy with 170 survivals.[21] Not every clinic shared the enthusiasm. Splenectomies were done at St. Bartholomew's Hospital in London during the latter years of the century. Yet Frederick Taylor makes no mention of the operation's having been done at Guy's Hospital in his discussion of "Some Disorders of the Spleen" seen at Guy's during the decade 1892–1901.[22] Hayem, regarded by some as the father and founder of hematology, took no notice of splenectomy in his book *Du Sang* published in 1889, the first detailed textbook of clinical hematology. Indeed, in this 1035-page tome, the spleen is dealt with in two pages.[23]

It is notable that during the first 50 years of splenectomy, little or no attention was given to the consequences of removal of the spleen except to note that the patient survived, was "relieved," or, as O'Brien put it, there was no "injury or derangement of the animal economy."[13]

In the early years of the twentieth century, series of cases began to be published.[24] But not until the 1920s does the *Quarterly Cumulative Index Medicus* begin to list such titles as "Indications for Splenectomy." Of course, by this time, contraindications had also become evident.

Micheli's splenectomy in a case of hemolytic anemia performed in 1910 appears to have inaugurated the modern era.[25] Prior to this time, hemolytic anemia had been identified by Hayem[26] and by Chauffard[27] (Chapter 8). This was one of the first entities to be lifted out of the "splenic anemia" catch basket and was defined as an anemia that is characterized by light jaundice, microspherocytosis, and reticulocytosis in addition to the splenomegaly. In Paris, several surgical attempts had been unsuccessful, the patients dying during or after splenectomy. Ferdinando Micheli was a professor of medicine at Turin and a hematologist. His patient, a man of 35, probably had a severe acquired hemolytic anemia. He survived and was cured of the anemia. Micheli published three reports of his success, two in Italian and one in German. There was enthusiastic editorial comment in English and French, and, thereafter, many spleens were removed from patients with hemolytic anemia. It is noteworthy, however, that a year before Micheli's paper, there was published in London by Sutherland and Burghard a report of two cases of successful splenectomy in girls with hereditary hemolytic anemia. Both patients were cured of the anemia. The authors commented:

> Our experience does not support the view that there is an inhibition of blood formation. We believe that the spleen is actively engaged in the destruction of blood cells. The yellowish tinge in the skin and in the conjunctivae is probably due to active haemolysis in the spleen—it is certainly not due to any disturbance of the liver function. The condition after splenectomy supports this view. The pigmentation of the skin and conjunctivae disappears within a week, and at the same time the number of red cells and the amount of haemoglobin increase with astonishing rapidity. If there had been inhibition of blood formation we should not have expected such a rapid return to normal, but if the blood-forming organs had been working at high pressure to make up for the destruction of red cells this rapid recovery, when haemolysis had ceased, is exactly what would have been expected.[28]

This sophisticated, clearly reasoned argument was years ahead of its time. It seems a pity that this publication was unnoted at the time and has never been cited since in any review or textbook.

Kaznelson's splenectomy in 1916 for idiopathic thrombocytopenic purpura (ITP, Chapter 16) was another success in a high-risk patient. The patient, a 36-year-old woman, had been afflicted with severe bruising and hemorrhages since her youth. Her spleen extended three fingerbreadths below the rib cage, and her platelet count was extremely low (300!). Paul Kaznelson, a medical student in Prague at the time, had been interested in the theories of Frank, which related thrombocytopenia to the spleen. This student had the temerity to propose that the bleeding woman's spleen be extirpated, and Professor Schloffer had the temerity to do it. The case was reported 4 weeks after the operation, when the platelet count was 500,000.[29] Five years later, the patient was in good health. Credit for the first surgical cure of chronic ITP clearly belongs to Kaznelson, although an American has been credited with *thinking* of it earlier and attempting the operation unsuccessfully. It has been written, "The first two cases, splenectomized at the suggestion of Hess (1915), were fatal."[30] The claim is a bit off the mark. Dr. Alfred Hess of New York City did make such a suggestion, but there was one case only, and the fatal splenectomy was done in August 1917, not 1915.[31]

Hematologic indications for splenectomy have broadened during the past 50 years.[32] Serious diseases in organs remote from the spleen have sometimes been cured after splenectomy. This topic will be discussed later in this chapter. Contraindications to splenectomy have also been perceived. Nowadays, another consideration is coming to the fore. Because the spleen is not an essential organ, surgeons have tended to regard it as useless. Morgenstern estimates that "accidental splenectomy," the removal of a normal spleen consequent to surgical injury, accounts for 20 to 40 percent of all splenectomies performed in the United States. "The morbidity rate resulting from this accident is well above fifty percent, and the mortality may be as high as fifteen percent."[33] Without supporting data, this estimate seems high. Morgenstern's scolding indicates, nevertheless, that an era of complacency is drawing to a close. Especially is there great concern for the severe, often fatal pneumococcal bacteremia that can occur in the absence of the spleen. Morgenstern further recommends repair of minor splenic injuries without removing the organ, and he has experimented with subtotal splenectomy. There are several reports by eighteenth century surgeons who removed portions of the spleen while repairing knife wounds to the abdomen, and the procedure has been recommended from time to time during the twentieth century.[34]

Anatomy of the Spleen[35] (Chapter Opening Photo)

When the spleen is slit open, its cut surface is dark and purplish and dotted with many light points. The darker fabric is called *red pulp* and the points are *white pulp*. Two historically resonant names have been attached to these tissues—Malpighi and Billroth. We speak of malpighian corpuscles and the cords of Billroth.

Marcello Malpighi, who lived during the seventeenth century, was the founder of microscopic anatomy. He discovered, for example, that glands are accumulations of cells surrounding central channels into which the cells empty their secretions. In describing the spleen, Malpighi interpreted as glandular the densely packed cells that comprise the *malpighian corpuscles.*[36] That the malpighian corpuscles are not glands was perceived in the eighteenth century by William Hewson, who probably was the first to group together, with some reason, the thymus, the lymph nodes, and the spleen.[37] He proposed that the lymph nodes and thymus produce lymphocytes, which he called *central particles:* "A due proportion of them is received by the spleen with its arterial blood, and that when arrived there, the spleen has a power of separating them from the other parts of the blood and depositing them in the cells (malpighian corpuscles) already described."[37] This amazing guesswork was neglected until after great advances in microscopic anatomy were made in 1837 by Johannes Müller. Müller's careful observations gave credence to the concept that the malpighian corpuscles are composed of a central arteriole which is encased in a sheath of lymphocytes ("irregular globular particles") of about the same diameter as red cells.[38] Evans in 1844, after an arduous study of the micro-anatomy of the spleen, concluded that the malpighian corpuscles are lymphatic glands that secrete lymph via the spleen's efferent lymphatic vessels.[39] For many early anatomists, the discovery of lymphatic vessels satisfied the longing for an excretory duct for this supposed gland, the lack of which had troubled Galen, as noted previously in this chapter.

In 1854, Theodor Billroth (Figure 5-2) provided the first adequate description of the red pulp and identified the splenic sinus, the vascular structure that is unique to the spleen.[40,41] It has been called the *sinus of Billroth,* and the red pulp, as already mentioned, is often referred to as the *cords of Billroth.*

The splenic sinus, like other vascular sinuses (in the liver and marrow, for example), is a large, specialized capillary; large, yet in the spleen, it is the smallest vessel of the venous collecting system. The splenic sinus differs from other sinuses because its cylindrical wall is discontinuous. Long, threadlike cells lie parallel to form the wall of the cylinder, inviting comparison with a loosely coopered barrel, hooped about by threads of a discontinuous basement membrane. The splenic sinus, thus, is slotted with apertures through which blood cells can move (Figure 5-3).

Functionally, the white pulp generates cells of the lymphocyte-plasmacyte series, which can synthesize the immunoglobulin antibodies. The red pulp, on the other hand, is a filter rich in phagocytes, which can trap and ingest "foreign" particles in the blood as well as old or inadequate blood cells.

The Spleen and the Circulation

MICROCIRCULATION OF THE SPLEEN[42-45] (Figure 5-4)

The discoveries that the white pulp is the arterial side of the splenic circulation and the red pulp is the venous side were the openers in a long game of speculation and observation relating to the flow of blood through the spleen. The microcirculation of the spleen is unlike that of any other organ. To understand the functions of the spleen requires some familiarity with the pattern of its circulation. First of all, for a little organ (0.1 percent of the total body weight), the volume of blood that passes through it is astonishingly large. Cardiac output at rest in an average-sized adult is about 5000 ml per minute. Of this, the spleen receives about 300 ml—more than 5 percent. Bear

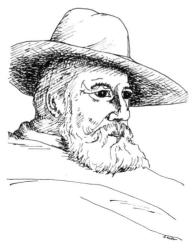

Figure 5-2 Theodor Billroth (1826–1894) was one of the greatest men of nineteenth century medicine. He is best known as the father of abdominal surgery. Even today, the standard operation for removing a portion of the stomach (to cure duodenal ulcer) is the *Billroth II*. He was a great teacher and a severe critic of the shabby curriculum of the contemporary medical schools. He was the first surgeon to make statistical analysis of the results of his surgery.

The other side of Billroth was his musical life. He might have become a professional musician. He was a pianist. He did compose. He wrote verse, musical criticism, and even attempted some musicology, which was gently criticized by his lifelong friend, Johannes Brahms. Their correspondence, "Letters of a Musical Friendship," has been published.

As a young man before he became a surgeon, Billroth carried out his study of the microanatomy of the spleen, describing the splenic sinuses in the red pulp, now called the cords of Billroth.

this in mind while considering the argument whether the splenic circulation is "open" or "closed" (Figure 5-3).

When histologists examine the microscopic anatomy of the spleen in fixed, stained tissue, it is evident that the small arterioles branching out from the malpighian corpuscles are not connected to capillaries, sinuses, or veins, as in any other tissue. They are open-ended so that the blood must flow into the swamplike meshes of the red pulp. The blood cells work their way across this splenic filter to enter the sinuses through the slits in the walls, thence to the veins and out of the spleen. This, simply put, describes the concept of *open circulation*.

According to proponents of the *closed circulation*, vascular channels directly connect the arterioles with the venous collecting system; blood cells enter the red pulp from the sinuses, moving *out of* rather than *into* them.

Experiments using brightly colored fluids perfused into the splenic artery gave contradictory results. Some experiments demonstrated direct channels

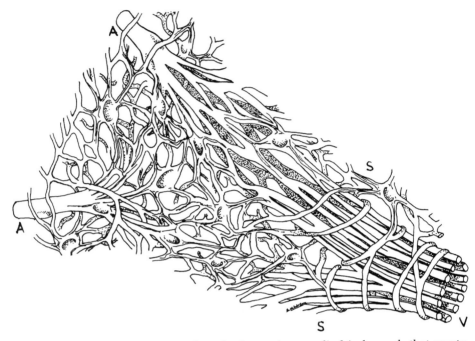

Figure 5-3   The splenic sinus. In the *red pulp* are shown cylindrical vessels that empty into the splenic veins (V). The walls of these sinuses are composed of parallel rods, which are extensions of endothelial cells. Blood cells can pass into the sinus through the spaces between these rods. Blood enters the red pulp from arterioles (A). Much of the blood flows rapidly from the end of the arteriole to the end of a sinus, as suggested by the arrangement at the top of the diagram. In the arrangement at the bottom, some blood flows into the tangled webs of the red pulp. Such blood cells flow slowly and escape through the slits in the sinus wall(s).

from the arterial to the venous side; in others, the perfusion fluid flowed into the red pulp.[42] Knisely examined living, transilluminated spleens of mice under the microscope and was able to demonstrate only direct streams of flow from arterial to venous vessels.[43] It stands to reason that this must be the way that blood crosses the spleen. After all, in every minute, blood equivalent in weight to twice the spleen's weight enters and leaves that little organ. Flow through the cords of the red pulp must be sluggish indeed. It is impossible for so much blood to flow sluggishly. The *logistics* of the situation demand a closed circulation. The spleen, however, is a filter and splenic *function* demands an open circulation. The paradox is easily resolved—the spleen has both open and closed circulations.

An experiment by McNee demonstrated the duality.[44] He injected yeast spheres the size of red cells into the splenic artery and promptly killed the anesthetized animal. When nerves to the spleen had first been stimulated by electricity, the spleen was firmly contracted and the yeast was present only in the sinuses, not in the pulp. In the contracted spleen, blood flowed directly from arteries to veins across "ad hoc" channels through the pulp. Knisely's observations were made upon living, tightly contracted spleens. Yet when his mice became moribund, the spleens expanded and the cords of Billroth filled with red cells. In McNee's experiments, on the other hand, when the spleen was not artificially contracted, yeast cells were present both in the sinuses and in the pulp, evidence for coexistence of both open and closed circulations.

Figure 5-4 Diagram of the spleen's circulation. The spleen is divided into compartments by thin fibrous walls or trabeculae (1) that are extensions of the fibrous capsule. Blood vessels, the trabecular arteries (2), and veins (3) penetrate the spleen along these walls. Central arteries (4) that branch into the splenic pulp are enclosed in a lymphatic sheath (5). The sheath is the white pulp (malpighian corpuscles). Arterioles (6) extend out of the white pulp and into the pulp cords (7), otherwise called red pulp or cords of Billroth. Blood flows from the open ends of these arterioles and into the venous system through the sinuses (8). See Figure 5-3. The sinuses empty into pulp veins (9), which empty, in turn, into the trabecular veins (3). The round body within the sheath (5) is a germinal follicle, where antibody synthesis takes place. (*Adapted from Klemperer, P: The spleen, in Downey H (ed): Handbook of Hematology. New York, Hoeber, 1938, vol III.*)

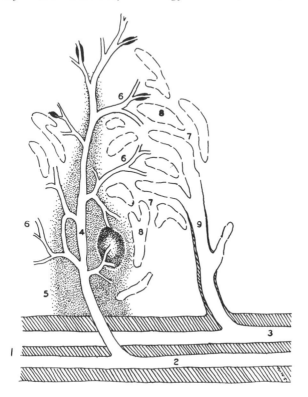

Some blood is shunted rapidly across the organ, some spins off into the sluggish morass of the splenic filter. Roy Williams, professor of anatomy at the University of Pennsylvania, transplanted tiny fragments of splenic tissue into windows planted in the ears of rabbits and, by direct microscopy, could demonstrate these two components of the circulation crossing the living splenic tissue at different velocities.[46]

RESERVOIR FUNCTION OF THE SPLEEN

It has been known for centuries that the spleen is an expansile-contractile organ. The "spongy" nature of its tissue and its ability to enlarge by filling with blood has provoked, over the years, repeated comparisons with the corpora cavernosa of the penis.[38,47,48] Contractions of the spleen have suggested an analogy to systole of the heart.[49,50] Benjamin Rush, a historical personage of Philadelphia during the early days of the Republic, was much interested in emotional stress and emotional illness. He proposed that the spleen is a "receptacle for the blood, when exerted in tumultuous motions," and the blood vessels thereby "protect themselves from destruction, by means of a temporary reservoir of their redundant motions, or quantity of blood." Rush was also a notorious proponent of phlebotomy (vein cutting) as a cure for diverse ills, and he bent the argument about splenic function to his purpose: "We are taught from the use assigned to (the spleen), the necessity of blood-letting in all those diseases in which it has been found to be unduly distended."[51]

These old opinions regarding the occasion and usefulness of the spleen's distention and contraction were based largely upon conjecture and post-mortem experience. Thus Henry Gray extrapolated his observations of dead horses to derive a vital function of the spleen: "The spleen also serves to regulate the amount of blood according to the nutrition of the animal . . . the spleen in well-fed animals always containing a much larger quantity of blood than in ill-fed or starved animals."[52] Gray also subscribed to the opinion that the spleen is a "reservoir for blood, a safety valve to the circulation which can, from its structure, be suddenly called into use, and as suddenly become quiescent, when the conditions under which its activity is excited subside."[53] This concept, as we shall see, is exactly the reverse of the spleen's behavior in living animals.

The first "modern" experiments upon the reservoir function of the spleen were conducted in 1881 by Charles Roy, a professor of physiology at Cambridge, who devised a plethysmograph that gently encased the spleen in situ and, with this apparatus, demonstrated that asphyxia or stimulation of splenic nerves causes an immediate reduction of splenic volume. He did not, however, come to the logical conclusion that the reduction of splenic volume must entail a reciprocal enlargement of circulating, extrasplenic blood volume,

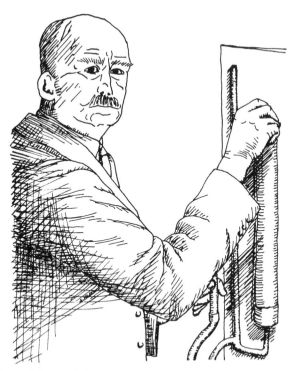

Figure 5-5 Sir Joseph Barcroft (1872–1947) was a physiologist whose primary interest was in respiratory function, especially the behavior of the hemoglobin molecule in the binding and release of oxygen. An interest in the spleen was aroused when he noted that mixtures of red cells, some containing oxygen, others carbon monoxide, behaved differently in the spleen than in other organs. This led him to the recognition of a "splenic reservoir function." Over a period of 10 years, 1923 to 1932, he wrote almost 30 papers on this topic, yet it was a relatively minor one in his investigative career.

His perception and perspective of the biological world can be seen in the observation, "Haemoglobin, by reason of the quantity of oxygen it can transport, has made life on the great scale possible to the mammalia."

although he did discuss the "amount of blood which the spleen is capable of expelling at each systole."[54]

In the 1920s, Sir Joseph Barcroft, also a professor of physiology at Cambridge, discovered a function of the spleen which he "described briefly as that of acting as a reservoir for erythrocytes."[55] Barcroft (Figure 5-5) did experimental studies by "exteriorizing" the spleens of rabbits, cats, and dogs and demonstrated expansion and contraction of the organ, the contractions occurring when the animals were alarmed or asphyxiated or subjected to blood loss.[56] These discoveries were published at a time when Cannon's theory of alarm reactions (reactions that prepare animals for "fight or flight") was a lively topic. The concept of a reservoir that could inject red cells into the circulation at the time of need fitted neatly into this scheme of things. Barcroft seems not to have been aware of Roy's experiments done in 1881, not so long before, indeed within Barcroft's lifetime.

Barcroft had no hesitation in extending, by analogy, the results of his dog experiments to humans: "Suppose (1) that the blood volume of a man is five litres, (2) that he can expel one litre of blood from his spleen, (3) that this can be expelled in 12 seconds. . . ."[55] Barcroft's extrapolation was accepted uncritically by many essayists discussing the functions of the spleen in humans. McNee, for example, stated in his Croonian lectures: "The chief function of the spleen, excluding that in which reticuloendothelial system is concerned, is its contractility."[57]

It was not until almost 20 years after Barcroft's first publication on the topic that Ebert and Stead demonstrated that the normal human spleen has no discernible reservoir function relative to erythrocytes.[58]

The normal human spleen does, however, sequester about one-third of the circulating platelets,[59] although few if any leukocytes.

RESERVOIR FUNCTION OF ABNORMAL HUMAN SPLEENS

Although normally weighing about 120 g in an adult, the spleen's size in chronic infection and hereditary hemolytic anemias not uncommonly increases by 10 to 20 times. Neoplastic spleens may be even larger; weights of almost 10 kg have been reported.[60,61]

The normal human spleen receives about 5 percent of the cardiac output. With massive splenomegaly, the spleen may receive more than 50 percent.[62] This places a heavy burden upon the circulatory system, not only upon the heart but also upon the portal circulation, into which the splenic venous blood must flow.

During the 1950s, experiments with radioisotopes showed that blood can be stored in the spleen when it is greatly enlarged. In such subjects, a tracer dose of radiolabeled red cells mixes rapidly with, say, 80 percent of the circulating red cells and then slowly mixes with the remaining 20 percent, while at the same time surface counts over the spleen gradually increase as radioactive red cells accumulate.[63,64] Some of the red cells within the spleen move slowly and mix slowly with the tracer. They do move, but their movement is slower than in the general circulation, and, so, they are said to be sequestered. Splenic sequestration of red cells from the circulating blood intensifies anemia in patients with large spleens.

Splenomegaly also causes an expansion of circulating plasma volume, a phenomenon best demonstrated in tropical splenomegaly, a condition in which the spleen sometimes becomes enormous without the patient becoming especially ill.[65] Such patients are anemic in that the concentration of red cells in the circulating blood is low, yet the total volume of red cells in the blood may be normal or even greater than normal. The "anemia" is a consequence of dilution by the expanded plasma volume as well as of sequestration of red cells in the spleen. It is noteworthy that the concentration of albumin in the expanded plasma is normal, which means that the total amount of albumin is increased; albumin production by the liver must, therefore, be increased. This suggests that the massive spleen somehow provokes the liver to produce more albumin. After splenectomy, the expanded plasma volume subsides very slowly. It is 6 months or a year before the normal volume is restored. During this lag time, the concentration of albumin remains normal, indicating that the excess production of albumin only gradually decreases.[66] This function of the spleen relative to production of plasma albumin is not yet understood.

The Spleen and the Blood Elements

There were many barriers to the comprehension of splenic functions. Some of its functions were unknowable to our forebears. For example, the concept of immunity, a process requiring the participation of tissues and organs of the immune system, began to take shape only at the beginning of the twentieth century. Furthermore, the spleen's participation in the turnover of blood cells could not be recognized until after the concept of normal cell destruction had been demonstrated and accepted. The first demonstrations of erythrophagocytosis, that is, one cell devouring another, were discovered histologically in splenic tissue by Kölliker[67] and by Ecker[68] in 1847. Kölliker proposed that this is a normal phenomenon. "For the present, therefore, so long as the pathological character of the phenomena in question is not conclusively demonstrated, I must claim their physiological nature and regard the disintegration of red corpuscles in the spleen as a normal occurrence."[69] This interpretation was challenged. Billroth, and others, suggested that the cell-within-a-cell configuration represented erythropoiesis, the production of red cells. The mighty Virchow recognized that phagocytosis is evidence of cell destruction, but refused to believe it to be a normal activity.[70] Kölliker recanted and accepted Virchow's opinion, omitting discussion of "physiological or pathological" in later editions of his handbook.[71] Such are the uses of authority. Kölliker's view was the correct one.[72]

The barrier to understanding in this dispute was that a living animal was not yet perceived to be a sort of "biological vortex." A vortex is a mass of fluid whirling around a funnel-shaped cavity. Fluid flows into it, over the shoulder of the vortex, and out through the narrow tip. The shape of the spinning vortex remains constant, but its constituent fluid is continually changing. The animal body is also a vortex, its shape constant, its cellular constituents forever changing. All of its organs also are vortices. The blood is a vortex. Constituent cells of the blood are maintained as a mass of constant volume, but the cells are continually being destroyed and replaced. This concept of normal hemolysis and compensatory hematopoiesis was slow to be perceived. Vanlair and Masius may have been first to propose that chronic anemia might be the result of abnormally rapid destruction of red blood cells.[73] Gowers in 1877 came close to grasping the concept of blood cell turnover:

> What are we to conclude is the fate of the white blood corpuscles? It appears probable that a few of them persist and perish, as such, in the blood. Many of them pass out of the blood into the tissues, and there subserve processes of growth in a manner at present ill-understood. They also, without doubt, leave the vessels wherever inflammation is going on, and appear in the inflammatory products as pus corpuscles. Other white blood corpuscles probably divide and give rise to similar cells. . . . Lastly, it is now believed that a large number of white corpuscles are transformed into red ones . . . mainly in the tissues of certain organs, especially the spleen and the medulla of the bone."[74]

Only with the recognition of normal splenic destruction of normal red cells has the balance that the spleen and marrow maintain finally been placed in a proper perspective. This has permitted development of a mathematical model of the *vortex* that is the body's red cell mass.[75]

Other impediments to the understanding of splenic functions developed as more was learned of the spleen. Animal studies provided many insights but were sometimes misleading. In some animals, the spleen is an important adjunct to the marrow in the production of blood cells, but this is not true in humans. In some animals, the spleen is distensible and provides a normal reservoir capacity wherein red blood cells can be stored, but not in humans. When a dog is killed with an overdose of barbiturate, the spleen is distended; with an overdose of ether, it is contracted. Disease of one sort or another can result in a spleen that is 10, 20, 30 times normal size or a spleen that is completely atrophied.

Removal of the spleen results in a multitude of subtle changes in the blood cells, in blood volume, and in the immune system. Some of these changes differ from species to species and may vary according to the age and the health of the animal.

All of these variables had to be sorted out in order to achieve a clear picture of splenic function. These matters have, by now, been clarified, yet we still do not understand everything about the spleen.

SPLENIC ANEMIA

The discovery that ultimately removed the spleen from the ranks of the digestive organs and placed it with the blood system was reported simultaneously in 1845 by Craigie,[76] by Bennett,[77] and by Virchow,[78] when each described a patient with chronic leukemia and an enlarged spleen (Chapter 15). This disease came to be called "splenic leukemia."

However, because in many diseases besides leukemia, anemia is associated with a large spleen, a new nosologic concept was required, "splenic anemia." This term was coined by Gretsel in 1866 to name the disease of a 1-year-old anemic infant with massive splenomegaly.[79] It was not until 1882 that Banti defined and used this term for anemia in adults.[80] Thereafter, it caught on and was widely and variously assigned to any anemia not evidently leukemic in origin. The diagnosis of splenic anemia was popularized in America by Osler, who tried to bring some sort of clinical order to an accumulating hodgepodge of cases. He failed, after publishing a half-dozen papers, because his cases of splenic anemia were no more homogenous than any other collection of the time.[81] As the clinical, histological, and laboratory experiences converged in the early years of this century, the need for the term evaporated. More precise diagnoses such as hemolytic anemia and Hodgkin's disease came into use.

BANTI'S SYNDROME

Guido Banti (Figure 5-6) made the first effort to separate out a definite entity from the catch basket of "splenic anemia." He collected a series of cases of

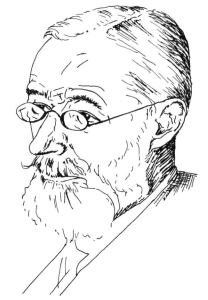

Figure 5-6 Guido Banti (1852–1925) was one of the first physicians who might properly be called a hematologist. A contemporary of Osler, he worked at a time when the methods and laws of biological research were just developing. Medical discovery was commonly a consequence of clinical insight aided only by physical examinations and necropsy. The titles of Banti's earliest publications give the direction of his lifelong interests: "Splenic anemia" and "Enlargement of the spleen with cirrhosis of the liver." His efforts to define these conditions as entities came to nothing, but the discussions about them did much to demonstrate the essentialness of method in clinical research.

chronic anemia with splenomegaly that terminated with cirrhosis of the liver.[82] Splenomegaly with cirrhosis is common, but Banti asserted that in *morbus Banti*, splenomegaly comes first with an associated anemia. Then comes a transitional phase with enlargement of the liver, pigmentation of the skin, and decreased urine output, and, finally, comes a third phase, cirrhosis with ascites. A long and acrimonious debate ensued.[83-85] Is there a Banti's syndrome or isn't there? Recall that Banti published his first description in 1894. In 1920, Eppinger declared that Banti's syndrome was one of the most discussed problems of internal medicine.[86] In 1951, Di Guglielmo wrote an impassioned argument concluding that a pure Banti disease does exist even though its pathogenesis may not yet be established.[87] The story of Banti's syndrome is instructive as an example of the futility of argument without evidence, a common pastime of medical scientists, we who are doomed to work with information that is slippery and volatile. Here are some of the problems that beset the students of what may have been a phantom disease:

1 Banti stipulated three clinical stages of his disease, the spleen involved in the first, the liver in the third. Without liver biopsy or liver function tests, it was not possible to know when the liver first became involved.

2 An illogical claim by Banti was that the disease could be cured if the spleen were removed during the first stage. Because the syndrome could only be established by its ultimate progression to cirrhosis, how could Banti be sure of the diagnosis in a cured patient?

3 Late in his career, Banti attempted to clinch his argument on histologic grounds. He assembled a collection of microscopic sections of the spleens from typical cases and pointed out that they had in common a fibrotic reaction surrounding the small arteries, "fibroadonia." These sections were sent to outstanding pathologists, who were unimpressed, pointing out that the changes were those found in association with ordinary cirrhosis of the liver.[84] This settled nothing. Histologic appearances may be unexceptional when the spleen is on its worst behavior, in immune hemolytic anemia or thrombocytopenia for example. Banti had chosen an inappropriate method to resolve the problem. With methods unimagined during the heat of the Banti debate, it has now been suggested that cirrhosis may sometimes result from autoimmune disease[88,89] Thus, Banti may have been correct in saying that disease of the spleen may precede disease of the liver, but he did not have the investigational tools to demonstrate it.

4 With many authorities redefining the syndrome, each in a different way, the waters grew murky. Banti's syndrome became the same sort of waste basket as the term *splenic anemia*. Some have said that Banti contributed to the confusion by changing his definition of the disease. Others replied that with experience, he was able to refine the definition. At the present time,

the term Banti's syndrome is still used to some extent and is applied to splenomegaly associated with cirrhosis, even in experimental animals. It seems an irony that in some contemporary index, we find it listed as a synonym of the catch-basket term *splenic anemia.*

The scientific method requires that one construct the hypothesis that best fits all available data pertaining to a phenomenon. Experiments are then devised to challenge the hypothesis. If the experiments fail to destroy it, the hypothesis is strengthened (not proved; hypotheses never can be proved). When an experiment destroys the hypothesis, a new one is constructed to fit the new data. In the case of *morbus Banti,* the long effort was to *prove* the hypothesis.

As I have said, the misfortune of the Banti episode is that his hypothesis stimulated argument rather than research, a phenomenon not unique in medical history. In this regard it is appropriate to mention Castle's law (after William B. Castle), "There is nothing like a fact to stop an argument."

Red Cells and the Spleen

The normal human spleen plays many roles in the life cycle of normal human red cells.

ERYTHROPOIESIS

Red cell production is a normal function of the human spleen only around the time of the fifth fetal month. Then the marrow takes over this function. In tiny mammals, the marrow cavity of the bones is relatively small and provides insufficient room for blood formation. In these animals—mice, for example—the spleen shares in this function. In some lower vertebrates with cartilaginous bones, the spleen does the entire job.

Removal of the spleen from dogs and other mammals in which the spleen has a massive reservoir capacity results in a gradual onset of anemia. The total red cell volume shrinks during a period of 30 to 40 days to about 65 percent of its normal size. Then, after several months, it gradually regains its presplenectomy volume. This anemia was a puzzle to those who studied the phenomenon early in this century. Was it caused by blood destruction? Did the spleen have a blood cell preserving function? Or does the spleen have a marrow stimulating function? During the early days of splenic surgery, surgeons frequently noted that human patients were anemic postsplenectomy. They attempted to correlate this with the anemia of dogs, but we now suspect that postsplenectomy human anemia was a consequence of blood loss during surgery. The removal of a normal human spleen nowadays does not cause anemia. The postsplenectomy anemia in dogs is caused not by bleeding or hemolysis but by a temporary reduction in the formation of red cells. Some suspect that in such animals the spleen may be a producer of the hormone that stimulates the marrow's red cell production, *erythropoietin.*[90]

SPLENIC REMODELING OF THE RED CELL SURFACE

In the early twentieth century, investigators noted several postsplenectomy changes in the red cells circulating in the blood. The most consistent were the phenomena of increased osmotic resistance and the presence of granules within the cells.

Increased osmotic resistance as a consequence of splenectomy was first reported by Chalier and Charlet[91] and was promptly confirmed by Karsner and Pearce[92] and by many others. This phenomenon concerns the behavior of red blood cells suspended in a dilute solution of sodium chloride, the concentration of which is less than that of the blood itself. In order to establish equilibrium between the internal milieu of the red cell and the dilute solution, the cell accepts water, thereby diluting its own salt concentration. The disc-shaped red cell swells, becoming more spherical to accommodate the water. When the solution is excessively dilute, the cell first becomes a perfect sphere and then it bursts. The dilution at which bursting occurs determines the cell's osmotic resistance. The cause of increased osmotic resistance postsplenectomy was not established until 1942, when Miller, Singer, and Dameshek[93] noted *target cells* in the blood of splenectomized dogs. Target cells are abnormally thin red blood cells. Their thinness gives them a more-than-normal capacity to accept water from the dilute salt solutions. This change has been interpreted as an indication that the spleen somehow modifies the maturation of young red cells in the circulation. Red cells as delivered from the marrow are considerably larger than mature red cells. During the first day or two of its life, the cell becomes smaller in volume (from approximately 120 μm^3 [fl] to approximately 90 μm^3 [fl]) and in surface area (from 200 μm^2 to 135 μm^2).[94] In the absence of the spleen, the mean surface of mature red cells may be larger than normal (150 μm^2) while the volume still remains a normal 90 μm^3 (fl). The surface of the red cell is composed, for the most part, of lipid. How the spleen controls the loss of surface lipid remains a topic of conjecture.[95]

PITTING FUNCTION OF THE SPLEEN (Figure 5-7)

The Howell-Jolly body is a small dark-staining granule that is found in the red cells of the blood after splenectomy. In a normal person after splenectomy, the inclusion is present in about 1 percent of the red cells. It is found with such consistency in splenectomized humans that we regard it as an indication of the absence of the spleen. The Howell-Jolly body is a fragment of the nucleus of the progenitor erythroblast from which the red cell is derived. Only a few cells escape from the marrow with this remnant. For years it was believed that the

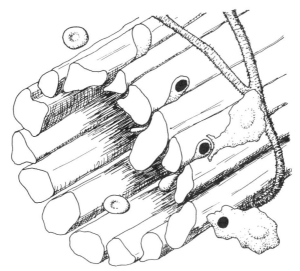

Figure 5-7 "Pitting" function of the spleen. Circulating red blood cells sometimes contain small, abnormal granules. These may be remnants of the precursor cell's nucleus or grains of iron not used for hemoglobin. They may be organisms of infections such as malaria or bits of destroyed hemoglobin. The spleen can remove such granules at the wall of the splenic sinus.

Red cells are pliant, almost fluid in their deformability. Above, in clockwise progression, a granule-containing red cell pours itself through a slit in the sinus wall. Because the inclusion body is not deformable, it cannot get through the slit. The granule, then, is simply amputated, the red cell goes its way essentially unharmed, while a phagocyte ingests the amputated "pit."

spleen recognizes these cells as decadent and destroys them, while in the absence of a spleen the inclusion-containing red cells continue to circulate.

The siderocyte is another inclusion-containing red cell that appears in the blood in large numbers after splenectomy in patients with hemolytic anemia. Fifty percent or more of the red cells may contain these iron-loaded granules. McFadzean and Davis, who studied the siderocytes in patients cured of hemolytic anemia by splenectomy, proffered that "a red cell containing inclusion bodies is a defective cell fated to rapid elimination from the circulation, a process in which the spleen plays a major part."[96]

However, when siderocyte-rich blood was transfused into recipients with normal spleens, it was learned that the granules rapidly disappeared, but the red cells did not. In transfusion recipients who had no spleen, both the granules and the red cells remained in the circulation. It was concluded that the spleen is somehow able to bring about the removal of siderin inclusion bodies without destroying the red cells that contain them.[97] This led to speculation concerning splenic function:

After splenectomy, in certain conditions other intra-erythrocytic inclusion bodies may become more numerous: red-cell nuclei, Howell-Jolly bodies, malarial plasmodia, organisms of bartonellosis, Heinz bodies. Is it possible that a normal function of the spleen is to assist the circulating red cells to rid themselves of any inclusion bodies, as it does the siderocyte? If true, this might be called the "pitting function" of the spleen.[97]

The *Heinz body*, just mentioned, is a red cell inclusion composed of degraded hemoglobin. It results from the poisoning of red cells by oxidative injury. Irreversibly damaged hemoglobin molecules aggregate, forming small granules. The mystery of the removal of red cell granules was solved with experiments involving Heinz bodies in rat spleens. Electron micrographs show that the inclusion is removed at the wall of the splenic sinus, the sinus of Billroth. Cells in the pulp cords enter the sinuses by squeezing through slits between the endothelial "staves" of the sinus "barrel." The Heinz body is a hard little "clinker" and, although the easily deformable red cell slithers into the sinus, it stops when the rigid inclusion stops, like a dog with its tail caught in a spring-loaded screen door. At this juncture, the red cell simply amputates its inclusion body and proceeds into the splenic vein. The Heinz body, sheathed in red cell membrane, is ingested by a phagocyte.[98]

This *pitting function* of the spleen, reminiscent of a housewife squeezing the pits out of cherries, removes the siderin granules and Howell-Jolly bodies as well as the infectious inclusion bodies of such diseases as malaria and babesiosis. In our arbitrary division of splenic function into two categories, *hematologic* and *immune*, pitting serves both categories—it cleans up circulating red cells and it helps fight infection.

DESTRUCTION OF RED CELLS BY THE SPLEEN

Virchow wrote that the "heretical thought of the continued reproduction of cells" had gradually germinated in his mind in the late 1840s, but he did not make the "first hesitant attempts" to proclaim it until 1852.[99] Except as a pathologic phenomenon, Virchow seems not to have examined the other side of the concept, i.e., cell death. He perceived "the continued reproduction of cells" as the means for repairing the ravages of disease. Cell regeneration implies cell death. He seems to have rejected the normal destruction of normal cells. When Kölliker bowed to authority concerning Virchow's opinion that erythrophagocytosis is a pathologic phenomenon, he was implicitly accepting a concept that cells, unless damaged by disease, might live forever. Virchow was correct in his opinion that phagocytosis is the fate of damaged red cells, but this is also the way in which normal cells die at the end of their life cycle.

With hereditary abnormalities of red cells and when red cells are damaged by chemicals, infections, or antibodies, the number of phagocytic cells in the spleen is vastly increased, and the size of the spleen is abnormally large.[100] When the blood contains a mixture of normal and abnormal red cells, the spleen is able to distinguish between them and destroys only the defective ones.[101] This discernment is the so-called culling function of the spleen.[102]

In humans, the spleen is the normal site of red cell destruction. However, after removal of the spleen, this function is performed in other parts of the body. The spleen is not an essential organ. Red cells not destroyed by the spleen do not pile up in the blood. The life span of normal red cells is not extended after splenectomy.[103]

When red cells are destroyed, the constituent materials become waste products, of which the phagocytes and the body as a whole must make some disposition. Hemoglobin provides, by far, the greatest problem, comprising one-third of the red cell's mass. (Most of the remaining two-thirds is water.) The protein portion, the globin, is degraded into its constituent amino acids, which reenter the body's amino-acid pool to be reutilized. The heme molecule is composed of a porphyrin ring encircling an iron atom. These two constituents are dealt with in vastly different ways. The porphyrin is degraded to bile pigment and excreted from the body in its entirety. Iron, on the other hand, is not excreted at all; it is available for reuse, and in the normal situation about 90 percent of it is incorporated into the hemoglobin of a new generation of red cells (Chapter 7).

THE SPLEEN AND BILE PIGMENT

It is fitting that the spleen, antiquity's center of the black bile, should have been discovered by modern physiology to participate in bile-pigment metabolism. Some anatomists of the prephysiology era surmised from the arrangement of the splenic vein's draining into the liver that the spleen is somehow related to the liver's secretion of bile. Rejecting the Ancients' belief that the spleen "attracted to itself" the black bile, these later commentators framed other equally lurid concepts: that the blood by its retardation in the spleen is rendered thicker and consequently more fit for the excretion of the bile—or that the spleen assists in the secretion of the bile by diluting the thicker blood brought in from the intestines to the liver with the thinner blood from the splenic vein—or that the spleen serves as auxillary to the formation of the bile, producing changes in the venous blood traversing it, which acquires some peculiar property from the action of the splenic nerves. All of these are described in Henry Gray's superb historical introduction to his 1854 treatise on the spleen.[104]

Kölliker was the first to propose, in 1847, that "the blood corpuscles undergo dissolution in the spleen, and that their colouring matter is employed in preparing the colouring matter of the bile." This, too, is a quotation from Henry Gray, who then added disparagingly "but this is certainly not the case."[105] They were both guessing, but Kölliker guessed right. Vanlair and Masius, who in 1871 published the first description of the hemolytic anemia now called hereditary spherocytosis, correctly identified their patient's enlarged spleen as the center of the mischief in this disease and proposed that the patient's jaundice was a reflection of the excess bile pigment formed when hemoglobin was released from the "senile" red cells.[73] However, the concept of splenic origin for bile pigment was challenged by many experimenters for many years. They removed spleens, they created bile fistulae in order to recover bile pigment without its traversing the intestine, and they induced hemolytic anemia.[106] They measured the concentration of bile pigment in blood from splenic arteries and veins.[107] The results were variable and confusing.[108] Some reported that removal of the spleen had no effect upon bile-pigment excretion, some found that it was decreased, and some found cycles of high bile-pigment output alternating with low bile-pigment output.[106] But pigment output did not cease when the spleen was removed. This was confusing to those who believed the spleen to be the source of bile pigment. It is now appreciated that hemoglobin is the single great source of bile pigment and *all* the porphyrin in hemoglobin is excreted as bilirubin. Although most red cells are normally destroyed in the spleen, they are destroyed in other organs when the spleen is absent,[109] and all of the hemoglobin porphyrin is still degraded to bilirubin and excreted in the bile. Increased red cell destruction results in increased amounts of bile pigment. When splenectomy causes anemia because of the diminished production of red cells, as it does in normal dogs, bile pigment output decreases. When splenectomy results in hemolytic diseases, as it does in dogs infected with *Bartonella*, bile pigment output increases. Working backward from quantitative knowledge of hemoglobin production and destruction, we can compute what amount of bile pigment must be produced, and, thus, we can estimate the magnitude of this splenic function; the normal daily destruction of 20 g of old red cells in an adult human results in the degradation of 6.25 g of hemoglobin (3.7 percent porphyrin), yielding 230 g of bilirubin, all excreted in the bile. This neat calculation was evolved in a brilliant series of chemical and animal experiments by the great student of pigment metabolism, Cecil Watson.[110]

THE SPLEEN AND IRON METABOLISM

Early histologists recognized the spleen's participation in iron metabolism by the accumulation of iron pigment (siderin) within phagocytes after the ingestion of red cells.[69,111] It was also noted that when circulating red cells had been damaged, the siderosis became very conspicuous.[111,112]

In the early twentieth century, extracellular accumulations of iron pigment within the red pulp of human spleens, *Gandy-Gamna nodules*, were found in cases of chronic splenomegaly. Their significance was a topic of considerable attention.[111] Histologists thought them to be the remnants of hemorrhages. Threadlike mycelial projections from these ferruginous lumps were thought by others to be fungi; Nanta "identified" them as *Aspergillus nigricans* and believed them to be the cause of Banti's disease.[113]

Some iron deposits in the spleen were probably artifacts, resulting from the use of acid fixatives that leach iron from its anatomical locations and permit it to collect upon collagen fibers. Hence, this vagrant iron was observed not only as mycelia, but also as ferruginous deposits in the capsule of the spleen, in the trabeculae, and in the fibrillar reticulum.

The central importance of the spleen to the internal exchanges of iron within the body was not appreciated until about 25 years ago, when the life span of the red cell became a topic of intense interest. Then it was finally appreciated how much iron must move each day through the hemoglobin-iron cycle. Prior to this, and unmindful of the necessity to reutilize iron, Rous (Chapter 8) in his classic review of 1923 on the splenic destruction of the red cells wrote:

> The prevailing view of the normal fate of hemoglobin is that it is broken up into globin and hematin, which latter in turn yields hematoidin—thrown off in the bile and bilirubin—and iron-containing materials of uncertain chemical constitution which are retained.[114]

Krumbhaar, however, in 1926, in his classic review on the functions of the spleen, asked:

> Is it possible that the spleen is needed in iron utilization from the point of view not so much of preventing its loss by excretion as of so acting upon the iron that it becomes available to the bone marrow for building up the hemoglobin molecule?[107]

Krumbhaar's prescient question went unanswered and unnoted. The concept of ecologic cycles of red cells and of iron was not so easily perceived. As late as 1936 Klemperer wrote:

> The quantity of hemosiderin observed under normal and pathological conditions, also after blood transfusion, is not wholly accounted for by the destruction of erythrocytes phagocytosed within the spleen.[111]

Klemperer's conclusions, congruent with those of others before his time and since, were based upon the appearance of phagocytosis of red cells in tissues fixed for microscopic examination. What actually occurs during the life of the spleen is obscured in such material by the failure of phagocytes to die immediately after blood flow stops. They continue to digest the red cells they have ingested. Unless the spleen is fixed promptly, the true picture of its phagocytic activity is lost.[115]

In the normal adult, about 20 g of red cells is destroyed each day. Most of this destruction occurs within the spleen, whence the iron is quickly returned via the plasma to the marrow, there to be used for the synthesis of new hemoglobin. About 20 mg of iron per day travels through this hemoglobin cycle, and none of this iron accumulates in the spleen. If even a fraction were retained in the spleen each day, in time a heavy accumulation would result. In hemolytic anemia, where many blood cells are prematurely destroyed, the spleen may turn over 100 mg—or even 200 mg—of iron per day, resulting from the destruction of 5 to 10 times the normal amount of hemoglobin.[75]

The Reticuloendothelial System[116-118]

The phenomenon of phagocytosis received vast attention during the second half of the nineteenth century. Dozens of researchers were occupied with the description and location in the body of the kinds of cells that are able to ingest particulate matter. Studies were made of individual cells, of bits of tissue, of perfused organs, and of entire animals.[116] The last sort of experiment involved injection of tiny particles into the bloodstream; this permitted the cartography of a widespread system of phagocytic cells. The early study of Ponfick[119] in 1885, using the mineral cinnabar, and the definitive study in 1904 by Ribbert,[120] using carmine, established the locations of these clusterings of phagocytes. But, as Krumbhaar pointed out, it was not until 1913 that Aschoff and Landau proposed "to group together a special type of cells of wide distribution in the mammalian organism as a system of reticuloendothelial cells."[121]

The reticular cells, which are fixed cells that extend many long threads into surrounding tissue, are those of the splenic pulp, the lymphoid tissue, and the marrow. Endothelial cells are those that line the sinuses of the spleen, liver, and marrow. Also included in the *reticuloendothelial system* (RES) are macrophages of the spleen, the marrow, the liver (Kupffer cells), and the lungs as well as the blood monocytes (see Chapter 13). Krumbhaar (Figure 5-8), who had done much to draw the RES to the attention of American biologists, concluded a discussion of the spleen and immunity with this comment: "It is the reticuloendothelial system that is here concerned, and the spleen's importance is due to the fact that it is the chief habitat of that system."[122]

The RES is not only phagocytic, but it participates in the immune reactions of the body—one of the primary functions of the spleen.

The Spleen and Immunity

Long before the functions of the spleen could be comprehended, it was recognized that the spleen is involved with infections. The large spleen in malaria was recognized by Hippocrates. The term *ague cake* (ague, malarial fever; cake, a mass or concretion), an obsolete English vulgarism for malarial splenomegaly, indicates that the laity has long known of the relationship. After discovery of the bacterial basis for infectious disease 100 years ago, it

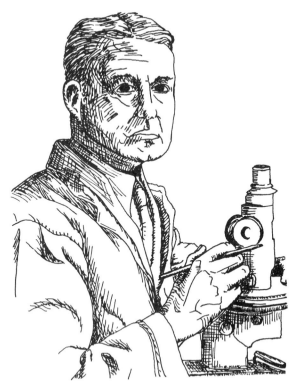

Figure 5-8 Edward B. Krumbhaar (1882–1966) was a young member of a large team of investigators at the University of Pennsylvania under the leadership of R. M. Pearce. During the early years of this century, they performed extensive experimental work on the functions of the spleen. This research was a model of animal experimentation performed in an era when most such work was rather squalid. Dozens of papers were published, most of them in the *Journal of Experimental Medicine,* and, in 1918, the work was synthesized and summarized in a valuable book, *The Spleen and Anaemia.*[83] Krumbhaar was the member of that team who attempted to translate the experimental work in terms of clinical application. Even after the team ceased its experimental work, Krumbhaar continued to discuss the role of the spleen in the blood and immune systems.

became possible to clarify the relation between a variety of infections and the spleen.

In 1904, the Royal College of Physicians of London invited Frederick Taylor to deliver the annual Lumlian Lectures. Dr. Taylor, Senior Physician to Guy's Hospital, after a "feeling of despair as to the choice of a subject," presented a series of three lectures on "Some Disorders of the Spleen," based upon ten years of experience at Guy's Hospital, 1892 to 1901, concerning the state of the spleen in 4762 necropsy examinations.[22]

Much of his discussion was concerned with the causes of splenomegaly, and first among these was infection—typhus, enteric fever, relapsing fever, malaria, measles, scarlet fever, variola, glandular fever, Malta fever, diphtheria, influenza, Weil's disease, anthrax, dysentery, beri-beri [sic], tuberculosis, syphilis, actinomycosis, and pneumonia. I give his entire list because the topic of infection pervades the lectures.

The other causes of splenomegaly that received extensive coverage were the splenomegaly of cirrhosis, Banti's disease (the two considered separately), splenic anemia, von Jaksch's anemia (a "splenic anemia" of infants), pernicious anemia, and, finally, leukemia. In each discussion of these several causes of splenomegaly, Dr. Taylor comes to a consideration of infection and toxin. He does not state his own conjectures, but in each case he was able to quote authorities who emphatically believed that the disease in question was caused by infection.

We must remember that these scientists had become authorities during the time when bacteriology was being discovered. Small wonder they were trying to push every illness into this dazzling new category. We do the same. Today, *immune reaction* is our pathogenic shibboleth.

Experimental studies on the role of the spleen in infection began with the beginning of bacteriology. Enlargement of the spleen was noted after animals were inoculated with virulent organisms. In 1886, Wyssokowitsch injected bacteria intravenously. They disappeared rapidly from the blood and appeared in great numbers in the spleen.[123] Bardach demonstrated that an intravenous dose of anthrax bacilli insufficient to kill a normal animal would kill a splenectomized dog.[124] Tizzioni and Cattani took this sort of investigation a step further by measuring the immune response in rabbits after vaccination with tetanus organisms. Unlike normal animals, the splenectomized animals did not become immune and died when challenged with injections of tetanus culture.[125] Since then, it has been amply demonstrated that removal of the spleen impairs the ability to produce antibodies to *particulate* antigens. There is no such effect upon the response to soluble antigens.[126]

The production of antibodies after a challenge by particulate antigen appears to require a nice collaboration of the red and white pulp of the spleen.[127,128] When radioactive antigenic particles are injected into the bloodstream, the radioactivity is immediately captured by the phagocytes of the red pulp. Within a few hours, radioactivity has been transferred to cells of the germinal follicles of the white pulp (Figure 5-5). These cells enlarge, proliferate, and become producers of the protein antibodies. The enlargement of the spleen associated with many acute infections is caused not by congestion with blood but by the swelling of the corpuscles of Malpighi. When antibody production has passed its peak, the corpuscles subside to normal size, as does the spleen itself.

OVERWHELMING POSTSPLENECTOMY INFECTION

In 1929, O'Donnell reported the case of a 6-year-old boy whose spleen was removed in 1926 for "early Banti's disease." "The operation checked his downhill course at the time, and subsequently he improved greatly." In June 1928, he developed a headache, fever, and vomiting, and he died within 48 hours "from an acute septicemia, possibly fulminating cerebro-spinal fever, but the case also had features of purpura fulminans." The boy's father had had his spleen removed in 1919 and had later "died of septic pneumonia, manifesting a similar lack of resistance to the disease."[129]

This may be the first report (and the second case) of a dreadful sequela of splenectomy now nicknamed OPSI, an acronym for *overwhelming postsplenectomy infection*. The case report, the warning that such a disease might occur, went unnoted. OPSI did not come to medical attention again for 23 years, when King and Shumacker described its occurrence in patients who had undergone splenectomy in infancy.[130] Now much has been learned and written about OPSI.[131] Those most at risk are the very young and those with severe diseases. But it does occur uncommonly in healthy older children and, rarely, in healthy adults. The infecting agent is usually the pneumococcus or *H. influenzae,* which are encapsulated organisms. The cause of the "lack of resistance" to the disease is not known. Is it the absence of the splenic filter, the lack of spleen-produced antibodies, the diminished numbers of *suppressor T-lymphocyte cells,* which are "conditioned" in the spleen? Or some post-splenectomy changes not yet perceived?

THE SPLEEN AND AUTOIMMUNITY

Paul Ehrlich, while studying immune responses to antigenic stimulation, noted a most significant *negative* phenomenon, the most difficult kind to perceive. Tissue antigens, foreign red blood cells for example, might stimulate antibody production in a recipient animal, but an animal's own red cell antigens never provoke immune reactions in the animal itself. Ehrlich named this phenomenon *horror autotoxicus*. In autoimmune disease, however, the immune system does make antibodies against one or another of the body's own tissues. The first demonstration of this was in 1904 with the Donath-Landsteiner test, a hemolytic reaction that is characteristic of cold hemoglobinuria (Chapter 8). Soon afterward, agglutinating antibodies, which cause red cells to clump, were implicated in acquired hemolytic anemia, and Micheli demonstrated in 1910 that splenectomy could cure this form of autoimmune disease.[25]

Hematologists accepted the concept of autoimmunity to explain these phenomena, but immunologists tended to take an orthodox view with regard to Ehrlich's law: the body, because of *horror autotoxicus*, could not injure itself;

the phenomena of hemolysis and agglutination could *resemble* but could not *be* immune reactions. Sir John Dacie provided the common sense to resolve the dilemma by commenting that *horror autotoxicus* describes the normal posture of the immune system, while autoimmunity is a disease. Now the concept of autoimmunity has extended beyond the red cells to include diseases of platelets, leukocytes, marrow, thyroid gland, kidney, eye, gut, perhaps disease of any tissue.

Involvement of the spleen in autoimmune diseases of the blood cells is evident because splenectomy often cures these diseases. The pathogenic mechanism may be twofold. First, the spleen may be a source of autoantibody, in some cases the only source. Following splenectomy, the antibodies gradually disappear. Second, the spleen may destroy antibody-sensitized blood cells.

HYPERSPLENISM[132–135]

Following is the introduction to an article on hypersplenism published in 1961:[132]

> The word "hypersplenism" appeared in Paris early in the 20th century, used first by Chauffard, or perhaps by Gilbert, to describe the role of the spleen in hereditary spherocytosis. But the word did not catch on. In the forty years from 1907 to 1947 it was used less than a dozen times, although countless papers on splenic disease appeared. Except for an occasional speculative comment, it was used only with reference to anemia. Hypersplenism today has a broader connotation of exaggerated or perverted splenic activity which may be directed against many parts of the blood and marrow. This present use of the word, together with a definition, appeared in 1941 in an obscure paper by Dameshek. In discussing "hypersplenism" he wrote:

> The normal spleen may be said to be interposed between the bone marrow on the one hand and the blood on the other . . . the spleen may have effects on delivery and maturation of cells in the bone marrow. The large spleen . . . is usually associated with anemia, leukopenia, granulopenia and thrombopenia in the blood, while at the same time there is hyperplasia of the bone marrow. Following splenectomy the blood picture usually becomes normal. . . . These phenomena suggest that the large spleen has a "hypernormal" inhibitory effect on the bone marrow.

> The word "hypersplenism" did not achieve wide usage until 1947, after Dameshek and Estren had published a fascicle, "The Spleen and Hypersplenism." Then the word and the concept immediately came into vogue, and a flood of publications began.

> Early in the contemporary hypersplenic era, the lines of an argument were drawn which stimulated interest in the subject and served as a frame for most of the published discussions. The debate was Doan versus Dameshek, with few taking

sides and most reserving judgment. Doan declared that hypersplenism results from sequestration and destruction of blood cells in the spleen. Dameshek declared that hypersplenism results from inhibition of bone marrow by humoral factors from the spleen. This was the argument, with hedgings and qualifications on both sides, but this was its essence. One day in Dameshek's laboratories a platelet transfusion was given to a girl with idiopathic thrombocytopenic purpura undergoing splenectomy. During the transfusion, blood was taken simultaneously from her other arm and from her splenic vein. There were many platelets in the arm blood, few in the splenic blood, as though the transfused platelets had been lost in the spleen. Dameshek was shown the two tubes of clotted blood: good clot retraction in the arm blood, none in the splenic blood. After an explanation of the experiment he stood silent for a moment; then he said with a smile, "Well, it looks as though Charley Doan is right"—but, he added, "in some cases." Everyone laughed, Dameshek included.

The argument is almost burnt out by now. Most would agree that Dameshek was correct when he said, "It looks as though Charley Doan is right." Recently there have appeared reports which state that "we have not detected such an (impairing) effect of the spleen on erythropoiesis," and reviews which conclude that there is no evidence for "depressive hypersplenism." At present, the preponderance of evidence favors splenic sequestration and lysis of blood elements as the mechanism of hypersplenic cytopenias.[132]

However, the story of hypersplenism had not ended in 1961, when this was written. A summary is provided by the history of ITP (*idiopathic thrombocytopenic purpura*, more recently, *immune thrombocytopenic purpura*). Recall Kaznelson's first successful splenectomy for ITP in 1916.[29] The arguments about the cause of ITP began at that time. In 1915, Frank had proposed that the spleen can cause aplastic anemia and, further, that thrombocytopenia results from a sort of aplastic (empty) marrow, the spleen inhibiting platelet production by megakaryocytes in the marrow.[136] Kaznelson, on the other hand, believed that the "diseased spleen" removed platelets from the blood.[29] Such differences of opinion thrived in the absence of information. Marrow biopsy was rarely performed before the 1940s, so that the response of the marrow to hypersplenism and splenectomy could only be surmised. Yet, even when marrow biopsy became a commonplace procedure and *increased* numbers of megakaryocytes were found in all cases of ITP, it was argued that the thrombocytopenia is a consequence of "maturation arrest."[137] Only when the spleen in ITP was shown to remove platelets from the circulating blood[138] and an abnormally brief life span for the platelets was demonstrated,[139] did the debate lose its head of steam.[135]

Yet, some have clung to the concept of splenic inhibition of the marrow megakaryocytes. True, platelet life span is brief in ITP, yet the compensatory response of platelet production appeared to be absent or inadequate.[140] In one of his last papers, Dameshek (Figure 5-9) demonstrated in animals that

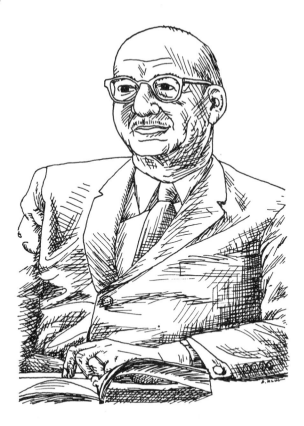

Figure 5-9 William Dameshek (1900–1969) was my mentor and friend of 20 years. His wisdom and enthusiastic personality provided stimulation for the more than 200 fellows he trained. From about 1940 until his death, one of his primary interests was the spleen and both of its prime functions—that relating to blood cells and that relating to the immune reactions. His teaching stressed the significance of disordered splenic function, and he popularized the term *hypersplenism*. His perspective was clinical: how will this information help us to care for patients?

Dameshek's life was hematology. Once I said that he should spell his name Domeshek. In Hebrew, *dom* is the blood.

antibodies prepared against platelets not only wiped out platelets when injected intravenously but also injured the megakaryocytes.[141] There is, however, a profound abyss between autoimmune diseases and experiments using antibodies from one species of animal to cause reactions in another. Autoimmunity is usually a chronic, subtle disorder, while the experiment is an acute explosion. In the case of ITP, McMillan has been working to close the gap. He has demonstrated, as have others, that the platelets of patients with ITP are coated with autoantibodies, immune globulins of the G variety, so-called IgG. He estimated the number of molecules of IgG on each platelet. Using spleens removed to cure ITP, he demonstrated that splenic "immunocytes" can produce IgG in test tubes. He found that the IgG on the blood platelets of his patients disappeared after splenectomy cured the disease.[142-144] Thus, in ITP the circle linking spleen-generated autoimmunity to platelet injury and demise has been closed.

More recently, McMillan has demonstrated that the IgG of ITP can fix upon the surface of marrow megakaryocytes. Whether it causes injury resulting in reduced platelet production remains to be seen, but the implication is there.[145] This appears to be a most significant observation, indicating the ability and the means by which a deranged spleen may injure a remote organ, the marrow.

THE SPLEEN'S INVOLVEMENT WITH DISEASES
REMOTE FROM THE SPLEEN

Splenectomy performed for hematologic diseases has unexpectedly cured disorders in other organs.

Chronic, intractable leg ulcer is sometimes associated with splenomegaly; removal of the spleen has been followed by prompt healing of the ulcers.[132] Cause of the splenomegaly seems not to be significant; hereditary spherocytosis, tropical splenomegaly, Felty's syndrome, hemoglobinopathy, and myeloid metaplasia have all been associated with leg ulcer cured after splenectomy.

Felty's syndrome (rheumatoid arthritis, splenomegaly, low white blood cell count) may be complicated by recurrent, severe infections. Although the white blood cell count is low, it is adequate. Splenectomy is often followed by the cessation of serious infection,[146] and, sometimes, the arthritis goes into remission.

Pulmonary siderosis is a disease of small blood vessels of the lung, which leak red blood cells into the lung tissues. The phagocytes of the lung ingest the red cells, degrade the hemoglobin, but are unable to yield the hemoglobin iron to the plasma. Iron accumulates in the phagocytes, and the iron-loaded phagocytes accumulate in the lung, gradually destroying pulmonary function while the patient has severe iron-deficiency anemia. In some patients, cure of the pulmonary siderosis has followed splenectomy.[147] The pulmonary vessels evidently stop leaking.

Thrombotic thrombocytopenic purpura (TTP) is another disorder of small blood vessels. The body's smallest arteries become almost occluded by accumulations of plasma clot and platelet debris. There is a serious lack of platelets, and there is hemolytic anemia associated with red cell fragmentation. This often fatal disease is sometimes cured by splenectomy.[148]

In some of these diseases of organs remote from the spleen, there is evidence of autoimmunity. In TTP, antibodies against platelets have been demonstrated.[149] In Felty's syndrome, the white cells are loaded with IgG.[150] The existence of these abnormally placed antibodies suggests the presence of autoimmune reactions, but it does not explain the basic lesions in these disorders. It does not explain, for example, how in TTP, small blood vessels are injured by something of splenic origin. It does not explain the leg ulcers of chronic splenomegaly or the susceptibility to purulent infections in people with Felty's syndrome. It does not explain how these diseases can be cured by splenectomy.

We suspect that these are immunologic reactions with the spleen producing antibodies that move through the blood to injure distant organs. But, especially in biologic systems, circumstantial evidence is not to be taken as a matter of fact.

Conclusion: the spleen has not yet yielded all of its mystery. Nor, for that matter, has any other organ.

References

1   Crosby WH: Hyposplenism: An inquiry into normal functions of the spleen. *Annu Rev Med* 14:349–370, 1963.
2   Herrlinger R: Die Milz in der Antike. *Ciba Zeitschr* 8:2982–3012, 1958.
3   Gray H: *On the Structure and Use of the Spleen.* London, John W Parker, 1854, 380 pp.
4   May MT (trans): Galen: *On the Usefulness of the Parts of the Body.* Ithaca, Cornell University Press, 1968, 801 pp, pp 232–233.
5   Vesalius A: *Opera Omnia Anatomica.* Leiden, 1725, 20 p 1, 1156 pp, pp 437–440.
6   Gray: op. cit., p 7.
7   Rosner F: The spleen in the Talmud and other early Jewish writings. *Bull Hist Med* 46:82–85, 1972.
8   Gould GM, Pyle WL: *Anomalies and Curiosities of Medicine.* Philadelphia, Saunders, 1900, 968 pp, p 461.
9   Krumbhaar EB: The history of extirpation of the spleen. *NY Med J* 101:232–234, 1915.
10 Major RH: *A History of Medicine.* Springfield, Thomas, 1954, 1155 pp, p 516.
11 Adelmann G: Die Wandlungen der Splenectomie seit dreissig Jahren. *Arch klin Chir* 36:442–492, 1887.
12 Pohl JC: Casum anatomicum de defectu lienus sistitet de liene, in *Genere Quaedam Disserit Simulque Collegium Disputatorium Publicum Indicit,* Lipsiae, 1740, XIV pp, p 3.
13 O'Brien E: Case of removal of the human spleen, without injury or derangement of the animal economy. *Med Chir J Rev (London)* 1:8–10, 1816.
14 Gooch B: *A Practical Treatise on Wounds.* Norwich, Chase, 1767, vol 1, 459 pp, pp 102–103.
15 Fioravanti L: *Il Tesoro della Vita Humana (Libro Secondo).* Venice, Melchior Sessa, 1570, 327 pp, pp 25–27.
16 Franzolini F: Della splenectomia. *Gaz Med Torino* 33:337–348, 1882.
17 Stukeley W: *Of the Spleen its Description and History, Uses and Diseases, Particularly the Vapors, with their Remedy. To Which is Added Some Anatomical Observations in the Dissection of an Elephant.* London, privately printed, 1723, 108 pp, p 26.
18 Wells TS: Remarks on splenectomy with a report of a successful case. *Med Chir Trans* 71:255–263, 1888.
19 Dawson BE: Haemolytic icterus. *Br Med J* 1:921–928, 963–966, 1931.
20 Dawson BE: Indications for, and results of, removal of the spleen. *Br Med J* 2:699–700, 1932.
21 Vanverts J: De la splénectomie. *Gaz Hop Paris* 71:245–250, 1898.
22 Taylor F: *Some Disorders of the Spleen.* London, Churchill, 1904, 94 pp.
23 Hayem G: *Du Sang et de ses Alterations Anatomique.* Paris, Masson, 1889, 1035 pp, pp 199, 607.

24 Mayo WJ: Principles underlying surgery of the spleen, with a report of ten splenectomies. *JAMA* 54:14–18, 1910.

25 Micheli F: Effetti immediati della splenectomia in un caso di ittero emolitico splenomegalico acquisito tipo Hayem-Widal (ittero splenoemolitico). *Clin Med Ital* 50:453–468, 1911.

26 Hayem G: Sur une variété d'ictère chronique. Ictère infectieux chronique splénomégalique. *Presse Méd* 6:121–122, 1898.

27 Chauffard AME: Des hepatites d'origine splenique. *Sem Méd* 19:177–178, 1899.

28 Sutherland GA, Burghard FF: The treatment of splenic anaemia by splenectomy. *Lancet* 2:1819–1823, 1910.

29 Kaznelson P: Verschwinden der hämorrhgischen Diathesis bei einem Falle von "essentieller Thrombopenia" (Frank) nach Milzexstirpation. Splenogene thrombolytische Purpura. *Wien klin Wochenschr* 29:1451–1454, 1916.

30 Rosenthal N: Hemorrhagic diatheses, in Downey H (ed): *Handbook of Hematology*. New York, Hoeber, 1938, vol I, 698 pp, p 513.

31 Whipple AO: Splenectomy as a therapeutic measure in thrombocytopenic purpura haemorrhagica. *Surg Gynecol Obstet* 42:329–341, 1926.

32 Crosby WH: Splenectomy in hematologic disorders. *N Engl J Med* 286:1252–1254, 1972.

33 Morgenstern L: The avoidable complications of splenectomy. *Surg Gynecol Obstet* 145:525–528, 1977.

34 Morgenstern L: The surgical inviolability of the spleen: Historical evaluation of a concept. *Proc XXIII Congr Hist Med* 62–68, 1972.

35 Weiss L: The spleen, in Greep RO, Weiss L (eds): *Histology*, 3d ed. New York, McGraw-Hill, 1973, pp 445–478.

36 Malpighi M: *De Viscerum Structura Exercitatio Anatomica*. Bonn, De Liene, 1666, 172 pp, Ch IV, pp 101–150.

37 Hewson W: In Falconar M (ed): *Experimental Inquiries, Part the Third, Containing a Description of the Red Particles of the Blood in the Human Subject and Other Animals, with an Account of the Structure and Offices of the Lymphatic Glands, of the Thymus Gland, and of the Spleen*. London, T. Longman, 1777, 218 pp, pp 133–134.

38 Müller J: Über die Struktur der eigenthümlichen Körperchen in der Milz einiger planzenfressender Säugetiere. *Arch Anat Physiol* 1:80–90, 1834.

39 Evans WJ: Anatomy of the spleen in man. *Lancet* 1:63–67, 1844.

40 Billroth T: Beiträge zur vergleichenden Histologie der Milz. *Arch Anat Physiol* 24:88–108, 1857.

41 Billroth T: Neue Beiträge zur vergleichenden Anatomie der Milz. *Z Wissenschr Zool* 11:325–340, 1861.

42 Klemperer P: The spleen, in Downey H (ed): *Handbook of Hematology*. New York, Hoeber, 1938, vol III, 773 pp, pp 1587–1754; Ref cit pp 1621–1624.

43 Knisely MH: Spleen studies. I. Microscopic studies of the circulatory system of living unstimulated mammalian spleens. *Anat Rec* 65:23–50, 1936.

44 McNee JW: The spleen. *Trans Med Soc Lond* 54:185–236, 1931.

45 Björkman SE: The spleen's circulation with special reference to the function of the splenic sinus wall. *Acta Med Scand* 128(suppl 141): 1–89, 1947.

46 Williams RG: Microscopic structure and behavior of spleen autografts in rabbits. *Am J Anat* 87:459–503, 1950.
47 Stukeley: op. cit., p 53.
48 Bechard PA: Additions à l'anatomie générale de Xavier Bichat, ca 1820. Cited by Gray H op. cit., p 37.
49 Leeuwenhoek A van: Microscopical observations on the structure of the spleen. *Philos Trans R Soc Lond (Biol)* 25:2305, 1708.
50 Stukeley: op. cit., p 42.
51 Rush B: An inquiry into the functions of the spleen, liver, pancreas and thyroid gland. *Phila Med Museum* 3:9–29, 1806.
52 Gray: op. cit., p 346.
53 Gray: ibid., p 350.
54 Roy CS: The physiology and pathology of the spleen. *J Physiol (Lond)* 3:203–228, 1881.
55 Barcroft J, Harris HA, Orahovats D, Weiss R: A contribution to the physiology of the spleen. *J Physiol (Lond)* 60:441–456, 1925.
56 Barcroft J, Stephens JG: Observations upon the size of the spleen. *J Physiol (Lond)* 64:1–22, 1927.
57 McNee JW: Liver and spleen: their clinical and pathological associations. *Br Med J* 1:1017–1022, 1068–1073, 1111–1116, 1932.
58 Ebert RV, Stead EA: Demonstration that in normal man no reserves of blood are mobilized by exercise, epinephrine, and hemorrhage. *Am J Med Sci* 201:655–664, 1941.
59 Aster RH: Pooling of platelets in the spleen. Role in the pathogenesis of "hypersplenic" thrombocytopenia. *J Clin Invest* 45:645–665, 1966.
60 Browne HL: Rapid hypertrophy of the spleen; excision. *Lancet* 2:310, 1877.
61 Gould GM, Pyle WL: op. cit., p 657.
62 Garnett ES, Goddard BA, Markby D, Webber CE: The spleen as an arteriovenous shunt. *Lancet* 1:386–388, 1969.
63 Rothschild MA, Bauman A, Yalow RS, Berson SA: Effect of splenomegaly on blood volume. *J Appl Physiol* 6:701–706, 1954.
64 Jandl JH, Greenberg MS, Yonemoto RH, Castle WB: Clinical determination of the sites of red cell sequestration in hemolytic anemias. *J Clin Invest* 35:842–867, 1956.
65 Pryor DS: The mechanism of anaemia in tropical splenomegaly. *Q J Med* 36:337–356, 1967.
66 Hess CE, Ayers CR, Sandusky WR, Carpenter MA, Wetzel RA, Mohler DN: Mechanism of dilutional anemia in massive splenomegaly. *Blood* 47:629–644, 1976.
67 Kölliker A: Über den Bau und die Verrichtungen der Milz. *Mitt Züricher naturf Ges*, 1847, p 120. Cited in Kölliker A: *Manual of Human Microscopical Anatomy*. Philadelphia, Lippincott, 1854.
68 Ecker A: Über die Veränderungen welche die Blutkörperchen un der Milz erleiden. *Verh Schweiz Naturf Ges* 32:115–119, 1847.
69 Kölliker A: *Manual of Human Microscopical Anatomy*. Philadelphia, Lippincott, 1854, pp 561, 562.
70 Virchow R: Über blutkörperchenhaltige Zellen. *Virchows Arch* 4:515–540, 1852.

71 Kölliker A: *Handbuch der Gewebelehre des Menschen* (5th edition). Leipzig, Egelmann, 1867, 749 pp, pp 452, 453.

72 Kusnezoff A: Über blutkörperchenhaltige Zellen der Milz. *Sitzungsb Akad Wissensch Wien* 67:58–67, 1873.

73 Vanlair CF, Masius JB: De la microcythémie. *Bull Acad R Méd Belg* 5:515–613, 1871.

74 Gowers WR: Splenic leucocythaemia, in *Reynolds' System of Medicine*. London, Macmillan, 1866, vol 5, 1040 pp, pp 274, 275.

75 Crosby WH, Akeroyd JH: The limit of hemoglobin synthesis in hereditary hemolytic anemia. Its relation to the excretion of bile pigment. *Am J Med* 13:273–283, 1952.

76 Craigie D: Case of disease and enlargement of the spleen in which death took place in consequence of the presence of purulent matter in the blood. *Edinburgh Med Surg J* 64:400–413, 1845.

77 Bennett JH: Case of hypertrophy of the spleen and liver, in which death took place from suppuration of the blood. *Edinburgh Med Surg J* 64:413–423, 1845.

78 Virchow R: Weisses Blut. *Neue Notiz Geb Natur Heilk* 36:151–156, 1845.

79 Gretsel: Ein Fall von Anaemia splenica bei einem Kinde. *Berl klin Wochenschr* 3:212–214, 1866.

80 Banti G: *Dell'Anemia Splenica*. Firenze, Le Monnier, 1882, 70 pp, p 5.

81 Osler W: Anemia splenica. *Trans Assoc Am Physicians* 18:429–461, 1902.

82 Banti G: La splenomegalia con cirrosi del fegato. *Sperimentale Sez Biol* 48:407–432, 1894.

83 Pearce RM, Krumbhaar EB, Frazier CH: *The Spleen and Anaemia, Experimental and Clinical Studies*. Philadelphia, Lippincott, 1918, 419 pp, pp 248–253.

84 Klemperer: op. cit., pp 1716–1722.

85 Wagley PF: A consideration of the Banti syndrome. *Bull Johns Hopkins Hosp* 85:87–114, 1949.

86 Eppinger H: *Die Hepato-Lienal Erkrankungen*. Berlin, Springer, 1920. Cited in Klemperer: op. cit., p 1718.

87 Di Guglielmo G: Il morbo di Banti. *Progresso Med* 7:289–293, 1951.

88 Ruggieri P, Bolognesi G: Anemia emolitica acquisita autoimmune e cirrosi epatica. *Policlinico Sez Prat* 62:1605–1614, 1955.

89 Wands JR, Dienstag JL, Bhan AK et al: Circulating immune complexes and complement activation in primary biliary cirrhosis. *N Engl J Med* 298:233–237, 1978.

90 Arias Elenes N, Ewald RA, Crosby WH: The reservoir function of the spleen and its relation to postsplenectomy anemia in the dog. *Blood* 24:299–304, 1964.

91 Chalier J, Charlet L: État de la résistance globulaire chez l'animal normal et splenéctomizé. *J Physiol Pathol Gén* 13:728–734, 1911.

92 Karsner HT, Pearce RM: The relation of the spleen to blood destruction and regeneration and to hemolytic jaundice. IV. A study by the methods of immunology, of the increased resistance of the red blood corpuscles after splenectomy. *J Exp Med* 16:769–779, 1912.

93 Miller EB, Singer K, Dameshek W: Experimental production of target cells by splenectomy and interference with splenic circulation. *Proc Soc Exp Biol Med* 49:42–45, 1942.

94   Crosby WH: The pathogenesis of spherocytes and leptocytes (target cells). *Blood* 7:261–274, 1952.

95   Crosby WH: Splenic remodeling of red cell surfaces. *Blood* 50:643–646, 1977.

96   McFadzean AJS, Davis LJ: Iron-staining erythrocytic inclusions with especial reference to acquired haemolytic anaemia. *Glasgow Med J* 28:237–279, 1947.

97   Crosby WH: Siderocytes and the spleen. *Blood* 12:165–170, 1957.

98   Rifkind RA: Heinz body anemia: An ultrastructual study. II. Red cell sequestration and destruction. *Blood* 26:433–448, 1965.

99   Virchow R: Über die Standpunkte in der Wissenschaftlichen Medicin. *Virchows Arch* 70:1–10, 1877.

100 Jandl JH, Files NM, Barnett SB, MacDonald RA: Proliferative response of the spleen and liver to hemolysis. *J Exp Med* 122:299–325, 1965.

101 Emerson CP, Shen SC, Castle WB: Osmotic fragility of the red cells of the peripheral and splenic blood in patients with congenital hemolytic jaundice transfused with normal red cells. *J Clin Invest* 26:922 (abst), 1946.

102 Crosby WH: Normal functions of the spleen relative to red blood cells. A review. *Blood* 14:399–408, 1959.

103 Singer K, Weisz L: The life cycle of the erythrocyte after splenectomy and the problems of splenic hemolysis and target cell formation. *Am J Med Sci* 210:301–323, 1945.

104 Gray: op. cit., pp 1–53.

105 Gray: ibid., pp 51 and 365.

106 Inlow WD: The spleen and digestion. Study IV. The spleen and biliary secretion. The reaction in bile-pigment secretion following splenectomy. *Am J Med Sci* 167:10–29, 1924.

107 Krumbhaar EB: Function of the spleen. *Physiol Rev* 6:160–200, 1926, p 175.

108 Pearce et al: op. cit., pp 58–86.

109 Pearce RM, Austin JH: The relation of the spleen to blood destruction and regeneration and to hemolytic jaundice. V. Changes in the endothelial cells of the lymph nodes and liver in splenectomized animals receiving hemolytic serum. *J Exp Med* 16:780–788, 1912.

110 Watson CJ: Pyrrol pigments and hemoglobin catabolism. *Minn Med* 39:294–300, 403–412, 467–474, 1956.

111 Klemperer: op. cit., pp 1640–1644.

112 Ponfick E: Studien über die Schicksale körniger Farbstoffe im Organismus. *Virchows Arch* 48:1–55, 1869.

113 Nanta A: Une mycose splénique. *Ann Anat Pathol (Paris)* 4:573–585, 1927.

114 Rous P: Destruction of the red blood corpuscles in health and disease. *Physiol Rev* 3:75–105, 1923.

115 Rappaport H: The pathologic anatomy of the splenic red pulp, in Leunert K, Harms D (eds): *Die Milz The Spleen.* New York, Springer-Verlag, 1970, pp 24–41.

116 Krumbhaar EB: The so-called reticulo-endothelial system. *Int Clin* 2:280–293, 1925.

117 Jaffé RH: The reticulo-endothelial system, in Downey H (ed): *Handbook of Hematology.* New York, Hoeber, 1938, vol II, 885 pp, pp 973–1271.

118 Weiss L: *The Cells and Tissues of the Immune System.* Englewood Cliffs, NJ, Prentice-Hall, 1972, 252 pp.

119 Ponfick E: Über Hämoglobinämie und ihre Folgen. *Berl klin Wochenschr* 20:389–392, 1885.

120 Ribbert H: Die Ausscheidung intravenös injizierten gelösten Carmins in den Geweben. *Z Allg Physiol* 4:201–210, 1904.

121 Aschoff L, Landau M: Cited in Krumbhaar: The so-called reticulo-endothelial system, p 280.

122 Krumbhaar: Function of the spleen, p 181.

123 Wyssokowitsch W: Über die Schicksale der in's Blut injizcirten Mikroorgismen im Körper der Warmbluter. *Z Hyg* 1:3–45, 1886.

124 Bardach G: Recherches sur le rôle de la rate dans les maladies infectieuses. *Ann Inst Pasteur* 3:577–603, 1889.

125 Tizzioni G, Cattani G: Über die Wichtigkeit der Milz bei der experimentellen Immunisierung des Kaninchens Gegen den Tetanus. *Zentralbl Bakteriol* 11:325–327, 1892.

126 Likhite VV: Immunological impairment and susceptibility to infection after splenectomy. *JAMA* 236:1376–1377, 1976.

127 Nossal GJV, Austin CM, Pye J, Mitchell J: Antigens in immunity. XII. Antigen trapping in the spleen. *Int Arch Allergy Appl Immunol* 29:368–383, 1966.

128 Langevoort HL: The histophysiology of the antibody response. I. Histogenesis of the plasma cell reaction in rabbit spleen. *Lab Invest* 12:106–118, 1963.

129 O'Donnell JF: The value of splenectomy in Banti's disease. *Br Med J* 1:854, 1929.

130 King H, Shumacker HB: Splenic studies. I. Susceptibility to infection after splenectomy performed in infancy. *Ann Surg* 136:239–242, 1952.

131 Bisno AL: Hyposplenism and overwhelming pneumococcal infection. A reappraisal. *Am J Med Sci* 262:101–107, 1971.

132 Crosby WH: Hypersplenism. *Annu Rev Med* 13:127–146, 1962.

133 Doan CA: Hypersplenism. *Bull NY Acad Med* 25:625–650, 1949.

134 Dameshek W: Hypersplenism. *Bull NY Acad Med* 31:113–136, 1955.

135 Crosby WH: Is hypersplenism a dead issue? *Blood* 20:94–99, 1962.

136 Frank E: Die essentielle Thrombopenie. *Berl klin Wochenschr* 52:454–485, 490–494, 1915.

137 Dameshek W, Miller EB: The megakaryocytes in idiopathic thrombocytopenic purpura, a form of hypersplenism. *Blood* 1:27–51, 1946.

138 Wright CS, Doan CA, Bouroncle BA et al: Direct splenic arterial and venous blood studies in the hypersplenic syndromes before and after epinephrine. *Blood* 6:195–212, 1951.

139 Hirsch EO, Gardner FH, Thomas ED: Isolation and concentration of human blood platelets: Their properties in vitro and in vivo. *J Clin Invest* 31:638–639, 1952.

140 Baldini M: Platelet production and destruction in idiopathic thrombocytopenic purpura: a controversial issue. *JAMA* 239:2477–2479, 1978.

141 Rolovic Z, Baldini M, Dameshek W: Megakaryocytopoiesis in experimentally-induced immune thrombocytopenia. *Blood* 35:175–188, 1970.

142 McMillan R, Smith RS, Longmire RL et al: Immunoglobulins associated with human platelets. *Blood* 37:316–322, 1971.

143 McMillan R, Longmire RL, Yelenosky R et al: Immunoglobulin synthesis in vitro by ITP splenic tissue. *N Engl J Med* 286:681–684, 1972.

144   McMillan R, Longmire RL, Yelenosky R et al: Quantitation of platelet-binding IgG produced in vitro by spleen from patients with idiopathic thrombocytopenic purpura. *N Engl J Med* 291:812–817, 1974.

145   McMillan R, Luiken GA, Levy R et al: Antibody against megakaryocytes in idiopathic thrombocytopenic purpura. *JAMA* 239:2460–2462, 1978.

146   Crosby WH: What to treat in Felty's syndrome. *JAMA* 225:1114, 1973.

147   Steiner B: Essential pulmonary haemosiderosis as immunohaematologic problem. Improvement following splenectomy. *Arch Dis Child* 29:391–397, 1954.

148   Amorosi EL, Ultman JE: Thrombotic thrombocytopenic purpura. *Medicine (Baltimore)* 45:139–159, 1966.

149   Morrison J, McMillan R: Elevated platelet-associated IgG in thrombotic thrombocytopenic purpura. *JAMA* 238:1944–1945, 1977.

150   Logue G: Felty's syndrome: Granulocyte-bound immunoglobulin G and splenectomy. *Ann Intern Med* 85:437–442, 1976.

CHAPTER 6

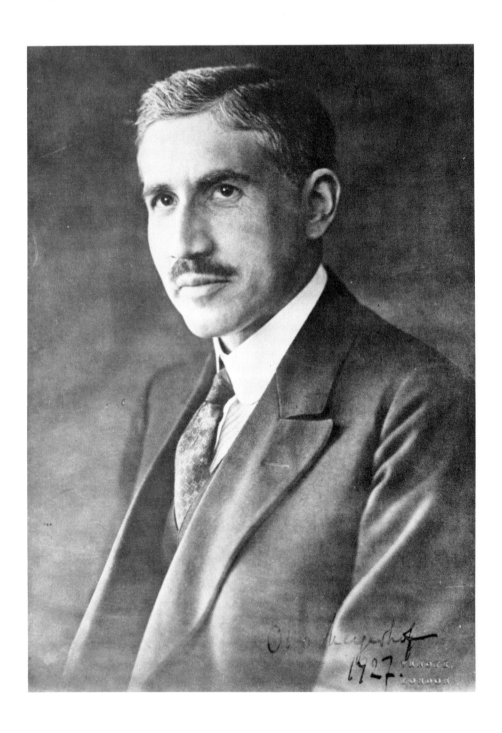

THE RED CELL: A TINY DYNAMO

Ernest Beutler

F or more than 2 centuries following the discovery of the red cells, the erythrocytes were considered to be inert and possibly unimportant physiologically. One hundred fifty years after their discovery, the *Dictionaire des sciences medicales*[1] quoted Peichel: "So there is nothing positive as to the shape, volume, and the changes that the globules may undergo—which is happily of no importance." Indeed, in the nineteenth century, even the very existence of red cells was questioned. The father of modern pharmacology, Francois Magendie (1783–1855), used water to dilute blood and, as a result in 1817 claimed that the red blood cells drawn by others might actually be air bubbles.[2] By 1839, however, Magendie had obviously recognized his error. He then provided an excellent morphologic description of the erythrocyte:

> The term globule is inappropriately applied to these bodies for their form is not spherical but lenticular. What proves this, and the fact can easily be ascertained, is that when they roll under the microscope they turn their edge to the eye of the observer. This edge generally measures in point of thickness the fifth or sixth part of their superficial extent; seen in this manner the globule appears thicker than at

Chapter Opening Photo Otto Meyerhof (1884–1951). (*Courtesy National Library of Medicine, Bethesda, Md.*)

141

its middle, which part has the appearance of being slightly depressed, and, as it were, excavated; this is, however, the case only with the globules of mammiferous animals, for those of others, such as reptiles and fishes, present a real swelling in their centre. . . . It is possible (but I would not affirm that such is the case) that these bodies are provided with an investment which tears. Observers are, indeed, generally of the opinion that they are surrounded with a very delicate pellicle; and this idea receives some support from the fact that in the globules of dead subjects there is a sort of puckering visible, such as is presented by membranes of extreme thinness when they begin to dry; for instance, the outer skin of onions.[3]

Toward the end of the nineteenth century, some appreciation of the functions of red cells first began to emerge. The studies of Hoppe-Seyler in 1865 established the role of the red pigment of erythrocytes as a carrier of oxygen, as described in an earlier chapter. By the end of the century, the osmotic properties of red cells began to be understood. Hedin[4] demonstrated that the volume of red cells increased in hypotonic solutions or in solutions such as urea, ethylene glycol, or glycerol, but that solutions of sodium chloride, sucrose, or mannitol produced shrinking of erythrocytes. It also became apparent that the permeability of the red cells to solutes was highly selective—some molecules were able to pass readily through the red cell membrane while others could not do so. Relatively sophisticated studies of the oxygen-binding properties of red cells and of their osmotic behavior were carried out at the turn of the century. The results of these investigations suggested that the red cell possessed a degree of complexity undreamed of only 60 years earlier, when the globules had been considered to be bubbles of air. It was ultimately realized that erythrocytes are living cells, which consume sugar and produce lactic acid.

This chapter deals primarily with the remarkable metabolic activity of this highly specialized cell. Devoid of nucleus and of many other minute organelles which other cells possess, it has, nonetheless, retained a variety of active metabolic pathways vital to its function. In these pathways, highly specialized protein molecules known as enzymes transform sugar molecules into smaller fragments. In breaking down the sugar molecules, energy is extracted. It is by the use of this energy that the red cell is able to maintain its shape and function. In addition, the red cell has retained as metabolic remnants certain enzymes that are no longer required for its function; these have proved invaluable, nevertheless, in gaining an understanding of or in the diagnosis of human diseases such as acatalasemia and galactosemia.

Understanding Red Cell Metabolism: How the Red Cell Burns Sugar

Interest in the metabolic activities of tissues was awakened in the latter part of the nineteenth century and culminated only a half century later through the brilliant experimentation, scholarship, and insight of such giants as Warburg,

Embden, Meyerhof, and Krebs who unravelled the chemical steps of inter-mediary metabolism; that is, the intracellular transformation of foodstuffs within the body, particularly that of the simple sugar glucose.

CONFUSION ABOUT RED CELL SUGAR CONSUMPTION

The early studies of the metabolic activities of red cells were hampered by failure to recognize the link between glucose and oxygen consumption. The fact that this simple sugar disappears from shed blood was recognized in the latter half of the nineteenth century by the great French physiologist Claude Bernard, and it was generally believed that the disappearance of glucose from blood resulted from the action of "a ferment." Yet, great confusion prevailed regarding the relative roles of plasma, red cells, and white cells in this process. In particular, the need for the structural integrity of the red cells in the disappearance of sugar from blood was not appreciated.

The understanding of natural phenomena requires the collection of accurate observations. Since the measurement of sugar concentration was technically relatively simple and was feasible at the turn of the century, it seems surprising that, even some 25 years later, such a body of data had not been developed.

In 1925, H.J. John,[5] in a thorough but uncritical review, cited contradictory data indicating:

1 That the rate of glycolysis (sugar breakdown) in blood has a direct rela-tionship to the sugar content of the blood and that it is unrelated to the sugar content of the blood

2 That the power of glycolysis is retained in laked (hemolyzed) blood and that it is lost when blood is hemolyzed

3 That blood can be kept at room temperature for 24 hours without the loss of sugar content and that sugar disappears completely from blood in this period of time

4 That red cells are unable to consume glucose when suspended in a bal-anced salt solution and that they can consume glucose in an artificial salt solution

5 That plasma can consume glucose and that plasma cannot consume glu-cose

6 That the destruction of glucose in the blood is due primarily to the action of red cells and that destruction of glucose in blood is due primarily to the white cells

7 That the plasma glucose penetrates into the erythrocytes and that there is no glucose to be found within erythrocytes

8 That destruction of blood sugar is simply due to the action of alkali in the plasma on glucose and that fluids with the same pH as blood do not de-stroy glucose

9   That alcohol is formed during glycolysis of blood and that alcohol is not formed during glycolysis

10 That blood contains an enzyme identical to "the widely distributed oxidizing ferment" and that it does not contain this ferment

John concluded from his review that "a definite and uniformly progressive glycolysis takes place in blood in vitro. The cause of glycolysis is still undetermined."

Today we recognize that all blood cells consume glucose, but that, because of the much larger number of erythrocytes in whole blood, glucose consumption by other blood cells is quantitatively unimportant. We know that hemolysis, the breaking of the red cell membrane, immediately arrests sugar consumption. Plasma does not have the capacity to break down glucose. Much of the confusion regarding glucose metabolism in blood seems to have arisen because investigators did not appreciate the importance of maintaining sterility during long-term incubations of blood; in many of their experiments it was bacterial fermentation rather than fermentation by blood cells that was actually occurring. Earlier investigators, who perceptively recognized this contingency and cautioned that only sterile incubations should be carried out, unfortunately were largely ignored. Even those who professed to use sterile techniques and who carried out apparently meticulous investigations sometimes achieved results which today appear bizarre. Thus, Slosse[6] proposed the scheme, shown in Figure 6-1, by which blood was presumed to decompose glucose. Ignorant of the 10 intervening steps, he believed that the 6-carbon sugar glucose is cleaved directly into two molecules of the 3-carbon compound lactic acid. Lactic acid, now recognized to be the final product of red cell metabolism of glucose, was thought to be cleaved further into 1- and 2-carbon fragments. Today Slosse's view of the catabolism of glucose by blood seems analogous to that of the flat earth reflected in the maps produced by early

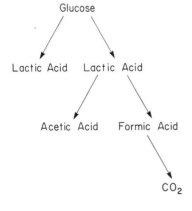

Figure 6-1 The concept of glucose catabolism proposed by Slosse.[6] This early, naive conception of intermediary metabolism bears little relationship to the scheme of glucose catabolism as we know it today (see Figure 6-3).

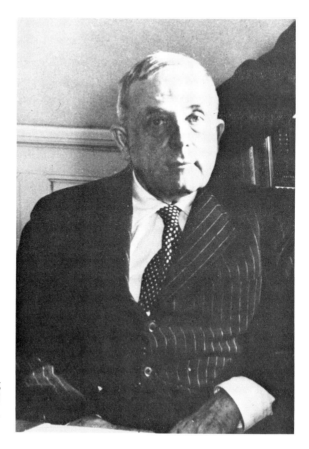

Figure 6-2 Otto Warburg (1883–1970). *(Courtesy National Library of Medicine, Bethesda, Md.)*

cartographers, who imagined sea serpents in unexplored oceans and sharp precipices where the sea seemed to meet the sky.

YOUNG WARBURG STUDIES THE RESPIRATION OF BLOOD

Against this dismal background, the extraordinary accuracy of the early observations on red cell oxygen consumption by the great biochemist Otto Warburg (Figure 6-2) are especially notable. Born in 1883 the son of a prominent physicist, Warburg studied under Emil Fischer, probably the greatest chemist of all time. Although half-Jewish, Warburg was able to continue working in Germany during World War II; his genealogy was conveniently rearranged so that he was classified as only one-quarter Jewish. This seems to have been accomplished through personal connections with high-ranking military officers.[7] Hitler's obsession that he might have cancer of the throat may also have played a role in the contrivance since the metabolism of tumor cells was one of Warburg's long-standing interests.[8] His scientific work astonishingly spanned a period of 67 years. Although best known for showing that heme compounds are involved in respiration, for which he was awarded the Nobel Prize in 1931, and for his isolation of the flavin enzymes, some of Warburg's earliest work concerned the respiration of erythrocytes.

Warburg was a meticulous investigator, who prepared his own reagents and performed his experiments with his own hands, even after achieving world renown. In his early studies of red cell respiration in 1909, Warburg took special care to ensure that his preparations were sterile, not only by examining them microscopically but, in most cases, by preparing cultures.[9] He was also aware of the possible effects of platelets and white blood cells on his measurements and took pains to enumerate contaminating cells. He carefully ruled out the formation of methemoglobin, an oxidation product of hemoglobin. Warburg in fact observed that the oxygen consumption of the red cells of healthy human subjects was so low that he considered it possible that it represented respiration by contaminating white cells. He found considerably greater oxygen consumption in rabbit red cells than in those of humans and observed the greatest oxygen consumption in the nucleated erythrocytes of birds. He noted that red cell samples containing many bluish-staining (young) erythrocytes consumed more oxygen and concluded that oxygen consumption was highest in young red cells.

Perhaps because of the relatively scanty oxygen consumption of mammalian red cells, Warburg turned his studies of respiration to other tissues.

DYES MAKE BLOOD BREATHE FAST AND REAWAKEN INTEREST

In the meantime, George Harrop, Jr.,[10] a pioneer endocrinologist working at the Johns Hopkins University, confirmed that the consumption of oxygen by red cells was scanty. Together with E.S.G. Barron,[11] he studied the effect of dyes on the oxygen consumption of red blood cells; they discovered that methylene blue, in particular, had the capacity to greatly augment the respiration of erythrocytes. Barron demonstrated his findings to Warburg when the latter visited Johns Hopkins.

This reawakened Warburg's interest in red cell respiration 20 years following the meticulous investigations which he had carried out in his youth. Although he misinterpreted some of his findings, Warburg's research nevertheless culminated in the discovery of an important pathway in red cell metabolism. As the result of a series of experiments, he proposed that methylene blue reacts with hemoglobin to form the brown oxidation product methemoglobin, and that in the presence of sugar, the methemoglobin is reduced back to hemoglobin. The reduced, colorless methylene blue formed in the reaction was reoxidized by molecular oxygen, accounting for the oxygen uptake.[12,13] Warburg considered the possibility, now recognized to be the correct one, that methylene blue was directly reduced inside the cell. However, the inhibition he observed with carbon monoxide seemed inconsistent with this course of events.[12] We now know that hemoglobin is not involved in the reaction and that methylene blue stimulates oxygen consumption without involvement of hemoglobin; it oxidizes NADPH to NADP$^+$ through NADPH diaphorase, thus hastening metabolism by way of the hexose monophosphate pathway (see Figure 6-3).

Warburg's renewed interest in red cell metabolism quickly led him to discover two important enzymes: glucose-6-phosphate dehydrogenase, which he dubbed "Zwischenferment" (between-enzyme), and "coenzyme II" (TPN, NADP). He found that while hemolyzed red cells could not oxidize carbohydrates, the sugar phosphates (glucose 6-phosphate + fructose 6-phosphate), which had been discovered in yeast by Robison in 1922,[14] were oxidized by such hemolysates when either methemoglobin or methylene blue was present.[15] The oxidation of sugar phosphate failed to occur if the hemolysate had been absorbed with aluminum hydroxide, and Warburg concluded from this and other observations that a "ferment" and a "coferment" were involved. He was able to isolate the "ferment" because it could be adsorbed to rat hemoglobin crystals and then could be removed from the crystals with water. The coferment was prepared from horse erythrocytes after the hemoglobin had been precipitated with alcohol-chloroform and the supernatant treated with alcohol-ether and washed with alcohol. Oxygen consumption occurred when the ferment and coferment solutions were incubated together with sugar phosphate, particularly when methylene blue was added. This enzyme presumably was contaminated with NADPH diaphorase, the enzyme which mediated the reaction between his reduced coferment, NADPH, and methylene blue. In later studies,[16] the versatile Warburg elucidated the structure of the coferment as a triphosphopyridine nucleotide.

THE TRUTH OF HOW SUGAR IS BROKEN DOWN BY RED CELLS
IS GRADUALLY UNCOVERED

As Warburg initiated understanding of the hexose monophosphate pathway, other investigators were busy unraveling the mystery of the many steps which intervene between the entry of sugar into the erythrocyte and the formation of lactic acid. Because of its complexity, the sequence of events is perhaps best followed if presented retrospectively from the end, as it is understood today, to the beginning. The now well-established metabolism of glucose by erythrocytes is depicted in Figure 6-3. The complex series of reactions shown in this figure differs strikingly from the simple, but incorrect, scheme shown in Figure 6-1.

In the 1920s it became apparent that the formation of phosphorylated intermediates plays an important role in red cell glycolysis. Diphosphoglyceric

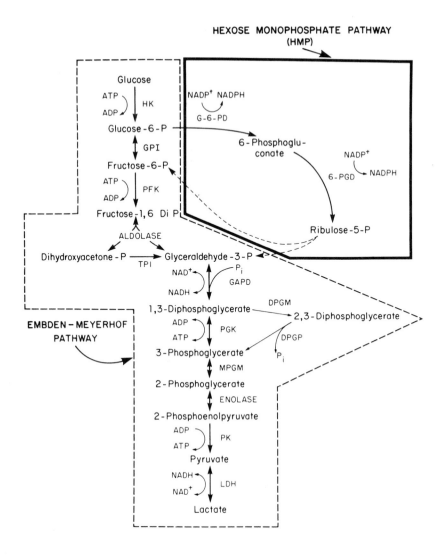

Figure 6-3 Glucose metabolism by the red cell. The enzymes which catalyze the breakdown of glucose are abbreviated as follows: HK = hexokinase, GPI = glucose phosphate isomerase, PFK = phosphofructokinase, GAPD = glyceraldehyde phosphate dehydrogenase, DPGP = diphosphoglycerate phosphatase, PGK = phosphoglycerate kinase, MPGM = monophosphoglycerate mutase, PK = pyruvate kinase, LDH = lactate dehydrogenase, G-6-PD = glucose-6-phosphate dehydrogenase, 6-PGD = 6-phosphogluconic dehydrogenase. The following abbreviations are used for some of the small molecules (coenzymes) which participate in the reactions: ATP = adenosine triphosphate; ADP = adenosine diphosphate; $NADP^+$ = nicotinamide adenine dinucleotide phosphate (formerly known as coenzyme II or TPN); NADPH = nicotinamide adenine dinucleotide phosphate, reduced form; NAD^+ = nicotinamide adenine dinucleotide (formerly coenzyme I or DPN); NADH = nicotinamide adenine dinucleotide, reduced form. P_i is inorganic phosphate. The dotted lines between replace a series of complex interconversions of 3-, 4-, 5-, 6-, and 7-carbon sugars.

148

acid (DPG), the major organic phosphate compound in red cells, was correctly identified in pig erythrocytes by Greenwald in 1925.[17] Two years later, Jost[18] showed that there was a close relationship between glycolysis and the formation and breakdown of organic phosphates.

Embden and Meyerhof Two major contributors to the understanding of the use of sugar by the red cell were Gustav Embden and Otto Meyerhof. Born in 1874 the son of a Hamburg lawyer, Gustav Embden studied medicine at the Universities of Freiburg, Munich, Berlin, and Strasbourg. When he was only 30 years of age, he was made director of the newly organized chemistry laboratory at the Municipal Hospital of Frankfurt Sachsenhausen, and within a few years, this laboratory was expanded into an outstanding Physiological Institute. Embden studied muscle extracts, much as yeast extracts had been investigated earlier. By June 1933, he and his assistants had succeeded in isolating most of the metabolic intermediates from such extracts, and he left his institute on vacation. While his coworkers awaited his return, he died suddenly of a pulmonary embolism at age 59.[19] The last of his studies were published in 1934 as a group of papers completed by his assistants.

It has been claimed that "in the course of his last experiments, in 1932–1933, Embden and his assistants succeeded in tracing all stages of the breakdown of glycogen in muscle to lactic acid."[20] In point of fact, Embden's achievement fell short of this goal. He and his assistant Deuticke divided glycolysis into five phases,[21] which are illustrated in Figure 6-4.

Although Embden will be forever remembered, since his name is attached to the metabolic pathway through which cells break down glucose to lactic acid, a comparison of the pathway which Embden proposed (Figure 6-4) with the metabolic steps as we now know them to occur (Figure 6-3) reveals that a number of the metabolic steps were incompletely understood. For example, the first phase of glycolysis postulated to occur by Embden and Deuticke[21] actually consists of several separate enzymatic reactions: the phosphorylation of glucose to glucose 6-phosphate by the enzyme hexokinase and ATP (or its formation, in muscle, from glycogen), the isomerization of the glucose 6-phosphate to fructose 6-phosphate by glucose phosphate isomerase (GPI), and, finally, the phosphorylation of fructose 6-phosphate to fructose 1,6-diphosphate by phosphofructokinase and ATP. Although Embden's writings show that he apparently recognized that 1,3-DPG was metabolized to lactate, he did not know where to place it in the metabolic scheme. Neither did he recognize the role of 2,3-DPG in glycolysis. It was not until the pioneering studies of Rapoport and Luebering[22] in 1950 that this part of the metabolic cycle, so important in red cells, was clarified. Although Embden knew that phosphoglyceric acid was metabolized to pyruvic acid, he did not appreciate the existence of the intermediates 2-phosphoglycerate and phosphoenolpyruvate and thought that the product of the reaction was inorganic phosphate rather than ATP.

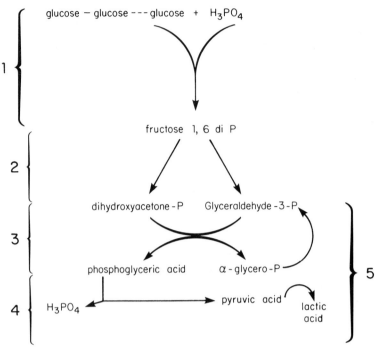

Figure 6-4 The five phases of glycolysis defined by Embden and Deuticke:[21] (1) the synthesis of hexose diphosphate from polysaccharide and phosphoric acid; (2) the cleavage of hexose diphosphate into dihydroxyacetone phosphate and glyceraldehyde phosphate; (3) the dismutation of these two trioses to α-glycerophosphate and phosphoglyceric acid; (4) the cleavage of phosphoglyceric acid into pyruvic acid and inorganic phosphate; and (5) reduction of pyruvic acid to lactic acid by α-glycerophosphate, which would be oxidized to glyceraldehyde 3-phosphate. This scheme is actually quite similar to glycolysis as it is known today (Figure 6-3). The α-glycerophosphate shown in this pathway does not appear in Figure 6-3 since it is a normal intermediate in many tissues, but not in erythrocytes.

Meyerhof (Chapter Opening Photo) was born in 1884. Ten years Embden's junior, he outlived him by 2 decades, long enough to see the glycolytic pathway understood in its final form. He came under Warburg's influence at the University of Heidelberg in 1909. In 1919 he demonstrated that during muscle contraction in the absence of oxygen, glycogen is converted to lactic acid. Meyerhof was awarded the Nobel Prize in physiology and medicine in 1922 for this achievement. Apparently considerable rivalry existed between Meyerhof and Warburg. Apprised on one occasion of a conversation regarding whether he or Meyerhof was the greater scientist, Warburg retorted hastily that this question really required no discussion. After some reflection, however, he commented, "Meyerhof may be smarter, but I can do more."[7]

Meyerhof extracted from muscle many of the enzymes responsible for the conversion of glycogen, through glucose 6-phosphate, to lactic acid. He subsequently investigated lactate formation in hemolysates prepared from goose and rat red cells and concluded that the same pathway of metabolism functioned in these cells as in muscle extracts.[23] Unlike Embden, Meyerhof seemed to understand that ATP is required for sugar consumption.[23] By the end of the 1940s, he was able to present the pathway of sugar breakdown by tissues complete in every detail save the involvement of 2,3-DPG.[24]

Hereditary Defects of Red Cell Metabolism

Thus, the stage was set for the discovery of hereditary abnormalities of red cell metabolism. A greater number of metabolic defects have been discovered in red cells than in any other tissue, and more has been learned about them. This is true for several reasons. First of all, human red cells are easily accessible; a "biopsy" is carried out with a minimum of pain and a minimum of risk. Secondly, the long nonnucleated life span of the erythrocyte makes it particularly susceptible to the effects of mutations which involve the stability of enzymes; such mutations are particularly apparent in erythrocytes since synthesis of new enzyme molecules is not possible. In contrast, other tissues are able to replace worn-out enzyme molecules rapidly, and mutations producing enzyme instability have little effect on such tissues. Finally, even mutations which drastically compromise red cell life span are not likely to be lethal early in life because of the enormous compensatory capacity of the bone marrow and because of the adaptive mechanisms which allow the organism to survive even when the hemoglobin level of the blood is much lower than normal. As a consequence, mutations which affect primarily the erythrocytes often come to the attention of the physician. Similar degrees of enzyme deficiency in other tissues could lead to intrauterine death.

HEREDITARY METHEMOGLOBINEMIA—CHANCE BRINGS THE PROBLEM TO AN IMAGINATIVE INVESTIGATOR

Hereditary methemoglobinemia is a disorder that had been observed sporadically over a long period of time, and its cause had been the subject of considerable speculation. It is characterized by a bluish tinge (cyanosis) that is particularly noticeable in the lips and fingernails. The reduction of the brown hemoglobin oxidation product methemoglobin by blood attracted the attention of leading biochemists for many years; Warburg and his colleagues[13] had shown that sugar is oxidized to pyruvate when methemoglobin is reduced to hemoglobin in red cells. Later, it was also demonstrated[25] that methylene blue accelerates the rate of methemoglobin reduction in red cells.

In an incisive, often overlooked study, Q. H. Gibson[26] defined the normal pathway of methemoglobin reduction, the pathway utilized when methylene blue is added, and correctly identified the site of the hereditary enzymatic lesion in hereditary methemoglobinemia. This achievement was particularly remarkable because it was accomplished at a time when the steps of sugar metabolism of the red cell had only just been defined and because the conclusions were reached through shrewd interpretation of studies of red cells treated with certain metabolic inhibitors.

Gibson at the time was under 30, a demonstrator in physiology at Queen's University in Belfast in the department headed by Henry Barcroft, the son of the famous hemoglobin physiologist Sir Joseph Barcroft. A country doctor, Dr. Deeny of Banbridge, Ireland, thought he had observed a beneficial effect of ascorbic acid on patients with congestive heart failure. Having been unable to convince his colleagues of the correctness of his observation, Deeny resolutely sought an opportunity for a dramatic demonstration of the efficacy of his treatment. One day he observed through his office window an intensely cyanosed man and, on inquiry, he learned that there were in fact two blue men in the town, the brothers Fred and Russell Martin. Deeny visited the Martins and offered to turn them pink. Giving ascorbic acid only to Fred, in three weeks Fred was indeed pink while his brother Russell remained a deep blue color. Armed with what he regarded as conclusive evidence, Dr. Deeny took his patients to Belfast. However, to the cardiologists there, it was immediately clear that the problem of the brothers was not one of heart failure.

Gibson had been investigating the problem of why hemoglobin levels seemed lower in the British than in Scandinavians and Americans (later found to be due to incorrect hemoglobin standards), and he was called upon to examine the brothers. With the support of Professor D. C. Harrison, Chairman of Biochemistry, and of Professor Barcroft, who arranged to have an artist make paintings of the skin color of the remaining blue brother at intervals during treatment with ascorbic acid, an exciting investigation was initiated. Much of the excitement of the project vanished, however, when the enthusiastic investigators found that others had already reported that ascorbic acid would reduce methemoglobin in a patient with familial methemoglobinemia.

Gibson, nevertheless, set to work to examine the reaction between methemoglobin and ascorbic acid in guinea pigs and in vitro. The in vivo experiments soon ended, however, because the heating system broke down during the Christmas holidays, killing the guinea pigs; the laboratory was too poor to replace the animals. Forced to concentrate his attention on the biochemistry of methemoglobin reduction, Gibson found that methemoglobinemic red cells, like normal ones, could rapidly reduce methemoglobin in the presence of methylene blue but sugar alone had scarcely any effect on them even though the rate of methemoglobin reduction in normal cells was greatly accelerated by sugar. This, it seemed to him, pointed toward a specific enzymatic defect. He reasoned that glucose might act either through the hexose monophosphate pathway, which had been described in the previous decade by Warburg[15] and elaborated by Dickens[27] or through the formation of triose phosphate and phosphoglycerate (the Embden-Meyerhof pathway) (see Figure 6-3). Distinguishing between these alternatives was not easy, and he wrote: "It is unfortunately impossible to test these reactions directly by trying out the intermediates postulated since the envelope of the erythrocyte is impermeable to phosphorylated compounds, and the reduction of methemoglobin effectively ceases on hemolysis."[26]

Gibson made a number of observations, however, which led him to correctly conclude that the Embden-Meyerhof pathway, and hence "coenzyme I" (DPN, NAD) was involved in methemoglobin reduction. He showed that the reduction of methemoglobin resulted in the accumulation of pyruvate but that phosphoglycerate accumulated instead when glycolysis was inhibited with fluoride. Moreover, iodoacetic acid, known to inhibit glyceraldehyde phosphate dehydrogenase, inhibited methemoglobin reduction when glucose was the substrate but not when lactate was substituted. He found that methylene blue greatly accelerated methemoglobin reduction in cells from patients with hereditary methemoglobinemia which were incubated with glucose but that no acceleration was observed in the presence of lactate. Since the methylene blue–catalyzed reaction was not associated with the accumulation of pyruvate, he concluded that it did not occur through the coenzyme I–linked reaction of the Embden-Meyerhof pathway, but rather through the coenzyme II–linked scheme. This led him to the conclusion that the defect in hereditary methemoglobinemia is in the enzyme which catalyzes the interaction between coenzyme I (NAD) and methemoglobin. His conclusion was amply confirmed by later investigators, who used more direct approaches to measure the relative effectiveness of NADH and NADPH as substrates for dye reduction in hemolysates.[28]

ACATALASEMIA

At about the same time that Gibson was unraveling the enzymatic basis of methemoglobinemia, a second hereditary enzyme abnormality was discovered in Japan by the serendipity of an otolaryngologist, Dr. Shigeo Takahara:[29]

> Toward the end of 1946, an 11-year-old, pale-looking girl came to our Ear, Nose and Throat Outpatient Clinic with high fever and complained of severe ulcers in her mouth. On examination, I found a peculiar type of gangrene starting around the neck of one of the molars of the right upper jaw and extending into the maxillary sinus and the nasal cavity. There was a foul-smelling and fetid granulation in her nose. Judging her condition to be very serious, I decided to remove the diseased part completely. After the radical operation, I poured hydrogen peroxide on the wound for cleansing. To my great surprise, the blood coming in contact with the

hydrogen peroxide immediately turned a brownish-black color and the usual bubbles did not appear. I thought that by mistake the nurse might have handed me a bottle of silver nitrate, commonly used in the ear, nose and throat clinics. So I at once poured saline solution into the wound to neutralize it. I was much relieved to know that nothing serious had happened. Then I applied hydrogen peroxide several times but obtained the same results. Thus, I came to believe that there was some abnormality in the blood of this patient.

She was the second child of seven siblings. Four of them had mouth gangrene of varying degrees, and their blood all reacted in the same manner as described. The other three had no oral lesions and their blood reacted to hydrogen peroxide in the normal fashion. Thus I presumed that there must be some close relationship between the blackening of the blood and the oral disease. Thereupon, I decided to study the blood samples of this patient and her siblings. It was demonstrated by a series of qualitative and quantitative analyses of the blood that catalase was lacking in the erythrocytes of these subjects.

At first, it seemed as though acatalasemia was a disease unique to the Japanese, 77 cases having been detected in 39 families in Japan by 1967.[29] Subsequently, Dr. Hugo Aebi, working in Bern, became interested in this defect, and, because of the difficulty in obtaining blood samples from Japan, he determined to find cases in Switzerland. He prevailed upon the Army Blood Group Laboratory of the Swiss Red Cross Transfusion Service to screen for acatalasemia samples from all Swiss Army recruits. After 15,000 samples were tested, not a single case of acatalasemia had been found, and discontinuing the seemingly fruitless screening program was contemplated. Just at this time, two unrelated cases were detected simultaneously. In subsequent screening, additional families were detected in Switzerland.[30]

Acatalasemia is a particularly interesting red cell enzyme defect because it demonstrates the capacity of individuals to survive the virtually total absence of a normally very active red cell enzyme. In the Swiss patients with acatalasemia, no untoward clinical consequences have been noted, but some of the Japanese patients, as described above, have oral ulcerations, presumably in response to decreased tissue catalase levels.

GALACTOSEMIA

In the case of the first two genetically determined enzyme abnormalities of red cells, hereditary methemoglobinemia and acatalasemia, it was obvious that the red cells were abnormal. In the case of hereditary methemoglobinemia, the erythrocytes were brown in color instead of red. In acatalasemia they turned brownish black when treated with hydrogen peroxide and failed to cause foaming of the peroxide solution. In the next hereditary abnormality of red cells to be discovered, galactosemia, the erythrocytes seem, superficially, not to be affected.

Galactosemia is an inborn error of metabolism in which galactose, a component of milk sugar, cannot be utilized by the body. Galactose accumulates in the blood and in the urine, and derivatives of galactose are formed in the tissues. Galactosemic infants do not take food well. They develop liver disease, and the abdomen swells. Cataracts form in the lens of the eye, and, if the child lives long enough, mental retardation becomes evident. Unless the disease is treated by withholding galactose from the diet, the child almost always dies within the first year of life.

The possibility that erythrocytes could serve as models in gaining understanding of metabolic processes such as sugar entry into cells had been emphasized earlier by Bartlett and Marlow.[31] In 1954, two leading biochemists, Leloir and Kalckar, were investigating the role of uridine nucleotide derivatives in the metabolism of glucose. At this time, a young scientist, Dr. Kurt Isselbacher, then at the National Institutes of Health (NIH), was pursuing quite a different problem. He was interested in the formation of glucuronides in steroid metabolism and, therefore, in the enzymatic oxidation of uridine diphosphate glucose to uridine diphosphate glucuronic acid. His desire to prepare glucuronides brought him into contact with Dr. Kalckar, also at the NIH, and excited his interest in the various conversions which occur in uridine bound sugars. Kalckar called Isselbacher's attention to an abstract by Schwarz,[32] which indicated that galactose 1-phosphate accumulates in the red cells of patients with galactosemia. This finding suggested to Isselbacher and Kalckar that galactose must be metabolized to galactose 1-phosphate in the red blood cell, and that further metabolism of galactose 1-phosphate might be impaired. It so happened that a pediatrician in the Bethesda area, where the NIH is located, had a son with galactosemia, and this provided a ready source of red blood cells. When it then was shown that the red cells lacked the enzyme galactose-1-phosphate uridyl transferase, it became possible to accurately diagnose not only the disease but also the carrier state.

Much later, applying the lessons learned from developing screening methods for glucose-6-phosphate dehydrogenase deficiency, which will be described shortly, the author directed his attention to finding a method for the detection of galactosemia. Effective treatment depends upon early detection, for which a means was now conceptually quite simple but in practice depended on an adequate supply of a very expensive sugar phosphate compound, galactose 1-phosphate. In about 1953, a drastic decrease in the price of this sugar made it possible to develop a practical screening procedure.[33] In the final phases of the studies, a sample of blood was drawn from the author's assistant, Mrs. Mary Ellen Baluda. To our dismay, an intermediate result was obtained. A quantitative assay for galactose-1-phosphate uridyl transferase carried out later revealed about one-half normal red cell enzyme activity. Although it appeared that we had identified a heterozygote for galactosemia, examination of parents and children revealed approximately three-quarters normal activity. With similar results in another family, it became apparent that another allele existed at the galactose-1-phosphate uridyl transferase locus. Using the fluorescence of NADPH as an indicator in the reaction sequence, it was possible to stain the enzyme and to demonstrate that the mutant form of enzyme, designated the Duarte variant, moved more rapidly than normal.[34] As a result of this experience, it seemed logical to consider that if fluorescence could be used as an indicator for enzyme activity after electrophoresis, it might also be a convenient indicator in the screening for enzyme deficiency. Thus, a fluorescent screening test for galactosemia[35] was designed, a test which is much easier to perform than the dye decolorization test, which had been described previously. It quickly became apparent that NADPH or NADH fluorescence can serve as a convenient indicator for many other enzymes, including G6PD, glucose phosphate isomerase, and triose phosphate isomerase.

Glucose-6-Phosphate Dehydrogenase Deficiency

THE ROAD FROM A CLINICAL PROBLEM TO BASIC SCIENCE

Glucose-6-phosphate dehydrogenase (G6PD) deficiency is the most prevalent of the metabolic defects of the red cell. Not only is this deficiency very common, but, because the gene for this enzyme is carried on the X chromosome and because electrophoretic variants of G6PD are easily found, it has been an invaluable tool in the study of basic mammalian genetics, as will be discussed later.

During World War II, the Allied forces fought in many areas in which malaria was endemic, but the Japanese had cut off the principal source of quinine. This stimulated the U.S. Army to sponsor an extensive search for other antimalarial drugs. Literally thousands of analogues of compounds known to have antimalarial activity were synthesized, tested in animal systems, and ultimately tested in human beings. One of the starting compounds for such syntheses was pamaquine (Plasmochin), a 6-methoxy-8-aminoquinoline, which had been introduced by Mühlens[36] in 1926. Although it was hailed as an effective, safe antimalarial, not a year had passed before it was recognized that this drug had dangerous toxic properties. Administered to workers on the United Fruit Company plantation, the drug produced severe and even fatal hemolytic anemia in some individuals.[37] Over the next decade, many additional cases of hemolytic anemia resulting from the administration of pamaquine were reported.[38] Moreover, it became apparent that pamaquine was not very effective in eradicating the erythrocytic stage of malaria, although it seemed to have considerable activity in preventing relapse of vivax malaria. As a result of Army-sponsored studies, various analogues of pamaquine were tested, and several of these, pentaquine, isopentaquine, and primaquine, proved to be more effective than pamaquine in the eradication of tissue stages of malaria.

Scarcely 5 years after the guns of the southern Pacific battles of World War II had been silenced, the Korean conflict erupted. A strain of vivax malaria with a long latent period was common in Korea. American soldiers returning from Korea often experienced attacks of malaria many months after their return to the United States. The need for a curative antimalarial was again as pressing as ever, and primaquine seemed to provide the best solution. But, like pamaquine, primaquine produced severe hemolytic anemia in certain subjects who ingested 30 mg of the drug daily, a dose which was innocuous to the vast majority of soldiers. Approximately 11 percent of black Americans were "primaquine sensitive."

STUDIES OF HEMOLYTIC ANEMIAS CARRIED OUT IN VOLUNTEERS LEAD TO DISCOVERY OF THE UNDERLYING DEFECT

The malaria project which had been initiated at Stateville Penitentiary in Joliet, Illinois under Army sponsorship during World War II had continued to function between the wars. Study of the hemolytic anemia induced by primaquine became an important objective of this project, which was operated by the University of Chicago under the directorship of Dr. Alf S. Alving. Alving had joined the University of Chicago in 1934 after working at the Rockefeller Institute for a number of years. The Army Research and Development Command assigned two medical officers to Stateville to investigate the therapeutic effect and toxicity of antimalarial drugs. The availability of prisoner-volunteers and the close association with the University provided a unique environment for the conduct of clinical research. Preoccupation with the ethical aspects of research has become so great in some quarters that it is unlikely that the studies carried out at the Stateville Penitentiary in the early 1950s would now be possible. Fortunately, a balanced view, which took into account both the individual rights and the needs of society, prevailed at that time, and, thus, it was possible to unravel the cause of primaquine-induced hemolysis. The volunteers who were studied were volunteers in the true sense of the word. No coercion of any type was applied to obtain their participation. Neither were undue inducements offered. Volunteers were paid 10 dollars for up to 1 year's participation in toxicity studies and 25 dollars for being infected with malaria. No commitments were made regarding shortening of prison sentences or granting of parole. The motivation of individual prisoners to take part in the investigations was undoubtedly complex. It is probable that some hoped that their willingness to participate in important scientific studies at some, albeit small, risk to themselves might favorably influence the parole board on their behalf. Certainly, the prison hospital environment was more pleasant than the various workshops and small cells between which the prisoners alternated their daily routine. The nature of the studies was fully explained to each potential volunteer; the agreement to participate was signed before witnesses.

Army officers assigned to this project generally were those members of the house staff at the University of Chicago Clinics who had a strong interest in research, and who were faced with a military service requirement. The first direct attack on the problem of primaquine-induced hemolytic anemia in drug-sensitive volunteers was carried out by one of these officers, Raymond J. Dern. Dern had received a Ph.D. in physiology prior to entering medical school and he directed his attention to the classical physiologic question which must be asked about any hemolytic disorder: was it due to an intrinsic abnormality of the red cell or were extracorpuscular factors the basic cause? In the past, it had been necessary to use the tedious Ashby technique (see Chapter 8), which measured the survival of type O cells in a type A, B, or AB recipient, to answer this question. However, Irwin M. Weinstein, another medical resident at the University of Chicago, had become interested in the ^{51}Cr red cell survival technique (Chapter 8). This new technique seemed ideally suited for studying the fate of red cells from primaquine-sensitive volunteers in the circulation of nonsensitive recipients.

The results of these investigations were clear-cut. In cross-transfusion experiments, red cells from primaquine-sensitive volunteers which had been labeled with ^{51}Cr were rapidly destroyed in the circulation of normal recipients when they were given primaquine, but cells from normal donors were not affected by primaquine administration even when circulating in primaquine-sensitive persons.[39] Primaquine sensitivity was clearly due to an intrinsic defect of the red blood cell.

But what was the defect? This was a question which was to occupy much of the author's attention when he joined the Army malaria research project. The circumstances were unusually propitious for the investigation of this problem. In the research laboratories at the Stateville Penitentiary, the laboratory assistants were men who had been convicted of major crimes, such as burglary, armed robbery, or murder, and our secretary was in prison because of his propensity to write checks on the bank accounts of others. These men were hard-working and loyal. Ponder's classic work *Hemolysis and Related Phenomena*[40] served as the text.

Using the techniques Ponder had described, we studied the lysis of red cells in vitro by such agents as saponin and by primaquine itself but were unable to detect an abnormality. Red cell antigens also were normal. The fact that sickle-cell disease was due to the inheritance of an abnormal hemoglobin had been discovered only a few years earlier. It seemed quite possible that primaquine sensitivity, like sickle-cell disease, might be due to an abnormal hemoglobin since both occurred most commonly in blacks. But the results of hemoglobin electrophoresis also were negative.

Dern suggested that the same defect that caused sensitivity to primaquine might also be responsible for hemolytic anemia resulting from ingestion of many other drugs, including sulfonamides and acetanilid, and even of fava beans. Using cross-transfusion studies with ^{51}Cr-labeled cells, we found that this was indeed the case; primaquine sensitivity was actually a manifestation of sensitivity to many drugs.[41] Our observation that small doses of phenylhydrazine destroyed a large proportion of primaquine-sensitive red cells drew our attention to the possible role of Heinz body formation in the hemolytic process. Heinz bodies are particles of denatured hemoglobin and stromal proteins which characteristically appear in erythrocytes after phenylhydrazine treatment.

Heinz bodies did, indeed, appear when primaquine was administered. The formation of Heinz bodies could also be effected by incubation of red cells with phenylhydrazine or its analogues, and soon it was possible to demonstrate that the pattern of Heinz body formation in primaquine-sensitive cells after incubation with acetylphenylhydrazine was quite different from that in normal cells[42] (Figure 6-5).

Figure 6-5 Heinz bodies formed by incubation of red cells with acetylphenylhydrazine. The erythrocytes have been stained with crystal violet. The enzyme-deficient cells form many small Heinz bodies (on the left), while only one or two large Heinz bodies are found in most of the normal cells (right). This test first made it possible to detect individuals who were sensitive to the hemolytic effect of primaquine without actually administering the drug. (*From Ref. 42, courtesy of Mosby and Co.*)

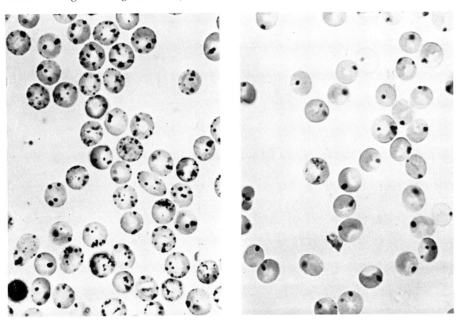

In the course of these investigations, Dern made a significant observation. He noticed that primaquine-induced hemolytic anemia was self-limited; the hemoglobin concentration of the blood reached a nadir and then rose to normal even when the dose of primaquine which had initially induced hemolysis was continued or increased.[43] Cross-transfusion studies with ^{51}Cr-labeled red cells provided an explanation for this phenomenon. Two types of red cells were present in the circulation of primaquine-sensitive individuals, sensitive and resistant cells. Inspection of some of our red cell survival curves suggested that this differential sensitivity might be a function of red cell age. The sensitivity of red cells of different ages could be studied by selectively labeling young erythrocytes with ^{59}Fe and challenging them with primaquine at different times in their life span. The results of such a study clearly showed that young cells were resistant to the hemolytic effect of primaquine while older cells were exquisitely sensitive.[44]

It had been known since the early part of the century that young red cells were metabolically more active than older cells; it seemed that the severe hemolysis of the older cells might reflect a metabolic defect. Although by 1953, all of the individual steps of red cell metabolism had been studied, there were few comprehensive accounts of the metabolic activities of erythrocytes. Indeed, Ponder's classic treatise,[40] which dealt in a remarkably prescient way with the physical properties of erythrocytes, made mere mention of the fact that red cells metabolize at all. The unique pattern of Heinz body formation observed in primaquine-sensitive cells provided the opportunity to investigate the effect of metabolic inhibitors on red cells to determine whether inhibition of metabolic pathways of normal cells might cause them to behave like primaquine-sensitive cells. Inhibition of glycolysis with fluoride failed to have this effect, but iodoacetate and arsenite produced "sensitive" cells from nonsensitive ones. Both of these poisons act on sulfhydryl groups. A chance discussion with Dr. Irving London, who, with Dimant,[45] had just been studying the turnover of glutathione (GSH) in erythrocytes, led to the suggestion that we examine the GSH content of the red cells since GSH is their main sulfhydryl compound. On the advice of E.S.G. Baron, the scientist whose studies of methylene blue catalysis of red cell oxygen consumption had stimulated Warburg to discover G6PD, a recently published method[46] for the measurement of GSH, suitably modified, was used to measure the GSH content of sensitive and nonsensitive cells. It was found that an abrupt fall in red cell GSH content occurred when primaquine was administered to sensitive subjects, and this GSH instability could be reproduced in vitro by exposing the red cells to acetylphenylhydrazine.

By this time, Dr. Paul E. Carson had been assigned to duty at the Stateville Penitentiary, and he began to study the pathways of GSH metabolism in primaquine-sensitive erythrocytes. At first, he focused his attention upon glutathione reductase, the enzyme which maintains GSH in the reduced state by reducing oxidized glutathione (GSSG). Since NADPH, the substrate for this enzyme, was quite expensive, he decided to generate NADPH from the less costly NADP utilizing glucose-6-phosphate dehydrogenase (G6PD), which is normally present in the hemolysate. Indeed, in this system, GSSG was not reduced to GSH. It therefore appeared, for the moment, that primaquine sensitivity might be due to a deficiency in glutathione reductase. However, when Carson supplied NADPH directly to the hemolysate, he discovered that the glutathione reductase activity of the cells was normal. This led him to conclude that the defect actually must be in the NADPH generating system, i.e., in G6PD.

After publishing these important findings,[47] Carson was dismayed to find that he could no longer reproduce them. The explanation soon became apparent. In carrying out his original investigations, Carson did not have access to a refrigerated centrifuge, with the result that during preparation of hemolysates the residual G6PD in G6PD-deficient cells was largely destroyed. His discovery that G6PD was deficient in primaquine-sensitive cells was rewarded by purchase of a refrigerated centrifuge. With the use of this instrument, the residual G6PD in the primaquine-sensitive cells was no longer destroyed, and the defect was no longer detected. Thus, had more advanced equipment been available to Carson, the defect of primaquine-sensitive cells would not have been discovered in the Stateville laboratories. Had the defect of G6PD deficiency not been found there, however, it would doubtless have been recognized elsewhere within a short period of time. Other laboratories were studying this enzyme, the "zwischenferment" of Warburg, in human red cells for other reasons. Dr. Paul Marks, for example, was measuring G6PD activity in red cells in studies of pentose metabolism and as a marker of red cell age.[48] He had noted that some samples seemed to lack G6PD activity but did not pursue this finding initially. At a German university, Waller and Löhr studied an Iranian student who had developed severe hemolytic anemia.[49] While routinely measuring a number of red cell enzymes in patients with hemolytic anemia, they discovered that his red cells were lacking in G6PD activity. They published their finding, apparently unaware of the significance of Carson's publication a year earlier.

With the discovery of the basic defect in primaquine-sensitive red cells and the development of simple screening tests for the detection of this abnormality, it soon became apparent that G6PD deficiency did not result in hemolytic anemia only when primaquine and related drugs were given but also under certain other circumstances. After a trip to Sardinia, Crosby[51] noted the similarity between the severe hemolytic anemia associated with the ingestion or even the inhalation of the pollen of fava beans and the hemolytic anemia induced by primaquine. Fava beans are a staple of the diet in many Mediterranean countries. Favism, as the disorder has been called, has been observed since antiquity; these beans are said to have been shunned by

Pythagoras and his followers.[50] It was soon discovered that persons with favism were invariably G6PD deficient.

Severe G6PD deficiency has been found to be very common in Mediterranean populations and has been shown to be responsible for severe and even fatal hemolysis in some newborns as well as for severe hemolytic episodes when deficient individuals acquire infections such as pneumonia or typhoid fever.

Genetic studies of families with G6PD deficiency have shown that this is a sex-linked abnormality: the gene for G6PD is carried on the X chromosome. Genetic mutations involving G6PD deficiency, not only those variants causing deficiency but others causing harmless changes in the electrical charge of the enzyme, are extremely common. They occur in about 11 percent of black males, thus explaining the high incidence of primaquine sensitivity in black U.S. troops. The G6PD marker has become an invaluable tool in the investigation of the activity of human genes. It was studies of G6PD which first led to the suggestions that only one of the two X chromosomes in the body cells of women is active.[52]

Enzyme Defects in Other Types of Hemolytic Anemia

Professor John Dacie at the Hammersmith Hospital in London called attention in 1953 to a group of hereditary hemolytic anemias which differed from the form of hemolytic anemia most commonly recognized at that time, hereditary spherocytosis (HS), in that they were nonspherocytic.[53] These *hereditary nonspherocytic hemolytic anemias* provided an interesting challenge to a number of hematologists. In 1958, Newton and Bass[54] discovered that a patient with this syndrome was G6PD deficient, but it was immediately evident that G6PD deficiency only accounted for a minority of patients with nonspherocytic hemolytic disease. In most of the patients, G6PD activity was normal.

In the 1950s, Dr. William Valentine and his associates at the University of California at Los Angeles were studying white cell enzymes in various disease states. Valentine reasoned that G6PD deficiency would very likely not stand alone as an enzyme defect associated with hemolytic anemia. It had become much easier than previously to assay a variety of glycolytic enzymes, pyridine nucleotide cofactors and purified enzymes that could be used in indicator systems having become available commercially. The studies of autohemolysis which had been carried out by Dacie and his collaborators led Valentine and his students to turn their attention to the glycolytic enzymes of patients with hereditary nonspherocytic hemolytic anemia. Working with Valentine in 1960 were Dr. Kouichi Tanaka and Dr. Shiro Miwa, both of whom in their own right subsequently became productive investigators in the study of red cell metabolic defects. Valentine and his two young colleagues soon discovered that patients with hereditary nonspherocytic hemolytic anemia from several different families had in common a deficiency of the enzyme pyruvate kinase. They submitted a report of this important finding to a prestigious journal (*Science*), but it was rejected as being insufficiently broad in its appeal. After their reports appeared in the *Transactions of the Association of American Physicians*[55] and in *Blood*,[56] many other cases of pyruvate kinase deficiency were reported from all over the world. Indeed, this enzyme deficiency ranks with G6PD deficiency as the most commonly recognized cause of hereditary nonspherocytic hemolytic anemia.

Subsequent studies in Valentine's laboratories soon implicated many of the other enzymes of the red cell glycolytic pathways in the etiology of hereditary nonspherocytic hemolytic anemias. Included were defects of glucose phosphate isomerase, triose phosphate isomerase, hexokinase, and phosphoglycerate kinase. In other laboratories, patients with defects of still other glycolytic enzymes were identified, including phosphofructokinase, aldolase, diphosphoglyceromutase, and lactate dehydrogenase. Defects in glutathione synthesis, in hydrolysis of phosphate from pyrimidine nucleotides, and in the enzyme adenylate kinase have been shown to be responsible for hemolysis in some families.[57] Even increased enzyme activity has been implicated in one family; a 45- to 70-times increase in adenosine deaminase activity, inherited as an autosomal dominant trait, was responsible for the hemolytic anemia in this family.[58] And yet, in spite of the many defects of red cell metabolism which have been implicated in the etiology of hereditary nonspherocytic hemolytic anemia, the cause of most cases still remains obscure. The elucidation of other causes of nonspherocytic hemolytic anemia remains a task for the future, one which may reward us with even better understanding of the normal metabolism of the red cell.

The Red Cell in the Diagnosis of Nonhematologic Disease

The identification of the basic defect in galactosemia in the red cell and the use of the red cell as a means for diagnosing this disorder have been described already. Since this classical achievement, the etiology of a number of other disease states has been characterized by using the red cell as a tool. Studies of pathways of purine biosynthesis in patients with mental retardation, self-mutilation, and hyperuricemia led to the discovery by Seegmiller, et al.[59] of hypoxanthine-guanine phosphoribosyl transferase deficiency in their erythrocytes. More recently, a deficiency of adenine phosphoribosyl transferase was found to be associated with a severe gouty disorder and 2,8-dihydroxyadenine urinary stones.[60]

Thanks to a chance finding by Dr. Eloise Giblett, totally unexpected abnormalities in nucleoside metabolism were discovered in the red cells of patients with immunodeficiency diseases. In examining a patient with combined immunodeficiency for various genetic red cell markers in preparation for bone marrow transplantation, she found that when the patient's hemolysate was subjected to electrophoresis, the stain for adenosine deaminase failed to develop. Suspecting a methodologic error, the studies were quickly repeated, with the same results. Quantitative estimation of the activity of this enzyme revealed that a severe deficiency did, indeed, exist.[61] A systematic study of the enzymes of purine metabolism was then carried out on other patients by Dr. Giblett and her associates, and a second defect, that of nucleoside phosphorylase, was discovered.[62]

Examination of the electrophoretic mobility of red blood cell enzymes has revealed marked inherited variability. Because of the many polymorphisms that exist and because of the ready availability of red cells, erythrocytes have been an extraordinarily fruitful resource for the population geneticist, in carrying out linkage studies, and in forensic medicine.

Red Cell Enzymes as Genetic Markers in the Study of Populations

Differences in the appearance of races and between persons of the same race are almost entirely genetically determined. They reflect the enormous diversity in the genetic constitution of human beings. Outward appearance provides anthropologists with a guide to population movements. The American Indian resembles Asians in facial appearance and in lack of body hair, and these characteristics may lend some support to the putative origin of the American Indian in Asia. But physical appearance is due to the combination of many different genes and, at best, is difficult to measure. The movement of genes from continent to continent is much more readily studied by tracing single, well-defined genes such as that for glucose-6-phosphate dehydrogenase deficiency. Chaim Sheba, in a private conversation, suggested that the distribution of genes such as that for G6PD deficiency around the Mediterranean basin reflects the movements of the seagoing Phoenicians. He also provided a plausible explanation for the fact that Middle Eastern Sephardic Jews manifest a high incidence of G6PD deficiency while the defect is relatively rare among their European offspring. Since G6PD deficiency is sex-linked, it is transmitted from mothers to sons but never from fathers to sons. Apparently, Jewish men taken captive by the Romans generally married non-Jewish slaves. Their sons, who carried on the Jewish faith and culture, carried the X chromosomes of non-Jewish mothers, and, thereby, the incidence of G6PD deficiency was sharply diminished.

The Consequences of the Study of Red Cell Metabolism

Within the past century, our conception of the red blood cell has changed from that of an inert corpuscle to that of a tiny dynamo of marvelously coordinated metabolic activity. Could Swammerdam and Leeuwenhoek possibly have believed that study of the tiny cells which they spied under their primitive microscopes might lead to the discovery of such a complex metabolic mechanism? Would it be possible to persuade Claude Bernard that the consumption of glucose by blood was the result of the complex series of steps which we now recognize? Even Warburg, who first studied erythrocyte respiration in 1909, is unlikely to have anticipated the intricacy of the reactions which he helped to unravel in these tiny structures. Who would have guessed that hereditary defects of red cell enzymes would provide the information needed to demonstrate the cause of conditions as diverse as oral ulcers, galactosemia, hemolytic anemias, self-mutilation and gout, kidney stones, and immunodeficiency? And who can dream today what the red cell may tell us in the future?

Acknowledgments

I am grateful to Dr. Irwin Haas, longtime associate of Professor Otto Warburg, to Dr. Quentin H. Gibson, Dr. Kurt Isselbacher, Dr. William Valentine, and Dr. Grant Bartlett, who shared with me some of their personal recollections, and to my wife, Bonnie, who provided invaluable editorial assistance.

References

1 Monfalcon: *Dictionaire des sciences medicales*. Paris, CLF Pankoucke, 1820, 582 pp, vol 49, pp 486–506.
2 Magendie F: *Precis Elementaire*. Paris, Mequignon-Marvis, Libraire pour la Partic de Medicine, 1817, 473 pp.
3 Magendie F: *Lectures on the Blood*. Philadelphia, Haswell Barrington and Haswell, 1839, 276 pp, p 252.
4 Hedin SG: Über die Permeabilitaet der Blutkörperchen. *Pflügers Arch* 68:229–338, 1897.
5 John HJ: Glycolysis. *Ann Clin Med* 3:667–696, 1925.
6 Slosse A: Étude sur la glycolyse aseptique dans le sang. *Arch Int Physiol Biochim* 11:154–190, 1911.
7 Krebs HA: Otto Heinrich Warburg. *Biogr Mem Fellows R Soc* 18:629–699.
8 Burk D: Warburg, Otto Heinrich, in Gillispie CC (ed): *Dictionary of Scientific Biography*. New York, Scribner, 1976, vol XIV, pp 172–177.
9 Warburg O: Zur Biologie der roten Blutzellen. *Hoppe Seylers Z Physiol Chem* 59:112–121, 1909.
10 Harrop GA Jr: The oxygen consumption of human erythrocytes. *Arch Intern Med* 23:745–752, 1919.
11 Harrop GA Jr, Barron ESG: Studies on blood cell metabolism. I. The effect of methylene blue and other dyes upon the oxygen consumption of mammalian and avian erythrocytes. *J Exp Med* 48:207–223, 1928.
12 Warburg O, Kubowitz F, Christian W: Über die katalytische Wirkung von Methylenblau in lebenden Zellen. *Biochem Z* 227:245–271, 1930.
13 Warburg O, Kubowitz F, Christian W: Kohlenhydratverbrennung durch

Methämoglobin. (Über den Mechanismus einer Methylenblaukatalyse.) *Biochem Z* 221:494–497, 1930.

14 Robison R: LXXXV. A new phosphoric ester produced by the action of yeast juice on hexoses. *Biochem J* 16:809–824, 1922.

15 Warburg O, Christian W: Ueber aktivierung der Robinsonchen Hexose-monophosphorsäure in roten Blutzellen und die Gewinnung aktivierender Fermentlösungen. *Biochem Z* 242:206–227, 1931.

16 Warburg O, Christian W, Griese A: Die Wirkungsgruppe des Coferments aus Roten Blutzellen. *Biochem Z* 279:143–144, 1935.

17 Greenwald I: A new type of phosphoric acid compound isolated from blood, with some remarks on the effect of substitution on the rotation of L-glyceric acid. *J. Biol Chem* 63:339–349, 1925.

18 Jost H: Über die biologische Bedeutung des Säurelöslichen organischen Blutphosphors. *Hoppe Seylers Z Physiol Chem* 165:171–214, 1927.

19 Thomas K: Gustav Embden. *Hoppe Seylers Z Physiol Chem* 230:3–11, 1934.

20 Schmauderer E: Embden, Gustav, in Gillispie CC (ed): *Dictionary of Scientific Biography*. New York, Scribner, 1976, vol IV, 624 pp, pp 359–360.

21 Embden G, Deuticke HJ: Über die Bedeuting der Phosphglycerinsaeure für die Glykolyse in der Muskulatur. *Hoppe Seylers Z Physiol Chem* 230:29–49, 1934.

22 Rapoport S, Luebering J: The formation of 2,3-diphosphoglycerate in rabbit erythrocytes: the existence of a diphosphoglycerate mutase. *J Biol Chem* 183:507–516, 1950.

23 Meyerhof O: Über die Abtrennung des milchsäurebildenden Ferments aus Erythrocyten. *Biochem Z* 246:249–284, 1932.

24 Meyerhof O: Glycolysis of animal tissue extracts compared with the cell-free fermentation of yeast. *Wallerstein Lab Communications* 12:255–265, 1949.

25 Cox WW, Wendel WB: The normal rate of reduction of methemoglobin in dogs. *J Biol Chem* 143:331–340, 1942.

26 Gibson QH: The reduction of methemoglobin in red blood cells and studies on the cause of idiopathic methemoglobinemia. *Biochem J* 42:13–23, 1948.

27 Dickens F: CCXI. Oxidation of phosphohexonate and pentose phosphoric acids by yeast enzymes. I. Oxidation of phosphohexonate. II. Oxidation of pentose phosphoric acids. *Biochem J* 32:1626–1644, 1938.

28 Scott E: The relation of diaphorase of human erythrocytes to inheritance of methemoglobinemia. *J Clin Invest* 39:1176–1179, 1960.

29 Takahara S: Acatalasemia in Japan, in Beutler E (ed): *Hereditary Disorders of Erythrocyte Metabolism*. New York, Grune and Stratton, 1968, City of Hope Symp Series vol 1, 343 pp, pp 21–40.

30 Aebi H, Bossi E, Cantz M, Matsubara S, Suter H: Acatalas(em)ia in Switzerland, in Beutler E (ed): *Hereditary Disorders of Erythrocyte Metabolism*. New York, Grune and Stratton, 1968, City of Hope Symp Series vol 1, 343 pp, pp 41–65.

31 Bartlett GR, Marlow AA: Enzyme systems in the red blood cell. *Bull Scripps Metabolic Clin* 2:1–17, 1951.

32 Schwarz V, Golberg L, Komrower GM, Holzel A: Metabolic observations on the erythrocytes from cases of galactosaemia. *Biochem J* 59:XXII, 1955.

33 Beutler E, Baluda M, Donnell GN: A new method for the detection of galactosemia and its carrier state. *J Lab Clin Med* 64:694–705, 1964.

34 Mathai CK, Beutler E: Electrophoretic variation of galactose-1-phosphate uridyl transferase. *Science* 154:1179–1180, 1966.

35 Beutler E, Baluda MC: A simple spot screening test for galactosemia. *J Lab Clin Med* 68:137–141, 1966.

36 Mühlens P: Die behandlung der naturlichen menschlichen malaria infektion mit plasmochin. *Naturwissenschaften* 14:1162–1166, 1926.

37 Cordes W: *Experiences with Plasmochin in Malaria.* Boston, United Fruit Co (Med Dept), 15th Annual Report, 1926, pp 66–71.

38 Beutler E: The hemolytic effect of primaquine and related compounds. A review. *Blood* 14:103–139, 1959.

39 Dern RJ, Weinstein IM, LeRoy GV, Talmage DW, Alving AS: The hemolytic effect of primaquine. I. The localization of the drug-induced hemolytic defect in primaquine-sensitive individuals. *J Lab Clin Med* 43:303–309, 1954.

40 Ponder E: *Hemolysis and Related Phenomena.* New York, Grune and Stratton, 1948, 398 pp.

41 Dern RJ, Beutler E, Alving AS: The hemolytic effect of primaquine. V. Primaquine sensitivity as a manifestation of a multiple drug sensitivity. *J Lab Clin Med* 45:30–39, 1955.

42 Beutler E, Dern RJ, Alving AS: The hemolytic effect of primaquine. VI. An in vitro test for sensitivity of erythrocytes to primaquine. *J Lab Clin Med* 45:40–50, 1955.

43 Dern RJ, Beutler E, Alving AS: The hemolytic effect of primaquine. II. The natural course of the hemolytic anemia and the mechanism of its self-limited character. *J Lab Clin Med* 44:171–175, 1954.

44 Beutler E, Dern RJ, Alving AS: The hemolytic effect of primaquine. IV. The relationship of cell age to hemolysis. *J Lab Clin Med* 44:439–442, 1954.

45 Dimant E, Landberg E, London IM: The metabolic behavior of reduced glutathione in human and avian erythrocytes. *J Biol Chem* 213:769–776, 1955.

46 Beutler E: The glutathione instability of drug-sensitive red cells. A new method for the in vitro detection of drug-sensitivity. *J Lab Clin Med* 49:84–94, 1957.

47 Carson PE, Flanagan CL, Ickes CE, Alving AS: Enzymatic deficiency in primaquine-sensitive erythrocytes. *Science* 124:484–485, 1956.

48 Marks PA: Red cell glucose-6-phosphate and 6-phosphogluconic dehydrogenases and nucleoside phosphorylase. *Science* 127:1338–1339, 1958.

49 Waller HD, Löhr GW, Tabatabai M: Hämolyse und Fehlen von Glucose-6-phosphat-dehydrogenase in roten Blutzellen (eine Fermentanomalie der Erythrocyten). *Klin Wochenschr* 35:1022–1027, 1957.

50 Sigerist HE: Early Greek, Hindu, and Persian medicine, in *A History of Medicine.* New York, Oxford University Press, 1961, vol II, 352 pp, p 96.

51 Crosby WH: Favism in Sardinia (newsletter). *Blood* 11:91–92, 1956.

52 Beutler E: Biochemical abnormalities associated with hemolytic states, in Weinstein I, Beutler E (eds): *Mechanisms of Anemia in Man.* New York, McGraw-Hill, 1962, 380 pp, p 195.

53 Dacie JV, Mollison PL, Richardson N, Selwyn JG, Shapiro L: Atypical congenital haemolytic anaemia. *Q J Med* 85:79–97, 1953.

54 Newton WA Jr, Bass JC: Glutathione sensitive chronic nonspherocytic hemolytic anemia. *Am J Dis Child* 96:501–502, 1958.

55 Valentine WN, Tanaka KR, Miwa S: A specific erythrocyte glycolytic enzyme defect

(pyruvate kinase) in three subjects with congenital non-spherocytic hemolytic anemia. *Trans Assoc Am Physicians* 74:100–110, 1961.

56 Tanaka KR, Valentine WN, Miwa S: Pyruvate kinase (PK) deficiency hereditary non-spherocytic hemolytic anemia. *Blood* 19:267–295, 1962.

57 Valentine WN: Metabolism of human erythrocytes. *Arch Intern Med* 135:1307–1313, 1975.

58 Valentine WN, Paglia DE, Tartaglia AP, Gilsanz F: Hereditary hemolytic anemia with increased red cell adenosine deaminase (45- to 70-fold) and decreased adenosine triphosphate. *Science* 195:783–785, 1977.

59 Seegmiller JE, Rosenbloom FM, Kelley WN: Enzyme defect associated with a sex-linked human neurological disorder and excessive purine synthesis. *Science* 155:1682–1684, 1967.

60 Cartier P, Hamet M: Une nouvelle maladie metabolique: le deficit complet en adenine-phosphoribosyltransferase avec lithiase de 2,8-dihydroxyadenine. *C R Acad Sci (Paris)* 279:883–886, 1974.

61 Giblett ER, Anderson JE, Cohen F, Pollara B, Meuwissen HJ: Adenosine deaminase deficiency in two patients with severely impaired cellular immunity. *Lancet* 2:1067–1069, 1972.

62 Giblett ER, Ammann AJ, Wara DW, Sandman R, Diamond LK: Nucleoside-phosphorylase deficiency in a child with severely defective T-cell immunity and normal B-cell immunity. *Lancet* 1:1010–1013, 1975.

CHAPTER 7

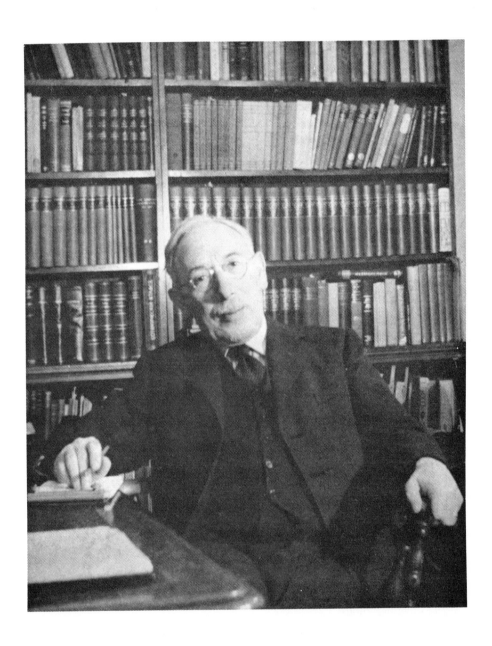

IRON AND HEME: CRUCIAL CARRIERS AND CATALYSTS
Irving M. London

In speculating on the origin of life on Earth and on the possibilities of life on other planets, we are struck by the central role of porphyrin compounds in metabolic processes. The green of plants and the red of blood are symbolic of living matter. Magnesium protoporphyrin is the essential component of chlorophyll, which, in the process of photosynthesis, is involved in the conversion of solar energy to chemical energy stored in plants. Iron protoporphyrin, or heme, serves in the transport of oxygen by hemoglobin and in the conversion of the chemical energy of food into the metabolic energy of living organisms by respiratory heme pigments. In the interplay of chance mutation and selective advantage that has occurred in the evolution of life on our planet, these porphyrin compounds have been chosen for leading roles. We shall focus our attention in this discussion on iron and heme, i.e., ferrous protoporphyrin IX. Heme is the prosthetic group of hemoglobin and myoglobin, of the respiratory heme pigments (the cytochromes), of enzymes involved in the activation (peroxidase) and splitting (catalase) of hydrogen peroxide, and of other enzymes in the liver required for the metabolic conversion or detoxifica-

Chapter Opening Photo   David Keilin (1887–1963).

171

tion of chemical agents or drugs. And recently heme has been found to have a new function in the regulation of the initiation of protein synthesis in animal cells. On this very broad canvas we shall not do more than sketch a somewhat impressionistic account which cannot do justice to the wide range of subjects nor to the numerous scientists and scholars who have made major contributions in these fields.

Iron and the Heme of Hemoglobin

In ancient times, as early as 1500 B.C., preparations of iron were used therapeutically in Egypt, and during the Roman Empire, iron was regarded as a panacea for a wide range of ailments.[1] With the clinical description of "the green sickness," chlorosis, in the sixteenth century and recognition of the value of iron in its treatment in the seventeenth, a remarkable period in the history of hematology began. For more than three centuries, not only physicians but painters and poets were captivated by this illness. In 1554, Johannes Lange provided this clinical description of the disorder in writing to a friend who had sought his advice:[2]

> You complain to me, as to a faithful Achates, that your eldest daughter, Anna, is now marriageable, and has many eligible suitors, all of whom you are obliged to dismiss on account of her ill-health, the cause of which no doctor can discover: for one calls it cardialgia, a second, palpitation, a third, dyspnoea, a fourth, hysteria, nor are there wanting who say that her liver is out of order. Wherefore you entreat me by our ancient friendship to give an opinion on her case, with advice as to marriage, and you send me an excellent account of her symptoms. Her face which last year showed rosy cheeks and lips, has become pale and bloodless, her heart palpitates at every movement, and the pulse is visible in the temporal arteries; she loses her breath when dancing or going upstairs, she dislikes her food, especially meat, and her legs swell towards evening, particularly about the ankles. I marvel that your physicians have not diagnosed the case from such typical symptoms. It is the affection, which the women of Brabant call the "white fever," or love sickness, for lovers are always pale, but there is very rarely any fever.

The green sickness or lovesickness found expression in paintings by members of the Dutch School, especially Jan Steen, and in plays of Shakespeare, which refer to its existence among males[3] as well as among females.[4]

It was Thomas Sydenham in 1681[5] who recognized the therapeutic value of iron in chlorosis:

> To the worn-out and languid blood, it gives a spur or fillip, whereby the animal spirits, which before lay prostrate and sunken under their own weight, are raised and excited. Clear proof of this is found in the effects of steel upon chlorosis. The pulse gains strength and frequency, the surface warmth, the face (no longer pale

and death-like) a fresh ruddy colour. Here, however, I must remark that with weak and worn-out patients the bleeding and purging may be omitted, and the steel be begun with at once.

Next to steel in substance, I prefer a syrup. This is made by steeping iron or steel filings in cold Rhenish wine. When the wine is sufficiently impregnated, strain the liquor; add sugar; and boil to the consistency of syrup.

As has often been the case in medicine, effective therapy was discovered long before rational understanding of the disease was achieved. In 1713, Lemery and Geoffroy[6] demonstrated the presence of iron in the ash of blood. More than a century later, in 1832, Pierre Blaud[7] reported success in the treatment of chlorosis with pills containing ferrous sulfate and potassium carbonate, each pill providing 64 mg of iron. He wrote, "the treatment is ferruginous preparations, modifiers of the organism, which return to the blood the exciting principle which it has lost, that is to say the coloring substance." The same year, Foedisch[8] showed that chlorotic blood had a diminished content of iron.

These clinical and laboratory findings were soon amplified by studies on the chemistry of the coloring substance of the blood. In 1838, Lecanu isolated hematin and analyzed its composition.[9] A decade later, Reichert crystallized guinea-pig hemoglobin,[10] and in 1851, Funke crystallized hemoglobin from horse blood.[11] Shortly thereafter, in 1857, Teichmann crystallized hemin free of protein.[12] It remained for Hoppe-Seyler in 1864 to show that the blood pigment, which he named hemoglobin, can be split into hematin and a protein.[13] In 1894, Hüfner established that the iron content of hemoglobin is 0.335 percent and, on the basis of an oxygen capacity of 1.34 ml per gram of hemoglobin, calculated that one molecule of oxygen is combined with one atom of iron.[14]

This greatly increased knowledge of the chemistry of hemoglobin was complementary to the studies of Hayem on erythrocytes and hemoglobin in chlorosis. He observed that the average size of the erythrocytes declines from a normal diameter of 7.5 μm to as little as 6 μm and that the amount of hemoglobin per cell is decreased in chlorosis.[15]

Despite these chemical and morphologic findings and the demonstrated effectiveness of iron in the treatment of chlorosis, the mechanism of action of iron was the subject of controversy. Bunge, who demonstrated the presence of iron in hemoglobin, believed that synthetic processes do not occur in animals and refused to credit the idea that iron is absorbed from the gastrointestinal tract and is utilized in the synthesis of hemoglobin.[16] Von Noorden in 1912 argued that iron served to stimulate hematopoiesis but that this effect was unrelated to its presence as a component of the hemoglobin molecule.[17] On the other hand, Stockman[18] demonstrated that in chlorotic women treated with iron parenterally or orally there was a significant increase in hemoglobin, whereas no response occurred to bismuth, arsenic, manganese, or hydrochloric acid; he also showed that the iron content in the diet of chlorotic girls was much less than that in a normal diet.[19]

The question of the therapeutic value of iron was addressed by G.H. Whipple and his associates, who studied the influence of various dietary factors on the regeneration of hemoglobin and erythrocytes in dogs made anemic by bleeding. These were mentioned in Chapter 1. In acute experiments in which dogs were bled one-fourth of their blood volume on each of 2 successive days, beef muscle, beef heart, and cooked liver were found to promote blood regeneration, whereas iron given as Blaud's pills had no favorable influence.[20] Their conclusion that iron was of no value in the treatment of simple anemia of blood loss was not long sustained, however. In 1925, they wrote, "The history of anemia treatment with drugs is indeed a tale to make the judicious grieve. A multitude of drugs have been proposed, enthusiastically supported, then questioned and finally abandoned. . . . On the whole, iron seems to enjoy the most constant favor by practicing physicians." They then reported that in chronic severe anemia of blood loss, iron was clearly of value. They declared, however, that it is probable that in human beings, food factors (by which they meant various meat products) will be found more efficient in the control of simple anemia than iron or other drugs. They also believed that even in complex anemias (human pernicious anemia, anemia with nephritis, and cancer cachexia) food factors deserve serious consideration in the clinical management of the blood condition.[21] The confusion which their studies made so evident is explained by the fact that their experiments were conducted before physicians learned to differentiate the various types of anemia (Chapter 1). Fortunately, however, their work had a profound influence in stimulating Minot and Murphy to study the effects of liver and beef muscle in patients with pernicious anemia.

It remained for Heath, Strauss, and Castle to provide clear evidence of a close correspondence between the amount of iron given parenterally to patients with hypochromic anemia and the amount of iron gained in the circulating hemoglobin; they concluded that the iron "is apparently utilized to a very large extent in the building of new hemoglobin." They showed, too, that only a very small fraction of an oral dose of iron is absorbed and utilized for hemoglobin regeneration since 32 mg of iron given parenterally as iron and ammonium citrate was equivalent in its therapeutic effect to 1000 mg given orally.[22] Other studies by Reimann, Fritsch, and Schick showed that normal subjects given 100 mg of added ferrous iron in the diet daily excreted 99 percent of the iron whereas anemic subjects retained almost half of the orally administered iron.[23] The evidence was clear that in these patients with iron-responsive anemia, there was increased utilization of iron.[23]

In 1937, McCance and Widdowson presented evidence, derived from studies on iron balance in humans, that established the very limited capacity of the human organism for excretion of iron.[24] Their studies were conceptually very important for they led to the conclusion that the iron content of the body was controlled by the regulation of iron absorption and not of excretion. But balance studies were soon to be replaced by investigations made possible by the advent of the isotopic age.

"With the production of radioactive isotopes by the physicists and the concentration of naturally occurring isotopes by the chemists, the grateful physiologists have been presented with what may prove to be the 'Rosetta Stone' for the understanding and study of body metabolism." This statement by Hahn, Bale, Lawrence, and Whipple[25] was to prove valid very soon thereafter. With the aid of radioactive iron, a host of scientists began to study the absorption, transport, storage, and excretion of iron, and they convincingly demonstrated the utilization of food iron in the synthesis of hemoglobin. A detailed discussion of these and related studies, which span the past half-century, is far beyond the limits of our space. But it may be worth noting some highlights.

IRON TRANSPORT

In a normal human being, there is only about 3 to 4 mg of iron in the plasma. This iron, however, is of major importance for it represents the transport of iron, especially from sites of storage or absorption to immature red blood cells in the bone marrow, where it is utilized in the synthesis of hemoglobin. In 1925, Fontés and Thivolle observed nonhemoglobin iron in serum and concluded that "there is a circulating form of iron, capable of transporting, from storage organs to hematopoietic cells, the mineral element indispensable to the synthesis of hemoglobin."[26] Barkan[27] in 1927 showed that at physiological pH, the serum iron was not dialyzable or ultrafiltrable but that at an acid pH, iron was easily split off and appeared in the ultrafiltrate. The iron-binding protein was found in the globulin fraction on ammonium sulfate precipitation. Holmberg and Laurell[28,29] and Schade and Caroline[30] independently observed that the addition of iron to serum produces a salmon-pink color which is maximal when the iron-binding capacity is saturated. Although other metal ions, such as copper, can also combine with the iron-binding protein, the high affinity for iron prompted Holmberg and Laurell to name the protein transferrin. The authoritative review by Laurell on the transport and metabolism of iron proved to be highly influential in drawing the attention of scholars in this field to the physiologic significance of transferrin.[31] After the earlier plasma fractionation studies of Surgenor et al.,[32] Koechlin succeeded in crystallizing human transferrin in 1952.[33] Laurell and Ingelman[34] and Laurell[35] were similarly successful in isolating and crystallizing transferrin from swine serum.

The past three decades have witnessed an extraordinary range of studies on transferrin, including its physical and chemical properties (it has a molecular weight of 77,000, is a single polypeptide chain, has two iron-binding sites, and binds the anions, preferably carbonate, concomitantly with iron); the genetic polymorphism of human transferrins with at least 19 known genetic variants; its biosynthesis, principally in the liver; its almost equal distribution between the plasma and interstitial fluid; and the concentrations of transferrin and its degree of saturation with iron in various human diseases, especially in iron-deficiency anemia and in iron storage excess. These studies are summarized in numerous reviews and monographs.[36–39]

The studies of Jandl and his colleagues on the mechanism of transfer of iron from plasma transferrin to immature erythroid cells established the concept of specific receptors for transferrin on the surface of these cells.[40,41] Much work in recent years has addressed the question of whether this transfer involves the entry of transferrin into the cell[42] or whether the transferrin releases its iron at the receptor site and is then dissociated from the receptor; this question remains a subject of debate. Rapid progress, however, has been made on the chemical characterization of the transferrin receptors. Aisen has found that the transferrin receptor of the rabbit reticulocyte is a glycoprotein, an asymmetric molecule, apparently composed of two subunits of approximately equal size, with a molecular weight of 175,000.[43,44]

FERROKINETICS

Ferrokinetic analysis was introduced by Huff and his associates in 1950[45] and has proved valuable in the study of various hematopoietic disorders, especially as the techniques of analysis have been progressively refined by Finch,[46,47] Pollycove,[48] Ricketts,[49] and their associates.

ABSORPTION

From the time the studies of McCance and Widdowson focused attention on the control of the iron content of the body by the regulation of absorption, this regulatory process has been the subject of extensive investigation by many workers, especially Moore and his colleagues,[50] Cook et al.,[51] Crosby,[52] Bothwell,[53] and Worwood et al.[54] These studies have been concerned with factors in the intestinal lumen affecting the absorption of food iron, control mechanisms in the intestinal mucosal cell, the exchange of iron between transferrin and iron stores, and the possibility that humoral factors signal the body's iron requirements. Despite a great deal of excellent work, the regulatory process remains to be elucidated.

IRON STORAGE

Approximately 25 percent of the body iron is stored as a complex of iron and protein. These iron-protein complexes exist in two principal forms, ferritin and hemosiderin. Ferritin is a red-brown protein, widely distributed in animal cells; in mammals it is especially abundant in the liver, spleen, and bone marrow. It serves to store iron for subsequent utilization in the synthesis of heme and iron compounds and to sequester iron, which, when free, may be toxic. In 1937, Laufberger[55] crystallized ferritin from horse spleen, established its high content of iron, and suggested its storage function. Granick subsequently isolated ferritin in crystalline form from various species and tissues, demonstrated the removal of iron on reduction to yield the iron-free apoferritin, and observed the increased presence of ferritin in response to an increased concentration of iron. Ferritin was found to contain 17 to 23 percent by dry weight of iron; apoferritin was shown to be a large molecule with a molecular weight of 460,000.[56]

These studies paved the way for extensive work by numerous investigators on the detailed structure of ferritin, the mechanisms of uptake and release of iron, the existence of multiple structural forms differing in amino-acid composition, the role of iron in the regulation of the biosynthesis of ferritin, and the presence and clinical significance of ferritins in serum. For reviews of these subjects, the reader is referred to Crichton,[57] Harrison et al.,[58] Drysdale,[59] and Munro and Linder.[60]

Hemosiderin is found in iron overload disorders, in which iron is accumulated, especially in the cellular organelles that contain various hydrolytic enzymes (lysosomes). Hemosiderin is insoluble and has the appearance of golden yellow granules on light microscopy. It is probably derived in part from ferritin, but it may also consist of other forms of colloidal iron.[61]

The understanding of diseases of excess iron stores, in which there is markedly increased deposition of ferritin and hemosiderin, was greatly advanced by the monograph of Sheldon published in 1935.[62] Therapeutic phlebotomy for the removal of excess iron was first introduced in 1947 by Finch[63] and was subsequently confirmed in many other studies.[64] An alternative approach to the removal of iron was made possible by the development of desferrioxamine, a powerful agent for the chelation of iron, prepared from the fermentation of *Streptomyces pilosus*.[65] The use of desferrioxamine, particularly in the treatment of tissue siderosis observed in thalassemic patients with chronic hemolytic anemia requiring blood transfusion, represents a significant recent advance in therapy.[66]

But what has happened to chlorosis, which provided the impetus for so much of modern hematology? In a thoughtful review, "Chlorosis—An Obituary," W.M. Fowler[67] noted the declining incidence of the disorder, which "seems destined to occupy only a niche in medical history rather than the prominent place among blood dyscrasias which it has held in the past." The reasons for the disappearance of the disorder are not clear, although better differentiation of iron deficiency from other causes of hypochromic anemia is certainly a factor. But the very existence of chlorosis was challenged by Richard Cabot:[68]

It takes the eye of faith to see any justification for the title of the disease. If one exercises a great deal of imagination, one may possibly see the slightest imaginable tint of olive green in the shadow beneath the chin, but that is all. To the ordinary eye, the color is a yellowish pallor in brunettes and a whitish, although extreme, pallor in blondes.

Nevertheless, iron deficiency and iron-deficiency anemia, the probable fundamental pathogenetic factors underlying the syndrome of chlorosis, although usually not as clinically obvious or as severe as they once were, still are among the principal chronic medical disorders of the present day, especially in the less developed regions of the world.

The Respiratory Heme Pigments

In primitive societies and from earliest antiquity, respiration has been recognized as a prime feature of living organisms. Not until the seventeenth century, however, did discoveries concerning the circulation of the blood and the function of air in combustion provide a clearer understanding of the processes of respiration.* As told elsewhere (Chapter 1), in 1628, William Harvey discovered that the heart propels the blood which circulates from the left side of the heart via arteries to various organs and returns via veins to the right heart, after which it passes through the lungs and returns to the left heart. Somewhat later, Malpighi in 1661 and Leeuwenhoek in 1668 demonstrated the existence of the capillaries that provide for continuity in the circulation of the blood from arteries to veins.

At approximately the same time, Robert Boyle found that air was required for both combustion and life; when he pumped air out of a vessel in which he had placed a burning candle or a mouse or sparrow, the flame was extinguished and the animal or bird died (1660). Robert Hooke in 1667 recognized that when blood is exposed to air it becomes very "florid," and he predicted that blood from the pulmonary vein would show this change. Within 2 years, Richard Lower demonstrated that such is the case and concluded that blood takes up air in the lungs and then as the arterial blood circulates through the tissues, it gives up the air and acquires a dark venous color.

John Mayow, who graduated in law at Oxford and studied medicine as well, was a student of anatomy under Lower. At age 25 in 1668 he published a book, *Tractatus duo Quorum prior agit De Respiratione: Alter De Rachitide*, in which he assembled findings drawn from Boyle, Hooke, and Lower and presented

---

* In this discussion of the development of knowledge of heme compounds involved in cellular respiration, I have tried to summarize the highlights, as presented in the superb *The History of Cell Respiration and Cytochrome* by David Keilin, the discoverer of the cytochromes.[69] In this work, the reader will find extensive bibliographic references to the contributions by the various scientists whose work is cited here.

them in a form which emphasized that respiration and combustion consist in the combination of combustible materials with a portion of the air, that when animals breathe they draw this portion from the air, and that this portion of air is essential to life. His work went largely unrecognized at the time. More recent historians of science have tended to credit him with the discovery of oxygen or at least with anticipating by many years the definitive discoveries of Scheele and Lavoisier. This view, however, is severely criticized by T.S. Patterson[70] but Keilin valued Mayow's contributions more highly and stated that "no one before Lavoisier gave as coherent and correct an interpretation of the general processes of respiration or formulated his views so clearly as did Mayow."[69]

After these important seventeenth-century advances, there was relatively little progress in understanding respiration until mid-eighteenth century, when Joseph Black in 1755 showed that burning charcoal and breathing animals give off "fixed air." When this "fixed air" was removed by caustic alkali or lime, a large fraction of the air remained, which did not sustain life or a flame. This residual air was named nitrogen by Chaptal and azote by Lavoisier. In 1771 Joseph Priestley discovered that when he put a sprig of mint into a quantity of air in which a wax candle had previously burned out, another candle would burn well in it, "the mint had somehow restored the air which had previously been injured" by the candle flame. Priestley was observing photosynthesis, but he did not recognize the part played by sunlight in his experiments. It remained for Ingen-Housz in 1779 and Senebier in 1782 to demonstrate the effect of light in the production of oxygen by plants.

In the course of extensive studies which overthrew the phlogiston theory, Lavoisier in 1777 showed experimentally that respiration involves only a portion of the air, the oxygen, and that the remainder, nitrogen, is unaltered.[69] He and Laplace in 1780 established the quantitative relationship between respiration and animal heat production, and in 1789, Seguin and Lavoisier correlated measurable physical activity and respiratory activity as estimated by oxygen uptake and carbonic acid output.

But still Lavoisier failed to recognize that respiratory activity occurs principally in peripheral tissues and not exclusively in the lungs and blood. It was Lazaro Spallanzini who first showed, at the eighteenth century's end, that organisms lacking lungs take up O_2 and give off CO_2 and that these processes occur in all tissues of the body.[69]

An important next step was the finding of Georg Liebig in 1850 that when a frog's leg muscle is separated from the body, it is capable of taking up oxygen and producing carbon dioxide in the absence of circulation. He concluded that the blood acts to transport the oxygen and carbon dioxide but that the respiration itself occurs in the tissues.[71]

Slightly more than a decade later, major progress in the chemistry of the pigment of red blood cells was achieved. As noted earlier, in 1862 and 1864,

Hoppe-Seyler discovered the absorption spectrum of the oxygen-carrying pigment and determined that it is a complex protein, which he named hemoglobin, and which can be split into hematin and a protein.[13]

The work of Hoppe-Seyler on the absorption spectrum of hemoglobin attracted the attention of George Gabriel Stokes, one of the triumvirate which also included James Clark Maxwell and Lord Kelvin and which established the fame of the University of Cambridge school of physics. Stokes found that hemoglobin "is capable of existing in two states of oxidation (i.e., oxygenation), distinguishable by a difference of colour and a fundamental difference in the action on the spectrum. It may be made to pass from the more to the less oxidized state by the action of suitable reducing agents and recovers its oxygen by absorption from the air." Stokes inquired whether the change of color from arterial to venous blood could be imitated chemically by reduction. He added ferrous ammonium tartrate (Stokes' solution) to blood and obtained a purple red color and a change in absorption spectrum from two dark bands to one broader band intermediate between the two. On exposure of the purple solution to air, it quickly returned to its original color and showed the original two bands again.[72]

With this added knowledge of the chemistry of hemoglobin and with the earlier studies of Liebig that demonstrated oxygen uptake and carbon dioxide production in muscle isolated from the circulation, Pflüger and his associates[73,74] carried out quantitative studies which demonstrated that the respiratory activity of an organism occurs in the cells and tissues. Oertmann in Pflüger's laboratory replaced the blood of a frog with physiologic salt solution and showed that the respiratory activity was unchanged.[75] They concluded that respiration is an intracellular process and that the principal function of hemoglobin is the transport of oxygen.

The mechanism of tissue respiration was considered by Claude Bernard in his *Leçons sur les phenomènes de la vié communs aux animaux et aux végétaux* (1878–1879).[69] He emphasized the relationship between respiration and fermentation and argued that the production of carbon dioxide is the result of a decomposition analogous to those which are produced by fermentations. He acknowledged that he could not explain the role of oxygen, but he criticized the simplistic idea that the function of oxygen is to sustain combustion because he claimed that respiration does not in fact involve true combustion.

It was shortly thereafter that a major discovery involving intracellular respiration occurred, but it was destined to be unappreciated for 40 years. This discovery was made by Charles Alexander MacMunn, a practicing physician in Wolverhampton, England. MacMunn was born in Ireland and received his medical education at Trinity College, Dublin. At the young age of 22 he began to practice medicine in Wolverhampton, where he stayed for the rest of his life. Shortly after starting in practice, he built a small laboratory in the hayloft over his stables. His large practice allowed little time for research—a half hour after lunch, a few minutes in the afternoon, but principally in the evenings after dinner. However, as his wife wrote:[76]

> His research problems were always on his mind and during his medical rounds he had the habit of writing down his ideas on his shirt cuffs so that he could try them out at the next opportunity. When, some time later, he received a grant from the Birmingham Philosophical Society to build a small laboratory in his garden, he had a small horizontal iron pipe built into the wall, the purpose of which was to enable him to see which patients were coming up the garden path so that if he did not wish to interrupt his work, he could warn the maid to say he was out.

In 1884, at the age of 32, and in further publications in 1886 and 1887, MacMunn described a pigment which he observed spectroscopically in the muscles and other tissues of invertebrates and vertebrates. In the reduced state, it showed four absorption bands; when oxidized, the absorption bands disappeared. He recognized that the pigment was a hemoprotein which he called "myohematin" when present in muscle and "histohematin" in other tissues. He appreciated the importance of his finding and wrote:

> These respiratory proteids, detected in the solid organs and tissues of animals by means of the microspectroscope . . . are so important as haemoglobin, if not more so in some animals, and they have the right of priority in time, as they were developed at an earlier period than haemoglobin, speaking from a phylogenetic point of view. Even in the lowest of metazoa—the sponges—I have met histohaematins, where they are also capable of oxidation and reduction and are therefore respiratory.

And then he added:[77]

> If iron is necessary for the formation of myohaematin and the histohaematins, an interesting medical point is raised: and another equally interesting question is this: May not oxygen starvation of the tissues occur from a deficiency of the respiratory proteids? And if these are not present in quantity or quality sufficient for the discharge of tissue—or internal respiration, then metabolism cannot be properly performed in the various organs and tissues, and these may become laden with products of incomplete metamorphosis leading to the production of disease. These are not mere hypotheses, for I have definitely proved that myohaematin and the histohaematins are not themselves products of the metabolism of haemoglobin, but are mother substances of great importance from a physiological point of view.

MacMunn's work was challenged by Hoppe-Seyler (1825–1895),[78] who pointed out that MacMunn was in error in claiming that there was no hemoglobin in pigeon breast muscle, and he concluded that the spectrum observed by MacMunn was produced by hemoglobin and some hemochromogen. Hoppe-Seyler ignored, however, the abundant evidence of MacMunn that these respiratory pigments are present in the muscles of invertebrates, such as insects, which are devoid of hemoglobin.

So great was Hoppe-Seyler's authority that MacMunn's own confidence was shaken. Furthermore, the significance of MacMunn's findings was not appreciated by his contemporaries, in part because of the lack of evidence that these pigments undergo oxidation and reduction in living tissues untreated with oxidizing or reducing agents. The lack of acceptance of MacMunn's work was bitterly disappointing to him, and this disappointment, together with failing health due to malaria contracted during the Boer war, destroyed his confidence in his work and the incentive to continue it.[76]

For more than 30 years, MacMunn's findings lay dormant until they were rediscovered and fully appreciated by David Keilin of the Molteno Institute at the University of Cambridge. Keilin (1887–1963) (Chapter Opening Photo) was born in Moscow of Polish-Jewish parents. After attending the gymnasium in Warsaw, he pursued premedical studies in Liège and then moved to Paris, where he studied parasitology under Maurice Caullery in the Laboratoire d'Evolution des Etres Organisés. In 1914 he was invited by Nuttall to join the Quick laboratory in Cambridge, and then, with the establishment of the Molteno Institute in 1921; he became a member of its staff. Primarily a parasitologist, Keilin was interested in respiratory systems of dipterous larvae. In 1924, while studying the life cycle of the horse parasite *Gasterophilus intestinalis,* he observed the presence of a pigment with an absorption spectrum of four bands in the insect's muscles and found a similar spectrum in the muscles of the adult wax moth and the adult blowfly as well as in the aerobic microorganism *Bacillus subtilis* and baker's yeast. The pigment's presence in organisms devoid of hemoglobin showed that it was independent of hemoglobin and its derivatives. But then came the discovery of its reversible oxidation and reduction:[69]

One day, while I was examining a suspension of yeast freshly prepared from a few bits of compressed yeast shaken vigorously with a little water in a test-tube, I failed to find the characteristic four-banded absorption spectrum, but before I had time to remove the suspension from the field of vision of the microspectroscope, the four absorption bands suddenly reappeared. This experiment was repeated time after time and always with the same result: the absorption bands disappeared on shaking the suspension with air and reappeared within a few seconds on standing.

I must admit that this first visual perception of an intracellular respiratory process was one of the most impressive spectacles I have witnessed in the course of my work. Now I had no doubt that cytochrome is not only widely distributed in nature and completely independent of haemoglobin but that it is an intracellular respiratory pigment which is much more important than haemoglobin. On the other hand, the nature of the pigment showing four distinct absorption bands when it was in the reduced state, but none when it was oxidized, still remained very obscure. Although I had by this time a first-hand knowledge of the absorption spectra of haemoglobin and of all its derivatives, I could not find among them a compound which in the reduced state showed four characteristic absorption bands (a–d) occupying the following approximate positions: a, 604 mμ; b, 564 mμ; c, 550 mμ; and d, 521 mμ.

However, a careful spectroscopic study of yeast cells and of the thoracic muscles of insects under a great variety of conditions soon revealed that the complex spectrum of cytochrome is that of a mixture of three distinct haemochromogen-like compounds, the absorption bands, a, b and c being their α-bands while band d represents their β-bands fused into one complex absorption band showing several reinforcements (or maxima). Thus cytochrome was resolved into three haemochromogen components designated cytochrome a, cytochrome b and cytochrome c.

The realization that cytochrome must play an important part in cellular respiration induced me to put off further studies of the respiratory systems and respiratory adaptations in dipterous larvae and to enter a new field of research—that of the mechanism of intracellular oxidation.

Keilin's discovery of the cytochromes succeeded in synthesizing the conflicting views of Thunberg and Wieland, who were working with dehydrogenases, and those of Otto Warburg, who emphasized the activation of oxygen by an iron-containing enzyme which he called "respiratory ferment." Keilin provided experimental evidence that the cytochromes serve as the link between the dehydrogenases and the activation of oxygen—the three components of cytochrome act as hydrogen acceptors in relation to the dehydrogenases and their substrates and as hydrogen donors to cytochrome oxidase and oxygen.

The Structure of Heme and of Hemoglobin

Work on the structure of porphyrins began at the end of the nineteenth century. It has been summarized in the works of Willstäter and Stoll,[79] Hans Fischer,[80] and Lemberg and Legge.[81]

In 1913, Küster first suggested that the structure of heme is a cyclic tetrapyrrole joined by four methene bridges[82] (Figure 7-1). At that time, however, multimembered ring systems were not yet known, and this suggested structure was not accepted, but by 1929, Hans Fischer and his coworkers had achieved a complete synthesis of protoporphyrin and hemin. It was Willstäter who recognized that hemin is a complex iron salt of protoporphyrin and that chlorophyll is a complex magnesium salt of protoporphyrin. The synthesis of porphyrin compounds and the establishment of their definitive structure were major achievements of modern organic and biological chemistry and engaged the interest and effort of several of the world's outstanding organic biochemists.

The twentieth century has seen the definitive elucidation of the structure

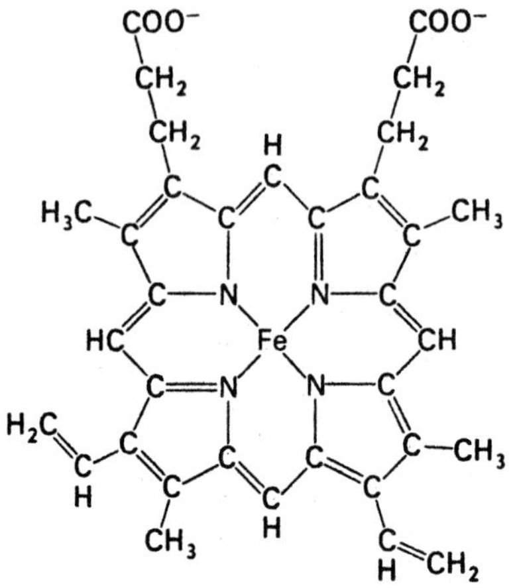

Figure 7-1 Heme.

of hemoglobin. On the basis of its iron content, the equivalent weight of hemoglobin was calculated to be 16,700, but this value provided only a minimum estimate of the size of the hemoglobin molecule. In 1924, G.S. Adair measured the osmotic pressure of hemoglobin solutions at low temperature with careful control of pH and obtained a molecular weight of 68,000, comprising four subunits of 16,700 each.[83] This was confirmed by Svedberg and Fåhraeus, who used the ultracentrifuge to establish the molecular weight.[84] After the development by Frederick Sanger of methods for determining the amino-acid sequence of proteins, the composition and amino-acid sequence of the human hemoglobins were established in studies in many laboratories. The shape and structure of the hemoglobin molecule were definitively established by the classical x-ray crystallographic studies of Max Perutz.[85]

The Biosynthesis of Heme and Porphyrin Compounds

Once the tetrapyrrole ring structure of heme was established, it was not unexpected that precursor compounds of somewhat similar ring structure would be proposed. Indeed, proline and glutamic acid, whose anhydride, pyrrolidone carboxylic acid, has a ring structure, were suggested as likely precursors. It was not until the advent of the isotopic age, however, that definitive determination of the biological precursors and the biosynthetic sequence in the formation of protoporphyrin and heme could be achieved.

When Harold Urey, of Columbia University, discovered the heavy stable isotope of hydrogen deuterium, the potential utility of this isotope for biochemical investigation was soon apparent to Rudolph Schoenheimer, who was working in the Department of Biochemistry at the College of Physicians and Surgeons of Columbia University. Schoenheimer (1898–1941) was a refugee from Nazi Germany who was welcomed into the hospitable department led by Hans T. Clarke. In a happy combination of humanitarianism and wise scientific judgment, Clarke gathered many outstanding biochemists fleeing from Nazi tyranny. When Schoenheimer approached Urey with the suggestion that deuterium be used in biochemical investigation, Urey proposed that one of his recent Ph.D. graduates, David Rittenberg (1906–1970) (Figure 7-2), be invited to join Schoenheimer in a collaborative effort. So was born a school of biochemistry which was to change our conceptions of the metabolic behavior of the body's constituents.

The principal contribution of Schoenheimer, Rittenberg, and their collaborators was the discovery that the body's constituents are continually being synthesized, converted, and degraded along specific pathways. After the untimely death of Schoenheimer in 1941, Rittenberg assumed the leadership of the laboratory. Among the gifted investigators who joined him were David Shemin (1911–   ) (Figure 7-3) and Konrad Bloch. Shemin and Rittenberg

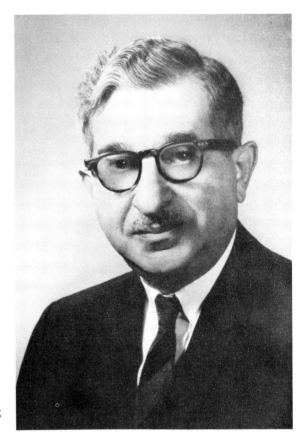

Figure 7-2 David Rittenberg (1906–1970).

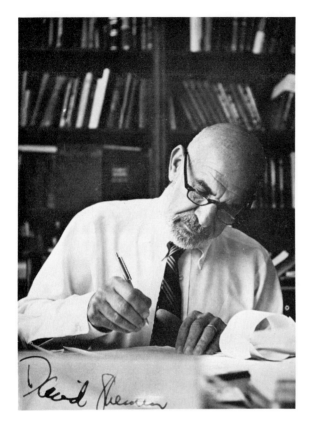

Figure 7-3   David Shemin (1911–   ).

were especially interested in studying the interconversions of amino acids. For this purpose, they employed amino acids labeled with ^{15}N, the heavy, stable isotope of nitrogen. In an experiment that was to prove extraordinarily important, Shemin ingested 66 g of the amino acid glycine labeled with ^{15}N.[86–87] The purpose of this experiment was to study the extent to which glycine serves as a nitrogenous precursor for other amino acids by its deamination or transamination. It was the basic principle of the laboratory that all biological specimens would be saved should they be needed for subsequent analysis during or after the experiment. The principal focus was on the isolation of various plasma proteins and the determination of the ^{15}N concentration in their constituent amino acids. The red blood cells which were saved were not analyzed until several weeks after the ingestion of the labeled glycine. Whereas the incorporation of glycine into the plasma proteins behaved in the classical manner of the dynamic state, i.e., it rose rapidly following ingestion to a peak concentration after which it declined in accordance with a first-order rate reaction, the incorporation of isotopic nitrogen into hemin demonstrated a strikingly different curve. The ^{15}N concentration rose to a peak after about 20 days and then maintained a plateau for several weeks following which it declined along an S-shaped curve (Figure 7-4). Two principal conclusions could be derived from this work. First, the isotope concentration in the heme derived from ^{15}N-labeled glycine was so high as to indicate clearly that glycine was serving as a specific nitrogenous precursor of the protoporphyrin of heme. The second conclusion was that the curve of isotope incorporation into the heme of hemoglobin was strikingly different from that of the isotope concentration in plasma proteins and indicated a quite different pattern of behavior metabolically; whereas plasma proteins are continually being synthesized and degraded, and the degradation is random and unrelated to the age of the plasma protein molecules, the heme of hemoglobin, once formed, remains stable during the life of the red blood cell and is degraded or disappears from the circulation only when the erythrocyte itself is destroyed. This conclusion was not reached without some difficulty, however. When one reviews the findings in this experiment, one observes that between the twenty-first and seventy-seventh day there were no other points on the curve. As Shemin recounts:[87a]

> The hemin isolated from the blood sample taken on the 77th day was analyzed and, much to our surprise, the ^{15}N concentration was very similar to that taken on the 18th day; that is, it had much more ^{15}N than we had anticipated. Since both Rittenberg and I were programmed to the concept that body constituents are in a continuous state of flux, we were indeed astonished to find that the ^{15}N analysis of

Figure 7-4 Labeling of cells with ^{15}N in the human subject. The abscissa gives the proportion of ^{15}N in the total nitrogen of heme; time is given in days. ^{15}N-labeled glycine was fed for 3 days at the beginning of the experiment.

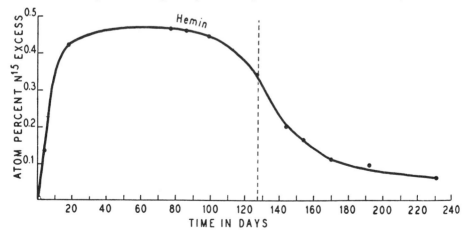

the hemin sample taken on the 77th day was similar to the one taken on the 18th day. We then had a serious discussion in which he more than mildly suggested that I either mixed up the samples or somehow contaminated the sample and I, offended by such an implication on my impeccable technique, suggested that his mass spectrometer was returning incorrect data. To settle the matter another hemin sample from the blood was isolated and the same result was found. We then realized hemoglobin, in contrast to all other proteins previously examined by these techniques, was not in the dynamic state and that its ^{15}N concentration over a period of time would reflect the life span of the red blood cell.

Some assurance of the correctness of this interpretation of the ^{15}N-hemin curve, which yielded an erythrocyte life span of 120 days, was derived from the earlier studies of Winifred Ashby,[88] as described in Chapter 8, and by the studies of Mollison and Young[89] and Callender, Powell, and Witts[90] on the survival of transfused cells in humans. Conclusive evidence that a plateau is maintained between approximately days 20 and 90 in normal humans was then provided in further experiments, which were conducted after I joined Shemin and Rittenberg in this work.[91] This method of biosynthetic labeling of erythrocyte hemoglobin was, and remains, the most physiologic of the techniques for the determination of the life span and pattern of survival or destruction of mammalian erythrocytes.

At about the same time, Konrad Bloch and David Rittenberg were studying the biosynthesis of cholesterol for which they employed isotopically labeled acetate. As a by-product of this work, they also examined the hemin of hemoglobin and noted a marked isotope incorporation into hemin from acetate.[92] This finding was subsequently to lead to the demonstration that the immediate precursor of heme in addition to glycine is succinyl coenzyme A.

A further step in the evolution of knowledge on the biosynthesis of heme derived from the demonstration that heme synthesis occurs in vitro in immature erythrocytes. After joining Rittenberg's laboratory in 1946, I studied the life span of the erythrocyte not only in normal humans but also in patients with pernicious anemia, sickle-cell anemia, and polycythemia vera. These studies provided further evidence that the normal human erythrocyte life span is approximately 120 days; but in addition, they demonstrated that in sickle-cell anemia, there is an accelerated random destruction of erythrocytes, in pernicious anemia there is a significant measure of random accelerated destruction of erythrocytes, and in polycythemia vera there is an increased formation of erythrocytes with a normal life span. The curve of isotope incorporation into the erythrocytes of normal humans indicated that heme was synthesized in erythrocyte precursors in the bone marrow after which it remained stable within the mature erythrocyte throughout the life span of the cell. In the course of discussing these studies with Clement Finch and Charles Rath, then in Boston, they raised the question of whether the reticulocyte might still be able to synthesize heme. Since reticulocytes were readily available in the peripheral blood of patients with sickle-cell anemia, I incubated the blood of such patients in vitro with isotopically labeled glycine. The hemin indeed became labeled, thus indicating the synthesis of heme from glycine in vitro. Mature human erythrocytes incubated under the same conditions did not synthesize heme in vitro.[93] To have a more readily available source of reticulocytes, I took advantage of a method described by Cecil Watson, who used acetylphenylhydrazine to produce hemolytic anemia in animals and, thereby, evoke an increased production of reticulocytes. Rabbit reticulocytes produced in this manner or by repeated bleeding synthesized heme in vitro at a very appreciable rate.[94]

The demonstration that the nonnucleated, immature erythrocyte is capable of synthesizing heme was contrary to the usually accepted belief that hemoglobin formation was complete prior to the loss of the nucleus from the erythroid cell in the bone marrow. In seeking a biological system which might be even more active in synthesis of heme in vitro, Shemin and I turned to the nucleated erythrocytes of birds because large amounts of blood would be readily available and it was possible that the nucleated cells would be more active than the nonnucleated reticulocytes of mammals. We found that the nucleated erythrocytes of the duck not only synthesize heme but also synthesize globin, with the synthesis of the protein occurring at approximately the same rate as that of heme.[95,96] This biosynthetic capacity, however, appears to derive from a normal reticulocytosis, up to 20 percent, in the blood of ducks and not from the fact that the erythrocytes are nucleated. It is perhaps amusing that as city dwellers we were bleeding ducks in the mistaken notion that they were geese. Thanks to Dr. G.L. Foster, the correct identification of the source of the avian blood was made. In these experiments, peptide bond synthesis was demonstrated for the first time in vitro. In subsequent years, the reticulocyte and reticulocyte lysate would prove to be the most productive system for the study of protein synthesis in animal cells.

In complementary experiments, Finch and his associates demonstrated that reticulocytes are capable of incorporating radioactive iron into the heme of hemoglobin in vitro.[97]

The in vitro system of heme synthesis made it possible to perform large numbers of experiments under carefully controlled conditions utilizing relatively small amounts of expensive isotopically labeled compounds. In the course of the next decade, Shemin and his graduate students and postdoctoral fellows carried out a classic series of experiments, which determined several of the principal elements of the biosynthetic sequence of heme[98] (Figure 7-5). They demonstrated that the amino group of glycine was equally utilized for all four pyrrole units of heme. Furthermore, they found that whereas the alpha carbon atom of glycine is utilized for porphyrin synthesis, the carboxyl group is not so utilized. This negative finding was an important clue to the mechanism by which glycine was utilized. With doubly labeled glycine

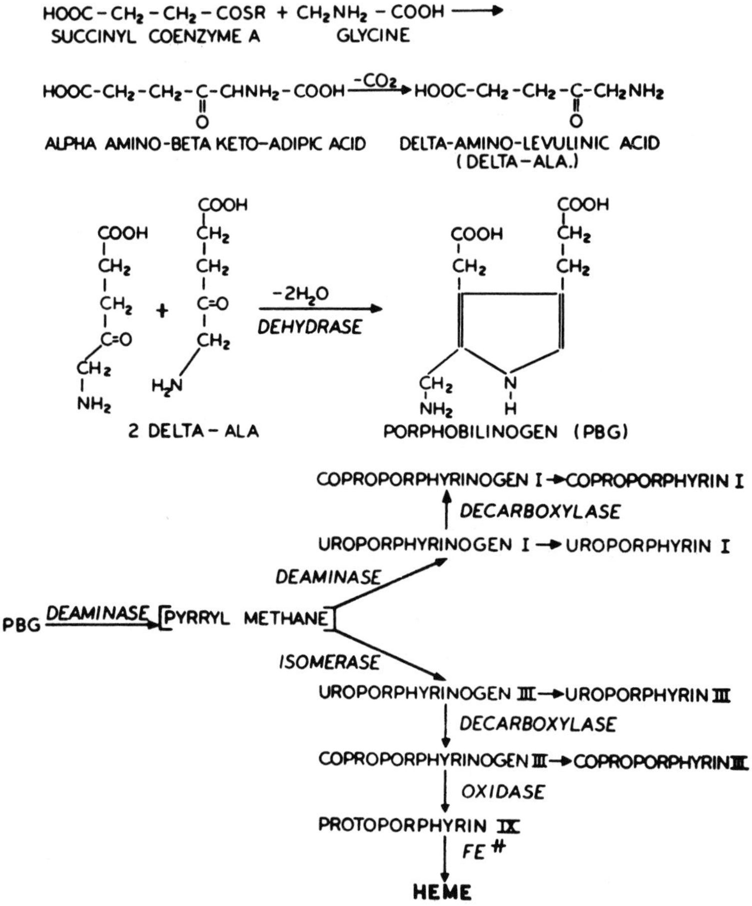

Figure 7-5 The biosynthesis of heme.

($^{15}NH_2{}^{14}CH_2COOH$), they found that the dilution of the nitrogen atom was twice that of the alpha carbon atom, i.e., for each nitrogen atom utilized, two carbon atoms from the alpha carbon atom of glycine entered the porphyrin molecule. To locate the positions in the porphyrin molecule of the carbon atoms derived from the alpha carbon atom of glycine, a procedure for the chemical degradation of protoporphyrin was developed which made it possible to identify the individual carbon atoms. The alpha carbon atom of glycine was found to serve as the source of the four methene bridges, and one carbon atom in each pyrrole ring was also derived from the alpha carbon atom of glycine, in each case in the alpha position under the vinyl and propionic acid side chains. These findings supported the proposal that a common precursor pyrrole was first formed and that the vinyl side chains arose from propionic acid side chains by decarboxylation and dehydrogenation. The next step was to determine the origin of the remaining 26 carbon atoms of the porphyrin ring. Konrad Bloch and Rittenberg had earlier shown that acetic acid labeled with deuterium led to the synthesis of hemin containing deuterium. This finding indicated that at least some of the carbon atoms of side chains of the porphyrin ring were derived from the methyl group of acetate. To determine how many of the carbon atoms might be derived from acetate, duck erythrocytes were incubated with either ^{14}C methyl-labeled acetate or with ^{14}C carboxyl-labeled acetate, and the resulting ^{14}C-labeled hemin samples were degraded chemically. All the carbon atoms were shown to be derived from acetate. The pattern of isotopic labeling of the carbon atoms of heme indicated that the acetic acid enters as a unit and that the utilization of acetic acid for pyrrole formation is by way of a 4-carbon compound. This 4-carbon compound was shown to be succinate, derived from acetate by the tricarboxylic acid cycle. The next question was to determine how all four atoms of succinate are utilized and yet only the amino group and alpha carbon atom of glycine are used. This consideration led to the hypothesis that succinate and glycine condense to form a 6-carbon compound, α-amino-β-ketoadipic acid, which then undergoes decarboxylation to yield δ-aminolevulinic acid. This hypothesis was proved to be correct, and it was shown that all the carbon atoms of protoporphyrin are derived from δ-aminolevulinic acid.[98] These findings were soon confirmed by Neuberger and Scott[99] and by Dresel and Falk.[100]

Independently, an organic chemist, R.G. Westall, succeeded in isolating and crystallizing porphobilinogen,[101] the product first shown by Waldenström and Vahlquist to be excreted in the urine of patients with acute intermittent porphyria.[102] Cookson and Rimington[103] then determined that porphobilinogen has a structure identical with that postulated for the precursor pyrrole derived from the condensation of glycine and succinate, namely, a monopyrrole with acetic acid and propionic acid side chains. Neuberger and Scott showed that δ-aminolevulinic acid and porphobilinogen are equally well utilized for heme synthesis.

In our initial studies on the biosynthesis of heme in duck erythrocytes and rabbit reticulocytes, the synthesis of heme from glycine was observed only in intact cells or in cells gently hemolyzed with water but not in preparations homogenized in a blender. Sano and Granick[104] studied the localization of porphyrin biosynthetic enzymes and found that the first enzyme in the series, δ-aminolevulinic acid synthetase, is bound to mitochondria. They found that the enzyme responsible for the oxidation of coproporphyrinogen to protoporphyrin, coproporphyrinogen oxidase, also is a mitochondrial enzyme. The enzymes responsible for the steps intermediate between δ-aminolevulinic acid and coproporphyrinogen are found in the soluble portion of the cell. The final enzyme in the pathway, which is responsible for the insertion of iron into protoporphyrin, called ferrochelatase or heme synthetase, also is a mitochondrial enzyme, which has been found in several tissues and micro-organisms.[105–107]

During the past two decades and more, the individual steps in the biosynthesis of heme have engaged the attention of numerous workers in laboratories throughout the world and are discussed in several excellent reviews.[108–111] A few points deserve particular mention. Uroporphyrins and coproporphyrins were recognized early in the twentieth century as excretion products in the urine of patients with porphyria. It remained for Neve, Labbe, and Aldrich[112] and then, Bogorad[113] to recognize that the colorless reduced forms of uroporphyrin and coproporphyrin, namely, uroporphyrinogen and coproporphyrinogen, are the true metabolic intermediates between porpho-bilinogen and protoporphyrin IX.

The conversion of porphobilinogen to uroporphyrinogen I and to uro-porphyrinogen III deserves special attention. In 1953, Bogorad and Granick[114] (Figure 7-6) demonstrated that at least two enzymes are involved in the

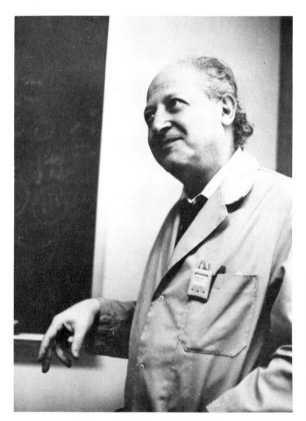

Figure 7-6 Sam Granick (1909–1977). Granick was a product of New York City public schools and earned degrees in physical chemistry and biochemistry from the University of Michigan. His doctoral thesis in plant physi-ology foreshadowed his sub-sequent work on chlorophyll.

synthesis of uroporphyrinogen III from porphobilinogen and that the two enzymes can be differentiated on the basis of their susceptibility to heat. Uroporphyrinogen I synthetase (porphobilinogen deaminase) is heat-stable and results in the formation from porphobilinogen of uroporphyrinogen I. Uroporphyrinogen III cosynthetase (porphobilinogen isomerase) is heat-labile; when it is incubated with porphobilinogen alone, there is no utilization of the porphobilinogen. However, on incubation of the uroporphyrinogen III co-synthetase with uroporphyrinogen I synthetase and porphobilinogen, uro-porphyrinogen III is produced. Clearly, the joint action of the two enzymes is required for the conversion of porphobilinogen to uroporphyrinogen III, the intermediate which is required for the formation of coproporphyrinogen III and, then, protoporphyrin IX.

Granick and Urata[115] carried out a detailed study of the enzymes of porphyrin biosynthesis in normal liver. They found that while the activity of δ-aminolevulinic acid synthetase (ALA synthetase) could barely be detected, considerable quantities of the other enzymes of the biosynthetic chain were present; ALA synthetase appeared to be rate limiting in porphyrin synthesis. Support for this view was provided by showing that in a chemical porphyria induced in guinea pigs by feeding a compound abbreviated DDC[115] the overproduction of porphyrin and porphyrin precursors in the liver resulted from a specific increase in the activity of ALA synthetase, which, as noted above, is a mitochondrial enzyme. Since incubation of the mitochondria from normal guinea pig liver with porphyria-inducing chemicals did not enhance the activity of this enzyme, it appeared that the increased activity was due to a de novo synthesis of the enzyme rather than to the activation of the inactive enzyme. In subsequent work, Granick[116] showed that an increase in the activity of ALA synthetase resulting in increased porphyrin formation could be induced in liver parenchyma cells in vitro by porphyria-inducing chemicals. The action of these chemicals is, therefore, a direct one on the liver cells rather than an indirect one through hormone action. The key to the mechanism of action of the porphyria-inducing chemicals was found in studies utilizing inhibitors of nucleic acid and protein synthesis which prevented the induction of ALA synthetase by DDC. These findings indicate that the porphyria-inducing drugs depress the formation of ALA synthetase by interfering in an as yet undetermined manner with the repressor control mechanism.

There is evidence from the work of several laboratories that heme controls its own synthesis by end-product inhibition of the activity of ALA synthetase. The first evidence for this mechanism derived from studies in the bacterium *Rhodopseudomonas spheroides* by Lascelles,[117] Gibson et al.,[118] and Burnham and Lascelles.[119]

To determine whether a similar mechanism obtains in mammalian erythroid cells, Doris Karibian and I studied the effect of hemin on the synthesis of heme in rabbit reticulocytes.[120] We found that whereas glycine utilization was inhibited by approximately 50 percent in the presence of $10^{-4}M$ added hemin, the utilization of δ-aminolevulinic acid was inhibited only slightly or not at all. This finding indicated that heme was inhibiting the formation of δ-aminolevulinic acid, a finding amply confirmed by Freedman et al.[121] Since the mammalian reticulocyte has no nucleus and is not capable of synthesizing ribonucleic acid, the effect of heme could not be ascribed to repression. It seemed most likely that heme was inhibiting the activity of ALA synthetase. Such inhibition of the enzyme was subsequently demonstrated in several studies,[122-124] although results in other laboratories have sometimes not been confirmatory, probably because of the difficulty in dealing with this mitochondrial particulate enzyme. With evidence that heme can repress the synthesis of ALA synthetase and that it can inhibit the formation of ALA, Donald Tschudy and his colleagues were prompted to investigate the effect of administration of hematin by intravenous infusion in a patient with acute intermittent porphyria. Although no clinical improvement occurred, there was an impressive decline in the excretion of plasma porphyrin precursors.[125] Subsequently, Cecil Watson (Figure 7-7) and his associates demonstrated in several patients with acute intermittent porphyria not only a marked decline in the production of ALA and porphobilinogen but also a marked amelioration of the neurological symptoms and signs in these patients.[126-128] Subsequently, Watson and his associates also demonstrated the repression by hematin of porphyrin biosynthesis in erythroid precursors in congenital erythropoietic porphyria.[129]

The Conversion of Heme to Bile Pigment

During the first decades of this century, bile pigment in the mammal was assumed to be derived exclusively, or very nearly so, from the hemoglobin of mature circulating erythrocytes. Indeed, measurements of bile pigment excretion in the feces were used to calculate a hemolytic index of erythrocyte destruction.[130] G.H. Whipple suggested that bile pigment is derived to a significant extent from sources other than the hemoglobin of circulating erythrocytes,[131] but conclusive evidence to support this suggestion was not available. The findings that glycine is specifically utilized in the synthesis of heme and that the administration of ^{15}N-glycine affords a method for determining the life span and pattern of destruction of erythrocytes made it possible to investigate the problem of the biologic origin of bile pigment in human beings. From our previous studies, it appeared that very few of the mature circulating erythrocytes are destroyed before day 40 and that maximal destruction occurred between approximately 100 and 145 days. Accordingly, if bile pigment were derived solely from the hemoglobin of mature circulating erythrocytes, no significant concentration of ^{15}N should be observed in the bile pigment during the first 6 weeks after the administration of ^{15}N-glycine. It was important that the bile pigment be pure, for otherwise erroneous conclu-

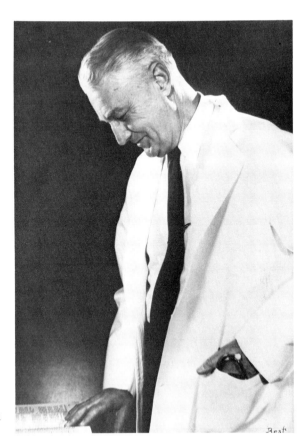

Figure 7-7 Cecil J. Watson (1901—   ).

sions might be drawn from isotopically labeled contaminants. Fortunately, Cecil Watson, who first successfully isolated stercobilin in Hans Fischer's laboratory,[132] had perfected the method of its isolation and crystallization from feces. During a very pleasant week in his laboratory in 1947, I learned the method and came to appreciate his admiration for Fischer, of whom it was said, "Er spuckt in die Hand, es kristalliert sofort aus."*[133]

Our studies in normal humans revealed that during the first 8 days after the administration of ^{15}N-glycine, when there is apparently no destruction of mature circulating erythrocytes containing labeled hemoglobin, the ^{15}N concentration in the stercobilin is very high[134] (Figure 7-8). A portion of the stercobilin, at least 11 percent, must be derived from sources other than the hemoglobin of mature circulating erythrocytes. This "early labeled" bile-pigment fraction is found greatly increased in pernicious anemia[135] and

---

* "He spits in his hand, and it crystallizes!"

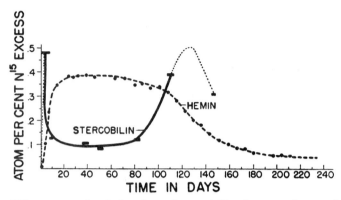

Figure 7-8   [15]N concentration in hemin and stercobilin of a normal man after the start of feeding ^{15}N-labeled glycine for 2 days.

congenital erythropoietic porphyria[136] and in hematologic disorders characterized by ineffective erythropoiesis. The hemoglobin of newly formed erythrocytes destroyed in the bone marrow was recognized as a likely source of bile pigment, and the respiratory heme pigments, as well as myoglobin, were considered as additional possible sources.[134] The demonstration that heme, not bound to globin, is readily converted to bile pigment[137] lent support to the idea that free heme, or heme compounds other than hemoglobin, can serve as precursors of bile pigment. Subsequent studies in several laboratories have shown that heme production in the liver can serve to increase the early labeled pigment fraction.[138] Whereas in normal humans, the hemoglobin of mature circulating erythrocytes is the source of about 85 percent of bile pigment, in hematologic disorders characterized by ineffective erythropoiesis and in conditions of increased formation of hepatic heme, the early labeled pigment fraction is greatly increased.

The mechanism of conversion of hemoglobin to bilirubin has been shown to involve a microsomal enzyme, heme oxygenase, which splits out the α-methene carbon atom of heme, yielding carbon monoxide and biliverdin.[139]

The Role of Heme in the Regulation of Protein Synthesis

During the past 15 years, there has been gradual elucidation of a new role of heme in metabolic processes, the regulation of the initiation of protein synthesis in eukaryotic cells. These studies began with an attempt to answer an apparently simple clinical question—in patients with iron-deficiency anemia, the administration of iron is followed not only by an increase in the hemoglobin of circulating erythrocytes but there is also a reticulocytosis, i.e., the delivery of an increased number of immature erythrocytes to the peripheral blood from the bone marrow. Although the reticulocytosis could result in part from a diminution in the destruction of erythroid cells in the bone marrow, it seemed reasonable to investigate the question of whether the administration of iron or of heme was affecting other processes, such as the synthesis of nucleic acids or the synthesis of protein. Previous studies by Kruh and Borsook,[140] by Kassenaar, Morell, and Savoie in our laboratory,[141,142] and by Nizet[143] had shown that the synthesis of protein by reticulocytes and by bone marrow erythroid cells is greatly enhanced by the addition of iron to the incubation medium. Iron also promotes the synthesis of heme by serving as a substrate for incorporation into protoporphyrin and by serving as a cofactor in the synthesis of δ-aminolevulinic acid. Evidence that the synthesis of heme and the synthesis of globin proceed at parallel rates, i.e., one heme molecule for each α or β chain of globin, raised the question of the existence of a mechanism for the coordination of the synthesis of heme and of globin.

In collaboration with Dr. Gail Bruns and Doris Karibian, I investigated the effect of heme not only on its own synthesis but also on the synthesis of protein in rabbit reticulocytes.[144] We found that heme regulates its own synthesis by inhibition of the formation of δ-aminolevulinic acid, but, quite remarkably, heme promotes the synthesis of the protein of the reticulocyte (Figure 7-9).[145] Since the reticulocyte contains no nucleus and does not synthesize ribonucleic acid, this effect on protein synthesis could not be at the level of the transcription of DNA, i.e., the synthesis of messenger RNA, but must be at the level of the translation of messenger RNA into protein. Since translation occurs at the level of the ribosome, the patterns of ribosomes in reticulocytes with iron or heme deficiency and in reticulocytes replete with

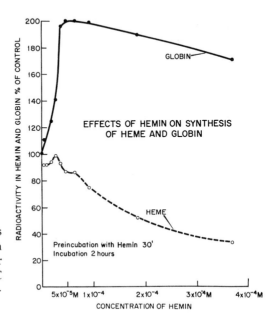

Figure 7-9 The effects of various concentrations of added hemin on the utilization of glycine-2-^{14}C for heme synthesis and of 1-valine-^{14}C for globin synthesis in rabbit reticulocytes.

heme were studied. These findings demonstrated that in heme deficiency there is a significant diminution in the number and size of polyribosomes, an indication of a defect in the initiation of protein synthesis.[146] Since added iron as well as added hemin serves to stimulate the synthesis of globin, it was important to differentiate between these effects. Accordingly, reticulocytes were incubated with added iron or hemin in the presence of the iron-chelating agent desferrioxamine. This agent inhibits globin synthesis and causes disaggregation of polyribosomes. These effects can be prevented by the simultaneous addition of hemin but not of iron. The results demonstrate that hemin acts directly to stimulate globin synthesis and does not serve merely as a source of iron.[146]

The study of this effect of heme on protein synthesis was greatly facilitated by the development by Zucker and Schulman[147] of a very active reticulocyte lysate protein synthesizing system responsive to hemin. The preparation contains no mitochondria, and, consequently, there is no heme synthesis. This system for the synthesis of protein is absolutely dependent on the presence of heme; in the presence of optimal concentrations of added hemin, linear synthesis is maintained for at least 60 minutes at 30°C, whereas in the absence of added hemin, maximal synthesis is maintained for only the first several minutes, following which there is an abrupt decline in the rate of synthesis. The shutoff of protein synthesis that occurs in heme-deficient lysates can be reversed if hemin is added soon after the start of incubation, but there is diminishing effectiveness of reversal by hemin with time. Legon et al.[148] observed a marked diminution in the 40S ribosomal subunit–met-tRNA$_f$ initiation complex. Since the binding of met-tRNA$_f$ to the 40S ribosomal subunit occurs early in protein chain initiation, a diminution in this complex might account for the observed decrease in protein synthesis. The next step was the finding that the shutoff which occurs in heme deficiency can be prevented or reversed by the specific initiation factor, a protein, eukaryotic initiation factor 2 (eIF-2), which is responsible for the binding of met-tRNA$_f$ and forms a ternary complex with met-tRNA$_f$ and guanosine triphosphate and is involved in the binding of this ternary complex to the 40S ribosomal subunit.[149,150]

The significance of the 40S-met-tRNA$_f$ complex as a site of regulation of protein synthesis is reflected in the effects of hemin or of heme deficiency on the synthesis of alpha and beta chains of globin. When hemin is present in optimal concentrations, equal numbers of alpha and beta chains are synthesized. In heme deficiency, the formation of 40S-met-tRNA$_f$ complexes is diminished, and the availability of these complexes becomes rate limiting. Since the beta globin messenger RNA has a greater affinity for the 40S-met-tRNA$_f$ complex than does the alpha globin messenger RNA, the decline in protein synthesis is much more marked for alpha chains than for beta chains and the ratio of alpha to beta globin chain synthesis falls. The effect of eIF-2 is to promote the formation of active 40S-met-tRNA$_f$ complexes and, consequently, to promote the synthesis of both alpha and beta globin chains in a ratio close to unity.

Further insight into the mechanism by which heme regulates the synthesis of protein was provided by Maxwell, Kamper, and Rabinovitz[151] and by Herbert, Adamson, and their colleagues.[152] They showed that an inhibitor is formed in the ribosome-free supernatant of reticulocyte lysates incubated in the absence of hemin. Clues to the mechanism of action of the inhibitor were provided by the findings that the inhibition observed in a heme-deficient lysate is enhanced by adenosine triphosphate.[153,154] During the past few years, we and others have shown that the isolated and purified inhibitor is a protein kinase which specifically phosphorylates the small subunit (38,000 daltons) of eIF-2.[155-157] The heme-regulated inhibitory protein kinase, isolated in its heme irreversible form by Dr. Rajinder Ranu[158] and in its heme reversible form by Dr. Hans Trachsel in our laboratory,[159] has a molecular weight of approximately 140,000 daltons and, on activation, undergoes autophosphorylation. Its activation occurs in heme deficiency, on treatment with sulfhydryl reagents, such as N-ethylmaleimide, or on prolonged heating at 37°C. The phosphorylation of eIF-2 appears to cause inhibition of the interaction of eIF-2 with other initiation factors required for the formation both of the ternary complex of met-tRNA-GTP-eIF-2[160-162] and for the binding of the ternary complex to the 40S ribosomal subunit.[160]

Since the inhibition which occurs in heme deficiency involves the mechanism of protein synthesis generally, it is to be expected that deficiency of heme or deficiency of iron will result in inhibition of protein synthesis generally. This, indeed, is the case with respect to all of the proteins in the reticulocyte. The generality of the phenomenon is demonstrable in the effects of heme on protein synthesis in ascites tumor cells and HeLa cells and in the finding of a cyclic-AMP-independent protein kinase in liver which has properties similar to those of the inhibitory protein kinase of the reticulocyte.[163]

These findings in protein synthesis help to explain the widespread systemic effects of iron deficiency, but there are surely other mechanisms that are also involved in iron deficiency. The requirement of iron for the activity of ribonucleotide reductase in the synthesis of DNA focuses attention on the role of iron in cell proliferation. The essentiality of the cytochromes for cell respiration raises the obvious question of the extent to which iron deficiency in humans leads to impairment of this vital process of energy production. And it is likely that still undiscovered functions of iron and heme will be found to be significant factors in the clinical manifestations of iron deficiency.

Summary

In the evolution of life on Earth, iron and heme have been selected to serve many critical functions. While we have discussed several of these functional roles, we should emphasize that there are still other metabolic activities which are dependent on iron or heme, e.g., ferredoxin-mediated electron transport in bacteria, metabolic detoxification by the hepatic cytochrome P_{450} system, and optimal activity of a growing list of enzymes. For some of these biological reactions, inorganic iron appears to serve optimally; for others, heme is far more effective. When iron or heme is an integral part of a complex with protein, the specificity of the function is determined by the structural characteristics of the protein and its relations to the heme or iron which it binds. In evolution's never-ending experimentation with living matter, mutations in the protein components of the complexes may afford selective advantages for known functions or may make new functions possible. Accordingly, the iron and heme compounds provide an especially fruitful field for the study of comparative molecular biology and biochemistry. Furthermore, it is quite likely that there are existing metabolic activities of iron and heme which await discovery. As for the future, is it not reasonable to expect these versatile actors to be chosen for additional new roles in the drama of evolution?

References

1   For an engaging and informative account of the early history of iron in medicine, the reader is referred to: Beutler E, Fairbanks VF, Fahey JL: *Clinical Disorders of Iron Metabolism*. New York and London, Grune and Stratton, 1963, 267 pp, p 1–18.

2   Lange J: *De Morbo Virgineo, Medicinalium Epistolarum Miscellanea*. Basle, 1554, Major RH (trans): *Classic Descriptions of Disease*. Baltimore, Thomas, 1932, 630 pp, p 445.

3   Lepidus, in *Antony and Cleopatra*, Act III, Scene 2, line 6; Prince John, in *King Henry IV*, part II, Act IV, Scene 3, line 90.

4   Juliet, in *Romeo and Juliet*, Act III, Scene V, line 154; and Marina, in *Pericles*, Act IV, Scene 6, line 13.

5   Latham RG: *The Works of Thomas Sydenham, M.D.* London, C and S Allard, 1850, vol II, 395 pp, p 98.

6   Reference to Lemery and Geoffroy, in Christian HA: A sketch of the treatment of chlorosis with iron. *Med Lib Hist J* 1:176–180, 1903.

7   Blaud P: Sur les maladies chlorotiques, et sur un mode de traitement specifique dans ces affections. *Rev Med Franc Étrang* 45:341–367, 1832.

8   Reference to Foedisch F, in Allg. Med. Ztung von Pierer 1832 in Immermann H: *Cyclopedia of the Practice of Medicine*, Am. ed., New York, 1877, 16:497.

9   Lecanu LR: Etudes chimiques sur le sang humain. *Ann Chim (Phys)* 67:54–70, 1838.

10 Reichert KB: Beobachtungen über eine eiweissartige Substanz in Krystallform. *Arch Anat Physiol* 197–251, 1849.

11 Funke O: *Atlas of Physiological Chemistry* (Suppl to Lehmann's *Physiological Chemistry*). London, Printed for the Cavendish Society by Harrison and Sons, 1852, 38 pp.

12 Teichmann L: Über das Hämatin. *Z Rat Med NF* 8:141–148, 1857.

13 Hoppe-Seyler F: Ueber die chemischen und optischen Eigenschaften des Blutfarbstoffs. *Virchows Arch* 23:446–449, 1864.

14 Hüfner G: Neue Versuche zur Bestimmung der Sauerstoffcapacität des Blutfarbstoffs. *Arch Anat Physiol* 130–176, 1894.

15 Hayem L: *Du Sang et ses Altérations Anatomiques*. xxvi, Paris, G Masson, 1889, 1035 pp.

16 Bunge F: Uber die Assimilation des Eisens. *Z Physiol Chem* 9:49–56, 1855.

17 Noorden CV von: *Die Bleichsucht*, 2d ed. Leipzig, A. Holder, 1912, 302 pp, p. 185.

18 Stockman R: Treatment of chlorosis by iron and some other drugs. *Br Med J* 1:881–885; 942–946, 1893.

19 Stockman R: On the amount of iron in ordinary dietaries and in some articles of food. *J Physiol* 18:484–489, 1895.

20 Whipple GH, Robscheit FS, Hooper CW: Blood regeneration following simple anemia. IV. Influence of meat, liver and various extractives, alone or combined with standard diets. *Am J Physiol* 53:236–262, 1920; V. The influence of Blaud's pills and hemoglobin. *Am J Physiol* 53:263–282, 1920.

21 Whipple GH, Robscheit-Robbins FS: Blood regeneration in severe anemia. III. Iron reaction favorable-arsenic and germanium dioxide almost inert. *Am J Physiol* 72:419–430, 1925.

22 Heath CW, Strauss MB, Castle WB: Quantitative aspects of iron deficiency in hypochromic anemia (the parenteral administration of iron). *J Clin Invest* 11:1293–1312, 1932.

23 Reimann F, Fritsch F, Schick K: Eisenbitanzversuche bei Gesunden und bei Anamischen 11. Untersuchungen uber das Wesen der eisenempfindlichen Anamien. ("Asiderosen") und der therapeutischen Wirkung des Eisens bei diesen Anamien. *Z Klin Med* 131:1–50, 1936.

24 McCance RA, Widdowson EM: Absorption and excretion of iron. *Lancet* 233:680–684, 1937.

25 Hahn PF, Bale WF, Lawrence EO, Whipple GH: Radioactive iron and its metabolism in anemia. Its absorption, transformation and utilization. *J Exp Med* 69:739–753, 1939.

26 Fontés G, Thivolle L: Sur la teneur du sérum en fer non hémoglobinique et sur sa diminution au cours de l'anémie expérimentale. *C R Soc Biol (Paris)* 93:687–689, 1925.

27 Barkan G: Eisenstudien. Die Verteilung des leicht abspaltbaren Eisens zwischen Blut Korperchen und Plasma und sein Verhalten under experimentellen Bedenplingen. *Hoppe Seylers Z Physiol Chem* 174:194–221, 1927.

28 Holmberg CG, Laurell C-B: Studies on the capacity of serum to bind iron. A contribution to our knowledge of the regulation mechanism of serum iron. *Acta Physiol Scand* 10:307–319, 1945.

29 Holmberg CG, Laurell C-B: Investigations in serum copper. I. Nature of serum copper and its relation to the iron-binding protein in human serum. *Acta Chem Scand* 1:944–950, 1947.

30 Schade AL, Caroline L: An iron-binding component in human blood plasma. *Science* 104:340–341, 1946.

31 Laurell C-B: Studies on the transportation and metabolism of iron in the body. *Acta Physiol Scand* 14 (suppl 46):1–129, 1947.

32 Surgenor DM, Koechlin BA, Strong LE: Chemical, clinical, and immunological studies on the products of human plasma fractionation. XXXVII. The metal-combining globulin of human plasma. *J Clin Invest* 28:73–78, 1949.

33 Koechlin BA: Preparation and properties of serum and plasma proteins. XXVIII.

The β_1-metal-combining protein of human plasma. *J Am Chem Soc* 74:2649–2653, 1952.

34 Laurell C-B, Ingelman B: The iron-binding protein of swine serum. *Acta Chem Scand* 1:770–776, 1947.

35 Laurell C-B: Isolation and properties of crystalline Fe-transferrin from pig's plasma. *Acta Chem Scand* 7:1407–1412, 1953.

36 Jacobs A, Worwood M (eds): *Iron in Biochemistry and Medicine*. London and New York, Academic Press, 1974, 317 pp.

37 Porter R, Fitzsimons (eds): *Symposium on Iron Metabolism*. Ciba Foundation Symposium 51 (new series), Elsevier, Excerpta Medica, North Holland, 1977, 375 pp.

38 Aisen P, Brown EB: Structure and function of transferrin, in Brown EB (ed): *Progress in Hematology*. New York, Grune and Stratton, 1975, vol 9, 336 pp, pp 25–56.

39 Aisen P, Brown EB: The iron-binding function of transferrin in iron metabolism. *Semin Hematol* 14:31–53, 1977.

40 Jandl JH, Inman JK, Simmons RL, Allen DW: Transfer of iron from serum iron-binding protein to human reticulocytes. *J Clin Invest* 38:161–185, 1959.

41 Jandl JH, Katz JH: The plasma-to-cell cycle of transferrin. *J Clin Invest* 42:314–326, 1963.

42 Morgan EH: Transferrin and transferrin iron, in Jacobs A, Worwood M (eds): *Iron in Biochemistry and Medicine*. New York, Academic Press, 1974, 317 pp, pp 29–71.

43 Leibman A, Aisen P: Transferrin receptor of the rabbit reticulocyte. *Biochemistry* 16:1268–72, 1977.

44 Aisen P, Hu H, Leibman A, Skoultchi AI: The transferrin receptor of erythroid cells, in Seventh Annual Symposium on Molecular and Cellular Biology. *J. Supramol Struct* (suppl 2, abst 495):198, 355 pp, 1978.

45 Huff FL, Hennessy TG, Austin RE, Garcia JF, Roberts BM, Lawrence JH: Plasma and red cell iron turnover in normal subjects and in patients having various hematopoietic disorders. *J Clin Invest* 29:1041–1052, 1950.

46 Giblett ER, Coleman DH, Pirzio-Biroli G, Donohue DM, Motulsky AG, Finch CA: Erythrokinetics: quantitative measurements of red cell production and destruction in normal subjects and patients with anemia. *Blood* 11:291–309, 1956.

47 Finch CA, Deubelbeiss K, Cook JD, Eschbach JW, Harker LA, Funk DD, Marsaglia G, Hillman RS, Slichter S, Adamson JW, Ganzoni AG, Giblett ER: Ferrokinetics in man. *Medicine (Baltimore)* 49:17–53, 1970.

48 Pollycove M, Mortimer R: The quantitative determination of iron kinetics and hemoglobin synthesis in human subjects. *J Clin Invest* 40:753–782, 1961.

49 Ricketts C, Cavill I, Napier JAF, Jacobs A: Ferrokinetics and erythropoiesis in man: an evaluation of ferrokinetic measurements. *Br J Haematol* 35:35–41, 1977.

50 Moore CV: Iron metabolism and nutrition. *Harvey Lect* 55:67–101, 1959–1960.

51 Cook JD, Layrisse M, Martinez-Torres C, Walker R, Monsen E, Finch CA: Food iron absorption measured by an extrinsic tag. *J Clin Invest* 51:805–815, 1972.

52 Crosby WH: The control of iron balance by the intestinal mucosa. *Blood* 22:441–449, 1963.

53 Bothwell TH, Charlton RW: Absorption of iron. *Ann Rev Med* 21:145–56, 1970.

54 Worwood M, Jacobs A, Cavill I: Iron absorption: Regulation by internal iron exchange, in Crichton RR (ed): *Proteins of Iron Storage and Transport in Biochemistry and Medicine*. Amsterdam, North Holland, 1975, 454 pp, pp 401–404.

55 Laufberger V: Sur la cristallisation de la ferritine. *Soc Chim Biol* 19:1575–1582, 1937.
56 Granick S: Structure and physiological functions of ferritin. *Physiol Rev* 31:489–511, 1951.
57 Crichton RR: Ferritin: structure, synthesis and function. *N Engl J Med* 284:1413–1422, 1971.
58 Harrison PM, Hoare RJ, Hoy TC, Macara IG: Ferritin and haemosiderin: structure and function, in Jacobs A, Worwood M (eds): *Iron in Biochemistry and Medicine.* London, Academic Press, 1974, 317 pp, pp 73–109.
59 Drysdale JW: Ferritin phenotypes: structure and metabolism, in Porter R, Fitzsimons DW (eds): *Iron Metabolism.* Ciba Foundation Symposium 51 (new series), Elsevier, Excerpta Medica, Amsterdam, North Holland, 1977, 375 pp, pp 41–67.
60 Munro HN, Linder MC: Ferritin: structure, biosynthesis and role in iron metabolism. *Physiol Rev* 58:317–396, 1978.
61 Harrison PM: General discussion I, in Porter R, Fitzsimons DW (eds): *Iron Metabolism.* Ciba Foundation Symposium 51 (new series), Elsevier, Excerpta Medica, Amsterdam, North Holland, 1977, 375 pp, p 69.
62 Sheldon JH: *Haemochromatosis.* London, Oxford, 1935, 382 pp.
63 Finch CA: Iron metabolism in hemochromatosis. *J Clin Invest* 28:780–781, 1949.
64 Bothwell TH, Finch CA: *Iron Metabolism.* Boston, Little Brown, 1962, 440 pp, pp 386–391.
65 Prelog V: Iron containing compounds in microorganisms, in Gross F (ed): *Iron Metabolism.* Berlin, Springer Verlag, 1964, 317 pp, pp 73–83.
66 Propper R, Cooper B, Rufo RR, Neinhuis AW, Anderson WS, Bunn HF, Rosenthal A, Nathan DG: Continuous subcutaneous administration of desferrioxamine in patients with iron overload. *N Engl J Med* 297:418–423, 1977.
67 Fowler WM: Chlorosis-an obituary, in Packard FR (ed): *Annals of Medical History, New Series VIII.* New York, Hoeber, 1936, vol 8, pp 168–177.
68 Cabot RC: Diseases of the blood, in *Osler and McCrae's Modern Medicine.* Philadelphia, Lea and Febiger, 1915, vol 4.
69 Keilin D: *The History of Cell Respiration and Cytochrome.* Cambridge, Cambridge University Press, 1966, 416 pp.
70 Patterson TS: in *John Mayow in Contemporary Setting.* A Contribution to the History of Respiration and Combustion. *Isis* 15:47–96, 504–546, 1931.
71 Liebig G: Ueber die respiration der muskelen. *Arch Anat Physiol* 393–416, 1850.
72 Breathnach CS: George Gabriel Stokes on the function of hemoglobin. *Ir J Med Sci* (sixth series) 484:121–125, 1966.
73 Pflüger E: Beiträge zur Lehre von der Respiration. I. Ueber die physiologische Verbrennung in den Ibendingen Organismen. *Pfluegers Arch* 10:251–367, 1875.
74 Pflüger E: Nachtrag zu meinem Aufsatz. Ueber die physiologische Verbrennung in den lebendigen Organismen. *Pfluegers Arch* 10:641–644, 1875.
75 Oertmann E: Ueber den Stoffwechsel entbluteter Frosche. *Pfluger Arch Ges Physiol* 15:381–398, 1877.
76 MacMunn CA, in Keilin D: *The History of Cell Respiration and Cytochrome.* Cambridge, Cambridge University Press, 1966, 416 pp, pp 355–357.
77 MacMunn CA: Further observations on myohaematin and the histohaematins. *J Physiol* 8:51–65, 1887.
78 Hoppe-Seyler F: Ueber Muskelfarbstoffe. *Z Physiol Chem* 14:106–108, 1890.

79   Willstäter R, Stoll A: *Investigations on Chlorophyll*. Lancaster, Ohio, Science Press, 1928, 389 pp.

80   Fischer H, Orth H: *Die Chemie des Pyrrols*. Leipzig, Akademische Verlagsgeselshaft, vol I, 1934; vol II, 1937, 399 pp.

81   Lemberg R, Legge JW: *Hematin Compounds and Bile Pigments. Their Constitution, Metabolism and Function*. New York and London, Interscience, 1949, 748 pp.

82   Küster W: Über die Konstitution des Hämins. *Hoppe-Seylers Z Physiol Chem* 88:377–388, 1913.

83   Adair GS: A comparison of the molecular weights of the proteins. *Proc Camb Philos Soc Biol Sci* 1:75–78, 1924.

84   Svedberg T, Fåhraeus R: A new method for the determination of the molecular weight of the proteins. *J Am Chem Soc* 48:430–438, 1926.

85   Perutz MF, Rossmann MG, Cullis AF, Muirhead H, Will G, North ACT: Structure of haemoglobin. A three-dimensional Fourier synthesis at 5.5 Å resolution obtained by x-ray analysis. *Nature* 185:416–422, 1960.

86   Shemin D, Rittenberg D: The biological utilization of glycine for the synthesis of the protoporphyrin of hemoglobin. *J Biol Chem* 166:621–625, 1946.

87   Shemin D, Rittenberg D: The life span of the human red blood cell. *J Biol Chem* 166:627–636, 1946.

87a   Shemin D: Glycine to heme, in *From Cyclotrons to Cytochrome*, a symposium held at the University of California at San Diego, August 27, 1978 (to be published).

88   Ashby W: The determination of the length of life of transfused blood corpuscles in man. *J Exp Med* 29:267–281, 1919; Study of the transfused blood: I. The periodicity in eliminative activity shown by the organism. *J Exp Med* 34:127–145, 1921.

89   Mollison PL, Young IM: On the survival of the transfused erythrocytes of stored blood. *Q J Exp Physiol* 30:313–327, 1940; *In vivo* survival in the human subject of transfused erythrocytes after storage in various preservative solutions. *Q J Exp Physiol* 31:359–392, 1941–1942.

90   Callender S, Powell EO, Witts L: The life span of the red cell in man. *J Pathol Bacteriol* 57:129–139, 1945.

91   London IM, Shemin D, West R, Rittenberg D: Heme synthesis and red blood cell dynamics in normal humans and in subjects with polycythemia vera, sickle cell anemia, and pernicious anemia. *J Biol Chem* 184:463–484, 1949.

92   Bloch K, Rittenberg D: An estimation of acetic acid formation in the rat. *J Biol Chem* 159:45–58, 1945.

93   London IM, Shemin D, Rittenberg D: The *in vitro* synthesis of heme in the human red blood cell of sickle cell anemia. *J Biol Chem* 173:797–798, 1948.

94   London IM, Shemin D, Rittenberg D: The synthesis of heme *in vitro* by the immature non-nucleated mammalian erythrocyte. *J Biol Chem* 183:749–755, 1950.

95   Shemin D, London IM, Rittenberg D: The *in vitro* synthesis of heme from glycine by the nucleated red blood cell. *J Biol Chem* 173:799–800, 1948.

96   Shemin D, London IM, Rittenberg D: The synthesis of protoporphyrin *in vitro* by red blood cells of the duck. *J Biol Chem* 183:757–765, 1950.

97   Walsh RJ, Thomas ED, Chow SK, Fluharty RG, Finch CA: Iron metabolism. Heme synthesis *in vitro* by immature erythrocytes. *Science* 110:396–398, 1949.

98   Shemin D: The biosynthesis of porphyrins. *Harvey Lect* 49:258–284, 1954–1955.

99   Neuberger A, Scott JJ: Aminolevulinic acid and porphyrin biosynthesis. *Nature* 172:1093–1094, 1953.

100   Dresel EIB, Falk JE: Conversion of delta aminolevulinic acid to porphobilinogen in a tissue system. *Nature* 172:1185, 1953.

101   Westall RB: Isolation of porphobilinogen from the urine of a patient with acute porphyria. *Nature* 170:614–616, 1952.

102   Waldenström J, Vahlquist B: Studien ueber die Entstehung der roten Harnpigmente (Uroporphyrin und Porphobilin) bei der akuten Porphyrie aus ihrer farblosen Vorstufe (Porphobilinogen). *Z Physiol Chem* 260:189–209, 1939.

103   Cookson GH, Rimington C: Porphobilinogen. *Biochem J* 57:476–484, 1954.

104   Sano S, Granick S: Mitochondrial coproporphyrinogen oxidase and protoporphyrin formation. *J Biol Chem* 236:1173–1180, 1961.

105   Goldberg A: The enzymic formation of haem by the incorporation of iron into protoporphyrin; importance of ascorbic acid, ergothioneine and glutathione. *Br J Haematol* 5:150–157, 1959.

106   Schwartz HC, Cartwright GE, Smith EL, Wintrobe MM: Studies on the biosynthesis of heme from iron and protoporphyrin. *Blood* 14:486–497, 1959.

107   Labbe RF, Hubbard N: Preparation and properties of the iron-protoporphyrin chelating enzyme. *Biochim Biophys Acta* 41:185–191, 1960.

108   Bogorad L: The biosynthesis of protochlorophyll, in Allen MB (ed): *Comparative Biochemistry of Photoreactive Systems*. New York, Academic Press, 1960, 325 pp, pp 227–256.

109   Granick S, Mauzerall D: The metabolism of heme and chlorophyll, in Greenberg DM (ed): *Metabolic Pathways*. New York, Academic Press, 1961, vol 2, 227 pp, pp 525–616.

110   Burnham BF: Metabolism of porphyrins and corrinoids, in Greenberg DM (ed): *Metabolic Pathways*, 3d ed. New York, Academic Press, 1969, vol 3, 235 pp, pp 403–537.

111   Marks GS: *Heme and Chlorophyll*. London, Van Nostrand, 1969, 208 pp, pp 121–162.

112   Neve RA, Labbe RF, Aldrich RA: Reduced uroporphyrin III in the biosynthesis of heme. *J Am Chem Soc* 78:691–692, 1956.

113   Bogorad L: The enzymatic synthesis of porphyrins from porphobilinogen. III. Uroporphyrinogens as intermediates. *J Biol Chem* 233:516–519, 1958.

114   Bogorad L, Granick S: The enzymatic synthesis of porphyrins from porphobilinogen. *Proc Natl Acad Sci USA,* 39:1176–1188, 1953.

115   Granick S, Urata G: Increase in activity of δ-aminolevulinic acid synthetase in liver mitochondria induced by feeding of 3,5-dicarbethoxy-1,4-dihydrocollidine. *J Biol Chem* 238:821–827, 1963.

116   Granick S: Induction of the synthesis of δ-aminolevulinic acid synthetase in liver parenchyma cells in culture by chemicals that induce acute porphyria. *J Biol Chem* 238:2247–2249, 1963.

117   Lascelles J: The synthesis of porphyrins and bacteriochlorophyll by cell suspensions of Rhodopseudomonas spheroides. *Biochem J* 62:78–93, 1956.

118   Gibson KD, Neuberger A, Scott JJ: The enzymic conversion of δ-aminolaevulinic acid to porphobilinogen. Proc. of the Biochemical Society, *Biochem J* 58:xli–xlii, 1954.

119 Burnham BF, Lascelles J: Control of porphyrin biosynthesis through a negative-feedback mechanism. Studies with preparations of δ-aminolaevulate synthetase and δ-aminolaevulate dehydratase from *Rhodopseudomonas* spheroides. *Biochem J* 87:462–472, 1963.

120 Karibian D, London IM: Control of heme synthesis by feedback inhibition. *Biochem Biophys Res Comm* 18:243–249, 1965.

121 Freedman ML, Wildman JM, Rosman J, Eisen J, Greenblatt DR: Benzene inhibition of *in vitro* rabbit reticulocyte haem synthesis at delta aminolaevulinic acid synthetase: Reversal of benzene toxicity by pyridoxine. *Br J Haematol* 35:49–60, 1977.

122 Scholnick PL, Hammaker L, Marver HS: Soluble hepatic δ-aminolevulinic acid synthetase: end-product inhibition of the partially purified enzyme. *Proc Natl Acad Sci USA* 63:65–70, 1969.

123 Scholnick PL, Hammaker L, Marver HS: Soluble δ-aminolevulinic acid synthetase of rat liver. II. Studies related to the mechanism of enzyme action and hemin inhibition. *J Biol Chem* 247:4132–4137, 1972.

124 Kaplan BH: δ-Aminolevulinic acid synthetase from the particulate fraction of liver of porphyric rats. *Biochim Biophys Acta* 235:381–388, 1971.

125 Bonkowsky HL, Tschudy DP, Collins A, Doherty J, Bossenmaier I, Cardinal R, Watson CJ: Repression of the overproduction of porphyrin precursors in acute intermittent porphyria by intravenous infusions of hematin. *Proc Natl Acad Sci USA* 68:2725–2729, 1971.

126 Watson CJ, Dhar GJ, Bossenmaier I, Cardinal R, Petryka ZJ: Effect of hematin in acute porphyric relapse. *Ann Intern Med* 79:80–83, 1973.

127 Dhar GJ, Bossenmaier I, Petryka ZJ, Cardinal R, Watson CJ: Effects of hematin in hepatic porphyria. *Ann Intern Med* 83:20–30, 1975.

128 Peterson A, Bossenmaier I, Cardinal R, Watson CJ: Hematin treatment of acute porphyria. Early remission of an almost fatal relapse. *JAMA* 235:520–522, 1976.

129 Watson CJ, Bossenmaier I, Cardinal R, Petryka ZJ: Repression of hematin of porphyrin biosynthesis in erythrocyte precursors in congenital erythropoietic porphyria. *Proc Natl Acad Sci USA* 71:278–282, 1974.

130 Miller EB, Singer K, Dameshek W: Use of the daily fecal output of urobilinogen and the hemolytic index in the measurement of hemolysis. *Arch Intern Med* 70:722–737, 1942.

131 Whipple GH: Pigment metabolism and regeneration of hemoglobin in the body. *Arch Intern Med* 29:711–731, 1922.

132 Watson CJ: Über Stercobilin und Porphyrine aus Kot. I. Mitteilung. *Hoppe-Seylers Z Physiol Chem* 204:57–67, 1932.

133 Watson CJ: Urobilin and stercobilin. *Harvey Lect* 54:41–83, 1948–1949.

134 London IM, West R, Shemin D, Rittenberg D: On the origin of bile pigment in normal man. *Fed Proc* 7:169, 1948; *J Clin Invest* 27:547, 1948; *J Biol Chem* 184:351–358, 1950.

135 London IM, West R, Shemin D, Rittenberg D: The formation of bile pigment in pernicious anemia. *J Biol Chem* 184:359–364, 1950.

136 London IM, West R, Shemin D, Rittenberg D: Porphyrin formation and hemoglobin metabolism in congenital porphyria. *J Biol Chem* 184:365–373, 1950.

137 London IM: The conversion of hematin to bile pigment. *J Biol Chem* 184:373–376, 1950.

138 Robinson SH: Bilirubin production from non-erythroid sources, in Goresky CA, Fisher MM (eds): *Jaundice.* New York, Plenum Press, 1975, 422 pp.

139 Tenhunen R, Marver HS, Schmid R: The enzymatic conversion of heme to bilirubin by microsomal heme oxygenase. *Proc Natl Acad Sci USA* 61:748–755, 1968.

140 Kruh J, Borsook H: Hemoglobin synthesis in rabbit reticulocytes *in vitro. J Biol Chem* 220:905–915, 1956.

141 Kassenaar A, Morell H, London IM: The incorporation of glycine into globin and the synthesis of heme *in vitro* in duck erythrocytes. *J Biol Chem* 229:423–435, 1957.

142 Morell H, Savoie J-C, London IM: The biosynthesis of heme and the incorporation of glycine into globin in rabbit bone marrow *in vitro. J Biol Chem* 233:923–929, 1958.

143 Nizet A: Recherches sur les relations entre les biosynthèses de l'hème et de la globine. *Bull Soc Chim Biol* 39:265–277, 1957.

144 London IM, Bruns GP, Karibian D: The regulation of hemoglobin synthesis and the pathogenesis of some hypochromic anemias. *Medicine (Baltimore)* 43:789–802, 1964.

145 Bruns GP, London IM: The effect of hemin on the synthesis of globin. *Biochem Biophys Res Comm* 18:236–242, 1965.

146 Grayzel A, Horchner P, London IM: The stimulation of globin synthesis by heme. *Proc Natl Acad Sci USA* 55:650–655, 1966.

147 Zucker W, Schulman H: Stimulation of globin-chain initiation by hemin in the reticulocyte cell-free system. *Proc Natl Acad Sci USA* 59:582–589, 1968.

148 Legon S, Jackson RJ, Hunt T: Control of protein synthesis in reticulocyte lysates by haem. *Nature* 241:150–152, 1973.

149 Beuzard Y, London IM: The effects of hemin and double stranded RNA on α and β globin synthesis in reticulocytes and Krebs II ascites cell free systems and the reversal of these effects by an initiation factor preparation. *Proc Natl Acad Sci USA* 71:2863–2866, 1974.

150 Clemens MJ, Henshaw EC, Rahamimoff H, London IM: Met-tRNA$_f^{Met}$ binding to 40S ribosomal subunits: a site for the regulation of protein synthesis by hemin. *Proc Natl Acad Sci USA* 71:2946–2950, 1974.

151 Maxwell CR, Kamper CS, Rabinovitz M: Hemin control of globin synthesis: an assay for the inhibitor formed in the absence of hemin and some characteristics of its formation. *J Mol Biol* 58:317–327, 1971.

152 Adamson SD, Herbert E, Kemp SF: Effects of hemin and other porphyrins on protein synthesis in a reticulocyte lysate cell-free system. *J Mol Biol* 42:247–258, 1969.

153 Balkow K, Hunt T, Jackson RJ: Control of protein synthesis in reticulocyte lysates: the effect of nucleotide triphosphates on formation of the translational repressor. *Biochem Biophys Res Comm* 67:366–375, 1975.

154 Ernst V, Levin DH, Ranu RS, London IM: Control of protein synthesis in reticulocyte lysates: effects of 3':5' cyclic AMP, ATP and GTP on inhibitions induced by heme deficiency, double-stranded RNA and a reticulocyte translational inhibitor. *Proc Natl Acad Sci USA* 73:1112–1116, 1976.

155 Levin DH, Ranu RS, Ernst V, London IM: Regulation of protein synthesis in reticulocyte lysates: phosphorylation of methionyl-tRNA$_f$ binding factor by protein kinase activity of the translational inhibitor isolated from heme-deficient lysate. *Proc Natl Acad Sci USA* 73:3112–3116, 1976.

156 Kramer G, Cimadevilla JM, Hardesty B: Specificity of the protein kinase activity associated with the hemin-controlled repressor of rabbit reticulocyte. *Proc Natl Acad Sci USA* 73:3078–3082, 1976.

157 Farrell P, Balkow K, Hunt T, Jackson RJ, Trachsel H: Phosphorylation of initiation factor eIF-2 and the control of reticulocyte protein synthesis. *Cell* 11:187–200, 1977.

158 Ranu RS, London IM: Regulation of protein synthesis in rabbit reticulocyte lysates: purification and initial characterization of the cyclic 3':5'-AMP independent protein kinase. *Proc Natl Acad Sci USA* 73:4349–4353, 1976.

159 Trachsel H, Ranu RS, London IM: Regulation of protein synthesis in rabbit reticulocyte lysates: purification and characterization of heme-reversible translational inhibitor. *Proc Natl Acad Sci USA* 75:3654–3658, 1978.

160 Ranu RS, London IM, Das A, Dasgupta A, Majumdar A, Ralston R, Roy R, Gupta NK: Regulation of protein synthesis in rabbit reticulocyte lysates by the heme-regulated protein kinase: inhibition of interaction of Met-tRNA$_f^{Met}$ binding factor with another initiation factor in formation of Met-tRNA$_f^{Met}$-40S ribosomal subunit complexes. *Proc Natl Acad Sci USA* 75:745–749, 1978.

161 deHaro C, Datta A, Ochoa S: Mode of action of the hemin-controlled inhibitor of protein synthesis. *Proc Natl Acad Sci USA* 75:243–247, 1978.

162 Ranu RS, London IM: Regulation of protein synthesis in rabbit reticulocyte lysates: additional initiation factor required for formation of ternary complex (eIF-2-GTP-Met-tRNA$_f$) and demonstration of inhibitory effect of heme-regulated protein kinase. *Proc Natl Acad Sci USA* 76:1079–1083, 1979.

163 Delaunay J, Ranu RS, Levin DH, Ernst V, London IM: Characterization of a rat liver factor which inhibits initiation of protein synthesis in rabbit reticulocyte lysates. *Proc Natl Acad Sci USA* 74:2264–2268, 1977.

CHAPTER 8

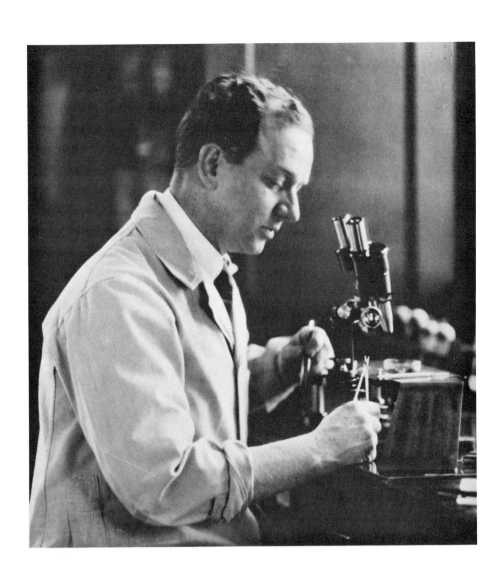

THE LIFE SPAN OF THE RED BLOOD CELL AND CIRCUMSTANCES OF ITS PREMATURE DEATH

John V. Dacie

P eyton Rous (1879–1970), of the Rockefeller Institute in New York, whose pioneer work on cancer as a young man was belatedly recognized by the award of the Nobel Prize for Medicine in 1966 (with Dr. Charles Huggins) 56 years after his first paper on a transmissible sarcoma of the fowl, switched his attention to the blood and its preservation under the impact of World War I.[1] As recounted on p. 217, the Rous-Turner preservative solution was the starting point for the work of a subsequent generation of research workers, who were faced in World War II with a similar urgent problem—how best to preserve blood for transfusion. In 1917, Rous' partner in the research on the normal fate of red cells, O. H. Robertson, a Canadian, operated the world's first blood bank in Belgium near the front line.[2]

In 1923, in a review which listed 245 relevant papers, Rous (Chapter Opening Photo) summarized knowledge and opinion about the destruction of the red blood corpuscles that extended back into the nineteenth century.[3] He also included his own succinct and penetrating and, sometimes, picturesque comments.

The questions that Rous attempted to answer in his review were many and searching. First and foremost was whether the red cells had a definite, as

Chapter Opening Photo   Peyton Rous (1879–1970). (*The Rockefeller University Archives.*)

opposed to an almost indefinite, sojourn in the blood (i.e., "life span"), and, if finite, how long was their life span. Rous found that: "So subtly is normal blood destruction conducted and the remains of the cells disposed of that were it not for indirect evidence one might suppose the life of most red corpuscles to endure with that of the body." In fact, he did not doubt that their life span was limited, and he listed a number of cogent arguments in favor of this view. For example, he cited the "continuous activity of broadly distributed hematopoietic tissue" and the "daily excretion through the bile of a pigment nearly if not precisely identical with one of the pigmented derivatives of hemoglobin."[3]

The question as to how long red cells circulate before undergoing destruction had been a vexing question for many years. A variety of methods and calculations had been employed to come up with some answers, ranging from observations of the time it took for the red cell count in a hypertransfused animal to be restored to normal to calculations based on bile excretion. The conclusions drawn from these studies were inevitably erroneous, and Rous[3] stated that the general view in the early 1920s was that about one-fifteenth of the red cell mass was normally destroyed each day, regardless of the species of animal.

Regarding increased blood destruction (hemolysis) in disease, he concluded that "much of the blood destruction of disease states is consummated by processes that themselves are normal." On the role of the spleen, he wrote, "by some hook or crook of function or morphology the spleen often serves as a midden for damaged erythrocytes." In referring to the possibility that the red cells might be mechanically damaged whilst circulating, he added: "The view that corpuscles may be normally threshed to pieces in the circulation is not new (Meltzer, 1900), nor will it seem strange to anyone who has watched in the living animal a red cell saddle-bagged at a capillary fork, and pulled well-nigh in two, with its bagging portions continually belabored and dragged upon by its passing fellows."

The observations just quoted are probably those of Rous himself, but "threshed to pieces in the circulation" is a paraphrase of what Meltzer,[4] of Baltimore, actually had said. He had been carrying out experiments on the effect of shaking and defibrination, followed by incubation, on the integrity of the red cells of various animals and had written: "It appears to me that a study of the effects of shaking upon the blood is desirable from many points of view. With each heart beat the blood cells receive a mechanical shock: in rapidly moving forward they hit upon one another and they hit upon the arterial walls, at least at each arterial bifurcation."

The Data of Winifred Ashby

The conclusions of only one observer stood out in striking contrast to the above observations—those of Winifred Ashby, whose first papers[5,6] were published in 1919. Dr. Winifred Ashby (1879–1975) (Figure 8-1) was born in

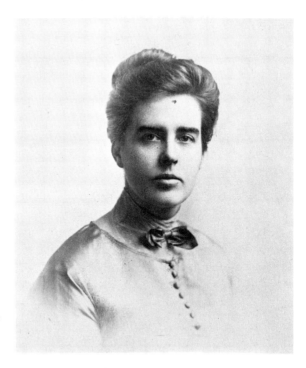

Figure 8-1 Winifred Ashby (1879–1975). (*Courtesy of Mayo Clinic.*)

London, England but moved with her family to Chicago when she was 14 years of age.[7] After obtaining B.S. and M.S. degrees at Northwestern and Washington Universities and after a period of teaching physics and chemistry and working in medical laboratories, she was awarded a Mayo Clinic Fellowship in immunology and pathology in February 1917. It was there that she carried out her pioneer work on the life span of red cells. She was awarded the Ph.D. degree by the University of Minnesota in 1921 and in 1924 joined the laboratory staff of St. Elizabeth's Hospital in Washington, D.C., where she supervised the serology and bacteriology laboratories until she retired in 1949. She died in 1975 at the age of 95.

Ashby can be regarded as a real pioneer, although the idea of transfusing red cells which were compatible with but nevertheless serologically distinct from those of the recipient, and the subsequent counting of their number after differential agglutination, may have stemmed from the work of Todd and White[8] in Cairo; in 1911 they had used isohemolytic sera in an attempt to trace the fate of blood cross-transfused between pairs of bulls.

Ashby[5] described in her first paper how she had transfused group IV (type O) blood to seven group II (type A) recipients who were suffering from various anemias, and how she had been able to count the free (unagglutinated) type O cells by making suspensions of posttransfusion blood in an anti-A serum (Figure 8-2). She concluded that transfused red cells live a long time—30 days

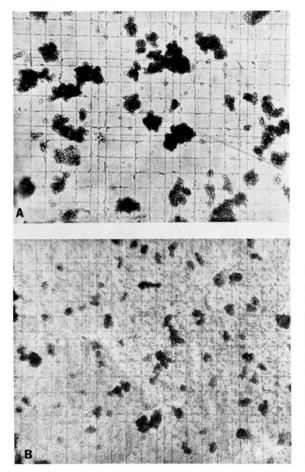

Figure 8-2 Reproduction of one of Ashby's original figures. (*A*) A suspension of group II (type A) red cells in an anti-A serum. Relatively few cells are free and unagglutinated. (*B*) A similar preparation after the transfusion of group IV (type O) red cells. Many of the cells are now free and unagglutinated, the great majority being transfused cells. (*From Winifred Ashby,*[5] *1919.*)

or more (Figure 8-3)—and that the beneficial results of blood transfusion are not due to the stimulation of the bone marrow (a view held by some at the time) but to the functioning of the transfused cells. In her second paper, Ashby[6] reported that in 10 patients who were not suffering from an idiopathic blood disease, 40 to 50 percent of the transfused cells had survived an average of 37 days.

By 1921, Ashby[9] was able to report on more than 100 patients. In eight of them, as illustrated in a figure, the period for complete elimination ranged from 28 to 30 days in a patient with cancer to 100 days in a healthy man. She also studied a long series of patients with pernicious anemia but was unable to find the intensive blood destruction she had expected.[10] Thus, in four patients who were followed until the elimination of the transfused cells was complete or almost complete, this did not take place until 83 to 100 days after transfusion.

Rous[3] was well aware of Ashby's work, in particular her tracing of blood that had been transfused to a healthy man for as long as 100 days. His comment was a cautious one: "the crying need . . . is not for a reconciliation of figures but for more facts."

One of the difficulties inherent in Ashby's work, which she could not circumvent, was that she was not measuring the life span of the red cells in their own environment. The long life spans she had observed were those of normal blood cells transfused from one subject to another. This raised the question of whether the foreign cells might survive longer than those of the host, a point which she was unable to resolve.

Ashby's data and conclusions are now known to be generally correct. But she was ahead of her time; her papers remained on library shelves largely unread and her technique was relatively unused until the late 1930s. However, it was not entirely overlooked. For, Wearn, Warren, and Ames,[11] of Boston, using her method, found that in four patients with pernicious anemia and four with other forms of anemia the transfused red cells could be traced between 59 and 113 days in both groups. In an extensive study, Jervell,[12] of Oslo, similarly observed that in nine patients suffering from various forms of anemia the transfused blood survived from more than 12 days to more than 8 weeks.

In Oslo, Dedichen[13] conceived the idea that it might be possible to obtain evidence by transfusion experiments as to which of the two current theories about the pathogenesis of "ictère hémolytique" (hereditary spherocytosis) was correct; hyperactivity of the organs of hemolysis (particularly the spleen) or production of cells with less than normal resistance. With this in mind, he

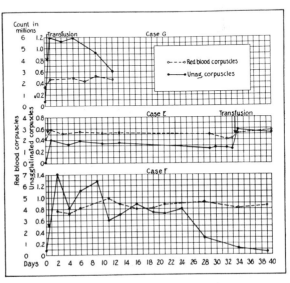

Figure 8-3 Reproduction of one of Ashby's original figures, illustrating the survival of transfused (unagglutinated) red cells. The early termination of observations in case G was caused by the patient's death from influenza. (*From Winifred Ashby,*[5] 1919.)

transfused two patients with citrated type O blood (no added glucose) and found that all the transfused blood had disappeared by the seventh post-transfusion day in one and by the fourth in the other. He remarked that his researches were "defective," that the concordance between duplicate counts was not good and that he could not obtain a good type B (anti-A) serum; he did not mention whether the blood that was transfused was fresh. He did, however, record that in the patient in whom the blood had the shortest survival (4 days) symptoms of hemolysis increased after the transfusion and that these were accompanied by fever. This unfortunate experience led him to discontinue his experiments.

Dedichen also considered the practicability of carrying out the reverse experiment; transfusing patient's blood into a normal recipient. He did not, however, pursue the idea because it was suggested to him that there might be an infectious element to the disorder as well as a congenital disposition. It is sad that, probably for technical reasons, Dedichen's experiments led him to the wrong conclusion; that is, that his results supported the theory that the shortened survival of the red cells was due to hyperactivity of the hemolytic organs. He, too, was ahead of his time, and more than a decade was to pass before similar (but more successful and decisive) experiments were again undertaken[14,15] (Figure 8-4).

In 1928, differential agglutination was also employed in the reverse (that is, the direct) way by Landsteiner, Levine, and Janes[16] at the Rockefeller Institute and by Wiener, of Brooklyn, New York. Wiener, in a letter[17] to the *Journal of the American Medical Association*, mentioned that he had detected blood group M (or N) cells, using anti-M (or anti-N) sera, in the circulation of

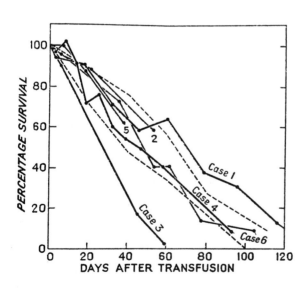

Figure 8-4 Survival of blood from normal donors after transfusion to six patients with hereditary spherocytosis. Although not shown in the figure, survival in cases 2 and 5, followed to completion, exceeded 100 days in each case. The dotted lines indicate the limits of survival found by Mollison in a group of normal recipients. The shortened survival in case 3 was probably because the patient, subsequently shown to be Rh-negative, received Rh-positive blood. (*From Dacie and Mollison*,[14] 1943.)

N (or M) recipients for between 80 and 120 days after the transfusion. Wiener also used the Ashby method, employing anti-M (or anti-N) sera to agglutinate the recipient's cells, and observed that between one-third and one-fourth of the transfused cells disappeared each month; he remarked that this continuous decrease in numbers was to be expected on the assumption that all the cells had approximately the same life span. He concluded: "Curiously enough, despite all this work, most textbooks still give the life of the erythrocyte as thirty days."

The direct method, using anti-M or anti-N sera, was also used by Dekkers,[18] of Amsterdam. In a paper published in 1939, he described how he had transfused 32 patients suffering from various types of anemia. The series included one patient, a young woman aged 18 years, who was thought to have an acquired hemolytic anemia. She was found to destroy the transfused cells "rapidly." Dekkers deduced that the patient's red cells were also being destroyed at a rapid rate and wrote, "these data demonstrate that this method of investigation is suitable to examine this intriguing group of anaemias."

Later work has amply confirmed Dekkers' prediction (see below). However, before being employed extensively in the investigation of patients with hemolytic anemias, the value and relative accuracy of the Ashby method was brilliantly vindicated in relation to the viability of blood that had been stored prior to transfusion. In the United Kingdom, after the outbreak of war with Germany in 1939, the question of how best to store blood for transfusion to military casualties and to the thousands of civilian air raid casualties that were expected in London and in the other major cities became a very urgent one. The only practical solution available at the time was to use the Ashby method to study the survival of blood stored under different conditions.

It is a sad commentary on the state of prewar hematology and blood transfusion in the United Kingdom to have to write that the method does not seem ever to have been used there prior to 1940. Nevertheless, under the stress of war, the method was quickly mastered and the technique improved.[19]* Much was learned about the optimum conditions for the storage of blood and, in particular, of the value of citrate as an anticoagulant and of glucose as a metabolic life preserver.[21]

The importance of dextrose (glucose) for the preservation of blood had, in fact, been demonstrated by Rous and Turner[22] as far back as 1916. They described the effect of the addition to blood of various substances, including sugars, on the preservation in vitro of the red cells of several animal species, including man. The blood was kept at 1 to 3°C, and sodium citrate was used as the anticoagulant; the degree of preservation was assessed in terms of the rapidity of onset of hemolysis. Although human blood to which sodium

---

*According to Dr. Hugh Chaplin, Dr. Winifred Ashby spoke of Dr. Mollison as "the man who resurrected me."[20]

citrate and Locke's salt solution had been added started to hemolyze after 1 week's storage, this did not happen for 4 weeks when isotonic dextrose was included in the preservative mixture.

Rous and Turner did not carry out any transfusions of stored blood in humans, although they did so in rabbits. They remarked, however, that if human red cells were kept in vitro before transfusion, it would be preferable to suspend them in a citrate and salt solution containing dextrose. In discussing their results, it is interesting to record that they did not mention the possibility that dextrose might be a substance the metabolism of which was essential for the continued viability of the cells; instead, the sugars were considered, perhaps, to retard proteolytic digestion or to protect the cells from injury from the salt solution in which they were suspended. The significance of this work appears not to have been generally appreciated, for Wiener and Shaeffer,[23] in reporting in 1940 on the use of stored blood for transfusion, emphasized the limitations rather than the practical value of the method. They followed the survival of the transfused red cells by the Ashby method, but they used citrated blood to which no glucose had been added prior to storage!

The tracing by the Ashby method of the survival of blood transfused into patients with anemia due to increased destruction of red cells (hemolytic anemia) was found to distinguish clearly between two major groups of cases—those in which the normal transfused blood survived normally and those in which it was destroyed along with the patient's own blood. These observations supported the idea that there might be "intrinsic" and "extrinsic" mechanisms for increased hemolysis. Later, the distinction was used as a rational basis for classification of the hemolytic anemias.

The Experiments of Hawkins and Whipple

The next major event in the story of red cell life span measurements, following the use of Ashby's method, was the advent of radioactive chromium (^{51}Cr), but before describing the impact and advantages of ^{51}Cr and other isotopic methods, one pioneer experimental method deserves mention.

In 1938, Hawkins and Whipple[24] described how they had created biliary fistulae in dogs so that all the bile excreted could be collected. Anemia was then produced by means of acetylphenylhydrazine, a hemolytic agent, or venesection, and the amount of bile pigment that was excreted daily was measured. In 110 to 130 days after anemia had been produced, there was a temporary increase in the excretion, and this was interpreted as being due to the breakdown of the hemoglobin released from the large cohort of red cells that had been formed in response to the acute anemia produced (Figure 8-5). Subsequent data on the life span of dog red cells, using differential agglutination and isotopic methods, have shown that Hawkins and Whipple's experiment had given the correct result.

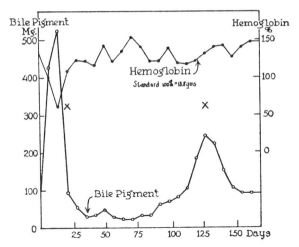

Figure 8-5 The figure shows how the production of anemia by the administration of acetylphenylhydrazine to a dog with a biliary fistula resulted in a large increase in the excretion of bile pigment and how this was followed by a second peak of excretion about 100 days later. This secondary peak was interpreted by Hawkins and Whipple as being due to the expiration of the life span (within a relatively short period of time) of the large cohort of cells formed in response to the stimulus of the acute anemia which had been produced about 100 days previously. (*From Hawkins and Whipple,*[24] 1938.)

Other early experimental methods were described and evaluated in Berlin, Waldmann, and Weissman's[25] valuable review published in 1959, but none had the simplicity of Hawkins and Whipple's classic experiment, nor was any other as free from difficulties of interpretation.

Radioactive Chromium (^{51}Cr)

The first studies using ^{51}Cr were reported by Gray and Sterling[26] in 1950 from Boston. The value of the isotope as a harmless label of red cells was soon confirmed in many centers throughout the world, and, because the ^{51}Cr could be used to label patients' own corpuscles and to study their survival in their own circulation, as well as to label transfused blood, Ashby's elegant but laborious technique, with its inherent limitations and technical difficulties, soon became obsolete.

^{51}Cr is still widely used in studies of red cell life span and in the measurement of blood volume. It is, however, not an ideal label, for the chromium slowly elutes from the red cells whilst they are still circulating. Nevertheless, because ^{51}Cr emits gamma rays, it is possible to count the radiation over, for instance, the area of the spleen and liver of the living patient and, thereby, to detect the site of blood destruction and to predict the likelihood of benefit from splenectomy. ^{51}Cr has, thus, been used extensively in the investigation of patients with hemolytic anemias. The results obtained for the normal red cell life span, 108 to 120 days,[25] have matched up well with the Ashby data.

^{51}Cr remains the most practical label for studies of red cell life span. Its nearest rival has been ^{32}P, used to label the cholinesterase inhibitor diisofluor-ophosphonate (DFP). DF^{32}P was first reported in 1954 to be a potentially satisfactory label for red cells by Cohen and Warringa,[27] of Rijwijk, Nether-lands, who were studying the metabolism of DFP, then in vogue as a possible means of treatment of myasthenia gravis and other disorders associated with atonia. A small fraction of the DF^{32}P ingested was found to be irreversibly bound to red cells, and in two patients studied, in whom there was no evidence of hemolytic anemia, the decline in ^{32}P radioactivity indicated red cell life spans of 116 and 129 days. The DF^{32}P technique has the advantage over ^{51}Cr in that the DF^{32}P, once attached to the red cells, is not eluted. But it has the great disadvantage that the limited penetration of its beta radiation does not allow for in vivo surface counting.

Mechanisms of Red Cell Destruction in Health

Granted that the red cells in man, and other mammals, have a relatively long life span in health, why do they die? Is this an age-related process or a random one? And where does the death take place? These questions have interested physiologists and others for many decades, and it is an interesting fact, but perhaps not a surprising one, that more is known about the causes and mechanisms of the abnormal shortening of red cell life span in the hemolytic anemias than about what happens in health.

Research workers in the early years of this century had established the course of events following the administration of anti–red cell sera or hemolytic chemicals to laboratory animals and had satisfied themselves that a regular and striking consequence was extensive phagocytosis of the red cells by "hema-tophages" (blood scavengers) in the spleen, as well as in the liver, bone marrow, and lymph nodes. As Rous[3] put it, "an immense number of auxiliary hematophages start into being." There is certainly no doubt that red cells damaged by a variety of means are eliminated from the circulation and destroyed in this way. But there is still doubt as to the role of phagocytosis in the removal from the circulation of normal red cells in a healthy subject. Rous considered that the ingestion of red cells (erythrophagocytosis) was not a conspicuous feature in any organ in health and that in some species, e.g., the cat, it was difficult to find any erythrophages.

The idea that red cells normally break up into pieces in the circulation received some support from the work of Rous and Robertson[2] published in 1917; this indicated that in several species of animals, fragments of red cells could be found in the peripheral circulation in small numbers and that the fragments might accumulate in the spleen. But is fragmentation caused by mechanical stresses or by age-determined changes? There is by now abundant evidence that regular and progressive biochemical changes take place as red cells become older. In general terms, the enzymes with which they are endowed, the synthesis of which ceases after the cells mature beyond the early reticulocyte stage, gradually cease their activity; the cells become slightly less disclike, and their flexibility diminishes. These processes continue steadily until the cells are no longer viable.

But it still is uncertain whether senescent cells are removed from the circulation intact or only after they have broken up into several fragments. It is, however, generally believed that the cells or their fragments are taken up by erythrophages in the spleen and elsewhere, although it is still not known what exactly the changes are on the cells' surfaces that the phagocytic cells recognize as characterizing senescent red cells and that trigger the process of phagocytosis.

In humans, at least, the elimination curve of normal red cells in a healthy recipient, as demonstrated by the Ashby method or by the use of DF[32]P, is virtually a straight line, and this is consistent with the concept of gradually increasing senescence (of metabolic origin) rather than of random elimination in which the cells would be destroyed indiscriminately regardless of age. The distinction between these two methods of elimination was clearly made and was illustrated by Schiodt of Copenhagen in 1938;[28] its validity was vindicated when cases of hemolytic anemia came to be studied during the next decade. In fact, the analysis of survival curves contributed most significantly at that time to the understanding of the pathogenesis of increased hemolysis.[14,29,30]

Hemolytic Anemia: The Early Observations

It is remarkable that the earliest clear descriptions of hemolytic anemia published in the nineteenth century were of disorders that we now regard as relatively rare. But this is understandable when it is realized that these were based primarily upon one unmistakable sign of increased hemolysis, namely the passage of red or pink urine, in this instance due to the presence of hemoglobin (hemoglobinuria).

PAROXYSMAL COLD HEMOGLOBINURIA (PCH)

Dressler,[31] of Würzburg, is generally credited with being the first (in 1854) to give a clear description of this curious disorder and of clearly distinguishing intermittent "chromaturia" from "hematuria." His patient was a 10-year-old boy, who may have had congenital syphilis. PCH, however, seems also likely to have been the diagnosis in the patient described by Elliotson in the *Lancet* in

1832,[32] who had heart disease and cold "fits" and passed bloody urine "whenever the east wind blew."

Following Dressler's report,[31] several excellent clinical accounts by London physicians were published in the *Lancet* during the 1860s. The authors realized that exposure to cold precipitated the attacks and that the urine contained blood pigment, but no blood cells. The condition was described unfortunately as "intermittent or winter *haematuria*." Dickinson,[33] writing in 1865, concluded that the disorder was due to an alteration in the blood and likened the urine to that seen in arsine poisoning! In 1867, Wiltshire[34] described an infant—perhaps the youngest such patient ever recorded—who passed bloody urine, free from red cells in the sediment, when the "weather was particularly inclement."

The term *hemoglobinuria* seems to have been used first by Secchi, of Breslau, in 1872,[35] but it is not clear whether the patient he described had PCH.

Kuessner, of Halle, in 1879 made the important observation that serum obtained by "cupping" a patient during an attack of hemoglobinuria was tinged red.[36] This probably was the first piece of evidence that indicated that the hemoglobin in the urine was being derived from hemoglobin liberated into the plasma, rather than being, in some mysterious way, of renal origin. Several additional significant observations soon followed. Rosenbach,[37] of Breslau, demonstrated that hemoglobinuria could sometimes be provoked by chilling the patient locally, e.g., by placing the feet in ice water (Rosenbach's test), and Paul Ehrlich,[38] already mentioned several times in this book, showed that if a ligature was placed around a finger which was then chilled in ice water, serum subsequently obtained from the finger might be colored with hemoglobin (Ehrlich's test). It was at about this time, too, that the association between PCH and syphilis was recognized. In 1894, Chvostek[39] wrote a monograph entitled *Ueber das Wesen der paroxysmalen Hämoglobinurie,* and it seems possible that more was written about PCH in the latter part of the nineteenth century than about any other hemolytic anemia; it must have been one of the best known of all the blood diseases recognized at that time, perhaps due to the prevalence of congenital syphilis as well as its dramatic symptomatology. Now (in the 1970s), although well known and an admitted classic, PCH is one of the rarest of disorders.

PCH has the distinction of being the first hemolytic anemia in humans for which the mechanism of hemolysis was clearly established. In a series of papers, the first of which was published in 1904, Donath and Landsteiner,[40] of Vienna, established that hemolysis was probably due to an autolysin which united with the patient's red cells at low temperatures and that labile serum factors (alexin, i.e., complement) caused lysis of the sensitized cells if the temperature were subsequently raised. This was what experiments in the laboratory suggested, and it was inferred that this is what happened in vivo, too. Observations similar to those of Donath and Landsteiner were published in 1906 by Eason,[41] working in Leith, Scotland.

Eason's experiments were undertaken in 1903 and communicated to the Galenian Society in Edinburgh in January 1904; they were also written up in the form of a thesis for the degree of M.D. (University of Edinburgh), for which he received a Gold Medal. In his 1906 paper, Eason refers to Donath and Landsteiner as having independently confirmed the most important of his observations (10 months after he had communicated them!) and of proving that it is the "process of anchoring of the intermediary body to the red corpuscles which requires the low temperature."

Earlier, in 1899, Ehrlich and Morgenroth[42] had made a passing reference to the possibility that paroxysmal hemoglobinuria might be due to amboceptor (antibody)-alexin lysis. According to Bolduan's[43] translation of Ehrlich's papers, *Collected Studies on Immunity,* published in 1906, Ehrlich and Morgenroth had written, "It is very probable that certain forms of haemoglobinuria originate through analogous haemolysins." However, they somewhat diminished the value of this suggestion by adding: "Many years ago Ehrlich showed that haemoglobinuria *ex frigore* was caused not by any particular sensitiveness of the erythrocytes to cold, but by certain poisons produced, especially by the vessels, as a result of cold."

Donath and Landsteiner's[40] and Eason's[41] observations were quickly confirmed in many parts of the world, and the diagnostic cold-warm sequence for the demonstration of the hemolysin still bears the eponym *Donath-Landsteiner test,* and the antibody, the eponym *Donath-Landsteiner antibody.*

EXERTIONAL (MARCH) HEMOGLOBINURIA

In 1881, Fleischer[44] described from Berlin a "neue Form von Haemoglobinurie" in a soldier after a "feld" (field) march, and this is probably the first clear account to be published of exertional or march hemoglobinuria.

Many cases have since been described, and the disorder has an extensive literature. Dickinson's[45] account to the Clinical Society of London in 1894 is particularly interesting. In it are described keen observations made on three individuals—in two, hemoglobinuria followed running; in one, a game of tennis. The running-ground attendant was reported to have said: "it is not very uncommon for the urine to appear bloody after a severe run, especially at the beginning of training." Dickinson considered that the hemolysis was probably brought about by muscular exercise and concluded that it was "perhaps an exaggeration of the blood destruction which is the normal result of exercise."

Subsequent observations showed that varying degrees of hemoglobinemia and hemoglobinuria were not rare as an apparent immediate consequence of certain types of exercise, and many instances were reported, particularly from Germany in soldiers. It is remarkable that more than 80 years were to pass after Fleischer's[44] original description before Davidson[46] provided from Aberdeen in 1964 the elusive and, as it turned out, simple explanation. In a classic study, he showed that the intravascular hemolysis responsible for the hemoglobinuria was brought about by the mechanical trauma to the blood between the bones of the feet and the unyielding ground during the blood's passage through the blood vessels of the feet. All the victims had to do to prevent the hemolysis was to wear resilient insoles in their boots or running shoes! The association between marching on the barrack square in heavy boots or running on a hard surface, particularly if the runner had a high stamping gait, as well as the rarity of exertional hemoglobinuria in women, was, thus, easily explained.

PAROXYSMAL NOCTURNAL HEMOGLOBINURIA (PNH)

In 1882, Strübing,[47] of Greifswald, described how in his patient, sleep appeared to be a determining factor in producing the passage of dark urine containing hemoglobin; neither cold nor exercise was an immediate precipitating cause. Strübing's paper suffered, however, by having the uninformative title "Paroxysmale Haemoglobinurie" and was seldom referred to by subsequent writers until Crosby,[48] in a review of the early history of PNH, pointed out its importance. But Strübing's account was, in fact, not the first description of probable PNH in the literature. Gull,[49] writing from Guy's Hospital in 1866, described how the urine passed in the early morning by an anemic-appearing patient contained "haematin." In Gull's words, "it was usually the early morning urine which was abnormal. The urine after one or two o'clock in the afternoon presented the normal characteristics." Gull, however, thought the inciting cause for his patient's illness was cold and dampness, and he did not, as did Strübing, distinguish the disorder from PCH.

PNH has proved to be one of the most interesting of all blood diseases, and for a rather rare disorder it has a disproportionately large literature. After Strübing, the next important publication was that of Hijmans van den Bergh,[50] of Rotterdam, in 1911. Strübing had speculated that the red cells of his patient were probably defective and that the slowing of the circulation during sleep and the accumulation of carbon dioxide and lactic acid from the previous day's exertion led in some way to their hemolysis. Hijmans van den Bergh demonstrated that his patient's red cells actually underwent lysis in vitro in normal serum if the serum-cell mixture was exposed to carbon dioxide and came to the prescient conclusion that carbon dioxide revealed a diminution in the resistance of the cells to normal lytic substances present in normal serum.

Later work initiated by Ham,[51] of Boston, was to show that acidification of fresh normal serum to pH 6.5 to 7.0 provided a medium in which red cells from patients with PNH readily underwent lysis. This reaction (the *Ham test*) provides a simple and reliable way of diagnosing PNH, for it is now known that the essential abnormality of the disorder is a remarkable increase in the red cells' sensitivity to lysis by complement, whether the complement is attached to the red cells via the classical antibody-complement sequence or through the activation of complement by the alternate pathway. The fundamental lesion (or lesions) leading to the increased sensitivity to lysis by complement has, however, still not been clearly demonstrated.

Characteristic features of chronic intravascular hemolysis, as exemplified by PNH, are chronic hemoglobinemia, disappearance of the plasma hemoglobin-binding proteins (haptoglobins), possibly hemoglobinuria, depending on the rapidity of intravascular lysis, and continuous hemosiderinuria (granules of hemosiderin in the urine which are stained Prussian blue by acid-ferrocyanide and are easily visible under the light microscope). These granules of hemosiderin were first recognized and described as a granular form of hemoglobin by Marchiafava and Nazari,[52] of Rome, in 1911. Their constant presence, even in the absence of hemoglobinuria, was recognized by Ettore Marchiafava (1847–1916), the leading pathologist of Italy in his time, and, in a later paper,[53] he referred to PNH as "anaemia emolitica con emosiderinuria perpetua." The term *paroxysmal nocturnal hemoglobinuria* (haemoglobinuria paroxysmalis nocturna) seems first to have been used by Enneking,[54] of Amsterdam, in 1928, and this title, or, more frequently, its abbreviation PNH, is now universally employed.

Recent studies suggest that PNH is a clonal disease, developing as the result of somatic mutation. There is evidence, too, that the PNH "lesion" affects the white cells and platelets, in addition to the red cells; this would suggest that the mutation affects the stem cells. A remarkable feature is the frequency with which PNH appears to follow marrow aplasia; equally remarkable is that a small percentage of patients who develop PNH recover completely, after perhaps a decade or more of illness.

Hemolytic Icterus: Congenital and Acquired

It was not until the end of the nineteenth century that descriptions of hemolytic anemias not characterized by hemoglobinuria began to appear. It had clearly been more difficult for the nineteenth century physicians, handicapped by primitive or absent laboratory facilities, to distinguish between anemias due to increased hemolysis (without hemoglobinuria) from other causes of jaundice, notably disorders of the liver.

HEREDITARY SPHEROCYTOSIS (HS)

HS was the first hereditary hemolytic anemia to be defined; it did not at first, however, bear its present title. Two important accounts are to be found in the *Transactions of the Clinical Society of London* in the 1890s. Wilson[55] and Wilson and Stanley[56] described in six members of a family "a condition in which an enlarged spleen, accompanied by a sallow or subicteric complexion, appears as a hereditary condition." Anemia was recognized as an important feature; Wilson and Stanley concluded that "no doubt can be entertained that the splenic disease is accountable for this." One patient died; her spleen was found to be firm and dark on section and, microscopically, to be engorged with red cells. Death was considered to have been "due to active haemolysis of splenic origin." The diagnosis of HS in this family was confirmed 33 years later by Campbell,[57] who examined the sole survivor.

Wilson and Stanley did not remark on the blood picture in their cases, but Vanlair and Masius,[58] of Liège, writing in 1871, did do so. Their paper entitled *De la microcythémie* is the text of a lecture given to the Belgium Royal Academy of Medicine in June 1871. The text is lengthy, almost 100 pages!

In it is described the clinical history of a young woman who developed, soon after the birth of her first child, repeated attacks of abdominal pain, centered over the hypochondrium and the spleen, which were associated with prostration, vomiting, and jaundice. Later, she suffered from aphonia and, then, marked weakness of her arms and legs without sensory loss. Her blood was examined four times between January and August 1870, and each time it was noticed that the majority of the red cells were smaller than normal and spherical (4 μm in diameter). Vanlair and Masius called the cells *microcytes,* and they are illustrated in a delightful lithograph drawn and colored by Vanlair, alongside a drawing of normal blood (Figure 8-6). The microcytes are depicted a slightly deeper shade of yellowish gray than are the larger, more discoidal cells.

The patient was again seen in April 1871, after a lapse of 8 months, and Vanlair and Masius were surprised to find how much she had improved; the mucous membranes were red, jaundice was hardly appreciable, and she had regained much of her muscular strength. The blood had changed too; it no longer consisted almost entirely of 4-μm microcytes; instead, the majority of the red cells were 6 to 7 μm in diameter. The cells were still considered, however, to be abnormally small, and the spleen, too, remained enlarged.

Vanlair and Masius discussed at length the nature of the microcytes—whether they were forms transitional between white cells and red cells (!) or whether they were "globules atrophiques," senile discoidal cells on the way to complete dissolution. They thought the latter hypothesis the more likely. In a discussion on the spleen, they suggested that its main function was to prepare red cells for destruction, i.e., to make them old. They thought that red cells within the pulp of the spleen, "soustraits" (removed) from the active circulation, fall into obsolescence; the cells become spherical and lose volume; their substance becomes more dense; they become less "attackable," less "vivante"—i.e., they become microcytes. If the spleen were hyperplastic, as in the patient they were describing, then (they argued) the number of microcytes produced by the spleen would be greater than normal. Vanlair and Masius thought that the liver continued the work started by the spleen, i.e., it destroyed the microcytes it received from the spleen via the splenic vein. They considered that their patient's liver was atrophic and concluded that the large number of microcytes in the peripheral blood, the microcythemia, was the resultant of two factors—increased production of microcytes by the spleen coupled with decreased removal by the liver.

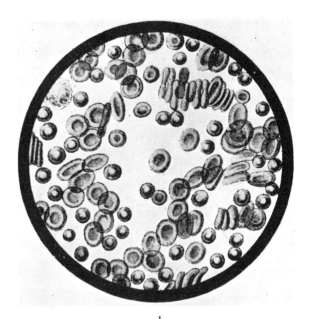

I

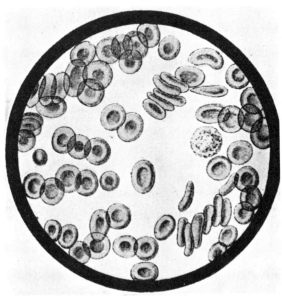

Figure 8-6 A reproduction of part of the tinted lithograph illustrating the paper by Vanlair and Masius (1871) entitled *De la microcythémie*. I is a drawing of the patient's blood. II is a drawing of control normal blood. (*From Vanlair and Masius,*[58] 1871.)

II

Vanlair and Masius believed that their patient's illness did not conform to any known disease. They mentioned (for the first time) in their concluding paragraphs that an elder sister of the patient had suffered from an illness which was so similar to that of their patient as to be described by them as "la production photographique la plus parfaite." The sister had suffered, in the same order, from pain in the hypochondrium, hypertrophy of the spleen, pain over the spleen, remittent icterus, transient aphonia, and paralysis of the arms and legs. She died after a "vomique," which had been preceded by pain in the splenic and diaphragmatic region. They added that the patient's mother was usually a little yellowish and was subject to jaundice!

Vanlair and Masius' keen observations and shrewd deductions were many years in advance of their time, and their paper has not received the attention it deserves. The present author's interpretation is that the two women (and their mother) had hereditary spherocytosis. That the disorder was usually well compensated is suggested by the fact that the younger of the two women had apparently not suffered from any serious illness until after the birth of her child. Then, for unknown reasons, she suffered from a prolonged hemolytic crisis with abdominal symptoms from which she eventually recovered. The onset of severe muscular weakness, which is described in great detail, and the report that her sister had had similar symptoms, makes the story all the more fascinating.

HS was at one time referred to quite widely by the eponym Minkowski-Chauffard. Oskar Minkowski (1858–1931) was born in Russia but was educated and spent the rest of his life in Germany. The renowned clinician, whose scientific work revolved about clinical chemistry and who was best known for his contributions to the understanding of diabetes mellitus, at the 18th German Congress of Internal Medicine held at Wiesbaden in April 1900 described eight members of a family, in three generations, living in Alsace who were affected.[59] The index patient (propositus) had had chronic jaundice since infancy. His general health was said not to be affected, and he did not attach any particular importance to the color of his skin as this was also present in other members of his family. His spleen was enlarged, and there was an increased amount of the pigment urobilin in the urine. No details of his blood picture were given. This patient died of pneumonia, and, at necropsy, no mechanical cause in the liver was found to account for the jaundice; the gallbladder, however, contained a pigment stone. The spleen weighed 1 kg; it was noticed to be hyperplastic and hyperemic, but microscopically nothing remarkable was noted. The kidneys (surprisingly) were reported to contain a great excess of iron. Minkowski[59] concluded that the most likely explanation for the disorder was a peculiar anomaly of the turnover of blood pigment, perhaps the consequence of a primary change in the spleen. This report, although better known, actually added little, if anything, to that of Wilson and Stanley.[56]

On the other hand, the contribution of Anatole Chauffard (1855–1932)

(Figure 8-7), published in 1907,[60] was a major one. Working in Paris in the heyday of French medicine, he used the technique of Ribierre[61] to measure quantitatively the osmotic resistance of red cells to lysis by hypotonic saline, and showed in three patients, who almost certainly had HS, that their red cells differed in two respects from those found in other types of jaundice—the cells were small (microcytic), and they were less resistant than normal to lysis in hypotonic saline, whereas in other types of jaundice the cells were larger than normal (macrocytic) and more resistant to lysis.

　　Chauffard's paper is a classic and contains a great deal of detail. His first patient was a male, studied when aged 24 years, who had become jaundiced on the day after his birth. Although he progressed well as an infant, jaundice persisted off and on, and, later, he suffered from crises of abdominal pain. When studied by Chauffard, his spleen was enlarged and the liver was just palpable. Chauffard considered that his patient had the same disorder as that of Minkowski's patients (an abstract[62] of Minkowski's report had appeared in *Semaine médicale* in 1900), and he concluded that "l'ictère congenital" of his patient could not be attributed to ascending "angiocholitis" or to biliary

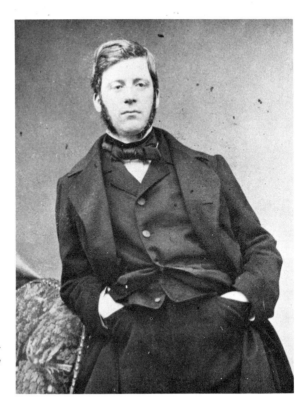

Figure 8-7 Anatole Chauffard (1855–1932). (*Courtesy National Library of Medicine, Bethesda, Md.*)

cirrhosis. The signs (he considered) pointed to a hemolytic pathogenesis despite a minor degree of anemia. Lysis in hypotonic saline was described as "précoce et prolongée" i.e., it began in more concentrated saline solutions than normally. The range was 0.62 to 0.36% NaCl (normal, 0.42 to 0.36 percent NaCl) (Figure 8-8), and the mean red cell diameter was given as 5.89 μm (normal, 7.6 μm). Chauffard obtained similar results with the blood of two other patients, a man and his daughter.

Chauffard noticed, too, that the red cells of his patients varied unusually in size, from 3 μm to 11 μm, and he concluded that it was probably the small cells which hemolyzed first. He stressed that the "inequality" in resistance to hypotonic saline was greater than in normal subjects or in patients jaundiced due to the retention of bile pigment. He could not decide whether the splenic reaction was the cause of the hemolysis or the effect, as seemed to be the case when hemolytic drugs were administered to animals. He concluded that in the patients he had studied, there was something special, something that was not operating in other anemias, this probably being "an active intervention of the splenic parenchyma." In Chauffard's view, the spleen, thus, played a "primordial and preponderant" role; the liver, on the other hand, was thought to play a passive role, by having to deal with the overabundant products of the

Figure 8-8   The figure illustrates the "precocious and prolonged" lysis in hypotonic saline of the red cells of a patient suffering from ictère congénital de l'adulte (hereditary spherocytosis). (*From Chauffard,*[60] 1907.)

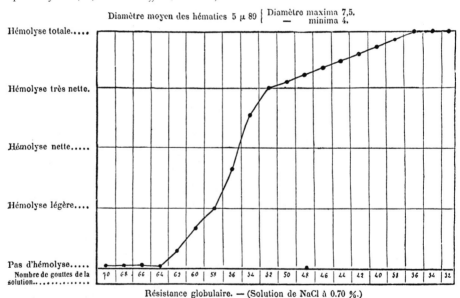

hemolysis. But he did not exclude the possibility of secondary lesions in the liver and of the possible formation of pigment gallstones. He did not speculate on the cause of the microcytosis or on the diminished resistance to hypotonic saline.

An interesting complication of severe HS is the occurrence of intractable ulcers on the lower part of the leg. This seems to have been reported for the first time in London in 1902 by Barlow and Shaw,[63] who thought that their patient had the same disorder as that of Wilson and Stanley's[56] patients.

Barlow and Shaw's patient was a boy, small for his age, who was "anaemic and yellow" and had a spleen extending below the umbilicus. Ulcers developed above both ankles when he was aged 10 years (a remarkably early age for this type of ulceration). Their report contains the details of numerous blood counts; the red cell count was said to average 2,603,753 (!) cells per mm^3 and the hemoglobin to average 41 percent. Nucleated red cells were nearly always present in blood films and "basophile cells" were frequently seen. When the patient was visited in the hospital by his mother, the house physician noticed that she had a yellowish complexion very similar to that of her son. He persuaded her to let him examine her; her spleen was palpable, and she was found to be anemic. She, too, had an ulcer on her right leg, which had been "discharging" for 27 years!

The main clinical features of HS had, thus, been described by the early years of the twentieth century, and the increased blood destruction had been linked with the enlargement of the spleen. It was not long before removal of the spleen was advocated, and several successful operations were referred to by Wynter[64] at a discussion held at the Royal Society of Medicine in London early in 1913. In fact, a successful splenectomy had been carried out many years before. According to Dawson[65] (Lord Dawson of Penn, Physician-in-Ordinary to H.M. King George V), writing in 1931, Spencer Wells had operated in 1887 on a woman aged 27 who had had attacks of jaundice since she was 9 years old. She had an abdominal tumor which had been diagnosed as a fibroid. But at operation, this was found to be a very large spleen; it was removed. When this patient was examined 40 years later, she was found to be in good health; her son had had his gallbladder and spleen removed when he was 14 years old, and Dawson found that his red cells had abnormal osmotic fragility.

The hereditary nature of HS, demonstrated by Wilson[55] in 1890 and Minkowski[59] in 1900, was fully evaluated by Meulengracht in 1921.[66] He found that the evidence clearly pointed to dominant inheritance, and in a study of seven Danish families, he was able to show, with one exception, that the disorder was inherited through an affected parent; he attributed the one exception to mutation. Thus, by the early 1920s, practically all the clinical phenomena of HS had been described, the spleen was suspected to be the cause of the hemolysis, and splenectomy had been found to be clinically curative. But nothing was known about the basis of the disorder and the mechanism of hemolysis was not understood.

ACQUIRED HEMOLYTIC ICTERUS

Parallel with the early observations on a hereditary type of hemolytic anemia (HS) were those on an acquired form. These originated in Paris. Hayem (1841–1935), the leading French hematologist of the time, in 1898 seems to have been the first physician to have differentiated anemia with jaundice from disease of the liver with jaundice,[67] but it was Widal, Abrami, and Brulé,[68] and their collaborators, in a series of papers published from 1908 onwards who first established "l'ictère hémolytique acquis" as a definite entity. The eponym *anemia of Hayem and Widal* was frequently used. Fernand Widal (1862–1929), another of the great pre-World War I French clinicians, is best known, however, for his agglutination test for typhoid fever.

Widal and his collaborators stressed that autoagglutination was characteristic of the cases they had studied, and Le Gendre and Brulé,[69] in contrasting the congenital and the acquired forms of hemolytic jaundice, stated that in the latter "auto-agglutination des hématies restait constamment intense et rapide, prenant une veritable valeur diagnostique."* Patients, too, were described, suffering from intense hemolysis, whose sera appeared to contain abnormal hemolysins. These studies, although we may now view them as incomplete and to some extent unsatisfactory, were pioneer ones well in advance of their time, and the idea that hemolytic anemia could occur apparently spontaneously in man in consequence of the development of abnormal agglutinins or hemolysins remained controversial for the next 30 years or so. It is remarkable, too, that in the few published accounts of apparently acquired acute hemolytic anemia, e.g., by Lederer[70] in 1925, no serologic studies were carried out or, at least, reported. Dameshek and Schwartz,[71,72] of Boston, deserve credit for their powerful championship of the importance of "hemolysins" in the pathogenesis of acquired hemolytic anemia, for they showed clearly that spherocytosis and increased osmotic fragility could develop in the course of an acquired hemolytic anemia in humans, as well as in experimental animals, and that these features were, thus, not specifically indicative of HS, a view which was current in England (at least) in the 1930s.

The difficulty in ascribing cases of acquired hemolytic anemia to the development of "hemolysins" was that they could not be demonstrated in the vast majority of cases by the serologic techniques then available, and it was not until the introduction of the antiglobulin (Coombs) test by Coombs, Mourant,

---

*The autoagglutination of the red cells is constantly pronounced and rapid, rendering it of true diagnostic value.

and Race[73] and its application to cases of hemolytic anemia by Boorman, Dodd, and Loutit[74] in 1946 that the matter was cleared up. It was then convincingly demonstrated that the common type of "hemolysin" was in fact an "incomplete" nonagglutinating and nonhemolytic antibody. The application of the antiglobulin test to cases of hemolytic anemia was, without doubt, a major landmark in the history of their investigation and understanding.

Changes in Red Cell Morphology in Hemolytic Anemia: Early Descriptions

SPHEROCYTOSIS

Spherocytes have already been mentioned in connection with HS and acquired hemolytic anemia in man and in experimental hemolytic anemia in animals. The term seems first to have been coined by Christophers and Bentley,[75] who were working in India, ostensibly on blackwater fever. In their report published in 1909, they described how, in order to improve their understanding of the mechanisms of hemolysis in general, they decided to study the hemolytic anemia produced in dogs by the injection of anti-dog red cell sera produced in goats.

In discussing their results, the authors referred to the small, darkly staining round cells, which had been described previously in blood diseases. Remarking that the term *microcyte* was unsuitable, they went on to write "[the] appearance [of spherocytes] is due mainly if not altogether to changes in their elasticity, which prevents them from becoming as flattened as are normal corpuscles." Because such cells are a "sign of most important pathological changes, we have thought it desirable to have a name to designate the condition and have termed them *spherocytes* [italics added]."

Rather similar experimental observations on rabbits were reported by Muir and McNee[76] of Glasgow in 1911. Their paper contains good photomicrographs, and, although they did not use the term spherocyte, they certainly described them. This is part of what they said: "as the anaemia progresses many of the old erythrocytes seem to diminish in size, so that corpuscles 3–5 μ in diameter, which stain deeply with eosin are present. At the same time, the larger newer formed corpuscles gradually lose their basophil reaction, and it would appear that some of them undergo contraction and diminution in size."

Muir and McNee's important contribution was followed by that of Banti,[77] of Florence, in 1913, who used both dogs and rabbits. Although he apparently did not study red cell morphology, he measured osmotic fragility and concentrated particularly on the role of the spleen. Like Christophers and Bentley and Muir and McNee, Banti was struck by the much greater potency in vivo of hemolytic antisera when compared with their ability to produce lysis in vitro. He rejected the hypothesis that the increased fragility was due to adsorbed antibody and suggested that the change more probably resulted from a "fragilizing activity" which the animal possesses or develops; he concluded that the severe anemia which the injection of a hemolytic antiserum might produce was in large part due to the hemolytic potentiality of the animal itself and that the spleen played an important role in bringing about the hemolysis.

These papers, published more than 60 years ago, are remarkable for the keenness of the authors' observations and the shrewdness of their deductions; another 25 years were to pass before Dameshek and Schwartz,[71] in 1938, reawakened interest in what could be learned from the experimental production by immune sera of hemolytic anemia. Their main message, as already referred to, was that spherocytosis could be acquired and that it could be produced in some way by the action in vivo of hemolytic antisera. Thirty years or so were to pass before the phenomenon was to be explained.

As already mentioned, spherocytes were, nevertheless, at one time considered not only to be characteristic but virtually pathognomonic of HS (despite the experimental studies referred to above, which had already been published and which had clearly indicated the contrary). This misconception seems to have stemmed largely from the powerful influence of Otto Naegeli (1871–1938), of Zürich. First referred to as Kugelzellen (globe cells) in the fourth edition of his *Blutkrankheiten und Blutdiagnostik*, the microcytes of HS were renamed "Sphärocyten" in the fifth edition, published in 1931.[78]

SCHISTOCYTOSIS

Reference in the literature to the presence of fragments of red cells in the blood in anemia stretches right back into the nineteenth century. They were, perhaps, first noted in patients with severe burns, and it was Paul Ehrlich[79] who introduced the term *Schistocyte* in a monograph published in Berlin in 1891. As already mentioned, Rous and Robertson[2] reported that "schizocytes" (schistocytes) could be found in small numbers in the blood of healthy animals and concluded that they represented effete red cells soon to be eliminated from the circulation. Subsequently, the presence of excessive numbers of schistocytes came to be accepted as a feature of the blood picture in thalassemia major and severe megaloblastic anemia and an indication that hemolysis was playing a part in the pathogenesis of these anemias. However, despite a general awareness of the occurrence and significance of fragmentation, it is a remarkable fact that it is only relatively recently that blood pictures in which fragmentation is a major feature and is largely responsible for hemolytic anemia have been recognized, as for instance in the microangiopathic hemolytic anemia of the hemolytic-uremic syndrome (p. 248) and in certain rare congenital hemolytic anemias.

HEINZ BODIES

Another phenomenon, first described in the nineteenth century, which recently has assumed considerable clinical importance, is the presence in red cells of denatured hemoglobin, which can be stained by basic dyes. Heinz,[80] of Breslau, described his eponymous bodies in 1890 in the blood of guinea pigs that had been poisoned with acetylphenylhydrazine; subsequently, it was established that the bodies could be produced in vivo (and in vitro) by the action of a wide range of aromatic nitro and amino compounds, as well as by inorganic oxidizing compounds such as potassium chlorate. The connection between chemical poisoning and Heinz-body formation became so firmly established that when Heinz bodies were found in the blood of patients thought to have a congenital hemolytic anemia their apparent spontaneous occurrence was at first viewed with considerable suspicion, and every effort was made to trace a chemical cause.

INTRAVASCULAR AND EXTRAVASCULAR HEMOLYSIS

It is noteworthy that the distinction between intravascular and extravascular hemolysis was made in the early years of this century. Hunter,[81] for instance, in 1901 wrote with reference to what he termed "chronic haematocytolysis": "They [the red corpuscles] become spherical, deeper in colour, and retain their haemoglobin to the last. In this form they continue to circulate until finally they are enclosed within the active cells of the spleen or in the capillaries of the liver." Later, in referring to "acute haematocytolysis," he wrote:

> The second process is marked by a different series of phenomena. The first of these is a liberation of haemoglobin from the corpuscle. It escapes from the corpuscle, either alone, or in combination with the albuminous stroma. Its fate is not, as in the former case, to be taken up by the splenic cells or leucocytes within the blood, but it is carried to the liver in the portal blood, where it is taken and broken up by the liver cells.

In 1909, Christophers and Bentley made a similar distinction; they concluded that hemoglobinemia resulted from intravascular hemolysis, "lysaemia," in contradistinction to erythrocyte destruction outside the bloodstream, which they referred to as "erythrocytolysis" and attributed to erythrophagocytosis without release of hemoglobin into the blood.

The distinction between intravascular and extravascular hemolysis has stood the test of time. The carriage of free hemoglobin in the plasma and its metabolism and fate, and its excretion by the kidney, have been particular subjects of study; the discovery of pseudomethemoglobin,[82] later named methemalbumin,[83] and of the hemoglobin-binding proteins (the haptoglobins) and of hemopexin has in each case been a minor landmark in the history of hematology.

State of Knowledge in the 1930s

The brief accounts in the foregoing pages illustrate how an understanding of the hemolytic anemias was gradually acquired, so that by the mid-1930s, when the present author first became aware of their existence (and fascination), most of the main syndromes had been recognized. The *mechanisms* of hemolysis were, however, poorly understood, and there was certainly no anticipation of the dramatic expansion of knowledge that was to come. The hemolytic anemias were regarded as a comparatively small group of disorders, worthy at the most of a separate chapter in books on hematology.

In the second edition of her classic textbook *The Anaemias,* published in 1936, Janet Vaughan[84] referred to six categories only: hemolytic anemias due to infection, chemical poisons, acholuric jaundice, sickle-cell anemia, paroxysmal hemoglobinuria, and acute hemolytic anemia (most cases of which she considered to be the result of an acute crisis occurring in latent or chronic acholuric jaundice). Castle and Minot,[85] also in 1936, in their article, *Pathological Physiology and Clinical Description of the Anemias,* classified the hemolytic anemias in a similar fashion. However, they admitted the existence of an acquired type of chronic hemolytic jaundice (Hayem-Widal). These accounts were written by physicians with a particular interest in hematology. In students' textbooks, the hemolytic anemias were dealt with still more cursorily.

At the present time—the late 1970s—we realize that very many types of hemolytic anemia exist and that they have many different causes, varying from subtle inherited defects of the red cell surface, its enzymes, or its hemoglobin to autoantibodies formed against red cell surface antigens. What is more, during the past 40 years or so, the hemolytic anemias have provided a rich field for research by clinical and laboratory-oriented hematologists, biochemists, geneticists, and immunologists. Together these investigators have built up a remarkable body of knowledge that has had repercussions well beyond the confines of hematology. For instance, it is difficult to overestimate the importance for the science of molecular genetics of the discovery that molecular variants of hemoglobin exist and for population genetics that one such variant, hemoglobin S, protects against malaria; or that the presence of a defective enzyme, e.g., G6PD, makes an individual unusually susceptible to the harmful effects of certain drugs, e.g., the antimalarials. These topics are discussed in Chapters 11 and 6, respectively.

The study of the acquired hemolytic anemias, too, has contributed powerfully to our understanding of the autoimmune disorders. Paroxysmal cold hemoglobinuria is the earliest recorded, and it remains perhaps the most dramatic, exception to Ehrlich and Morgenroth's[86] much quoted rule of *horror autotoxicus*.

Recent Developments: An Explosion of Knowledge

HEREDITARY ANEMIAS

Our knowledge has expanded in two main directions—many "new" diseases have been distinguished and much has been learned about their pathogenesis.

As already mentioned, the use of the Ashby method to trace the survival of normal red cells after their transfusion into patients with various types of hemolytic anemia in the 1940s enabled a clear distinction to be made between those disorders in which the normal cells survived normally and those in which they were eliminated abnormally rapidly. This led quite soon to the concept that increased hemolysis may be *intrinsic* or *extrinsic* to the red cell, a distinction that proved to be useful in classifying the hemolytic anemias. The inherited (familial and congenital) hemolytic anemias all belong to the first group (intrinsic abnormality) except for the rather special case of hemolytic disease of the newborn due to Rh (or other blood-group) incompatibility between mother and fetus. The acquired hemolytic anemias (noncongenital, nonfamilial) typically have an extrinsic pathogenesis, with the important exception of paroxysmal nocturnal hemoglobinuria.

So-called familial acholuric jaundice is now known to comprise several important groups of disorders due, respectively, to inherited defects of red cell membrane structure (probably) or of one of the red cell enzymes or of its hemoglobin. Hereditary spherocytosis remains the best known disorder of the first group and pyruvate kinase (PK) deficiency the most important enzyme deficiency.

It is a remarkable fact that, although it was known in the 1930s that patients with "acholuric jaundice" were occasionally not clinically cured by splenectomy, as in the typical disease, and that the blood of such patients might have a normal osmotic fragility, no one seems to have suggested at that time that these patients might have been suffering from a disorder of totally different pathogenesis. They were considered to be "atypical cases" and the matter was left at that point. It was not, in fact, until 1947 that Haden,[87] of Cleveland, published his well-known account of "A New Type of Hereditary Hemolytic Jaundice without Spherocytosis." Two families were described; in both, the anemia was macrocytic, osmotic fragilities were normal, and there was no spherocytosis. Splenectomy, carried out on one of the patients, did not alter the course of the disease.

Hereditary Spherocytosis and Allied Disorders It is now generally believed that the fundamental abnormality in hereditary spherocytosis (HS) resides within the red cell membrane; an abnormal structural protein, i.e., a molecular variant, may be present.[88] Spectrin is one such protein, and it seems possible that an abnormality within the molecule leads to a defect in its phosphorylation. Inefficient phosphorylation would have important biochemical consequences which lead ultimately to reduction in the flexibility of the cell, loss of membrane, and microspherocytosis, as well as a reduced capacity to withstand the metabolic consequences of stasis within the spleen. The analysis of membrane proteins and the assessment of their metabolism are technically difficult, and there seems, at the time of writing, no certainty that the spectrin story as recounted above is correct.[89] But the fact that HS is a clinical disorder that may be strongly expressed in heterozygotes does suggest that the basic abnormality is unlikely to be an abnormal enzyme.

A question that is often asked is whether HS is a single disease, i.e., whether a patient with trivial clinical manifestations and minor hematologic changes and another patient with major clinical and hematologic abnormalities, leading, perhaps, to severe neonatal jaundice and anemia, have one and the same disease, only variably expressed. This question can only be answered when the lesion in "typical" HS can be pinpointed in exact biochemical terms. This long-awaited advance is important, too, for the understanding of the rather rare patient who does not respond fully to splenectomy or who has an unusual blood picture. By analogy with the host of molecular variants of hemoglobin that are now known to exist, it seems likely that, if the basis of HS is an abnormal structural protein resulting from an amino acid substitution, HS may indeed be a group of disorders.

Hereditary Elliptocytosis (HE)   Hereditary elliptocytosis (HE) is the best known of the disorders allied with HS. It was first described in Ohio by Dresbach in 1904.[90] HE is not a rare disorder, and its relatively late description reminds us that blood was not examined under the microscope with any frequency until the beginning of the present century. This point is emphasized even more strongly by the fact that sickle-shaped cells were not described until 1910.[91]

HE presents an interesting contrast to HS in that there is no evidence of increased hemolysis in the majority of families affected. In the minority in which hemolysis is present, the spleen will be found to be enlarged, and splenectomy results in a clinical cure. This wide range of clinical expression suggests that HE, like HS, is a group of disorders and that, if its cause is the presence of a structural protein variant in the red cell membrane (which has not yet been demonstrated), then several, perhaps many, different variants exist. However, against this simple hypothesis are the findings of Jensson and colleagues in Iceland.[92] Although the clinical and hematologic expression varied considerably in the large number of HE patients studied, genetic detective work suggested that all the cases had originated from a single gene imported into Iceland many generations back.

HE has proved to be an exceptionally interesting disorder for several other reasons. In some families, but not in all, a linkage with the Rh genes has been established. Patients also have been described with severe hemolytic anemia and markedly abnormal red cells, both of whose parents have had mild HE. The red cell membranes of such patients, who are probably homozygotes, should be fascinating objects for study by protein chemists. Also, a few patients have been described with severe hemolytic anemia dating from birth; their blood films are characterized by a striking degree of fragmentation. Wiley and Gill[93] were able to show recently in one such patient that the red cells contained an excess of calcium; an inward calcium ion leak was postulated, with a consequent stiffening of the red cell membrane and proneness to fragmentation. The lesion responsible for the ingress of calcium ions was not defined. The work, however, has important implications, for it demonstrates a mechanism for fragmentation that may operate in other anemias.

There are other fascinating aspects of HE. For example, the reticulocytes are round in contour, and the cells become elliptic as they mature. The subtle reason for this is unknown. Moreover, there are some families in which the majority of mature cells are oval rather than elliptic—this is so-called *hereditary ovalocytosis* (HO).[94] Then, it has been recently realized that in the Far East, e.g., in Malaysia and Papua–New Guinea,[95] a form of HO exists, not accompanied by anemia, in which a rather characteristic morphological abnormality of the red cells is associated with diminished expression of certain red cell antigens.[96] This observation certainly points to a structural abnormality in or at the red cell surface.

The explanation of these remarkable variants once again awaits the definition of the causal lesion(s) in exact biochemical terms.

Hereditary Stomatocytosis (HSt)   The description of hereditary stomatocytosis (HSt) by Lock, Sephton-Smith, and Hardisty[97] in 1961 has proved to be another milestone in the history of the hemolytic anemias. The term *stomatocytosis* (Greek, $\sigma\tau o\mu\alpha$, mouth) was coined to describe the appearances of some of the red cells in the blood films of a small girl and her mother, both of whom had had their spleens removed for hemolytic anemia of uncertain diagnosis. In wet preparations, the cells tended to be cup-shaped. Neither patient responded fully to splenectomy.

A few other families have since been described in some of whose members a rather similar blood picture has been noted. It now appears that HSt comprises a rather rare but most interesting group of dominantly inherited hemolytic anemias of mild to moderate severity. A most interesting common feature has been the discovery by Nathan and his colleagues[98] in 1966 that the cation content of the red cells is abnormal; in particular, the Na^+ concentration has been found to be abnormally high and the K^+ concentration abnormally low—in some cases, the Na^+ concentration has even exceeded that of the K^+, particularly if the blood has been allowed to stand in vitro. The basic lesion thus appears once again to be a membrane abnormality which has a major effect on the function of the cation pumps and the regulation of the cells' content of water.

According to Wiley and coworkers,[99] there are two types of HSt—in one, the red cells are overhydrated, and stomatocytes can be seen in blood films; in the other, the cells are dehydrated, and target cells are present. The amount of cell water present parallels the sum of the intracellular $K^+ + Na^+$. Unfortunately, the nature of the primary biochemical lesion in the red cell membrane has not yet been determined.

The Hereditary Nonspherocytic Hemolytic Anemias (HNSHA): Enzyme-Deficiency Hemolytic Anemias   Although in 1947, Haden[87] had described a "new" type of hereditary hemolytic anemia, it was not until 1954 that there were any definite indications of the nature of the HNSHAs. It was then shown in two patients with severe congenital hemolytic anemia that the addition of glucose failed to reduce the rate of spontaneous lysis of sterile incubated blood, as it regularly does in normal subjects and in most cases of HS and in other cases of HNSHA;[100] the utilization of glucose by the red cells of the two patients was found to be only 25 percent and 30 percent, respectively, of that expected when allowance was made for the number of reticulocytes present. Selwyn and Dacie[100] concluded that "the greatly increased lysis of the cells in vitro, and probably in vivo, is related to their defective glucose utilization." The cases in which the addition of glucose failed to reduce (to "correct") the rate of spontaneous lysis of incubated blood (so-called autohemolysis) were referred to as type II and those in which partial correction was achieved, type I.

This work focused attention on the metabolism of red cells, an aspect of hematology that had been neglected by hematologists up to that time. A significant step forward was made by de Gruchy, Crawford, and Morton[101] in 1958 when they reported that in four type II patients, although adenosine triphosphate (ATP) was decreased in concentration, total organic phosphate was markedly increased, this being due largely to a major increase in 2,3-diphosphoglycerate (2,3-DPG). This work suggested that if the basis of the disorder was a defective enzyme, the enzyme would be one controlling a late rather than an early step in the Embden-Meyerhof pathway of glycolysis (Chapter 6). It was left to Valentine, Tanaka, and Miwa[102] in 1961 to pinpoint the putative defective enzyme in type II cases as pyruvate kinase (PK).

This discovery resulted in a further upsurge of interest and, as perhaps might have been anticipated, the HNSHAs have proved to be far more heterogeneous than was indicated by the tentative grouping into types I and II on the basis of the results in the autohemolysis test.

Although PK deficiency has been found to be by far the most common cause of HNSHA, it is not the only cause, and, in other patients, a variety of other enzymes have been found to be deficient.[103]

Another type of enzyme-deficiency hemolytic anemia has to be mentioned. At the same time as patients with *chronic* HNSHA were being studied, patients with a clinically different type of hemolytic anemia were under intensive study by members of the University of Chicago Army Malaria Research Unit, as described in Chapter 6. These were black American servicemen who had displayed an unexpected idiosyncrasy to the drug primaquine, used in the prophylaxis of malaria—they, a small minority, developed *acute* hemolytic anemia with hemoglobinuria. (According to Beutler,[104] this phenomenon had been observed by Cordes[105] as far back as 1926 when the first 8-aminoquinoline drug, Plasmochin, was used. A highly significant point in Cordes' first report was that all 72 patients who had developed acute hemolytic anemia were blacks!)

The University of Chicago Malaria Research Unit had the developing resources of modern biochemistry at their disposal, and the eventual outcome was that this peculiar idiosyncrasy, which seemed to be confined to black individuals, was shown to be due to the deficiency of an important enzyme in the hexose monophosphate shunt, namely, glucose-6-phosphate dehydrogenase (G6PD).[106] These observations provided yet another springboard for research into drug idiosyncrasy (for many other drugs are capable of acting like primaquine) and in population genetics and human polymorphisms. From the point of view of our present story, subsequent studies established that one type of chronic (not drug-induced) HNSHA[107] depended upon the presence of a defective type of G6PD. In fact, chronic G6PD-deficiency HNSHA, although a rare disorder, has proved to be exceptionally interesting, because, in almost every family studied, the defective enzyme has been shown by biochemical and biophysical means to have its own individual characteristics, i.e., many mutant types of G6PD exist, almost rivaling in number the host of molecular variants of hemoglobin. The severity of the hemolytic anemia depends upon how inefficient the mutant enzyme is, and, in this respect, its lability is a particularly important factor.

Inheritance of HNSHA The inheritance pattern of the HNSHAs contrasts sharply with that of the hemolytic anemias, such as HS, which appear to depend upon a structural defect of the red cell membrane. The HNSHAs are recessive disorders: that is, patients who have clinically obvious hemolytic anemia are homozygous for the enzyme defect or, more commonly, double heterozygotes for more than one variant of the same enzyme. Although heterozygotes often can be detected in the laboratory by means of enzyme assays, the presence of one normal gene usually provides sufficient enzyme activity for the metabolism of the red cell to proceed virtually normally. An exception to this is G6PD deficiency, which is sex-linked, i.e., the gene for the enzyme is carried on the X (sex) chromosome. Males, who are hemizygotes (XY), suffer from clinically obvious and often severe hemolysis if their X chromosome carries a defective gene, as they have no normal X chromosome.

The HNSHAs have provided interesting evidence on the cellular specificity of enzyme defects. Thus, in PK deficiency, it is the red cell enzyme that is the mutant; the isoenzymes present in leukocytes (and other tissues) usually are unaffected. In contrast, in G6PD deficiency, the enzyme that is affected is one which is common to both red cells and leukocytes and other tissues, although the clinical effect of having a defective enzyme in, for instance, leukocytes appears to be negligible. This probably is because leukocytes retain their ability to synthesize the enzyme throughout their life, whereas in red cells this is only possible in the early forms (erythroblasts and reticulocytes).

Recently, it has been recognized that in certain rare types of HNSHA the nervous system is also involved. This probably is the result of the deficiency of an enzyme that is not specific for the red cell. Triose phosphate isomerase (TPI) deficiency provides an example of this association,[108] for, in affected patients, a severe neurologic disease, characterized by generalized weakness and spasticity, has eventually developed. In relation to this, Schneider and his colleagues[108] have pointed out that TPI is involved in the metabolism of lipids: for example, 3-phosphoglyceraldehyde can act as a precursor of lipid only after isomerization to dihydroxyacetone phosphate, a reaction that is markedly limited in TPI deficiency.

The Unstable Hemoglobins; Congenital Heinz-Body Anemia   Before leaving the hereditary hemolytic anemias, reference must be made to a large and important group of disorders that have, so far, hardly been mentioned, namely, the abnormal hemoglobinopathies. This subject is covered in full by Dr. Conley in Chapter 11. However, one relatively recently recognized group of abnormal hemoglobins, the unstable varieties, deserves brief mention here as they can lead to chronic hemolytic anemia that mimics quite closely HNSHA due to an enzyme deficiency. The reason for this is that it is not until the spleen has been removed from a patient with a congenital Heinz-body anemia that the diagnostic large Heinz bodies can be seen in the majority of the patient's red cells.

The first certain case of unstable hemoglobin disease was described by Cathie[109] in 1952. The patient was a small boy whose spleen had been removed for an undiagnosed hemolytic anemia when he was 16 months old. After splenectomy, Heinz bodies were found in many of his red cells, and this led to a search for a noxious chemical or drug, but none was found. Eighteen years later, the presence of an unstable hemoglobin (hemoglobin Bristol) was demonstrated.[110]

Although other similar cases were reported, no real progress was made toward understanding their pathogenesis until, in 1960, Hitzig and coworkers[111] demonstrated an abnormal hemoglobin (hemoglobin Zürich) in the red cells of a young girl who had developed a severe Heinz-body anemia after sulfonamide therapy. The same hemoglobin was found later in several other members of her family. Ten years after Cathie's original report, Grimes and Meisler[112] made a key observation. They demonstrated that a hemolysate prepared from the red cells of a 10-year-old girl who was suffering from a severe congenital hemolytic anemia, with many Heinz bodies in her red cells after splenectomy, was unusually heat-labile: a reddish brown precipitate formed when a stroma-free hemolysate was heated at 50°C; this amounted to about 20 percent of the total hemoglobin present. The heme/globin ratio in the precipitate was found to be lower than in normal unheated hemoglobin, and it was concluded tentatively that the Heinz bodies which formed in vivo and the precipitate which was produced by heating in vitro were due to the presence of an unstable hemoglobin fraction.

A further important step forward was the demonstration in a case of unstable hemoglobin disease of an amino acid substitution in the hemoglobin molecule, i.e., methionine had replaced valine in position 98 of the β chain (FG5) (Hemoglobin Köln).[113]

Many different types of unstable hemoglobin have since been recognized, and the responsible amino acid substitution or deletion(s) pinpointed. Now it is realized that the unstable hemoglobin diseases comprise a large group of rather rare but most interesting inherited disorders which give rise to hemolytic anemia of variable severity.[114] The disorder is clearly expressed in heterozygotes, and splenectomy usually produces some alleviation but not a complete clinical cure. No homozygotes have yet been described, however, and it seems likely that with most substitutions, homozygosity would be lethal.

Severely affected patients often pass dark blackish urine, and it is remarkable that the striking syndrome of chronic anemia with jaundice and splenomegaly, and, perhaps, some cyanosis and blackish urine, and the characteristic blood picture after splenectomy was overlooked for so long.

The discovery of the unstable hemoglobins has had implications for science outside the field of clinical hematology and medicine. By demonstrating that the hemoglobin molecule could become unstable as the result of substitutions (or deletions) in key places in the amino acid chains, it focused attention on the molecular arrangements and on the forces that normally preserve the stability of the molecule—in particular, those that bind heme to the globin chains and prevent water from entering the heme pocket and those that link the chains together.

Not for the first time, observations made on patients suffering from "experiments of nature" have provided the stimulus for basic scientific work.

THE ACQUIRED HEMOLYTIC ANEMIAS

It was a report by Boorman, Dodd, and Loutit[74] in 1946 on the use of the antiglobulin (Coombs) test in the investigation of cases of hemolytic anemia

(p. 232) that showed without any possible doubt that acquired hemolytic anemias existed for which autoantibodies against red cells were responsible. Seventeen of the twenty-eight patients studied were considered to have congenital "acholuric jaundice," and in none of them were washed red cells agglutinated by a diluted antihuman globulin rabbit serum. In contrast, five patients were thought to have acquired "acholuric jaundice"; in each case, their red cells were agglutinated by the antiglobulin serum, although in another six patients, suffering from miscellaneous types of acquired hemolytic anemia, the results of the test were negative. Boorman, Dodd, and Loutit concluded (correctly) that the agglutination test "will discriminate the congenital from the acquired form [of haemolytic icterus], and that it indicates that the acquired form is due to a process of immunization, whereas the congenital form is not."[74]

The results obtained with antiglobulin serum agreed with the data on red cell survival which were being obtained at about the same time and which had clearly demonstrated that transfused normal red cells might survive for only a short time in patients suffering from acquired hemolytic anemias. Brown and his colleagues[29] made the additional point in 1944 that in such cases the elimination of the transfused cells, when plotted on graph paper, was markedly curvilinear rather than being almost linear, as in patients with hypochromic anemia. They concluded that the curvature indicated that the cells were being eliminated by "exponential" mechanisms which were different from the (linear) mechanism operating in health and that the exponential mechanisms are "probably of the nature of a process of destruction acting at random on the erythrocytes irrespective of their age or other characteristic." Mollison's more extensive data were published in 1947.[30]

The studies outlined above have made it clear that transfused normal red cells could be eliminated, at least in some patients who had acquired hemolytic anemia, by the same extrinsic mechanisms as were affecting the recipient's own cells and that one such mechanism was the development of autoantibodies. The existence of an autoimmune type of hemolytic anemia (AIHA) was, thus, firmly reestablished in the late 1940s.

Autoimmune Hemolytic Anemias: Warm-Antibody and Cold-Antibody Syndromes Subsequent developments form yet another fascinating story. It was soon recognized that patients with AIHA whose red cells gave positive antiglobulin (Coombs) tests could be separated serologically into two main groups according to whether the causal antibodies had "warm" or "cold" characteristics. The warm type reacted best at about 37°C; the cold type did not react at 37°C but became progressively more active as the temperature was lowered. It was recognized, too, that the type of antibody present had an important effect on the clinical syndrome; e.g., patients with cold autoantibodies, if of high thermal amplitude, usually suffered from acrocyanosis

(Raynaud's phenomenon) in cold weather; this caused their fingers and toes and, perhaps, nose and ears to become blue. They might also suffer from hemoglobinuria in cold weather. On the other hand, patients who had formed warm autoantibodies did not suffer from acrocyanosis and very seldom from hemoglobinuria, and their illness was not exacerbated by exposure to cold. The term *autoimmune hemolytic anemia* (AIHA) is now usually used to describe only the latter (warm-antibody) syndrome, i.e., the classical acquired hemolytic icterus of Hayem and Widal.

The *cold-antibody syndromes* were not widely recognized until the early 1950s. Nevertheless, isolated clinical accounts can be found in the literature of the 1920s and 1930s, and there is at least one nineteenth century account.

Druitt,[115] writing from Madras in 1873, described in detail the history of a doctor, aged 51 years, who over a period of at least 6 years had experienced attacks of numbness of the feet and a purplish blue discoloration of the hands on exposure to cold. These attacks might be followed by the passage of "haematinuria." The patient obtained relief from his symptoms when he went to live in a warm climate (India). Druitt believed that the nervous system and the blood were involved and suggested that the blood was undergoing "a haemolysis, a decomposition or necrosis of the blood globules."

The chronic form of cold-antibody hemolytic anemia, the *cold-hemag-glutinin disease* (CHAD), is now recognized to be a fairly common disorder, which has features in common with Waldenström's macroglobulinemia. It may, too, be associated with an underlying malignant lymphoma. An important transitory acute hemolytic anemia also has been recognized: this may follow nonbacterial pneumonia,[116] particularly that due to *Mycoplasma* infection or (rarely) infectious mononucleosis.[117]

The autoantibodies have been extensively studied in the laboratory. An important question that eluded solution for several years was their specificity, i.e., the identity of the antigen or antigens on the red cell surface with which the antibodies were reacting. At first, it seemed that the warm and cold antibodies were both "nonspecific," for they appeared to react with all human red cells (and some animal cells, too). This tentative conclusion was, however, eventually shown to be wrong, for in 1953, Weiner and his colleagues established in one case that the autoantibody had anti-e specificity.[118] It was subsequently discovered that the majority of warm antibodies reacted with an antigen associated with the Rh blood group antigen complex and that some had a definite and clear-cut specificity, the commonest being anti-e.

The cold antibodies, too, have been shown to have definite specificities. By far the commonest type of high-titer cold antibody reacts with the I antigen ("individual"), a small minority with the i antigen, and a few antibodies with an antigen outside the Ii system. It was Weiner and colleagues[119] in 1956 who named the Ii system of blood-group antigens. In attempting to find compatible blood for a patient who was severely anemic and had in her serum a very high-titer cold agglutinin, 22,964 blood samples were tested! Five were found to react extremely weakly and were designated I-negative or i, in contrast to the vast majority of cells which reacted strongly and were designated I-positive.

Another surprise was the demonstration that the powerful lytic antibody of paroxysmal cold hemoglobinuria—the classic Donath-Landsteiner (D-L) antibody described earlier—also had a peculiar and characteristic specificity, namely, anti-P.[120] The belief that the D-L antibody was nonspecific can be explained by the extreme rarity of phenotypes in the P blood-group system which do not react with anti-P, i.e., p and P^k cells.

The antibodies also have been studied by physical means. First, the use of the ultracentrifuge showed that in sera containing large amounts of a cold autoantibody, this would separate as a high-density protein and might also be visualized as a distinct sharp peak in the beta-gamma region on simple paper electrophoresis.[121] Subsequently, when methods of immunoelectrophoresis became available, it was clearly shown that not only were these protein peaks composed of macroglobulin (IgM) but that they were also monoclonal, and in this respect CHAD is analogous to Waldenström's macroglobulinemia in that the basis of both disorders is the formation by the patient of large amounts of an IgM paraprotein.

An interesting phenomenon observed in the 1950s was that the addition of gamma globulin to antiglobulin sera produced a reagent that could discriminate between the red cells of individual patients with AIHA.[122] Thus, although in many instances the positive antiglobulin reaction was abolished by adding the gamma globulin, this was not true in all cases. It seemed clear that in those cases in which the reaction was inhibited, the autoantibody on the cell was itself a gamma globulin, but that when the reaction was not affected, the material on the red cell surface could not be gamma globulin. The "nongamma protein" was eventually shown to consist of components of complement fixed to the cell as the result of antibody-antigen interaction.[123]

Treatment   The availability of ACTH and the synthetic corticosteroid drugs since the early 1950s has revolutionized the treatment of AIHA, and the more recent introduction of immunosuppressive drugs, e.g., Imuran, has provided a second line of attack. Splenectomy, formerly the only available treatment, still has its place, however, in patients who do not respond well to steroids or who develop serious side effects. Patients with chronic CHAD benefit from protection from the cold, and for them corticosteroid therapy is generally best avoided. Splenectomy, too, is less successful. Treatment with chlorambucil as for a lymphoma may, however, be helpful.

Pathogenesis and Etiology   Much has been learned in recent years about the way in which antibodies bring about red cell destruction, and the much greater effectiveness of antibodies in vivo compared with in vitro, which so puzzled the pioneer experimenters, has been explained. It is now known that phago-cytic cells have receptors for antibody molecules and also for the third com-ponent of complement. Antibody- or complement-coated red cells may, thus, adhere to macrophages and, if not phagocytosed, can sustain damage and loss of surface membrane at the site of adhesion.[124,125] If cells damaged in this way manage to escape from the macrophage and circulate once more, they do so as spherocytes.

The cause or causes of the development of the autoantibodies is not yet fully understood. Nevertheless, considerable progress has been made in the last 20 years or so. Of particular importance has been the discovery of an animal model of AIHA in certain strains of New Zealand mice,[126] and clinical observations in humans have also provided potentially important clues.

Three clinical clues deserve special mention: (1) the rare, but undoubtedly significant, development of AIHA in more than one member of the same family,[127] pointing to a genetic influence; (2) the association of AIHA with malignant lymphomas; and (3) the development of AIHA in patients receiving long-term treatment with the antihypertensive drug α-methyldopa (Aldo-met).[128] Then there is the quite common association between AIHA and idiopathic thrombocytopenic purpura (ITP) (Evans' syndrome)[129] and the frequent occurrence of low serum globulin concentrations, particularly of IgA, in patients with AIHA.[130] A real understanding of the mechanisms involved in these associations would surely go a long way to solve the riddle of the development of AIHA of apparent "idiopathic" origin.

Hemolytic Disease of the Newborn (HDN) Any account of the life and death of the red blood cell and of the hemolytic anemias would be incomplete without some reference to the type of hemolytic anemia of the newborn which is due to blood-group incompatibility between the fetus and its mother. The early history of HDN, the various novel methods of treatment that were devised, and the way its incidence has been sharply cut in recent years are described in Chapter 20. From our present point of view, HDN provided the stimulus that led to the elaboration of the antiglobulin test; for, after the original report of Levine and Stetson[131] in 1939, although it was soon widely accepted that in HDN antibodies were being formed in the mother against antigen(s) on the red cells of the fetus (antigens which had been derived from its father and which its mother lacked), the antibodies usually proved in practice to be remarkably difficult to demonstrate. The method of detecting weak and "incomplete" Rh agglutinins, which was described in 1945 by Coombs, Mourant, and Race,[73] provided a reliable means of diagnosing HDN and demonstrating the offending antibodies. The important consequences of applying the new test in other cases of hemolytic anemia have already been described.

Symptomatic Hemolytic Anemias   The life span of the red cell is decreased in many disorders that do not affect red cell production or the red cells primarily. In the literature, the terms *secondary*[132] and *symptomatic*[133] have been used to describe these hemolytic anemias. The intensity of increased hemolysis may be slight, and, in some cases, hemolysis is only detectable by measuring the life span of the red cells by an isotopic method; in others, it may be so severe as to dominate the clinical picture. The underlying disorders which may be accompanied by significantly increased hemolysis include infections, carcinoma, leukemia and allied disorders, collagen diseases, liver diseases, renal diseases, and vascular diseases. The mechanisms of hemolysis vary and are generally incompletely understood; they include, however, the effect on the red cell of products of bacterial metabolism (in infections), alterations in the chemical and physical environment of the red cell, and physical trauma.

The blood picture in most secondary hemolytic anemias is not particularly characteristic. However, there is one major exception. Almost the most remarkable feature of *microangiopathic hemolytic anemia*[134] (MAHA) is the fact that its characteristic blood film had been overlooked for so long: the bizarre-shaped, often sharply angled, cells and cell fragments together make an unmistakable picture. The cause of the hemolysis appears to be fragmentation of the red cells as the result of their being caught up and entangled in threads of fibrin deposited in the small blood vessels, through which, however, the circulation is maintained.[135] This seems to be the mechanism involved in various hemolytic-uremic syndromes, now widely known but previously unheard of (or at least unnamed) until 1955.[136] Apart from the hemolytic-uremic syndrome, MAHA is found in disseminated carcinoma—it is remarkable, too, how this association was overlooked for so long—and in the hemolytic anemia that follows cardiac surgery,[137] the usual cause of which is a malfunctioning valve prosthesis or a regurgitant jet of blood playing upon a fibrin-covered patch. It still is uncertain to what extent the fragmentation in the cardiac hemolytic anemias can be attributed to interaction between red cells and fibrin threads or whether excessive turbulence is also important.

Drug-Induced Hemolytic Anemias   The hemolytic anemias that follow drug therapy or the ingestion or inhalation of a hemolytic chemical are of great interest; they have thrown light on the mechanisms of drug sensitivity in general, as well as on red cell metabolism and human polymorphism. As already mentioned, it was the clinical observation that the acute hemolytic anemia with hemoglobinuria which sometimes followed the administration of antimalarial drugs and seemed almost always to affect black rather than white subjects that led to the classic series of researches which ultimately pinpointed the cause as red cell G6PD deficiency. This must be the most well-known and best worked out example of human idiosyncrasy.

Much less frequent as a cause of hemolytic anemia is the formation of antibodies against a drug or drug metabolite. Nevertheless, the classic study of Harris[138] on acute hemolytic anemia following the readministration of the drug Fuadin, used as treatment for schistosomiasis, has served as a model of the mechanism of immune hypersensitivity to drugs.

Finally, the formation of autoantibodies against red cells as the result of long-continued treatment with the antihypertensive drug α-methyldopa[139] deserves further mention. The remarkable feature of this association is that the antibodies that are formed are directed against normal red cell antigens and not against the drug. The drug, in some mysterious way, promotes or facilitates the formation of the antibodies, which are characteristically directed against Rh antigens. Clinically, in the patients who develop overt hemolysis,[128] the illness is exactly the same as AIHA of "idiopathic" origin; the difference is that in the α-methyldopa cases the patient recovers spontaneously upon stopping the drug.

In closing this account it is worthwhile, perhaps, to reiterate how the "explosion" in knowledge concerning the life span of the red cell and the anemias caused by increased red cell destruction has taken place: it is because those working in clinical and laboratory medical research have been quick to apply the great advances made in the biological and physical sciences, and the consequent advances of technology, to their own particular problems.

References

1   Andrews CH: Francis Peyton Rous, in *Biographical Memoirs of Fellows of the Royal Society of London.* London, 1971, vol 17, pp 643–662.

2   Rous P, Robertson OH: The normal fate of erythrocytes. I. The findings in healthy animals. *J Exp Med* 25:651–663, 1917.

3   Rous P: Destruction of the red blood corpuscles in health and disease. *Physiol Rev* 3:75–105, 1923.

4   Meltzer SJ: The effects of shaking upon the red blood cells. *Johns Hopkins Hosp Rep* 9:135–151, 1900.

5   Ashby W: The determination of the length of life of transfused blood corpuscles in man. *J Exp Med* 29:267–281, 1919.

6   Ashby W: Some data on the range of life of transfused blood-corpuscles in persons without idiopathic blood diseases. *Med Clin North Am* 3:783–799, 1919.

7   Fairbanks VF: In memoriam: Winifred M. Ashby. 1879–1975. *Blood* 46:977–978, 1975.

8   Todd C, White RG: On the fate of red blood corpuscles when injected into the circulation of an animal of the same species; with a new method for the determination of the total volume of the blood. *Proc R Soc Lond (Biol)* 84:255–259, 1911.

9   Ashby W: Study of transfused blood. I. The periodicity in eliminative activity shown by the organism. *J Exp Med* 34:127–146, 1921.

10 Ashby W: Study of transfused blood. II. Blood destruction in pernicious anemia. *J Exp Med* 34:147–166, 1921.

11   Wearn JT, Warren S, Ames O: The length of life of transfused erythrocytes in patients with primary and secondary anemia. *Arch Intern Med* 29:527–538, 1922.

12   Jervell F: Untersuchungen über die Lebensdauer der transfundierten roten blutkörperchen beim Menschen. *Acta Pathol Microbiol Scand* 1:155–185, 201–244, 1924.

13   Dedichen HG: Ictère hémolytique et ulcère de la jambe. *Acta Med Scand* 77:411–430, 1931–1932.

14   Dacie JV, Mollison PL: Survival of normal erythrocytes after transfusion to patients with familial haemolytic anaemia (acholuric jaundice). *Lancet* i:550–552, 1943.

15   Schrumpf CAA: Role of the spleen in familial spherocytosis, in *Proc 3rd Int Congr Int Soc Hemat, Cambridge 1950.* New York, Grune and Stratton, 1951, pp 94–95.

16   Landsteiner K, Levine P, Janes ML: On the development of isoagglutinins following transfusion. *Proc Soc Exp Biol Med* 25:672–674, 1928.

17   Wiener AS: Longevity of the erythrocyte. *JAMA,* 102:1779–1780, 1934.

18   Dekkers HJN: Fate of transfused red blood cells. *Acta Med Scand* 99:587–613, 1939.

19   Mollison PL, Young IM: On the survival of the transfused erythrocytes of stored blood. *Q J Exp Physiol* 30:313–327, 1940.

20   Mollison PL: Personal communication to the author. 1978.

21   Mollison PL, Young IM: *In vivo* survival in the human subject of transfused erythrocytes after storage in various preservative solutions. *Q J Exp Physiol* 31:359–392, 1942.

22   Rous P, Turner JR: The preservation of living red blood cells in vitro. I. Methods of preservation. *J Exp Med* 23:219–237, 1916.

23   Wiener AS, Shaeffer G: Limitations in the use of preserved blood for transfusion: a study of the fate of the transfused erythrocytes in the recipient's circulation. *Med Clin North Am* 24:705–722, 1940.

24   Hawkins WB, Whipple GH: The life cycle of the red blood cell in the dog. *Am J Physiol* 122:418–427, 1938.

25   Berlin NI, Waldmann TA, Weissman SM: Life span of red blood cell. *Physiol Rev* 39:577–616, 1959.

26   Gray SJ, Sterling K: Tagging of red cells and plasma proteins with radioactive chromium. *J Clin Invest* 29:1604–1613, 1950.

27   Cohen JA, Warringa MGPJ: The fate of P^{32}-labelled diisopropylfluorophosphonate in the human body and its use as a labelling agent in the study of the turnover of blood plasma and red cells. *J Clin Invest* 33:459–467, 1954.

28   Schiødt E: On the duration of life of the red blood corpuscles. *Acta Med Scand* 95:49–79, 1938.

29   Brown GM, Hayward OC, Powell OC, Witts LJ: The destruction of transfused erythrocytes in anaemia. *J Pathol Bacteriol* 56:81–94, 1944.

30   Mollison PL: The survival of transfused erythrocytes, with special reference to cases of acquired haemolytic anaemia. *Clin Sci* 6:137–172, 1947.

31   Dressler Dr: Ein Fall von intermittirender Albuminurie und Chromaturie. *Arch Pathol Anat Physiol* 6:264–266, 1854.

32   Elliotson J: Diseases of the heart united with ague. *Lancet* i:500–501, 1832.

33   Dickinson WH: Notes of four cases of intermittent haematuria. *Lancet* i:568–569, 1865.

34   Wiltshire A: Urine from a case of intermittent haematuria. *Trans Pathol Soc Lond* 18:180, 1867.

35   Secchi: Ein Fall von Hämoglobinurie aus der Klinik des Geh. Rath Prof. Dr. Lebert. *Berl Klin Wochenschr* 9:237–239, 1872.

36   Kuessner B: Paroxysmale Hämoglobinurie. *Dtsch Med Wochenschr* 5:475–478, 1879.

37   Rosenbach O: Beitrag zur Lehre von der periodischen Hämoglobinurie. *Berl Klin Wochenschr* 17:132–134, 151–152, 1880.

38   Ehrlich P: Über paroxysmale Hämoglobinurie. *Dtsch Med Wochenschr* 7:224–225, 1881.

39   Chvostek F: *Ueber das Wesen der paroxysmalen Hämoglobinurie.* Wien, Deuticke, 1894, 105 pp.

40   Donath J, Landsteiner K: Ueber paroxysmale Hämoglobinurie. *Münch Med Wochenschr* 51:1590–1593, 1904.

41   Eason J: The pathology of paroxysmal haemoglobinuria. *J Pathol Bacteriol* 11:167–202, 1906.

42   Ehrlich P, Morgenroth J: Ueber Haemolysine. Zwiete Mittheilung. *Berl Klin Wochenschr* 36:481–486, 1899.

43   Ehrlich P: *Collected Studies on Immunity,* Bolduan (trans). New York, John Wiley, 1906, 712 pp, p 15.

44   Fleischer R: Ueber eine neue Form von Haemoglobinurie beim Menschen. *Berl Klin Wochenschr* 18:691–694, 1881.

45   Dickinson W: Haemoglobinuria from muscular exertion. *Trans Clin Soc Lond* 27:230–233, 1894.

46   Davidson RJL: Exertional haemoglobinuria: a report on three cases with studies on the haemolytic mechanism. *J Clin Pathol* 17:536–540, 1964.

47   Strübing P: Paroxysmale Haemoglobinurie. *Dtsch Med Wochenschr* 8:1–3, 17–21, 1882.

48   Crosby WH: Paroxysmal nocturnal hemoglobinuria. A classic description by Paul Strübing in 1882, and a bibliography of the disease. *Blood* 6:270–284, 1951.

49   Gull WW: A case of intermittent haematinuria, with remarks. *Guy's Hosp Rep* 12:381–392, 1866.

50   Hijmans van den Bergh AA: Ictère hémolytique avec crises hémoglobinuriques. Fragilité globulaire. *Rev Med* 31:63–69, 1911.

51   Ham TH: Chronic hemolytic anemia with paroxysmal nocturnal hemoglobinuria. A study of the mechanism of hemolysis in relation to acid-base equilibrium. *N Engl J Med* 217:915–917, 1937.

52   Marchiafava E, Nazari A: Nuovo contributo allo studio degli itteri cronici emolitici. *Policlinico Sez Med* 38:241–254, 1911.

53   Marchiafava E: Anemia emolitica con emosiderinuria perpetua. *Policlinico Sez Med* 35:105–120, 1928.

54   Enneking J: Eine neue Form intermittierender Hämoglobinurie (Haemoglobinuria paroxysmalis nocturna). *Klin Wochenschr* 7:2045–2047, 1928.

55   Wilson C: Some cases showing hereditary enlargement of the spleen. *Trans Clin Soc Lond* 23:162–172, 1890.

56   Wilson C, Stanley DA: A sequel to some cases showing hereditary enlargement of the spleen. *Trans Clin Soc Lond* 26:163–171, 1893.

57   Campbell JMH: Early accounts of acholuric jaundice and the subsequent history of Wilson's patients. *Q J Med* 19:323–332, 1925–26.

58   Vanlair C, Masius: De la microcythémie. *Bull Acad R Med Belg* 5:3d series, 515–613, 1871.

59 Minkowski O: Ueber eine hereditäre, unter dem Bilde eines chronischen Ikterus mit Urobilinurie, Splenomegalie und Nierensiderosis verlaufende Affection. *Verh Kongr Inn Med* 18:316–319, 1900.

60 Chauffard A: Pathogéne de l'ictère congénital de l'adulte. *Sem Med (Paris)* 27:25–29, 1907.

61 Ribierre P: L'hémolyse et la mesure de la résistance globulaire; application à l'étude de la résistance globulaire dans l'ictère. Thèse de Paris, 1903, quoted by Chauffard (1907).

62 Minkowski M: Ictère chronique héréditaire avec splénomegalie. *Sem Méd (Paris)* 20:149, 1900.

63 Barlow T, Shaw HB: Inheritance of recurrent attacks of jaundice and of abdominal crises, with hepato-splenomegaly. *Trans Clin Soc Lond* 35:155–163, 1902.

64 Wynter WE: Case of acholuric jaundice after splenectomy. *Proc R Soc Med* (clin sect) 6:80–82, 1912–1913.

65 Dawson of Penn: The Hume lectures on haemolytic icterus. *Br Med J* i:921–928, 963–966, 1931.

66 Meulengracht E: Über die Erblichkeitsverhältnisse beim chronischen hereditären hämolytischen Ikterus. *Dtsch Arch Klin Med* 136:33–45, 1921.

67 Hayem G: Sur une variété particulière d'ictère chronique. Ictère infectieux chronique splénomégalique. *Presse Méd* 6:121–125, 1898.

68 Widal F, Abrami P, Brulé M: Les ictères d'origine hémolytique. *Arch Mal Coeur* 1:193–231, 1908.

69 Le Gendre P, Brulé M: Ictère hémolytique congénital et ictère hémolytique acquis. *Presse Méd* 17:70, 1909.

70 Lederer M: A form of acute hemolytic anemia probably of infectious origin. *Am J Med Sci* 170:500–510, 1925.

71 Dameshek W, Schwartz SO: Hemolysins as the cause of clinical and experimental hemolytic anemias. With particular reference to the nature of spherocytosis and increased fragility. *Am J Med Sci* 196:769–792, 1938.

72 Dameshek W, Schwartz SO: Acute hemolytic anemia (acquired hemolytic icterus, acute type). *Medicine (Baltimore)* 19:231–327, 1940.

73 Coombs RRA, Mourant AE, Race RR: A new test for the detection of weak and "incomplete" Rh agglutinins. *Br J Exp Pathol* 26:255–266, 1945.

74 Boorman KE, Dodd BE, Loutit JF: Haemolytic icterus (acholuric jaundice) congenital and acquired. *Lancet* i:812–814, 1946.

75 Christophers SR, Bentley CA: *Blackwater Fever. Scientific Memoirs by Officers of the Medical and Sanitary Depts. of the Government of India.* New Series, No 35, Calcutta, Government Printing, 1909, pp 76–77.

76 Muir R, McNee JW: The anaemia produced by a haemolytic serum. *J Pathol Bacteriol* 16:410–438, 1911–1912.

77 Banti G: Splenomégalie hémolytique anhémopoiétique: le rôle de la rate dans l'hémolyse. *Sem Méd (Paris)* 33:313–323, 1913.

78 Naegeli O: *Blutkrankheiten und Blutdiagnostik.* 5th ed, Berlin, Springer, 1931, 704 pp, p 292.

79 Ehrlich P: *Farbenanalytische Untersuchungen zur Histologie und Klinik des Blutes.* Berlin, Hirschwald, 1891, 137 pp, p 104.

80 Heinz R: Morphologische Veränderungen der rothen Blutkörperchen durch Gifte. *Virchows Arch (Pathol Anat)* 122:112–116, 1890.

81   Hunter W: *Pernicious Anaemia: its Pathology, Septic Origin, Symptoms, Diagnosis and Treatment.* London, C. Griffin and Co., 1901, 464 pp, p 363.

82   Fairley NH, Bromfield RJ: Laboratory studies in malaria and blackwater fever. Part III. A new blood pigment in blackwater fever and other biochemical observations. *Trans R Soc Trop Med Hyg* 28:307–334, 1934.

83   Fairley NH: Methaemalbumin. *Q J Med N.S.* 10:95–114, 115–138, 1941.

84   Vaughan JM: *The Anaemias.* 2d ed, London, Oxford University Press, 1936, 309 pp, pp 219–262.

85   Castle WB, Minot GR: *Pathological Physiology and Clinical Description of the Anemias.* New York, Oxford University Press, 1936, 205 pp, pp 29–38. (Reprinted from Oxford Loose-leaf Medicine, Christian HA [ed].)

86   Ehrlich P, Morgenroth J: Ueber Hämolysine. Fünfte Mittheilung. *Berl Klin Wochenschr* 38:251–257, 1901.

87   Haden RL: A new type of hereditary hemolytic jaundice without spherocytosis. *Am J Med Sci* 214:255–259, 1947.

88   Jacob HS: The abnormal red-cell membrane in hereditary spherocytosis: evidence for the causal role of mutant microfilaments. *Br J Haematol* 23 (Suppl.):35–44, 1972.

89   Valentine WN: The molecular lesion of hereditary spherocytosis (HS): a continuing enigma. *Blood* 49:241–245, 1977.

90   Dresbach M: Elliptical human red blood corpuscles. *Science* 19:469–470, 1904.

91   Herrick JB: Peculiar elongated and sickle-shaped red blood corpuscles in a case of severe anemia. *Arch Intern Med* 6:517–521, 1910.

92   Jensson Ó, Jónasson Th, Ólafsson O: Hereditary elliptocytosis in Iceland. *Br J Haematol* 13:844–854, 1967.

93   Wiley JS, Gill FM: Red cell calcium leak in congenital hemolytic anemia with extreme microcytosis. *Blood* 47:197–210, 1976.

94   Cutting HO, McHugh WJ, Conrad FG, Marlow AA: Autosomal dominant hemolytic anemia characterized by ovalocytosis. A family study of seven involved members. *Am J Med* 39:21–34, 1965.

95   Lie-Injo Luan Eng: Hereditary ovalocytosis and haemoglobin E-ovalocytosis in Malayan aborigines. *Nature* 208:1329, 1965.

96   Booth PB, Serjeantson S, Woodfield DG, Amato D: Selective depression of blood group antigens associated with hereditary ovalocytosis among Melanesians. *Vox Sang* 32:99–110, 1977.

97   Lock SP, Sephton-Smith R, Hardisty RM: Stomatocytosis: a hereditary red cell anomaly associated with haemolytic anaemia. *Br J Haematol* 7:303–314, 1961.

98   Nathan DG, Oski FA, Shaafi RI, Shohet SB: Congenital hemolytic anemia with extensive cation permeability. *Blood* 28:976, 1966 (abst).

99   Wiley JS, Ellory JC, Shuman MA, Shaller CC, Cooper RA: Characteristics of the membrane defect in the hereditary stomatocytosis syndrome. *Blood* 46:337–356, 1975.

100   Selwyn JG, Dacie JV: Autohemolysis and other changes resulting from the incubation in vitro of red cells from patients with congenital hemolytic anemia. *Blood* 9:414–438, 1954.

101   de Gruchy GC, Crawford H, Morton D: Atypical (nonspherocytic) congenital haemolytic anaemia. *VII Congr Soc Int Emat,* Roma. 1960, 2, Pt 1, 839 pp, pp 422–429.

102   Valentine WN, Tanaka KR, and Miwa S: A specific erythrocyte glycolytic enzyme

defect (pyruvate kinase) in three subjects with congenital non-spherocytic hemolytic anemia. *Trans Assoc Am Physicians* 74:100–110, 1961.

103 Valentine WN: Red cell enzyme deficiencies as a cause of hemolytic disorders. *Annu Rev Med* 23:93–100, 1972.

104 Beutler E: Glucose-6-phosphate dehydrogenase deficiency, in Stanbury JB, Wyngaarden JB, Fredrickson DS (eds): *The Metabolic Basis of Inherited Disease.* 2d ed, New York, Toronto, and London, McGraw-Hill, 1966, 1434 pp, p 1060.

105 Cordes W: Experiences with plasmochin in malaria. Preliminary reports. 15th Annual Report, United Fruit Co. (Med Dept), 1926, p 66. Quoted by Beutler (1966).

106 Carson PE, Flanagan CL, Ickes CE, Alving AS: Enzymatic deficiency in primaquine-sensitive erythrocytes. *Science* 124:484–485, 1956.

107 Newton WA Jr, Bass JC: Glutathione-sensitive chronic nonspherocytic hemolytic anemia. *J Dis Child* 96:501–502, 1958.

108 Schneider AS, Valentine WN, Hattori M, Heins HL Jr: Hereditary hemolytic anemia with triosephosphate isomerase deficiency. *N Engl J Med* 272:229–235, 1965.

109 Cathie IAB: Apparent idiopathic Heinz body anaemia. *Gt Ormond Str J* 3:43–48, 1952.

110 Steadman JH, Yates A, Huehns ER: Idiopathic Heinz body anaemia: Hb-Bristol (β67 (Ell) val → asp). *Br J Haematol* 18:435–446, 1970.

111 Hitzig NH, Frick PG, Betke K, Huisman THJ: Hämoglobin Zürich: eine neue Hämoglobinanomalie mit sulfonamidinduzierter Innernkörperanämie. *Helv Paediat Acta* 15:499–514, 1960.

112 Grimes AJ, Meisler A: Possible cause of Heinz bodies in congenital Heinz-body anaemia. *Nature* 194:190–191, 1962.

113 Carrell RW, Lehmann H, Hutchinson HE: Haemoglobin Köln (β-98 valine → methionine): an unstable protein causing inclusion-body anaemia. *Nature* 210:915–916, 1966.

114 White JM, Dacie JV: The unstable haemoglobins: molecular and clinical features, in Brown EB, Moore CV (eds): *Progress in Hematology.* New York and London, Grune and Stratton, 1971, vol VII, pp 69–109.

115 Druitt R: Two cases of intermittent haematinuria. *Med Times Gaz (Lond)* i:408–411, 461–462, 489–490, 1873.

116 Peterson OL, Ham TH, Finland M: Cold agglutinins (autohemagglutinins) in primary atypical pneumonias. *Science* 97:167, 1943.

117 Dameshek W: Cold hemagglutinins in acute hemolytic reactions in association with sulfonamide medication and infection. *JAMA* 123:77–80, 1943.

118 Weiner W, Battey DA, Cleghorn TE, Marson FGW, Meynell MJ: Serological findings in a case of haemolytic anaemia, with some general observations on the pathogenesis of this syndrome. *Br Med J* ii:125–128, 1953.

119 Wiener AS, Unger LJ, Cohen L, Feldman J: Type-specific cold auto-antibodies as a cause of acquired hemolytic anemia and hemolytic transfusion reactions: biologic test with bovine red cells. *Ann Intern Med* 44:221–240, 1956.

120 Levine P, Celano MJ, Falkowski F: The specificity of the antibody in paroxysmal cold hemoglobinuria (P.C.H.). *Transfusion* 3:278–282, 1963.

121 Christenson WN, Dacie JV: Serum proteins in acquired haemolytic anaemia (auto-antibody type). *Br J Haematol* 3:153–164, 1957.

122 Dacie JV: Differences in the behaviour of sensitized red cells to agglutination by antiglobulin sera. *Lancet* ii:954–955, 1951.

123 Dacie JV, Crookston JH, Christenson WN: "Incomplete" cold antibodies: role of complement in sensitization to antiglobulin serum by potentially haemolytic antibodies. *Br J Haematol* 3:77–87, 1957.

124 LoBuglio AF, Cotran RS, Jandl JH: Red cells coated with immunoglobulin G: binding and sphering by mononuclear cells in man. *Science* 158:1582–1585, 1967.

125 Brown DL, Lachmann PJ, Dacie JV: The *in vivo* behaviour of complement-coated red cells: studies in C6-deficient, C3-depleted and normal rabbits. *Clin Exp Immunol* 7:401–422, 1970.

126 Bielschowsky M, Helyer BJ, Howie JB: Spontaneous haemolytic anaemia in mice of the NZB/BL strain. *Proc Univ Otago Med Sch* 37:9–11, 1959.

127 Kissmeyer-Nielsen F, Bent-Hansen K, Kieler J: Immuno-hemolytic anemia with familial occurrence. *Acta Med Scand* 144:35–39, 1952.

128 Worlledge SM, Carstairs KC, Dacie JV: Autoimmune haemolytic anaemia associated with α-methyldopa therapy. *Lancet* ii:135–139, 1966.

129 Evans RS, Duane RT: Acquired hemolytic anemia. I. The relation of erythrocyte antibody to activity of the disease. II. The significance of thrombocytopenia and leukopenia. *Blood* 4:1196–1213, 1949.

130 Blajchman MA, Dacie JV, Hobbs JR, Pettit JE, Worlledge SM: Immunoglobulins in warm-type autoimmune haemolytic anaemia. *Lancet* ii:340–344, 1969.

131 Levine P, Stetson RE: An unusual case of intragroup agglutination. *JAMA* 113:126–127, 1939.

132 Watson CJ: Hemolytic jaundice and macrocytic hemolytic anemia: certain observations in a series of 35 cases. *Ann Intern Med* 12:1782–1796, 1939.

133 Singer K, Dameshek W: Symptomatic hemolytic anemia. *Ann Intern Med* 15:544–563, 1941.

134 Brain MC, Dacie JV, Hourihane DO'B: Microangiopathic haemolytic anaemia: the possible role of vascular lesions in pathogenesis. *Br J Haematol* 8:358–374, 1962.

135 Bull BS, Rubenberg ML, Dacie JV, Brain MC: Red-blood-cell fragmentation in microangiopathic haemolytic anaemia: in-vitro studies. *Lancet* ii:1123–1125, 1967.

136 Gasser C, Gautier E, Steck A, Siebenmann RE, Oechslin R: Hämolytisch-urämische Syndrome: bilaterale Nierenrindennekrosen bei akuten erworbenen hämolytischen Anämien. *Schweiz Med Wochenschr* 85:905–909, 1955.

137 Sayed HM, Dacie JV, Handley DA, Lewis SM, Cleland WP: Haemolytic anaemia of mechanical origin after open heart surgery. *Thorax* 16:356–360, 1961.

138 Harris JW: Studies on the mechanism of a drug-induced hemolytic anemia. *J Lab Clin Med* 44:809–810, 1954.

139 Carstairs KC, Breckenridge A, Dollery CT, Worlledge SM: Incidence of a positive direct Coombs test in patients on α-methyldopa. *Lancet* ii:133–135, 1966.

CHAPTER 9

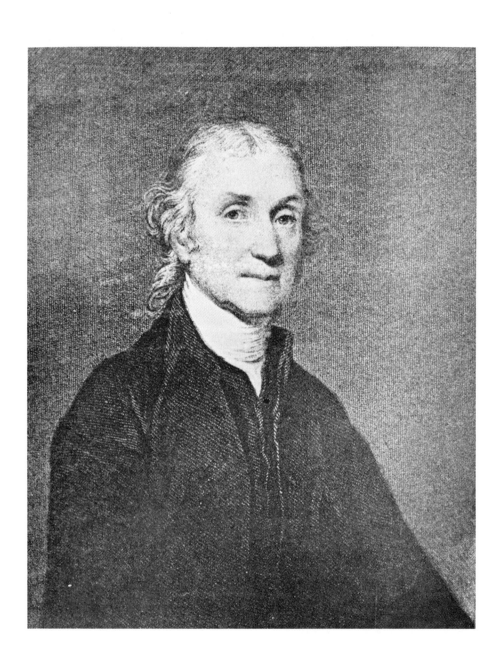

BLOOD AND MOUNTAINS
Allan J. Erslev

S ince time immemorial, the red cells in blood have provided color, drama, and poetic license to Goethe's "ganz besonderer Saft." However, the significance of these red cells has only recently been grasped despite the fact that malnutrition, malaria, and menstruation have made anemia the most common malady of man- and womankind. It was always taken for granted that the richness of blood plays a role in health and disease, but it was not until the end of the nineteenth century that the number of red cells in blood became firmly linked to our ability to bring oxygen from the air to the tissues. Much of this insight was derived from observations of life at high altitudes, and mountains and mountaineering have played major roles in our current understanding and management of anemias and polycythemias.

Mountains

Mountains are the harsh daily reality for about 25 million people who live and toil 10,000 feet or more above sea level. They undoubtedly appreciate the beauty of snowcapped peaks and marvel at breathtaking vistas, but throughout history, mountain dwellers have rarely been mountaineers. Prospectors,

Chapter Opening Photo   Joseph Priestley (1733–1804).[13]

crystal gatherers, and hunters may have reached some summits, but the intentional scaling of peaks is a physical and emotional challenge that the hardworking mountain dwellers could neither understand nor afford. The challenge may very well have little to do with mountains, beautiful views, or the fact that "they are there." It may have more to do with the feeling expressed in 1924 by Geoffrey Bruce, who, after another unsuccessful attempt at scaling Mt. Everest, shook his fist at the white monster and in the best Captain Ahab manner, shouted, "We'll get you yet."[1]

Regardless of the reasons for living in the mountains or for scaling their peaks, the experience gained from surviving at high altitude has taught us the importance of red cells and blood for survival at sea level.

In ancient times, no one lived in mountains but gods or trolls. Special dwelling places of gods were revered and given names such as Olympus, Parnassus, Sinai, or Jotunheim, and passes used for warfare or travel were also properly identified. However, spectacular peaks such as Monte Rosa, Matterhorn, and Mont Blanc remained unnamed and unadmired by our classic ancestors.[1]

The veil of superstition and religious awe that surrounded mountains was raised along with many similar veils towards the end of the Middle Ages and the beginning of the Renaissance. The first recorded scaling of a mountain top was made in 1339 by Petrarch,[2] whose lusty sonnets to his love Laura have been said to herald the Renaissance.[3] This was a period of emerging humanistic self-confidence, of pagan appreciation of physical beauty, and of boundless curiosity. Oswald Spengler, in his controversial but fascinating book on the life of cultures, *The Decline of the West,* has called this the "Faustian Period."[4] This was a time in which a man like Faust was willing to sell his soul so that he could explore science, art, and faraway places, reach beyond his grasp, and maintain the vigor of his youth: "Gib meine Jugend mir zuruck."[5] It was a tremendously dynamic and exciting period and a time when the climbing of mountains and the view from the top exemplified quest for achievement and search for infinity.

Many minor peaks were climbed during the Renaissance, but then, for unknown reasons, the Faustian quest ceased. After a final climb by Leonardo da Vinci in 1511,[2] only sporadic climbs in the Alps were recorded until the eighteenth century, when the Chamonix valley and Mont Blanc became the birthplace of modern mountaineering.

During this lull, the brutal conquest of the Inca empire by Spain had disclosed the existence of a culture adapted to altitudes unknown in Europe.[6] This Andean empire, spanning a distance longer than that of the Roman empire from Britannia to Persia (Figure 9-1), was strung together by a remarkable highway stretching from Quito at 9500 feet in Ecuador through the Inca capital Cuzco at 11,500 feet in Peru down into Bolivia and Chile.[7] Some of its passes reached an altitude of more than 17,000 feet, and its construction

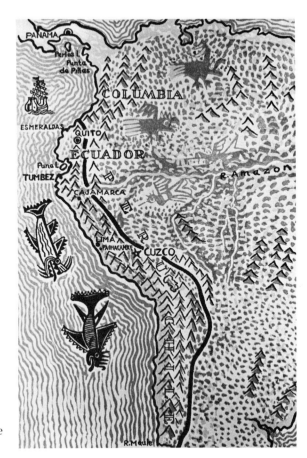

Figure 9-1 Inca Empire (1530).[6]

and maintenance by people who had not yet discovered the use of the wheel must be considered one of the great achievements of the ancient world. The warrior-emperors ruled absolutely, and the imperial court was as ceremonial and colorful as any medieval European court (Figure 9-2).[8,9] The subjects were strictly separated into high altitude dwellers serving as miners and keepers of vicunas and llamas and lowland natives working as farmers; imperial rules and regulations ensured that these two populations did not mix.[10]

MOUNTAIN SICKNESS

Francisco Pizarro, after his conquest in 1532, changed all this; everyone was called into action in search of gold and silver, and in expansion of Spanish rule. The results were devastating for the native population, the highlanders succumbing to seashore fever and the lowlanders to a mysterious

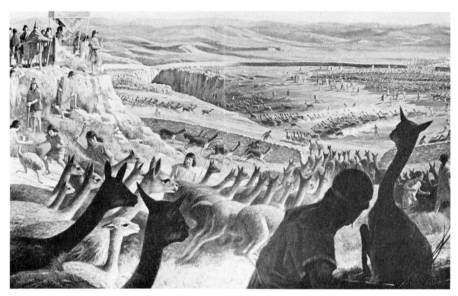

Figure 9-2 Imperial Inca vicuna hunt.[8]

and often fatal malady—*altitude sickness*. The Indians were familiar with this malady, called it "soroche" or "puna," and treated it by chewing coca leaves. However, the early Spanish settlers had only a vague feeling that altitude was responsible for some of their problems. One of the problems was infertility among the Spanish women, and infertility was eventually used as an excuse for moving the capital from Cuzco to a new city, Lima, at sea level.[10] The sufferings and loss of life by the troops crossing the Cordilleras were blamed on the snow, the freezing cold, and poor nutrition. It was not until 1569 that a Jesuit priest, Father Acosta (Figure 9-3), gave the first succinct description of the specific effects of altitude.[11] He described a strange and deadly syndrome of breathlessness, dizziness, vomiting, and fainting and most accurately related it to the fact that at high altitudes, "the elements of the air are in this place so thin and delicate that it is not suitable for human breathing."[12]

This remarkable deduction was made almost 100 years before Galileo and Torricello had discovered that air had weight and Pascal had shown that this weight, the so-called barometric pressure, decreased at high altitudes. However, until Priestley's discovery of oxygen 200 years later, Father Acosta's hypothesis did not appear to make much sense, and most observers, both in the Andes and the Himalayas, chose to believe that mountain sickness was caused by toxic emanations from minerals buried in the ground.

Joseph Priestley (Chapter Opening Photo) was a nonconformist, English minister, an admirer of the French revolution, and a remarkably gifted, self-taught chemist. He isolated and described a number of new chemicals and gases, using primitive measuring instruments with amazing accuracy.[13] In 1772, he directed a burning glass at red oxide of mercury and noted the release of a gas that made a candle burn with great vigor and kept mice from suffocating in a closed chamber. The potential importance of this gas, however, escaped him. Fortunately, during a visit to Paris he told Antoine Lavoisier about his new gas, and this brilliant chemist immediately grasped its significance. Lavoisier realized that the gas must be that part of the atmospheric air that Robert Boyle 100 years earlier had shown was necessary for combustion and respiration, and he named it *oxygen*. Sadly, the French revolution caught up with both. Lavoisier was sent to the guillotine, and Priestley had his church sacked by counterrevolutionaries. The latter fled to the United States, where he settled in Pennsylvania and is today recognized as one of the founders of the Unitarian Church there.

The stage was now set for an explanation of mountain sickness as a condition of relative suffocation caused by the inadequate content of oxygen in the rarefied atmosphere. Nevertheless, the theory of toxic emanations from the ground maintained its popularity, and the eminent and sophisticated scientist Alexander von Humboldt, who climbed in the Andes in 1799, even

Figure 9-3 Father José de Acosta and title page of his book on mountain sickness.[11]

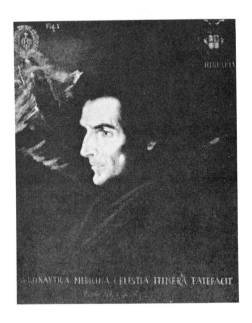

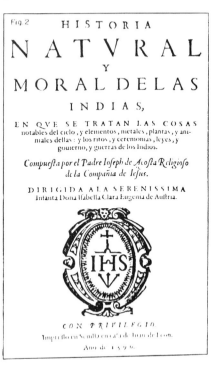

Fig. 2

HISTORIA

NATVRAL

Y

MORAL DE LAS

INDIAS,

EN QVE SE TRATAN LAS COSAS
notables del cielo, y elementos, metales, plantas, y animales dellas: y los ritos, y ceremonias, leyes, y
gouierno, y guerras de los Indios.

*Compuesta por el Padre Ioseph de Acosta Religioso
de la Compañia de Iesus.*

DIRIGIDA A LA SERENISSIMA
Infanta Doña Isabella Clara Eugenia de Austria.

CON PRIVILEGIO
Impresso en Seuilla en casa de Iuan de Leon.
Año de 1590.

believed that reduced climatic pressure on the joints caused most of the symptoms.[14] Charles Darwin, in his travel to these lofty altitudes in 1835, experienced respiratory oppression or "puna," as it was called by the natives. Some told him, "all the waters here have puna," others, "where there is snow there is puna." In his *Diary of the H.M.S. Beagle,* he wrote, however, that "there was a good deal of fancy even in this, for upon finding fossil shells on the highest ridge, in my delight I entirely forgot the 'Puna.' "[15]

MOUNTAIN CLIMBING

Meanwhile, in Europe, with its steep but only moderately high Alps, an emerging group of mountain climbers had become more interested in technical than in atmospheric difficulties. In 1741, after a lull of nearly two centuries, mountaineering was resumed by an English gentleman, William Windham, who, with a crew of eight well-armed masters and five servants, "discovered" the small alpine valley of Chamonix and its magnificent glaciers and snow-capped peaks.[16] We have to assume that the hardworking farmers of the valley had discovered it considerably earlier, but from the point of view of modern mountaineering, the year 1741 is considered its birth. A wealthy, science-oriented merchant from Geneva, Horace-Benedict de Saussure, followed up on this discovery and offered a reward equivalent to about $60 for the first to climb the valley's highest mountain, Mont Blanc. The reward was claimed in 1786 by the local physician Dr. Michel-Gabriel Paccard and his guide Jacques Balmart. Their memorable ascent of the highest mountain in Europe was observed through field glasses by the people in the valley; nevertheless it was never quite resolved whether Balmart had carried Dr. Paccard to the top or Dr. Paccard had forced a reluctant guide to follow him. In spite of this minor question of priority, Alexander Dumas the elder wrote a widely read article about it, and a British entertainer used the climb for a profitable show in London. De Saussure himself, after having presented the award to one or the other, made the third climb in the company of 1 servant and 18 guides, who were equipped with ladders and long poles (Figure 9-4). He measured pulse and respiration and made notes about fatigue and exhaustion, symptoms that at an altitude of 15,800 feet probably were due to a combination of hypoxia, poor conditioning, inadequate clothing, and lack of equipment.[16,17]

Over the next century, mountain climbing in the Alps became big tourist business. Each scaling of Mont Blanc was rewarded by certificate, cannon salute, and special dinner on the town. The guides organized into syndicates, and their reputations rested on how many "Herrens" they had guided up still uncharted peaks. As the number of such peaks decreased, the aura around the remainder increased, and the last unconquered peak, the Matterhorn, took on an almost magical quality. Edward Whymper, an English water

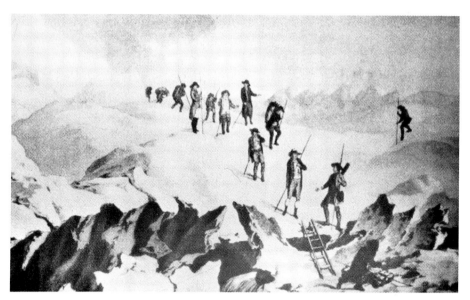

Figure 9-4 Climbing of Mont Blanc by de Saussure.[17]

colorist, fell under the spell and spent all his summers studying the approaches. Finally, in 1865, as the leader of an unwieldy group of experienced guides and frank novices, he tackled it and with remarkable ease brought all seven members of the group to the top. On the return, someone slipped and dragged down four members, including the young Lord Francis Douglas and the Reverend Charles Huston. The rope tying them together stretched and broke; Whymper and two guides watched in horror as the others fell to their deaths on a glacier thousands of feet below. The prominence of the victims and the broken rope led to a highly publicized inquest. Whymper and the guides were declared innocent but were never able to live down the suspicion that they had actually cut the rope.[18]

Altitude Physiology

With the Alps conquered and the Himalayas as yet beyond reach, the altitude enthusiasts and the amateur scientists turned to ballooning. Hot air balloons were first used in 1783 by the Montgolfier brothers but were soon replaced by the more manageable hydrogen balloons. The French, in particular, armed with élan and champagne, went higher and higher until the balloon Zenith (Figure 9-5) in 1875 reached a height of 26,000 feet, but at a cost of the lives of two of the three passengers.[19] This memorable ascent was made the more tragic because it had been commissioned by the French physiologist Paul Bert, who, as a result of his studies of low barometric pressure, had

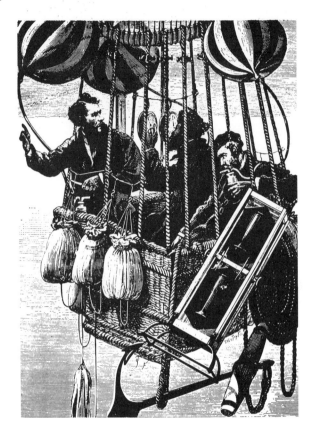

Figure 9-5 Balloon Zenith with crew and oxygen equipment.[19]

equipped the balloon with bags of oxygen. Unfortunately, these bags were not used, and the death of his friends convinced him that supplemental oxygen is necessary for survival at high altitudes. Paul Bert (Figure 9-6) began his career as an engineering student, became a lawyer, then a physician, then a physiologist, and, finally, a politician and resident-general of Indochina. As a physiologist, he was trained by Claude Bernard, in whose laboratory he developed the technique of parabiosis, a technique that, most appropriately, 100 years later would be used to provide fundamental new information about the control of oxygen transport. His main interest, however, was in respiratory physiology, and, as a gifted designer of complex apparatus, he succeeded in developing altitude chambers in which he could study the effect of both high and low air pressure (Figure 9-7). In his monumental book *La Pression barométrique*, published in 1878, he finally showed irrefutably that it is the lack of oxygen that causes altitude sickness.[19]

Paul Bert has been called the father of aviation medicine.[20] He did prove the essential role of oxygen for short-term survival on mountains and in balloons, but it was his older friend and mentor Dr. Dennis Jourdanet (Figure 9-8) who tied the evidence for long-term survival to blood. Dr. Jourdanet, a French physician, had lived for years in Mexico and had been especially interested in the blood of high altitude dwellers. He had noticed that the blood of his surgical patients was thick and flowed slowly, but he was also impressed by the fact that, despite this thick blood, patients with altitude symptoms had the same symptoms as patients with anemia. They were short of breath, had a rapid pulse, were dizzy, and prone to fainting spells. In his book *Anemia of Altitudes,* published in 1863, he coined the word *anoxemia* to express a lack of oxygen in arterial blood and explained that one could be anoxemic if there was not enough oxygen, as in high altitude dwellers, or not enough blood, as in patients with anemia.[21]

With oxygen and blood having been established as the limiting factors

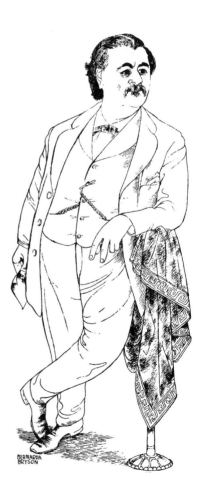

Figure 9-6 Paul Bert (1833–1886).[20]

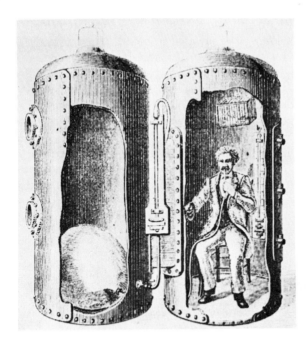

Figure 9-7 Altitude chamber designed by Paul Bert.[19]

in high altitude living, the question then became: how were the well-acclimatized natives able to overcome these limitations? The answer was to be found in the expansion of the lungs and in the increase in the volume of blood, both so characteristic of the deep-chested ruddy natives of the high Andes.

ACCLIMATIZATION

However, neither Bert nor Jourdanet believed that such acclimatization would take place until after generations of high altitude living. This belief in a slow inheritance of acquired adaptive traits had immediate political repercussions. At that time, Napoleon the Third was in the midst of establishing a French empire in Mexico, to be ruled by his puppet Maximilian. The idea that French troops and civilians would not be able to adapt to Mexico's high altitudes was obviously not very attractive to the government, and an obscure French Army physician, Dr. L. Coindet, was asked to disprove Dr. Jourdanet's hypothesis. Based on flimsy observations on pulse and respiration, the army physician concluded that any lowlanders could adapt to low barometric pressure and would be able in a relatively short period to establish a new equilibrium.[22] Rarely has the truth been expressed as clearly and yet based on fewer facts than in this politically motivated pamphlet on adaptive acclimatization.

Not surprisingly, Jourdanet and Bert held to their belief, and, when Bert found high oxygen-carrying capacities in animal blood sent from La Paz to Paris, he explained it on the basis that animals at high altitudes usually have lived there for generations.[23] However, the real blow to their hypothesis came in 1890, when E. Viault traveled by railroad from Lima to the little mining town Morococha at 15,000 feet. He found that his own red blood cell count increased in a few weeks from 5 million to 8 million per cubic millimeter and saw similar changes in his fellow travelers.[24] These observations showed that adaptive acclimatization occurs fairly soon after exposure to high altitude and that altitude polycythemia constitutes an important means of acclimatization.

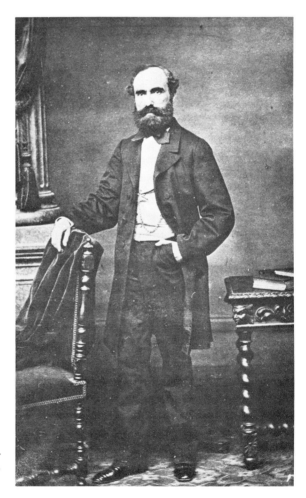

Figure 9-8 Dr. Dennis Jourdanet. (*Courtesy of the Wellcome Trustees.*)

Over the next 50 years, altitude polycythemia was established as the normal physiologic state for the millions of people who live and work at high altitudes in the Alps, Himalayas, and Andes. The degree of polycythemia was found to be roughly proportional to the altitude at which they lived. The capacity of the blood to facilitate oxygen transport and to supplement respiratory and cardiovascular adaptations was worked out in laboratories ranging in altitudes from Copenhagen, at sea level, to Monte Rosa, the peak of Teneriffe, Cerro de Pasco, Pikes Peak, and Morococha. Observations made by Alberto Hurtado (Figure 9-9) and his coworkers in the mining town of Morococha led to the publication in 1945 of the classic paper, "Influence of Anoxemia on the Hematopoietic Activity." There, the adaptation of the oxygen transport chain to atmospheric hypoxia was reviewed and the importance of altitude polycythemia was firmly established.[25]

Recognition of red cell mass as the most adaptable device for high altitude living does not, however, explain how it is made to expand in response to hypoxia. Friedrich Miescher, the famous Swiss physician and discoverer of DNA, was the first to suggest that a low oxygen pressure within the bone marrow itself would stimulate the marrow to produce more red blood cells.[26]

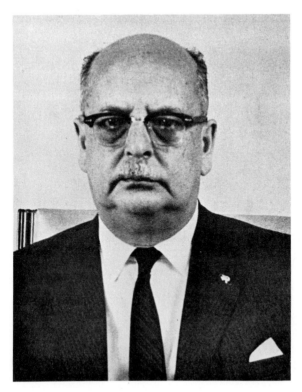

Figure 9-9 Dr. Alberto Hurtado (1901–   ).

This suggestion was made in 1893, at a time when patients with tuberculosis and other chronic illnesses, including Dr. Miescher himself, flocked to mountain sanatoriums. The proposed stimulation of the bone marrow was in accord with the presumed stimulation of other body functions that was thought to be induced by a stay in the high Alps. This idea was widely accepted and was not seriously challenged until 1948, when some investigators failed to find a direct relationship between bone marrow oxygen pressure (P_{O_2}) and red cell production.[27] Other investigators then resurrected an alternate hypothesis, one proposed only a few years after Miescher's work.

"HEMOPOIETINE" AND ERYTHROPOIETIN

In 1906, Paul Carnot, a professor of medicine at the University of Paris, and his assistant Mlle. Deflandre injected normal rabbits with serum obtained from anemic rabbits; they observed an immediate and rather unbelievable increase in the red cell count of the recipient animals.[28] Regardless of how they got their surprising results, they did formulate a hypothesis that has had a lasting impact. They proposed that the serum of anemic animals contained a factor, named by them *hemopoietine*, that was capable of stimulating bone marrow function. In other words, bone marrow control was more indirect than had been envisioned by Miescher. In subsequent studies by a number of other investigators, serum from rabbits kept at high altitude was also examined; in the hands of a few, these sera were found to stimulate bone marrow action.[29] However, the results from most studies were either too fantastic to believe or too insignificant to trust, and careful repetition of the Carnot and Deflandre study by Gordon and Dubin in 1934 led these investigators to doubt the existence of a hemopoietine.[30]

In 1950, Kurt Reissmann reawakened interest in the indirect stimulation of bone marrow by hypoxia. He used Bert's parabiotic technique and found that if two rats were joined by a nonvascular cutaneous connection and one was breathing air at low oxygen pressure, the hypoxic rat would transmit an erythropoietic signal to its normal partner.[31] Three years later, Erslev modified the Carnot experiment by infusing large, rather than small, volumes of plasma from anemic rabbits into normal ones.[32] As a result, he was able to show that Reissmann's erythropoietic signal is transmitted by a humoral factor or hormone, now known as *erythropoietin* (Figure 9-10). Subsequent studies have shown that erythropoietin appears in plasma soon after the oxygen-carrying capacity of the blood has been reduced (anemia) or the atmospheric oxygen tension has been lowered (altitude). In both cases, the tissue tension of oxygen is reduced, and this presumably stimulates the production of erythropoietin and in turn the production of red blood cells. These observations suggested that the rate of red cell production is controlled by a feedback system operating between the bone marrow and an oxygen

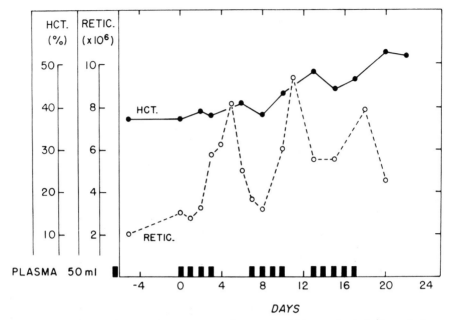

Figure 9-10 The erythropoietic response of normal rabbits to the infusion of plasma obtained from anemic rabbits. The reticulocyte count (Retic.) increased after each series of infusions (50 ml a day for four days), and the concentration of red cells (hematocrit, Hct.) rose gradually over this entire period.

sensor in the peripheral tissues and mediated in one direction by red cell oxygen and in the opposite direction by erythropoietin (Figure 9-11).

Although the concept of this simple feedback system has now been modified and elaborated, its basic structure has remained unchanged. In 1957, Jacobson and his coworkers showed that rats whose kidneys are removed (nephrectomized) fail to produce erythropoietin in response to anemia and proposed that the kidney is the site for oxygen sensing and erythropoietin production.[33] This important observation also suggested that impaired erythropoietin production may be responsible for the severe anemia present

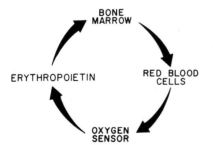

Figure 9-11 Basic feedback control system that adjusts the number of red cells in blood (red cell mass) to the needs for oxygen by the tissues.

in anephric patients or in patients with advanced kidney disease.[34] Conversely, the polycythemia found in some patients with kidney tumors could now be explained by the inappropriate overproduction of erythropoietin by neoplastic renal cells.[35]

The practical implications of these findings could be far reaching. About 30,000 to 40,000 patients with advanced kidney disease are kept alive today by a program in which hemodialysis three times a week replaces the failing excretory functions of the kidney. However, the capacities to sense hypoxia and to produce erythropoietin are not corrected by hemodialysis, and these dialysis patients are usually severely anemic. Replacement therapy with erythropoietin is clearly the answer, but this has proven to be more difficult to accomplish than anticipated.

Surprisingly, erythropoietin in significant amounts cannot be extracted from kidney tissue. Small amounts can be isolated from the plasma or urine of anemic patients, but these sources do not suffice for replacement therapy for the tens of thousands of patients needing it. The lack of extractable erythropoietin in kidney tissue has suggested to some that the kidney only senses oxygen pressure and that the production of erythropoietin occurs elsewhere.[36] Alternate possibilities are that erythropoietin inhibitors present in kidney tissue inactivate erythropoietin during the process of extraction[37] or that the kidney has no storage capacity for erythropoietin but secretes it into the bloodstream as soon as it is formed. In any case, we do not have enough erythropoietin and may have to await its molecular identification and synthesis before it can be packaged for clinical use.

It has been shown recently in adult anephric animals and humans that small amounts of erythropoietin are produced extrarenally, presumably by the liver, in response to hypoxia.[38] It appears that during fetal life, this extrarenal mode of production predominates[39] with a switch from extrarenal to renal production occurring shortly after birth. The question then becomes whether or not it would be possible to switch back again. It is a fascinating question for if this could be accomplished, it would solve the problem of inadequate renal production of erythropoietin in patients with chronic kidney disease. Unfortunately, this may merely be another wish for rejuvenation, like Faust's trade with the devil, Ponce de Leon's search for the fountain of youth, or the current excitement about cloning.

Although the exact source of erythropoietin is still debatable, the oxygen sensor is almost certainly located in the kidney and is triggered by the local tissue tension of oxygen. The amount of oxygen delivered to the kidney depends on the oxygen pressure in atmospheric air, the capacity of the lungs to bring oxygen to the alveoli and across the alveolar membrane to the pulmonary capillaries, the amount of hemoglobin in the blood and the affinity of this hemoglobin for oxygen, the capacity of the heart to pump blood from the lungs to the kidneys, the competency of the renal vessels, and the capacity of

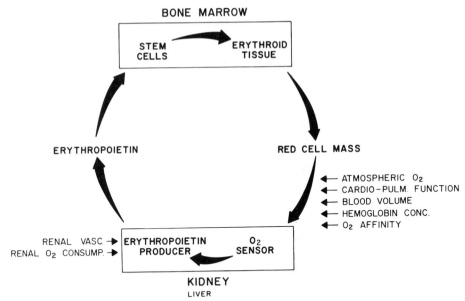

Figure 9-12 Current concept of the feedback circuit which controls the size of the circulating red cell mass. The red cell mass is loaded with oxygen in the lungs through the effects of atmospheric oxygen tension, pulmonary function, hemoglobin concentration, and oxygen affinity of hemoglobin. The oxygen-containing red cells are then brought to oxygen sensors located in the kidney and, possibly, also in the liver. This transport is affected by the cardiac output, blood volume, and peripheral resistance. If the oxygen supply is inadequate, the oxygen sensors transmit signals to erythropoietin producers, and the released erythropoietin is transported to the bone marrow, where it increases the rate of differentiation of stem cells to nucleated red blood cells. The resulting production of mature red cells swells the red cell mass and increases the oxygen supply to the oxygen sensors, which, in turn, decrease further erythropoietin production.

hemoglobin to unload oxygen at the threshhold of the renal oxygen sensor[40] (Figure 9-12).

At high altitude, this complex transport system is adjusted to facilitate the extraction of oxygen from the rarefied atmosphere. As mentioned previously, the two most important adjustments are (1) the augmented pulmonary activity with an increase in respiratory rate and volume and (2) the expanded red cell volume with an increase in oxygen-carrying hemoglobin. In addition, the heart can increase its pumping activity, but cardiac overactivity is costly and is usually reserved for brief periods of oxygen imbalance, such as during work or exertion.

A great deal of attention has recently been paid to the affinity of hemoglobin for oxygen or, in other words, to the capacity of hemoglobin to bind oxygen in the lungs and release it in the tissues. Around the turn of the century, Bohr, Hasselbalch, and Krogh, in Copenhagen,[41] demonstrated that the loading and unloading of oxygen could be graphically expressed by an oxygen dissociation curve (Figure 9-13). The shape of this curve depends on a number of variables including the hydrogen ion concentration (the pH) and the presence of certain organic phosphates in the red cells.[42] The potential significance of these findings for acclimatization to high altitudes is that hypoxia increases the intracellular concentration of these phosphates and thus causes a decrease in hemoglobin oxygen affinity, thereby facilitating the unloading of oxygen and tissue oxygenation. Unfortunately, such a decrease in oxygen affinity would also make it more difficult for hemoglobin to be loaded with oxygen in the lungs, and many investigators have questioned whether a decrease in its oxygen affinity really is an adaptive blessing.

This question appears to have been settled by some intriguing studies of llamas. Llamas and their close cousins the vicunas are indigenous to the

Figure 9-13 Oxygen dissociation curve relating oxygen tension in the blood to the capacity of hemoglobin to bind oxygen (percent saturation). At sea level, the oxygen tension in the pulmonary capillaries is high enough to saturate hemoglobin almost entirely with oxygen. At 3000 m, the oxygen tension in the lungs is much lower, resulting in incomplete oxygen saturation of hemoglobin. Since the tissue tension of oxygen has to be maintained at a fairly constant level regardless of altitude, less oxygen can be made available for the cells at high altitude. This can be overcome by increased blood flow to the tissues or by a shift in the oxygen dissociation curve to the right. Llamas, however, have a curve shifted to the left (see text).

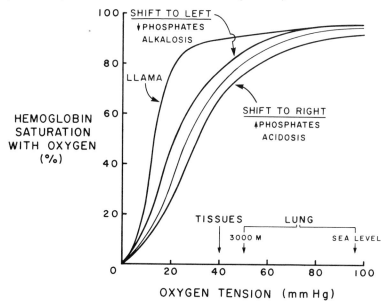

Andes and, surprisingly enough, have hemoglobins with oxygen dissociation curves shifted far to the left[43] (Figure 9-13). They are also not polycythemic, suggesting the presence of an efficient mechanism for the transport of oxygen from the thin atmospheric air. This could presumably be achieved by the high affinity of their hemoglobin for oxygen so that complete oxygen saturation takes place at even low atmospheric pressures. The problem of how these animals unload oxygen to the tissues is bothersome, however. First it was thought that unloading might be facilitated by some mechanism unique for llamas and vicunas. However, a recent study of a family with an inherited hemoglobin abnormality has suggested that this mechanism may not be so unique after all.[44] The abnormal hemoglobin of some members of this family has an affinity for oxygen similar to the one found normally in the llamas. This defect causes tissue hypoxia at sea level and the development of polycythemia. However, when affected family members were moved to an altitude of 3000 m and asked to perform vigorous tasks and tests, they were found to tolerate the altitude exceedingly well and performed far more efficiently than the normal family members, who were used as controls. The conclusion from these observations on "human llamas" was that the initial loading of hemoglobin in the lungs with oxygen is more critical for high altitude living than unloading in the tissues. It also appears that a chance mutation in the hemoglobin molecule of a llama ancestor may be responsible for the preference of todays llamas for high altitudes. It is almost a pity that Darwin, who saw and admired these graceful animals when he crossed the Andes, could not have used this striking example of adaptive evolution for his book *Origin of the Species*.

Stem Cells

Studies aimed at clarifying the bone marrow link in our feedback control system (Figure 9-14) have led to new concepts of cellular proliferation and differentiation and a better understanding of certain hematologic disorders, such as leukemia and aplastic anemia. Quite early, it was surmised that erythropoietin must act on very immature bone marrow cells because it always takes a number of days from the time of erythropoietin stimulation until the effect has been translated into the production of new mature red cells.[45] These erythropoietin-responsive cells were subsequently found to precede the earliest recognizable erythroblasts, and they were called *stem cells*[46] (Figure 9-14).

Stem cells are undifferentiated cells capable of indefinite self-renewal as well as transformation into further differentiated cells if exposed to a specific "poietin," such as erythropoietin. The differentiation induced by erythropoietin appears to be the last step in the gradual differentiation and maturation

ERYTHROPOIESIS

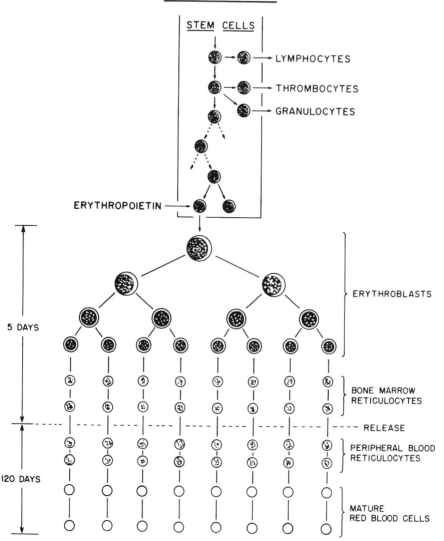

Figure 9-14 An outline of the cellular kinetics underlying the production of red cells. Stem cells become more and more differentiated and single-minded in their maturation from pluripotential to unipotential cells. Finally, triggered by erythropoietin, they undergo blast transformation to erythroblasts capable of hemoglobin synthesis. After a few mitotic divisions, they lose their nuclei and, via a reticulocyte stage, are released into the circulation and become mature, hemoglobin-containing red blood cells.

which characterize the transformation of the fertilized egg cell, the primordial stem cell, through a number of stem cells of ever diminishing potentials to the final functional cells. The stem cell responsive to erythropoietin is unipotential in that it can only differentiate into erythroblasts, while bone marrow stem cells a few steps further back are pluripotential and are capable of differentiating in several cellular directions, such as towards granulocytes, thrombocytes, and erythrocytes. Further back are stem cells capable of differentiation to lymphocytes. These bone marrow stem cells are all present and are potentially active in the adult. However, the earliest of the bone marrow stem cells are probably dormant, and only the final unipotential stem cells responsive to erythropoietin, granulopoietin, thrombopoietin, or lymphopoietin appear to remain active throughout life. Morphologically, all stem cells are small mononuclear cells resembling lymphocytes, and, so far, their uni- or pluripotential capacities can be recognized only by their growth characteristics in vivo or in vitro and not by their appearance.

The exact mechanism by which erythropoietin recognizes specific stem cells and transforms them into erythroblasts is not yet known. This mechanism must involve the activation of previously unused genetic segments which control cellular proliferation and hemoglobin synthesis. It is a process of fundamental biologic and clinical significance for normal and neoplastic growth but one which still has not been identified.

Mt. Everest

The realization that a renal hormone, erythropoietin, controls the size of the red cell mass has been of considerable importance for our ideas about high altitude acclimatization. It may also eventually have practical implications for mountaineering, which during the first half of this century was aimed at conquering Mt. Everest. Although individual fanaticism counted, it became increasingly a question of money, equipment, and oxygen. Climbers realized early that supplemental oxygen was a necessity, and the use of lightweight oxygen tanks, in addition to favorable weather and the organizational talents of Colonel Hunt, finally resulted in two climbers, Edmund Hillary and Tenzing Norkay, reaching the top of Mt. Everest in 1953 and "knocking the blighter off."[47] Since then, many more climbers, supported by paramilitary logistics, have scaled the peak and exulted about the view and the accomplishment. However, among the old mountain climbers, there still is a feeling that Everest, at 29,200 feet, really has not yet been climbed.[48] The ascents have been too artificial, too dependent on enormous logistic support, and on oxygen cylinders, which now can be found as discards all over the approaches to Everest.

The fascination of climbing the peaks unaided was expressed as early as 1799 by Alexander Humboldt[14] when he marveled at the condors soaring over the highest Andean peaks and by the British mountain climber George Lowe,[49] who in 1925 from the slopes of Mt. Everest watched a flock of bar-headed geese flying in echelon directly over the summit. It is known that the bar-headed geese start from the lakes of India at sea level and complete their spring migration to Tibet in a single majestic flight, but the mechanism of their adaptation is entirely unknown.

Hillary, who felt that the problem of climbing Everest unaided was a question of prolonged and intensive acclimatization, attempted to achieve such acclimatization in 1960 through a 6-month stay at 18,750 feet.[50] A quonset hut was erected (Figure 9-15), but the altitude was beyond that possible for adaptation. This limit was actually well known to the Andean Indians, who only have a few permanent settlements above 15,000 feet despite working intermittently in mines considerably higher. The highest inhabited village is probably Aucanquilcha in Chile at 17,500 feet, apparently the upper limit of human adaptation. A few birds, insects, and spiders live between 18,000 and 20,000 feet, but at this level, only transient visits by mammals are possible.[50] Not surprisingly, the attempt by Hillary failed, and members of his expedition were not able to adapt, but rather they developed symptoms of devastating chronic mountain illness and had to cancel all thoughts of climbing Everest without an oxygen mask that year.

Perhaps it is possible to climb Mt. Everest without supplemental oxygen, and perhaps further studies of blood production and blood transfusion will be

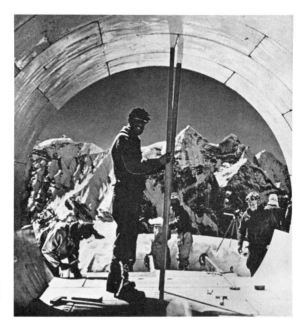

Figure 9-15 Quonset hut built at 18,750 feet by E. Hillary.[50]

of help for future mountain climbers.[51] However, there is little doubt that the observations made at high altitudes have been of practical importance for the survival of patients with too little or too much blood and have more than justified our admiration for blood and our love of mountains.

References

1   Ullman JR: *The Age of Mountaineering*. Philadelphia, Lippincott, 1954, 352 pp, p 16.

2   Rebuffat G: *Mont Blanc to Everest*. New York, Crowell, 1956, 158 pp.

3   Durant W: The Renaissance, in *The Story of Civilization*. New York, Simon and Schuster, 1935–1967, vol 5, 776 pp.

4   Spengler O: *Der Untergang des Abendlandes*. Munchen, CH Beck'sche Verlags-buchhandlung, 1918, vol I, 664 pp and vol II, 549 pp.

5   Goethe JW von: *Faust. Eine Tragoedie*. München: Hyperion verlag Hans von Weber, 1912, 198 pp. (First published 1808.)

6   Prescott WH: *The Conquest of Peru*. New York, The Heritage Press, 1957, 504 pp. (First published 1847.)

7   Hagen VW von: *Highway of the Sun*. Boston, Little Brown, 1955, 320 pp.

8   McIntyre L: Lost empire of the Incas. *Natl Geographic* 144:729–787, 1973.

9   McIntyre L: *The Incredible Incas and Their Timeless Land*. Washington, D.C., National Geographic Society Special Publication Division, 1975, 199 pp.

10 Monge C: *Acclimatization in the Andes: Historical Confirmations of "Climatic Aggression" in the Development of Andean Man*. Baltimore, Johns Hopkins Press, 1948, 130 pp.

11 Kellogg RH: Altitude acclimatization. A historical introduction emphasizing the regulation of breathing. *Physiologist* 11:37–57, 1968.

12 de Acosta J: *Historia natural y moral de las Inchas*. Seville, Juan de Leon, 1590, 535 pp. (Published in English by Val Sims for E. Blount and W. Aspley, 1604.)

13 Richardson BW: *Disciples of Aesculapius*. New York, Dutton, 1901, 424 pp, pp 344–361.

14 Humboldt A von: Notice sur deux tentatives d'ascension du Chimborazo. *Ann Chim Phys (Second Series)* 69:401–434, 1838.

15 Darwin C: *Diary of the Voyage of H.M.S. Beagle*. Barlow N (ed), Cambridge, Cambridge University Press, 1933, 442 pp, p. 292.

16 Bernstein J: *Ascent*. New York, Random House, 1965, 124 pp.

17 Clark RW: *A Picture History of Mountaineering*. New York, MacMillan, 1956, 352 pp.

18 Whymper E: *Scrambles amongst the Alps in the Years 1860–69*. London, John Murray, 1893, 468 pp. (First published 1871.)

19 Bert P: *La Pression Barometrique; Recherches de Physiologie Experimentale*. Paris, Masson; 1878, 1168 pp. (Translated by Hitchcock MA and Hitchcock FA, Columbus, College Book Co., 1943, 1055 pp.)

20 Olmstead JMD: Father of aviation medicine. *Sci Am* 186:66–72, 1952.

21 Jourdanet D: *De l'Anémie des Altitudes et de l'Anemie en Général dans ses Rapports avec la Pression de l'Atmosphère*. Paris, Bailliere, 1863, 44 pp.

22 Coindet L: De L'acclimatement sur les altitudes du Mexique. *Gaz Hebd Med Chir* 10:817–821, 1863.

23 Bert P: Sur la richesse en hemoglobine du sang des amimaux vivant sur les hauts lieux. *C R Acad Sci (Paris)* 94:805–807, 1882.

24 Viault F: Sur l'augmentation considérable du nombre des globules ranges dans le sang chez les habitants des hautes plateaux de l'amerique du sud. *C R Acad Sci (Paris)* 119:917–918, 1890.

25 Hurtado A, Merino C, Delgado E: Influence of anoxemia on the hematopoietic activity. *Arch Intern Med* 75:284–323, 1945.

26 Miescher F: Ueber die Beziehungen Zwischen Meereshohe und Beschaffenheit des Blutes. *Corr Bltt Schweizer Aerzte* 24:809–830, 1893.

27 Berk L, Burchenal JH, Wood T, Castle WB: Oxygen saturation of sternal marrow blood with special reference to pathogenesis of polycythemia vera. *Proc Soc Exp Biol Med* 69:316–320, 1948.

28 Carnot P, Deflandre C: Sur l'activité hémopoiétique de sérum au cours de la régenération du sang. *C R Acad Sci (Paris)* 143:384–386, 1906.

29 Thorling EB: The history on the early theories of humoral regulation of the erythropoiesis. *Dan Med Bull* 16:159–175, 1969.

30 Gordon AS, Dubin M: On the alleged presence of "hemopoietine" in the blood serum of rabbits either rendered anemic or subjected to low pressures. *Am J Physiol* 107:704–708, 1934.

31 Reissmann KR: Studies on the mechanism of erythropoietic stimulation in parabiotic rats during hypoxia. *Blood* 5:372–380, 1950.

32 Erslev AJ: Humoral regulation of red cell production. *Blood* 8:349–387, 1953.

33 Jacobson LO, Goldwasser E, Freed W, Plzak L: Role of the kidney in erythropoiesis. *Nature* 179:633–634, 1957.

34 Erslev AJ: Anemia of chronic renal disease. *Arch Intern Med* 126:774–780, 1970.

35 Thorling EB: Paraneoplastic erythrocytosis and inappropriate erythropoietin production. *Scand J Haematol* (suppl 17), 1972, 166 pp.

36 Gordon AS, Cooper GW, Zanjani ED: The kidney and erythropoiesis. *Semin Hematol* 4:337–358, 1967.

37 Erslev AJ, Kazal LA: Inactivation of erythropoietin by tissue homogenates. *Proc Soc Exp Biol Med* 129:845–849, 1968.

38 Fried W: The liver as a source of extrarenal erythropoietin production. *Blood* 40:671–677, 1973.

39 Zanjani ED, Peterson EN, Gordon AS, Wasserman LR: Erythropoietin production in the fetus: role of the kidney and maternal anemia. *J Lab Clin Med* 83:281–287, 1974.

40 Finch CA, Lenfant, C: Oxygen transport in man. *N Engl J Med* 286:407–415, 1972.

41 Bohr C, Hasselbalch K, Krogh A: Nebereinen in biologischer Beziehung wichtigen Eeinfluss, den die Kohlensähres-spannung des Blutes aufdessen Sanerstoffbindung ubt. *Skand Arch Physiol* 16:402–412, 1904.

42 Benesch R, Benesch RE: Effect of organic phosphates from human erythrocytes on allosteric properties of hemoglobin. *Biochem Biophys Res Commun* 26:162–167, 1967.

43 Hall FG, Dill DB, Barron ESG: Comparative physiology in high altitudes. *J Cell Comp Physiol* 8:301–313, 1936.

44 Hebbel RP, Eaton JW, Berger E, Zanjani E, Kronenburg RS, Moore L: Human llamas: adaptation to altitude in subjects with high hemoglobin affinity. *J Clin Invest,* 62:593–600, 1978.

45 Erslev AJ: The effect of anemic anoxia on the cellular development of nucleated red cells. *Blood* 14:386–398, 1959.

46 Filmanowicz E, Gurney CW: Studies on erythropoiesis XVI. Response to a single dose of erythropoietin in polycythemic mouse. *J Lab Clin Med* 57:65–72, 1961.
47 Hunt J, Hillary E: Triumph on Everest. *Natl Geographic* 105:1–63, 1954.
48 Smythe FS: The spirit of the hills, in Ullman JR(ed): *Kingdom of Adventure: Everest.* New York, William Sloane, 1947, 410 pp.
49 Swan LW: The ecology of the high Himalayas. *Sci Am* 205:68–78, 1961.
50 Bishop BC: Wintering on the roof of the world. *Natl Geographic* 122:503–547, 1962.
51 Pace N, Lozner EL, Consolazio WV, Pitts GC, Percora LJ: The increase in hypoxia tolerance of normal men accompanying the polycythemia induced by transfusion of erythrocytes. *Am J Physiol* 148:152–163, 1947.

CHAPTER 10

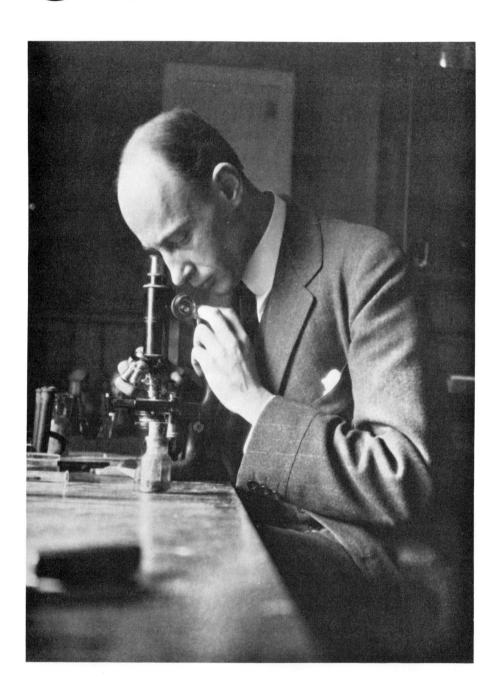

THE CONQUEST OF PERNICIOUS ANEMIA

William B. Castle

D uring the first quarter of the present century, there was seen with increasing ease of recognition in the wards of the hospitals in the large cities of North America, Great Britain, Western Europe, and Scandinavia a mysterious and fatal form of anemia. Its victims were usually past middle age, of varied economic status, and of either sex; the outlook for these sallow and exhausted patients, despite the hope engendered by an occasional temporary improvement, was little better with the ineffectual treatment then available than the prognosis of acute leukemia in the adult today. In 1908, a Boston physician, Richard C. Cabot,[1] analyzed the survival time of 1200 such patients seen in his own practice, in the practice of medical friends in various parts of the country, and as reliably reported in the medical literature. In summary, he found that survival after the onset of the disease was usually from one to three years, and in only six patients was permanent recovery known to have occurred. This anemia, by then appropriately called

Chapter Opening Photo   George R. Minot, M.D. (1885–1950), Assistant in Medicine, Harvard Medical School, in his laboratory at the Massachusetts General Hospital. (*Photograph by Miss Catherine Thacher in 1917, of which a copy was later given by Dr. Minot to W. B. Castle.*)

"pernicious," was not a new pathological condition. Like other historical examples of a new awareness of a common disease, it had gradually achieved clinical distinction during the last quarter of the nineteenth century, when its symptoms and physical signs, and especially its blood picture as seen under the microscope, together became clearly recognized as a distinct small constellation in the vast firmament of disease.

In 1926, two other Boston physicians, George R. Minot and William P. Murphy,[2] electrified the world of medicine with the announcement that they had abolished the anemia of a series of 45 pernicious anemia patients; these patients had been persuaded to eat for some months a special diet that contained up to half a pound of beef liver daily. The effect of this discovery was not only to commute a death sentence for these patients and for countless others to come but also to provide great expectations for hematology and to set in forward motion the frontiers of research concerning diseases of the blood.

Recognition and Description

Dr. Thomas Addison,[3] of Guy's Hospital, London, is customarily considered to have been the first to describe pernicious anemia in 1855. As a preface to his classic monograph *On the Constitutional and Local Effects of Disease of the Suprarenal Capsules*, he speaks of a "very remarkable form of general anemia, occurring without any discoverable cause whatsoever" during life or at postmortem examination. Consequently, he considered the condition to be "idiopathic" and merely speculated that it might be due to "some form of fatty degeneration." His account, in addition to being confused with his superb description of the destructive disease of the adrenal glands that today bears his name, included no microscopic examination of the blood, although it would have been possible at the time he wrote. Moreover, his description mentioned none of the characteristic signs and symptoms that surely would have been apparent then as now to such a keen bedside observer as Addison—the sore mouth or an inflamed or glassy-appearing tongue, slight jaundice of the eyes and skin, and a persistent numbness and tingling of the fingers and toes which sometimes progresses to unsteadiness or a spasticity of gait.

Today we know that these three manifestations together provide compelling evidence for a diagnosis of pernicious anemia. Actually, the sore mouth as a symptom had been briefly mentioned by A. W. Barclay[4] in 1851, but as his patient was a nursing mother, she more probably had a different kind of anemia, one that affected pregnant or recently delivered women in poor nutritional circumstances. After 1897, Dr. William Hunter,[5] a canny Edinburgh medical graduate who went to London to practice medicine, emphasized the prevalence of sore tongue in pernicious anemia, but he regarded it as evidence of oral sepsis, which he related to the cause of the disease. In 1908, Richard Cabot[1] reported that about 40 percent of his patients complained of a sore tongue that appeared red and ulcerated. He also stated that jaundice was apparent in most patients in whom the anemia was severe. In addition, Cabot noted that about 10 percent of his patients showed clinical evidence of spinal cord damage sufficient to cause the development of an ataxic or spastic gait; abnormalities of sensation in the hands or feet were even more common. Later, it was realized that in patients lacking the diagnostic triad, the more than chance occurrence of premature graying of the hair or of a patchy loss of skin pigment, known as vitiligo, is also suggestive of the diagnosis.

Unlike the sore tongue and mild jaundice, symptoms that also occur in other conditions, the demyelinating lesion of the spinal cord seen at autopsy is specific for pernicious anemia. Despite occasional reports of impaired sensibility of the extremities in association with the typical anemia, such as occurred in the patient described by Professors Osler and Gardner,[6] of McGill University, in Montreal in 1877, this particularity was only slowly realized. In 1883, at a medical meeting in Cologne, Otto Leichtenstern[7] reported the characteristic degeneration of the posterior (sensory) nerve tracts of the spinal cord observed at autopsy of two patients who during life had been diagnosed as having pernicious anemia and syphilis of the spinal cord. He expressed the unlikely belief that the anemia was a result of the nervous disease. In 1873, L. Lichtheim,[8] of Bern, clearly described the association of spinal cord lesions with pernicious anemia, and this was confirmed by others. Although in 1900 the British observers Russell, Batten, and Collier,[9] of Queen's Square Hospital, London, wrote a classical description with illustrations of the degeneration of both sensory and motor nerve tracts of the spinal cord, they were not convinced of its special relation to pernicious anemia. Thus, they pointed to the lack of anemia in some of their patients and the long antecedence of nervous symptoms in others. It remained for Hurst and Bell,[10] of Guy's Hospital, London, in 1922 to insist upon the specificity of the association with pernicious anemia. In additional support of this, they cited the consistent lack of the normal secretion of hydrochloric acid by the stomach in both conditions. Today it is clear that the immediate biochemical abnormality responsible for the anemia is not the same as that which produces the spinal cord degeneration; for this reason, these clinical manifestations may not necessarily occur simultaneously.

However suggestive of a diagnosis of pernicious anemia the triad of symptoms and physical signs was for the experienced bedside clinician at the end of the last century, the three were not always present even when the anemia was severe. Consequently, it was the discovery of ways to determine the number, size, and shape of the red cells and the amount of hemoglobin in a drop of blood that eventually supplied the crucial diagnostic criteria. In Chapter 1 are described these essential technical developments—the compound microscope, the ruled counting chamber of a uniform, known depth, and devices for the measurement of hemoglobin by the intensity of its color when released from the red cells. All these came into increasing clinical use after the introduction of dyes for staining the cells in films of dried blood made on glass slides.

Normally, the number of red cells in blood is about 5 million per cubic millimeter, and when an anticoagulated sample is subjected to an appropriate centrifugal force in a narrow tube (hematocrit), the corpuscles, which are normally in suspension in blood flowing in the body, settle and occupy a little less than half of the total volume of blood. The first reported red blood cell count of a patient with pernicious anemia was made by a Danish physician, S. T. Sörensen[11] in 1874. His very anemic patient had only 470,000 red cells per cubic millimeter or less than 10 percent of the normal. In an article published in 1877, the German clinician Heinrich Quincke[12] depicted the extreme variations in size and shape of many of the red cells of such patients, for which he used the term *poikilocytes,* and in 1876, Herrmann Eichhorst, professor of medicine at Jena,[13] published drawings of blood films showing rather too systematically a population of small round red cells or *microcytes.* However, it was soon found that both of these abnormal types of red cells were present in the blood in other kinds of anemia as well. Therefore, the Norwegian Sören Laache[14] in 1883 instead correctly emphasized the diagnostic importance for pernicious anemia of "giant" red cells, *macrocytes,* which had first been reported by Professor Georges S. Hayem,[15] of the University of Paris, in 1877. This perennial student of diseases of the blood had also noted the previous year the relatively greater reduction in the number of the red cells than of the hemoglobin content in the blood in a case of pernicious anemia; in his 1883 monograph, Laache[14] had insisted that this was a constant diagnostic feature. Conveniently, he proposed the term *color index* for the ratio of hemoglobin percentage to red cell percentage of normal. Thus, the normal color index was 1.0, while that of pernicious anemia was greater and that of chlorosis, an anemia in which the red cells contained less than the normal amount of hemoglobin, was less than 1.

In 1880, Paul Ehrlich[16] briefly reported a far more specific finding at a meeting of physicians in Berlin. He saw in the blood of certain pernicious anemia patients occasional large nucleated red cells that contained much cytoplasm and dispersed nuclear chromatin, the latter a recognized sign today of nuclear immaturity. These he called *megaloblasts* and correctly concluded that they were the escaped bone marrow precursors of Hayem's giant red cells. He contrasted these cells with nucleated red cells of a normal size that had condensed nuclear chromatin, which he called *normoblasts.* These occasionally are found in the blood in certain other severe anemias. Ehrlich's bone marrow megaloblast is, indeed, the hallmark of pernicious anemia, and its *raison d'être* was to become successively the central problem in the study of the morphology, the physiology, and the biochemistry of the marrow, the last now being explored at a molecular level.

In 1881 and 1885, using the dye methylene blue to stain samples of fresh blood, Ehrlich[17] described bluish particles and granules visible in a small percentage of normal adult red cells. He erroneously supposed these red cells, which, unlike the majority, accepted the stain, to be degenerating forms, an interpretation that was corrected in 1891 by the pioneer American bacteriologist Theobald Smith.[18] He was studying Texas cattle fever, research that provided the world with the first evidence for the transmission of disease by an insect, even before the mosquito vectors for malaria and yellow fever were discovered. Texas fever, an infection shown by him to be transmitted by ticks, caused a severe anemia in which the parasites were visible within the cow's red cells. By staining fresh blood with methylene blue, Smith saw that in addition to the parasites, "coccus-like particles" such as Ehrlich had observed appeared as the anemia deepened, as did nucleated red cells shortly thereafter. This chronological association led him to consider the particles to mark cells *younger* than the adult red cells, a conclusion that was fortified by similar appearances in the red cells of a healthy cow which had been rendered anemic by bleedings of 2 to 5 quarts daily for 6 days (thus, presumably, not on the Sabbath). With the passage of time, these young red cells, which in humans contained a more filamentous network, came to be called *reticulocytes,* a word coined by the Philadelphia pathologist Edward Krumbhaar[19] in 1922. By that time, the percentage of reticulocytes in the blood had already been recognized as a reliable indicator of the ability of the bone marrow to produce red cells. In 1913, Vogel and McCurdy,[20] of the pathological department of St. Luke's Hospital in New York City, expressed this view and published a graph showing a striking peak of reticulocytes at the time that the red cell count of a patient with pernicious anemia began a spontaneous and sustained increase. In 1916, Lee, Minot, and Vincent,[21] who were working in Boston at the Massachusetts General Hospital, found that surgical splenectomy sometimes produced a temporary remission in pernicious anemia. In the course of this work, they noted that "in the event of a persistent increase of the reticulated cells we found marked clinical improvement associated with an increased red count." This relationship was to prove to be of great value to Minot a decade later.

Much of the knowledge about the descriptive features of blood in pernicious anemia was acquired between 1875 and 1890, not by Addison's successors in Britain but by workers on the European continent. This came about in the accidental and circuitous fashion that sometimes characterizes progress in science. Thus, in 1868, Professor Anton Biermer, of Zürich, presented a preliminary report on the fatty degeneration of the heart and blood vessels associated with anemia. In 1872, he used the term "progressiver perniciöser Anämie" to describe a total of 15 cases, 14 of which were fatal.[22] He made no mention of Addison's work and stated that his anemia "was found amongst poor people, especially women about 30 years of age, among whom, in addition to poverty, puerperal conditions appeared to be a determining factor." The diagnosis of leukemia was excluded by the microscopic examination of unstained blood films, but cell counts were not made. In 1874, H. Immermann used the same descriptive term in his confirmation of Biermer's observations, and in 1876, an editorial in an English medical journal[23] reviewed the work of Biermer and of Immermann under the title "Pernicious Anaemia, a New Disease." In the meantime, in 1874, Addison's junior colleague Dr. Samuel Wilks[24] had come to the defense of Addison's priority, pointing out that he, Wilks, had published several reports of fatal cases of the kind about which he said Addison had lectured as early as 1843. And he added, "the most remarkable circumstance is its supposed recent discovery by these two foreign physicians." As a result of this editorial flurry over Biermer's work and terminology, his reports, as well as those of Addison and Wilks, received wider medical attention. In fact, as we shall see, the relatively recent growth of knowledge has made it almost certain that Addison and Biermer each described megaloblastic anemias, but from different biochemical causes.

By the turn of the century, the blood picture typical of Addison's pernicious anemia was well recognized in Britain and in America to be that of a frequently severe anemia in which the reduction of the number of red cells was relatively greater than that of the quantity of hemoglobin. Many of the red cells, as seen under the microscope, were large, oval, and well filled with hemoglobin, and there was often a moderate reduction in the number of white cells, especially the granulocytes, as well as of the platelets. An appreciation of the significance of the paucity of reticulocytes was yet to come, as was recognition of the diagnostic clue provided by the presence of the large multilobed granulocytes, first described by the German hematologist Joseph Arneth[25] in 1907. By then, the anemia, and its consequent reduction in the hemoglobin concentration of the blood, was understood to impose a limitation on the transport of oxygen from the lungs to body tissues and so was a cause of chronic fatigue and, on slight exertion, shortness of breath and pounding of the heart. On the other hand, the reduction in the number of white cells apparently gave rise to no clinical symptoms, and the reduction in the number of platelets, unless extreme, rarely led even to pinpoint bleeding. Nevertheless, the underlying cause of the anemia was still a mystery, and the nature of the pathological alterations in the bone marrow had already been the subject of futile discussion for a quarter of a century and would continue for many years to come.

Debated Mechanism

After 1875, with the bone marrow established as the source of the red corpuscles of the blood (Chapter 3), repeated efforts were made to understand the cause of the increased volume of red marrow and its primitive cellularity as seen at postmortem in pernicious anemia. Two principal difficulties confused that attempt for many years. First, especially on the continent, Biermer's dramatic term *progressive pernicious anemia* was often applied to any severe and fatal anemia, sometimes in clear association with another known disease, such as cancer or chronic infection. Even for Ehrlich, whose use of aniline dyes after 1880 provided easy identification of megaloblasts in blood or bone marrow, these cells were not the product of a specific disorder. Second, even after the turn of the century, when all competent pathologists agreed that the bone marrow of Addison's anemia contained a population of large red cell precursors with primitive nuclear structure, the so-called megaloblasts of Ehrlich, the functional interpretation of this appearance depended principally upon the prejudice of the particular observer, as indeed had been the case from the beginning.

Thus in 1875, William Pepper,[26] who had just returned from working with Julius Cohnheim in Germany, was the first in America to describe the microscopic appearance of the bone marrow in a fatal case of pernicious anemia in Philadelphia. Impressed by the intense cellularity that he thought was composed of lymphoid cells, he considered it to represent a form of "pseudo-leukemia." The following year, Cohnheim,[27] then professor of pathology at Breslau, recognized that such hypercellularity mostly involved the red cell precursors and suggested that the anemia was the result of a primary disorder of the blood-forming organs and was expressed as an unexplained reversion to the primitive type of red cell formation (erythropoiesis) seen in the human embryo.

Ernst Neumann,[28] brilliant pathological anatomist at Königsberg, Germany, next proposed the more understandable analogy of the increasingly immature type of red cell hypercellularity that had been observed to develop in the bone marrow of animals and patients as a response to repeated hemorrhage. Paul Ehrlich,[29] in 1880, found Cohnheim's somewhat mystical idea of embryonal reversion appealing and attributed it to an unknown poison or poisons that interfered with blood formation and also caused increased blood destruction. Thus, Ehrlich combined the contradictory interpretations of his predecessors.

However, as shown in Table 10-1, by deriving support from the clinical aspects of the disease, neither the thesis of decreased red cell production nor that of increased red cell destruction lacked suggestive evidence. By 1900, for example, the reports of Reyher and others of a cure for a similar anemia in Western Russia and Finland—by the expulsion of a fish tapeworm from the bowel—was thought to be due to the removal of the source of a red cell–destroying toxin.[30] There was a similarity in the role that Hunter[5] proposed for *Streptococcus longus* in producing a hypothetical blood-destroying toxin in stomach and intestine that was responsible, he thought, through the breakdown of hemoglobin, for the jaundice and increased iron deposits in liver and spleen.

Table 10-1 *Mechanism of anemia—dialectic vs. experiment (1875–1956)*

THESIS: SECONDARY TO HEMOLYSIS

Primitive erythroid marrow; jaundice and increased iron stores; correction by tapeworm removal.

ANTITHESIS: PRIMARY DECREASED ERYTHROPOIESIS

Primitive erythroid marrow; few reticulocytes, leukocytes, platelets; correction by liver feeding.

RESOLUTION: INEFFECTIVE MARROW ERYTHROPOIESIS

Erythroid precursor hemolysis *and* delayed DNA synthesis.

On the other hand, after the dramatic relief of the anemia by liver feeding, it seemed to Francis Peabody,[31] from his study of the bone marrow biopsies of patients treated in 1927 in Boston, that there was some factor in liver that "promotes the development and differentiation of mature red blood cells." To others also, the resulting increases in reticulocytes and adult red cells in the blood, as well as in white cells and platelets, suggested a similar abolition of prior defective marrow function.

The resolution of these opposing views was not advanced even by the ready availability of bone marrow for microscopic study during life by the introduction of sternal aspiration by needle and syringe by Mikhail Arinkin,[32] of Leningrad, in 1929. It only occurred many years later with the introduction of radioactive iron as a tracer of hemoglobin synthesis and destruction. In this way, in 1956, Clement Finch and his associates[33] at the University of Washington, in Seattle, were able to measure the rate of red cell (hemoglobin) production in the bone marrow and the rate of its delivery in new red cells to the circulating blood (Figure 10-1). This new method showed that in pernicious anemia, despite the rapid initial proliferation, many nucleated precursors of adult red cells died in the bone marrow. Much of the hemoglobin was released there prematurely, and fewer new red cells (reticulocytes) were launched into the bloodstream. There, as adult red cells, they also have a somewhat shortened life span. Actually, this explanation had been proposed in 1930 by Vladimir Jedlicka, of Prague,[34] and as early as 1922, George Whipple[35] had pointed out the discrepancy between the small amount of circulating hemoglobin in the anemia and the inordinately large amount of its usual pigmented breakdown products. Thus, the discovery of "ineffective erythropoiesis" within the bone marrow showed at long last that the champions of decreased production of red cells as well as those of increased destruction of red cells were both, in part, correct. A similar less easily defined process may account

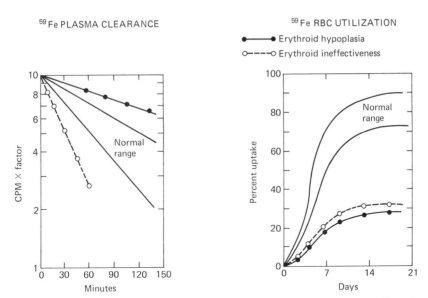

Figure 10-1 Initiating rate of hemoglobin production in the bone marrow (^{59}Fe plasma clearance) and subsequent rate of reappearance of ^{59}Fe-labeled hemoglobin in the blood (^{59}Fe RBC utilization). Values are shown for normal subjects and patients with erythroid marrow hypoplasia and pernicious anemia (erythroid ineffectiveness). Note that the ^{59}Fe plasma clearance is rapid in erythroid ineffectiveness and slow in erythroid hypoplasia, but that in both, ^{59}Fe utilization is markedly less than normal. (*From Erslev AJ, Gabuzda TG: Pathophysiology of Blood. Philadelphia, Saunders, 1975, p 33.*)

for the decreased numbers of white cells and platelets in the blood. Today we recognize that the characteristic macrocytosis of pernicious anemia is the result of altered red cell production, whereas the severity of the anemia is largely a reflection of the increased red cell destruction. The centrifugal extension of the hypercellular marrow to occupy most of the bones of the body is presumably the result of its effort to compensate for these aberrations.

Perhaps Something Is Missing

The prevailing concept about pernicious anemia at the turn of the century, that of being a toxic-hemolytic anemia, was consistent with the then recent discoveries of Pasteur, Koch, Ehrlich, von Behring, and others concerning diseases caused by bacterial infection and bacterial toxins. In contrast to their brilliant demonstration that certain diseases were due to such *positive* deleterious factors, evidence was shortly to be added that some morbid states could be the result of the *negative* qualities of defective nutrition. It turned out that, like bacteria, these defects could also be minute but critical. In 1897, Christian

Eijkmann,[36] a Dutch military doctor in Java and later professor of hygiene at Utrecht, in Holland, found that chickens experimentally fed the polished rice diet consumed by inmates of jails and hospitals developed a paralytic disorder that was similar to beriberi, a well-known affliction that appeared in some prisoners and patients. In the birds, as later in the patients, this condition was found to be curable and preventable by feeding whole unpolished rice. Eijkmann's interpretation was that the "silver skin" removed by the polishing process contained a natural antidote to a nerve poison produced in the intestine by an overly rich starch diet.

Five years later, this supposed link between the positive and negative theories of disease was eliminated by another Dutch scientist, G. Grijns,[37] who expressed for the first time the modern view that beriberi was due simply to the *lack* of an essential nutrient in the silver skin. The scientific basis for a theory of dietary deficiency was soon rapidly fortified by experimental work with animals in the laboratories of F. Gowland Hopkins in England, and, later, by Osborne and Mendel at Yale and by E. V. McCollum at the University of Wisconsin and, later, at Johns Hopkins. In 1912, another investigator, Casimir Funk,[38] published a review of the literature concerning beriberi, scurvy, and pellagra, which, well ahead of his time, he considered to be "deficiency diseases," and in it used the term "vitamine" for the first time.

It was now inevitable that the primordial notion that "good food makes good blood" should come under scientific scrutiny. This, in effect, was the purpose of an extensive series of experiments with dogs rendered anemic by systematic bleeding begun about 1918 by George Whipple (Figure 10-2). At first, he worked at the Hooper Institute in California and then, at the new School of Medicine and Dentistry of the University of Rochester, in New York, where in 1920 he became its first professor of pathology and dean. It was at Rochester that, with Frieda Robscheit-Robbins, the experimental design was perfected.[39] Over a period of weeks or months, the hemoglobin level of the blood of each dog was reduced at 2-week intervals to about half-normal by the removal of an appropriate and measured amount of blood. Eventually, when maintained on a basal diet of canned salmon and bread, very little blood needed to be removed to maintain this reduced level. However, when the basal diet was supplemented daily with a variety of animal or vegetable foods, such as liver, beef muscle, or spinach, hemoglobin production increased, and more blood had to be withdrawn. This was a measure of the effectiveness of the dietary supplements, of which liver was the most potent.[39] For reasons not entirely clear, the effect of inorganic iron was, at best, erratic. Consequently, Whipple advised clinicians in 1922[35] and again in 1925[39] to pay attention in the management of anemic patients to "diet factors proven to be potent in controlled experiments."

This advice, however, was not ahead of some physicians' clinical intuition. In 1871, Biermer had mentioned, among possible causes of his patients'

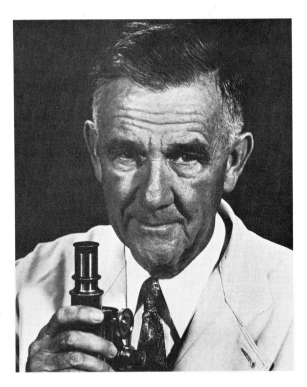

Figure 10-2 George H. Whipple, M.D. (1878–1976), Dean and Chairman of Department of Pathology, University of Rochester School of Medicine and Dentistry. (*Photograph by Ansel Adams, circa 1950, courtesy of Dr. Lawrence E. Young.*)

anemia, their "insufficient and unsuitable feeding."[22] Professor T. R. Fraser,[40] of Edinburgh, attempted a direct correction of bone marrow function in 1894 by feeding beef bone marrow daily in a well-conducted trial in a patient with "pernicious anemia." Although his patient's anemia was much benefited, this success could not be repeated by others. In 1917, Barker and Sprunt[41] reported a regimen "that had been found helpful" at Johns Hopkins Hospital; this included the feeding in frequent divided doses of up to 3 quarts of milk a day. Confirmation did not follow, but a few years later, Whipple's published experimental results caused a renewed interest in dietary therapy. This led several American clinicians to apply his experimental findings to various types of anemia, including pernicious anemia. Among the few who reported their results were Gibson and Howard,[42] of the State University of Iowa. As published in 1923, their primary interest was in the metabolic effects of a high protein diet that was low in fat and contained egg yolk and liver daily, rather than in its possible beneficial effect on anemia. However, in seven patients with pernicious anemia, moderate improvement in blood levels was observed. Indeed, it occurred rather promptly in four. Nevertheless, as "spontaneous remissions" of the anemia were well known to experienced clinicians, they did not consider this improvement as necessarily being related to the diet. Their considered advice was to try the diet "in the anemias," but not to neglect the time-honored remedies of iron and arsenic.

Victory over Death

There was in Boston in 1925 a practicing physician, George R. Minot, an assistant professor of medicine at Harvard, who had had a special interest in anemias and other disorders of the blood ever since he had been a medical student[43] (Chapter Opening Photo). He knew from his own experience that iron and arsenic were of little or no value in pernicious anemia. And he had also learned in 1916 that the surgical removal of the spleen,[21] although sometimes beneficial for a time, failed in the end to save the patient despite the help of transfusions, nor did the customary efforts to improve nutrition, and fresh air and bed rest, add much to the patients' outlook. However, while still a young medical "house pupil" at the Massachusetts General Hospital in 1912–1913, Minot[43] had been interested in learning at first hand the eating habits of pernicious anemia patients. In 1915, and later as a member of the hospital staff, his detailed questionings at the patients' bedside[44] seemed to Minot's interns merely a harmless eccentricity of a competent clinician. But from his interrogations, he gained the impression that these patients had often lived for some time on a limited and selective diet. A distaste for meat was sometimes strongly expressed. Consequently, Whipple's experiments seemed to confirm Minot's clinical suspicion of a possible dietary deficiency, and in about 1922, he began to advise his pernicious anemia patients to try to include meat and liver in their diets (Figure 10-3). Some improvement seemed to follow, and in 1925, Minot invited Dr. William P. Murphy, a member of the staff of the Peter Bent Brigham Hospital and of Minot's group practice, who had shown unusual interest in blood disorders, to join him in a rigorous trial of a special diet containing "an abundance of food rich in complete proteins and iron—particularly liver—and relatively low in fat." Originally, it was intended as a study of the effect in 10 patients with pernicious anemia, but because of its initial encouraging results and their access to patients at several Harvard teaching hospitals in Boston, the numbers studied rapidly increased.

On May 4, 1926, Minot and Murphy[2] were able to report to the distinguished audience of the Association of American Physicians the consistent clinical improvement and gain in red blood cell levels of a nearly consecutive series of 45 pernicious anemia patients. The special diet had contained from 120 to 240 g (about a half a pound) of lightly cooked beef liver daily. At first, for many of these ailing, dispirited individuals to "get it down," even in part, required the utmost patience, persuasion, and persistence by the principal investigators and their assistants and nurses. Finally, the prompt and quantitative increase of new red cells (reticulocytes) that consistently preceded the rise in the red cell level left no hiatus between apparent cause and effect. For

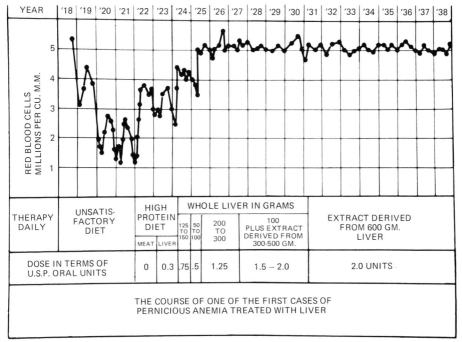

THERAPY DAILY	UNSATIS-FACTORY DIET	HIGH PROTEIN DIET		WHOLE LIVER IN GRAMS			EXTRACT DERIVED FROM 600 GM. LIVER
		MEAT 125 TO 150	LIVER 50 TO 100	200 TO 300	100 PLUS EXTRACT DERIVED FROM 300-500 GM.		
DOSE IN TERMS OF U.S.P. ORAL UNITS	0	0.3	.75 .5	1.25	1.5 – 2.0		2.0 UNITS

THE COURSE OF ONE OF THE FIRST CASES OF
PERNICIOUS ANEMIA TREATED WITH LIVER

Figure 10-3 Red cell levels in a patient with pernicious anemia treated by Dr. George R. Minot. Note early beneficial effect of addition of meat and liver to diet, later enhanced by more liver and sustained at a normal level by liver extract. (*From a chart, courtesy of Dr. Minot.*)

Minot, ever since 1916, this reticulocyte response had been a welcome harbinger of improvement.[21] And so, under close personal supervision, the life-saving discovery was made. For its inspiration, it was fortunate in retrospect that not until about 1936 did it become apparent that the efficacy of liver in Whipple's chronically bled dogs was mainly due to its available iron content.[45] Ignorance of this fact had encouraged the application of Whipple's work to a quite different type of anemia.

At first the reported success of liver feeding seemed far too simple to be credible, or at least sustainable, for some leading European medical authorities. But worldwide confirmation soon followed, and in 1934, when the Nobel Prize in Physiology and Medicine was rightly awarded Whipple, Minot, and Murphy, it seemed that an unknown biological requirement of blood formation had been discovered and its successful application to a fatal human anemia had been achieved.[46] The result of their work was so important for patients and for medicine that it matters little now that in fact the dogs responded to the iron and the patients to a then unknown vitamin in the liver. When in 1928, Minot was appointed professor of medicine at Harvard and the second director of the Harvard-affiliated Thorndike Memorial Laboratory of the Boston City Hospital, the opportunities were broadened for his important and continuing influence on the growth of American hematology.

Why was Minot successful in making this completely convincing demonstration, a discovery that others had so narrowly missed? The son of a physician on the staff of the Massachusetts General Hospital, his forebears, like those of other Boston medical families, had been significant contributors to the affairs of the Harvard Medical School and its affiliated hospitals.[43] Thus, his was an inheritance of typical Yankee traits—native optimism, intellectual curiosity, and a strong belief in rational causality and in the value of hard work. His special genius was for taking infinite pains. The discovery of insulin in 1922 by Banting and Best came in the nick of time to save Minot's life, for he had developed severe diabetes in the fall of 1921. Early in 1923, his physician Elliot P. Joslin, Boston's leading expert in diabetes, first obtained some insulin for his patient; and it was not without significance for the rigorous subsequent trial of "a special diet" that Minot had become, perforce, compulsively concerned with the details of his own.

Minot and Murphy[47] soon published a full account of their observations, and Minot discussed with Edwin J. Cohn, professor of physical chemistry at Harvard, the possibility of producing a clinically effective extract of liver and of identifying its active principle. This academic contact was logical because protein of high biologic quality in liver was thought by Minot to be the probable basis for the success of the special diet, and Cohn was known to have a special interest in research on proteins. A collaborative program was developed in which Cohn and his colleagues prepared successive fractions of liver—dichotomous chemical precipitates and filtrates—that were individually tested for potency in previously untreated patients with pernicious anemia by Minot, Murphy, and their associates.

In this evaluation, there now emerged the special advantage of daily reticulocyte counts of the blood, using a staining technique that had been taught Minot many years before by J. Homer Wright, pathologist at the Massachusetts General Hospital, in Boston. Individual liver fractions were now fed to patients in uniform daily amounts during successive 10-day periods.[48] If in a first period, no reticulocyte increase appeared, the fraction was provisionally judged to be inactive. Then, in a second period of daily administration of a different liver fraction, if a reticulocyte response indicated its activity, it also confirmed the lack of potency of the first. In this way, each patient could provide evidence of both a negative and a positive effect, and the delay in interpretation required by waiting for a substantial increase of the red cell level was avoided. Unexpectedly, but fortunately for the future development of concentrated liver extracts, almost at once, the bulky liver proteins were found to be inert, and by 1928, Cohn's water-soluble, alcohol-insoluble precipitate, the so-called liver fraction G, was shown to be consistently active in pernicious anemia. Then, with the collaboration of G. H. A. Clowes, of Eli Lilly and Company, who had been invited to participate, this liver fraction became commerically available to the medical profession in the form of a yellow powder, of which only 12.75 g had the clinical activity of 300 g of beef liver. The patent was given to the public.

When Cohn attempted to produce a more purified liver extract for clinical use by injection, the elimination of a contaminant that lowered blood pressure resulted in great losses of antianemic potency. In 1930, M. Gänsslen,[49] a professor of medicine in Germany, astonished the Boston workers with a report of a nearly protein-free liver extract that was fully active in pernicious anemia when injected daily in amounts derived from only 5 g of liver. This success was soon confirmed in Boston. When a sterile neutralized solution of liver fraction G derived from 10 g of liver was given daily by intramuscular injection,[50] it was found to be 30 to 60 times as potent as the parent substance, which had been given by mouth. This so-called crude liver extract was further refined by H. D. Dakin and Randolph West in New York, and by 1935, a purified liver extract was found to be fully active on injection in pernicious anemia.[51]

Another surprise came in 1938 when Lucy Wills and Barbara Evans,[52] two British physicians who were successfully treating the nutritional anemia of pregnant women in Bombay with a crude liver extract, reported that a more purified liver extract was ineffective. Their subsequent work on monkeys, kept on defective diets similar to those of the patients, led to the recognition of a macrocytic anemia different from that of pernicious anemia, although with similar blood and bone marrow characteristics. As was subsequently shown by the American workers Snell and Petersen[53] in 1940, the component missing from purified liver extract was a growth factor required for a lactobacillus when it was grown in the test tube. This finding quickly led to recognition of the fact that the growth factor was also present in yeast and green plants and so led to the name *folic acid* for the active chemical entity that was isolated from liver by Pfiffner et al.[54] and E. L. R. Stokstad in 1943.[55]

After World War II, the interrupted search for the substance in purified liver extracts that is active in pernicious anemia was resumed on both sides of the Atlantic. Progress was slow because of the necessity of conducting tests on a diminishing population of untreated patients. Possible guidance from studies on the growth of microbes had been delayed by preoccupation with the notion that pernicious anemia is a uniquely human disease. It was 1947 before the study of another lactobacillus by Mary Shorb[56] showed that the most purified liver fractions contained an essential growth factor for this bacterium. This information guided the final stages of its isolation, then made possible for the first time by the recent development of adsorption and partition chromatography. This, and the realization that the active liver fractions were red, brought about in 1948 the identification of the source of that activity as crystalline

Table 10-2 *Progress in concentration of antianemic principles of liver*

YEAR	SUBSTANCE	DRY WEIGHT (g)*
Clinical era		
1926	Whole beef liver (240 g)	60.0
1928	Liver fraction G (oral)	12.75
1930	Crude liver extract	0.35
1936	Refined liver extract	0.015
Microbiological era		
1945	Folic acid	0.001
1948	Vitamin B_{12}	0.000001

* Comparably effective therapeutic daily dosage when given by injection, unless otherwise indicated.

cyanocobalamin, termed *vitamin B_{12}* by Karl Folkers and his associates[57] at the Merck Laboratories, in the United States. The precious red material was supplied to Randolph West,[58] in New York, who had been a pioneer in the efforts for the identification of the source of the activity in liver. He now became the first to describe the extraordinary clinical potency of a few thousandths of a milligram of the new vitamin in pernicious anemia. Only a few weeks later, Smith and Parker,[59] at Glaxo Laboratories in England, reached the same goal guided entirely by clinical tests on patients.

So ended the long search for the unknown factor in liver that is active in pernicious anemia, which by its absence in the body was in some way presumably responsible for the development of the anemia and the other clinical features of the disease. The discovery of the life-saving effect of liver feeding by Minot and Murphy was as absolute a victory over death as medicine has known. Then, the development of liver extracts and, later, the availability of vitamin B_{12} allowed this victory to be repeated at will by any physician and the health of his patient to be sustained by monthly injections of amounts of cyanocobalamin averaging only a thousandth of a milligram a day—the most potent drug in the history of medicine.

Nevertheless, the availability of the remedy became a reality in practice only because industrial fermentations with molds and fungi, originally employed for the production of penicillin and other antibiotics, were adapted to the commercial production of cyanocobalamin. Remarkably enough, this came about in part as a result of a study of a wasting disease in sheep and cattle known as "bush sickness" or "pining" that develops in widely scattered areas of the globe. One such place was in South Australia, where the brilliant veterinary research work of Hedley Marston[60] and others at the University of Adelaide showed that a similar "coast disease" appeared in sheep pastured on land lacking in cobalt. After injection of cobalt failed to cure the disease, the natural fermentation of forage in the rumen (a specialized part of the stomach) of the sheep was shown to require cobalt to produce organic molecules with a central cobalt atom, such as vitamin B_{12}. In the absence of cobalt in the diet of the sheep, the disease could be cured experimentally by the injection of the vitamin or, in the practice commonly used today, by dosing the animal with a heavy cobalt pill and a gearlike steel "grinder" that remain in the rumen. Then, when activated by the digestive motions of the rumen, they together provide daily traces of cobalt.

It is now understood that the flesh or milk of ruminant animals is the ultimate source of vitamin B_{12} for all other animals, including humans. Today we know that in the pernicious anemia patient, the daily bacterial production of vitamin B_{12} in the colon, an organ distal to the absorptive area of the small bowel, would be sufficient (if only available) to prevent the disease! Not so silly the sheep, where first things come first, and so the vitamin produced in the rumen can subsequently be absorbed by the small intestine.

Following the isolation of vitamin B_{12} in 1948, a decade of chemical study by many investigators culminated in the resolution of the complete three-dimensional configuration of the cyanocobalamin molecule in 1956 and of the adenosyl cobalamin coenzyme in 1961. This was accomplished by the brilliant x-ray crystallographic work and exhaustive calculations of Dorothy C. Hodgkin's group[61] at Oxford University, for which she received the Nobel Prize in Chemistry in 1964. Similarly, many years of effort were required by the 1965 Nobel Laureate in Chemistry Robert B. Woodward,[62] of Harvard, working with Eschenmoser of Zürich and a host of collaborators to effect the total synthesis of vitamin B_{12} in 1973, another magnificent achievement.

Two New Vitamins and Their Shared Functions

In 1950, the preparation at the Merck Laboratories by Chaiet, Rosenblum, and Woodbury[63] of cyanocobalamin with a central radioactive cobalt atom provided a tracer for previously hidden biochemical pathways and greatly aided the search for the form, formation, and functions of vitamin B_{12}. Much of this information was now derived from studies of the metabolic activities of bacteria that require vitamin B_{12} for growth.

In 1958, the finding of an orange yellow cobalamin in the tetanus bacillus by H. A. Barker and his associates[64] at the University of California at Berkeley led quickly to the discovery of a related molecule that was biologically active in humans. In this vitamin B_{12} "coenzyme," the cyanide group of the usual therapeutic preparation was replaced by an adenosine moiety. About 1960, D. D. Woods' group[65] at Oxford and J. M. Buchanan's group[66] at the Massachusetts Institute of Technology independently concluded that in an unusual colon bacillus, a different coenzyme was metabolically involved. In 1962, Herbert and Zalusky,[67] working at the Thorndike Laboratory of the Boston

City Hospital, noted an increased level of the usual form of folic acid (subsequently identified as methyl tetrahydrofolate or methyl THF) in the blood serum of some patients with pernicious anemia; yet their serum vitamin B_{12} level was greatly diminished. They suggested that this "pile up" of methyl THF was due to its failure to be converted to methylene THF, as in the normal process. Methylene THF is a molecule uniquely essential for the subsequent fabrication of the "double helix" of DNA. In effect then, a deficiency of vitamin B_{12} "conditions" (sets up) a secondary defect in the metabolism of folic acid, whereas a deficiency of folic acid results more directly in a lack of the indispensable methylene THF. The conditioning defect in vitamin B_{12} metabolism is now known to be due to the lack of a second vitamin B_{12} coenzyme, methyl cobalamin, that functions as shown by Woods' group[68] in 1964 (Figure 10-4). This interpretation of the normal biochemical relationship between vitamin B_{12} and the folic acid derivatives and the effects of their respective deficiencies is fully consistent with recent studies of the altered metabolic activities of pernicious anemia bone marrow cells in vitro that were initiated by the Danish scientist S. A. Killmann[69] in the same year.

Modern molecular biology has shown us that DNA is an encyclopedia of the essential genetic information which is present in the nuclear chromosomes of all cells. However, each kind of body cell reads only the appropriate pages of three-letter "words" to find the directives for its growth and particular metabolic activities. For any cell to divide, it must at least double its nuclear

Figure 10-4 Essential biochemistry of vitamin B_{12}-folate interrelations with respect to DNA synthesis. Note that vitamin B_{12} is essential to the formation of tetrahydrofolate and, so, eventually of methylene tetrahydrofolate. (*From Waxman S, Metz J, Herbert V: J Clin Invest 48:485, 1969.*)

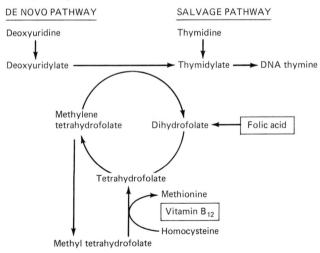

content of DNA, and, from the previous paragraph, it is apparent that a deficiency of either vitamin B_{12} or folic acid will delay or interfere with this doubling. The rapidly dividing cells of such organs as the bone marrow, the tongue, and the small intestine are the first to feel the pinch of this scarcity and, so, to develop the characteristic clinical signs and symptoms of these deficiencies. Under the microscope, the proliferating cells of these organs show the typical megaloblastic change.[70] This change, best seen in the erythropoietic cells of the bone marrow, represents a delay in the maturation of the nucleus relative to that of the cytoplasm.

The disclosure of the normal sequence of biochemical events in vitamin B_{12} and folic acid metabolism has clarified earlier confusing clinical observations. In 1945, Tom Spies,[71] of the University of Alabama at Birmingham, showed that large doses of folic acid caused a prompt blood-building response in pernicious anemia. Thus, it appeared for a time that the unknown factor lacking in pernicious anemia had been discovered. However, it was soon found that effective purified liver extracts contained little or no folic acid, and, as shown by Richard Vilter and his colleagues[72] at the University of Cincinnati in 1947, persistence in the treatment of pernicious anemia patients with only large doses of folic acid resulted in the development of the neurological signs that were characteristic of the untreated disease. With the demonstration by Marshall and Jandl[73] at the Thorndike Laboratory in 1960 that large doses of folic acid, much greater than the normal requirements for this vitamin, caused red cell responses in pernicious anemia, Spies' earlier work became comprehensible. A similar explanation presumably applies to the responses to large amounts of brewers yeast observed by Wintrobe[74] in 1939. Today, it is understood to indicate that in biochemical terms an excess of the folate substrate can sometimes partially compensate for a deficiency of the methyl cobalamin coenzyme and perhaps expose further a defect of the adenosyl cobalamin coenzyme function. Folic acid deficiency alone, although it causes a similar anemia, does not result in the neurological deficit. This clearly indicates that the neurological defect in vitamin B_{12} deficiency is not caused by a failure of the biochemical pathway that is normally shared with folic acid; instead a lack of the adenosyl cobalamin coenzyme may be involved. This coenzyme is essential for the final step of the fatty acid sequence from propionate through methylmalonate to succinate and might well be indirectly responsible for the integrity of the lipoid myelin sheaths of the nerves of the spinal cord. It is at least suggestive that E. P. Frankel[75] of Dallas has reported the finding of abnormal odd-numbered fatty acids in the myelin sheaths of the peripheral nerves of pernicious anemia patients.

Finally, the recognition of two biochemically different varieties of megaloblastic anemia and their different clinical presentations permits in retrospect an understanding of the probable nature of the anemia of some of the female patients reported by Biermer in 1872 as "progressiver perniciöser Anämie."

Thus, according to H. J. Huser,[22] Biermer's pupil H. Müller, using this title for his monograph, published the details of Biermer's original 15 patients in 1877. Ten were females, of whom six had been repeatedly pregnant. Müller confirmed the poor economic conditions that Biermer had mentioned and suggested that inadequate food was a possible cause of the anemia. Only one of Biermer's patients, a male aged 52, seems possibly to have had vitamin B_{12} deficiency. Instead, the clinical setting of the females, especially those who had been pregnant, bears a striking resemblance to that of the female patients studied by Wills and Evans[52] in India and now known to have suffered from a dietary deficiency of folic acid, which is recognized today as the most common vitamin deficiency of late pregnancy. There is a further semantic interest in the translation of the terminology, in which the name applied by Biermer to probable cases of folic acid deficiency crossed the English Channel to designate a condition described by Addison that was due instead to a deficiency of vitamin B_{12}.

Achylia Gastrica: Before, During, and After

Let us now leave the comfortable, although complex, knowledge of the present and return to the simpler but desperate uncertainties at the time Addison's anemia was first described. The disease was recognized, the patients died, and nobody knew why. Later, even the great debates of the morphologists were based on only more speculation. However, if the anemic patient described by J. S. Combe,[76] of Edinburgh, in 1824 was, as later believed by some, a case of pernicious anemia, he had correctly ascribed its cause to "some disorder of the digestive and assimilative organs." But as we shall see, it took more than 100 years for the accuracy of that surmise to be defined. In 1860, only 5 years after Addison's description, Austin Flint, Sr.,[77] a remarkable American physician and teacher, pointed the finger of suspicion at the stomach. Although in autopsies of a few patients with pernicious anemia, he had found no gross abnormalities of that organ, he was aware that Handfield Jones,[78] of England, had recently published an account of the microscopic examination of 100 human stomachs, in which he had found a considerable atrophy of the secretory glands in 14. Conscious of the unexpected revelations of the microscope in kidney disease, Flint[77] was led to remark in a lecture on anemia that such an important organ as the stomach might "undergo degenerative disease not rendered distinctly apparent to the naked eye." He further speculated "that [if] in these cases there exists degenerative disease of the glandular tubuli of the stomach . . . fatal anaemia must follow an amount of degenerative disease reducing the amount of gastric juice so far that assimilation of food is rendered wholly inadequate for the wants of the body." Here is a clear description of what later was called *achylia gastrica* and its consequences.

Ten years later, in 1870, Samuel Fenwick,[79] of the London Hospital, confirmed Flint's suspicion when he examined postmortem the mucosal lining of the stomach of a patient whom he considered to have died of Addison's "idiopathic anaemia." He saw with his microscope that the "glandular structure was in a state of atrophy." Scrapings of this withered lining to which hydrochloric acid had been added failed to digest hard-boiled white of egg, in contrast to the action of scrapings of normal gastric mucosa. Consequently, Fenwick concluded that "the progressive atrophy of the stomach had prevented the digestion of the albuminous material of the food." As we have seen above, during the exciting era of the discovery of bacterial disease, the time was not yet ripe for much attention to be given to these isolated promptings.

From the work of William Beaumont, United States Army doctor and pioneer physiologist, by 1822 it had become known that normal gastric juice contains hydrochloric acid. The first demonstration during life of a lack of such acid in the stomach was made by Cahn and von Mering[80] in Germany in 1886. In 1900, Faber and Bloch,[81] of Copenhagen, examined the gastric juice of 33 patients and found it to contain little or no acid. Thirteen of these patients had carried fish tapeworm in the intestine. In 1921, Levine and Ladd[82] completed a 6-year study of 150 pernicious anemia patients seen at the Peter Bent Brigham Hospital, in Boston. Using a flexible stomach tube of small diameter, they found no free hydrochloric acid in 99 percent of their patients after a test meal had been given to stimulate its secretion.

The idea fostered by such impressive evidence, that a lack of gastric acidity might play a causal role in pernicious anemia, owes much to Arthur Hurst, of Guy's Hospital, London. In 1901, William Hunter[5] had extensively documented his conviction that the anemia was the result of oral sepsis due to *Streptococcus longus* with a subsequent infection of the tongue, stomach, and intestine, where a hypothetical blood-destroying toxin was produced. Hunter had considered gastric anacidity to be an incidental result of the infection, whereas a quarter of a century later, Hurst[83] was convinced that an invariable *primary* failure of the antiseptic action of normal stomach acid permitted bacterial overgrowth in the small intestine of the pernicious anemia patient. The infection then produced "hemolytic and neurotoxic poisons." In further support of the primacy of gastric anacidity, Hurst emphasized that it was known to precede by a long period of time the development of the disease, to persist during its spontaneous remissions, and to be more common in the relatives of affected patients. Moreover, in a few instances, pernicious anemia had appeared after the surgical removal of the stomach as well as in patients with achlorhydria associated with cancer of the stomach.

These facts were known to William B. Castle, a young resident physician, who in 1927 was assisting Francis Peabody,[31] the first director of the recently established Thorndike Memorial Laboratory of the Boston City Hospital, in obtaining tibial bone marrow specimens from patients with pernicious anemia. The effectiveness of liver feeding that had been reported by Minot and

Murphy[47] the previous year relieved a desperate therapeutic need; it also suggested that in some way pernicious anemia might be a nutritional deficiency disease. The pertinent question which now arose was why normal persons did not need to eat half a pound of liver a day in order to stave off pernicious anemia. The promptness and regularity of the reticulocyte response induced by liver feeding seemed inconsistent with the idea that eating liver abolished intestinal sepsis. Was it possible that the stomach of the normal person could derive something from ordinary food that for him was equivalent to eating liver? Castle[84] wondered whether "by substituting some digestive process of the normal stomach . . . it might be possible to affect the patient's disease favorably." Although unknown to him at the time, this was in essence the same idea that Flint[77] and Fenwick[79] had expressed long before. But now there was a difference—the idea could be subjected to an experimental test. Castle had the advantage of knowing that the anemia was a potentially reversible condition and that a reticulocyte response would quickly indicate that the anemia was responding. In case of need, transfusions and liver extract were available.

The experimental procedure consisted of two consecutive periods of 10 days or more during which daily reticulocyte counts were made. During the first period of 10 days, the patient received 200 g of rare hamburg steak (lean beef muscle) daily as the only source of animal protein. There was no increase in the number of reticulocytes. Beef muscle was chosen because in 1925, C. Elders[85] had reported that a similar diet, useful in his experience in the treatment of sprue in Sumatra and especially rich in rare meat, had resulted in improvement in a case of pernicious anemia in Holland; naively, to Castle, meat seemed somewhat like liver. During the second period, the contents of the stomach of a healthy man were recovered daily 1 hour after the ingestion of 300 g of hamburg steak. (It was found that about 100 g of the beef muscle were not recovered.) The rest of the gastric contents was incubated for a few hours, until liquefied, and then administered on a daily basis to the anemic patient through a flexible stomach tube of small caliber. On the sixth day, a rise in the number of reticulocytes began, reached a peak on the tenth day, and then declined as an increase in the number of red cells in the patient's blood began and continued through a period of 30 days. These phenomena were similar in chronology and magnitude to those obtained for other pernicious anemia patients given moderate amounts of liver daily (Figure 10-5). So also was the improvement in the patient's sense of well-being. Similar observations on other patients were reported briefly in 1928 and more fully in 1929.[84] As a sideline experiment, other patients had similarly been tube-fed beef muscle digested by the acidified mucosal lining of the hog's stomach. There was no response; but shortly, Sturgis and Isaacs,[86] at the Simpson Memorial Institute at Ann Arbor, Michigan, found that desiccated and defatted hog stomach wall was therapeutically effective like liver, when eaten.

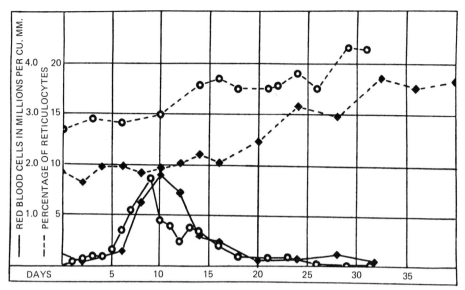

Figure 10-5 Erythropoietic effect in a case of pernicious anemia of the daily administration by flexible stomach tube of the contents of a normal human stomach recovered 1
hour after the ingestion of 300 g of beef muscle—reticulocytes (circles and solid lines)
and adult red cells (circles and broken lines). Note similar chronology and increases of
both cellular elements (diamonds) in another patient receiving daily a moderate amount
of liver. (*From Castle WB: Am J Med Sci 178:757, 1929.*)

The next question was whether the response observed with stomach
contents was due to the gastric juice alone or to its action on the beef muscle.
Similar observations on pernicious anemia patients showed that 150 cm³ of
human gastric juice given daily was, like 200 g of beef muscle, *ineffective unless
both were given together.* Thus, it was concluded that some essential interaction
was taking place between an unknown *intrinsic factor* in the gastric juice and an
unknown *extrinsic factor* in the beef muscle.[87] For the next 20 years, by means of
such laborious studies of reticulocyte responses or their absence in pernicious
anemia patients by Castle and his associates, as well as by others,[88–90] efforts
were made to determine the nature of each factor and the conditions essential
for their supposed interaction. The intrinsic factor (IF) was shown to be
secreted only by the human stomach. Like that of most enzymes, its activity
was readily destroyed by boiling, but it could not be identified with any known
enzyme. Moreover, no convincing evidence for the formation of a third factor
in the active digestion mixtures was obtained. Despite this, by analogy with
other known gastric functions, Castle clung to the mistaken idea of its existence.

The extrinsic factor was found to resist destruction by heat and to be
present in crude casein, eggs, and autolyzed yeast. As late as 1944, it could not

be identified with any of the known water-soluble vitamins, including a concentrate of folic acid. However, in 1948, shortly after the discovery that vitamin B_{12} was the anti-pernicious anemia "principle" of injectable purified liver extract,[57] Castle's associate Lionel Berk found that a small amount of such a liver extract became active when given by mouth with gastric juice. As a logical next step, he gave a small amount (5 μg) of vitamin B_{12} by mouth daily in a similar trial. This was without effect until given with gastric juice. Additional patients showed similar responses in work carried out in collaboration with Arnold Welch and his associates at Western Reserve University in Cleveland, Ohio.[91] Thus was established the nature of the extrinsic factor and its identity with the anti-pernicious anemia factor of liver extract, vitamin B_{12}. In retrospect, this conclusion was foreshadowed by the work of Helmer et al.[88] in 1933 when they showed that crude liver extract itself was a source of the extrinsic factor, but of course it could not be proved until the active principle in liver had been isolated.

The following year, 1949, Ternberg and Eakin,[92] at the University of Texas in Austin, showed that the addition of gastric juice to a culture of bacteria that require vitamin B_{12} for growth inhibited their multiplication. Prior heating of the gastric juice destroyed the inhibition. They proposed that this was due to a property of the gastric juice that interacted with the vitamin, was thermolabile, and had other properties similar to those of the intrinsic factor. Shortly afterward, it was confirmed that native intrinsic factor, as well as purified preparations thereof, possesses strong and specific "binding" capacity for vitamin B_{12}.

In 1956, Ralph Gräsbeck,[93] working in Helsinki, demonstrated with moist starch-block electrophoresis (in which the organic molecules migrate at different rates depending on their electric charge) that radioactive vitamin B_{12}, when added to human gastric juice, appeared in three separate peaks. Of these, the slowest moving was the one that was clinically active in pernicious anemia as intrinsic factor; the next was a degradation product of the first. The most rapid was inert as such but was subsequently identified as a transport protein for vitamin B_{12} in the bloodstream. In 1966, Gräsbeck and his associates[94] isolated the intrinsic factor from human gastric juice as a specific glycoprotein (i.e., protein molecule containing carbohydrate), of which 1 mg can bind about 30 μg of vitamin B_{12}. It is said that 40 liters of gastric juice yield only 8 mg of pure intrinsic factor! Meanwhile, taking advantage of its specific binding activity for radioactive vitamin B_{12}, P. J. Hoedemaeker,[95] working in Nieweg's laboratory in Groningen in Holland, showed by autoradiography that the parietal (acid-secreting) cells of the human stomach are the source of intrinsic factor.

Because 5 μg of vitamin B_{12} given daily by mouth with gastric juice were not as potent as 1 μg given by injection, it appeared that in some way the gastric juice merely facilitated the assimilation of vitamin B_{12} as such. In 1952,

Heinle, Welch, and their associates[96] at Western Reserve showed that when a tracer amount of radioactive vitamin B_{12} was given by mouth to a pernicious anemia patient, the simultaneous administration of gastric juice diminished its excretion in the feces (i.e., it increased its assimilation) over the next few days. The next year, Robert Schilling,[97] at the University of Wisconsin, improved the esthetics and convenience of the procedure by showing that gastric juice increased the assimilation of radioactive vitamin B_{12} as judged by its increased excretion in the next day's urine. Solubility studies indicated that the radioactivity was still present in the form of the intact vitamin. In 1957, Doscherholmen and Hagen,[98] at the University of Minnesota, using a more radioactive form of vitamin B_{12} that allowed its direct measurement in the blood, found that with a small tracer dose, the addition of intrinsic factor, as expected, enhanced its uptake in pernicious anemia; but that with a larger dose of 50 or 300 μg, absorption did not need the help of the intrinsic factor. This now explained the early success of liver feeding by Minot and Murphy.[2] In giving 240 g of liver a day, they had administered about 240 μg of vitamin B_{12}. That amount of the pure vitamin, even in the absence of the intrinsic factor in the pernicious anemia patient, was now shown to permit the passive assimilation of at least 2 μg of vitamin B_{12}, or more than twice the amount necessary for normal blood production. It thus appeared that the intrinsic factor is important only to assure the assimilation of enough of the small amount of vitamin B_{12} present in the usual diet of a normal person, i.e., perhaps only 2 to 5 μg a day.

Only after 1955 was it possible to apply experiments with laboratory animals to the details of vitamin B_{12} assimilation. In that year, Watson and Florey,[99] in Oxford, found that the surgical removal of the secretory portion of the rat stomach rendered the animal unable to assimilate tracer doses of radioactive vitamin B_{12} unless a source of rat intrinsic factor was given simultaneously. Shortly thereafter, H. O. Nieweg,[100] of Groningen, while working in Boston at the Thorndike Laboratory, demonstrated in gastrectomized rats enhancement of the uptake of radioactive vitamin B_{12} by isolated loops of intestine with intact blood supply perfused simultaneously in situ with rat intrinsic factor. The rapid disappearance of any residual native intrinsic factor was soon found to obviate the need for preliminary gastrectomy in devising even simpler systems for the study of intrinsic factor activity. Thus, rings and everted segments of rat, guinea pig,[101] or hamster intestine and even homogenates of rat[102] and human intestinal mucosa were so employed. The guinea pig intestine possessed the experimental advantage that, unlike that of the rat, it was responsive to human intrinsic factor. With tracer doses of radioactive vitamin B_{12} administered shortly before elective abdominal surgery, the site of its assimilation in humans by the distal small bowel was demonstrated by Booth and Mollin,[103] working in London.

It is notable that in 1971, P. P. Toskes et al.[104] began work which showed that a pancreatic enzyme (probably trypsin) normally serves as a "second

Table 10-3   *Phases of vitamin B$_{12}$ assimilation*

I	IF* competitively binds B$_{12}$ released from food, especially at acid pH values
II	IF-B$_{12}$ complex en route to ileum is resistant to pepsin, chymotrypsin, and parasites
III	IF-B$_{12}$ complex adheres to microvilli of distal ileal epithelial cells. Calcium ions, trypsin, and pH > 6.5 required
IV	Species-related release of B$_{12}$ to interior of ileal epithelial cells en route to blood

* IF = intrinsic factor.

intrinsic factor." As a result of numerous observations on animals and humans, a succinct description of the normal events in vitamin B$_{12}$ assimilation can be presented as in Table 10-3. Meanwhile, in addition to the effect caused by the surgical removal of the stomach and of various anomalies and diseases affecting the small bowel, rare congenital defects that involve intrinsic factor secretion in the stomach and of assimilation of vitamin B$_{12}$ in the distal small bowel have been described.

Striking is the modern revision of our understanding of the effects of parasitism of the intestine by the fish tapeworm or by bacterial overgrowth, at one time considered to be the sources of blood-destroying toxins in pernicious anemia. Today, the cause of their occasional mischief is understood to be successful local competition by the parasites for the available vitamin B$_{12}$ in the food, especially when, for some reason, gastric intrinsic factor is in short supply. Thus, in 1947 Bertel von Bonsdorff,[105] working in Helsinki, showed that anemic patients harboring the fish tapeworm may not respond to mixtures of beef muscle and gastric juice until the parasite has been eliminated. In 1951, vitamin B$_{12}$ was substituted for beef muscle with similar results, and in 1960, W. Nyberg[106] reported that the tapeworm in situ can absorb much of a tracer dose of radioactive vitamin B$_{12}$ whether the patient is anemic or not. In 1956, James Halstead and his associates[107] showed that in patients with various small bowel abnormalities, such as diverticula, partial obstruction, or a surgically created so-called blind loop, malabsorption of radioactive vitamin B$_{12}$ persisted until antibacterial therapy was applied. As R. M. Donaldson[108] has since shown experimentally, bacteria luxuriating in these piratical refuges can sally forth and seize vitamin B$_{12}$ in transit. Whether in cast-off segments of the tapeworm or in living bacteria, the vitamin is then carried in a packaged form beyond the site of its normal assimilation in the distal small bowel unless a vermifuge removes the tapeworm or an effective antibiotic kills the bacteria.[109]

Behind Gastritis

In Addisonian pernicious anemia, the villain of the piece is clearly the failure of gastric secretion. Microscopically perceived, there is atrophy of the secretory glands of the mucosal lining of the stomach, which is associated with an infiltration of white blood cells, including lymphocytes, plasma cells, and macrophages. A classical study at postmortem of the "gastritis" made by Magnus and Ungley[110] in Britain in 1938 showed that the process was largely confined to the main body of the stomach, where the parietal cells are found and which are now known to be the source both of hydrochloric acid and of intrinsic factor.[95] Cellular infiltration is eventually followed by glandular atrophy. This sequence was clarified when in 1949, the development of a stomach tube with a grasping mechanism activated by suction permitted Ian Wood and his associates[111] in Melbourne to carry out microscopic studies of small specimens of the gastric mucosa that were removed at intervals during life. Contrary to the earlier views of Hunter[5] and of others,[83] the gastritis did not seem to be the result of a visible invasion by bacteria and is now thought to be associated with some type of "autoimmunity."

The first intimation of this possibility came in 1958 when Michael Schwartz,[112] of Copenhagen, reported that the blood serum of certain patients with pernicious anemia who had become refractory to treatment with a refined preparation of hog stomach prevented the usual uptake of radioactive vitamin B_{12} when given by mouth with hog intrinsic factor. Confirmed by Keith Taylor[113] in Oxford the following year, but in patients who had never received hog stomach, the inhibitory effect was correctly ascribed to an antibody directed against human intrinsic factor as an antigen in an autoimmune reaction. Subsequent work by Roitt, Doniach, and Shapland[114] and others showed that there were two kinds of anti-intrinsic factor antibodies. One, found in almost 60 percent of pernicious anemia patients, *blocks* the binding of vitamin B_{12} by intrinsic factor in vitro. A second, found in about 30 percent of the patients, prevents the *binding* of the vitamin B_{12} intrinsic factor complex to the surface of the mucosal cells of specimens of small intestine in vitro. However, it was already suspected that unless such serum antibodies leak into the alimentary tract of the patient with pernicious anemia, they provide little or no antagonism to the assimilation of vitamin B_{12}.[115]

The idea of an autoimmune reaction as the cause of the gastritic process itself was strengthened by the study of Hashimoto's thyroiditis, in which a lymphoid infiltration of the thyroid gland leads to atrophy and to a failure of thyroid hormone secretion. In 1957, this condition was found by Deborah Doniach and her colleagues in England to be regularly associated with a serum antibody that was directed against the cytoplasm of the thyroid's secretory cells. Moreover, further suggesting a common cause for the more than coinci-

Table 10-4 *Autoantibodies in pernicious anemia and thyroiditis (patients and relatives)*

ANTIBODIES (IMMUNOFLUOR.)	PERNICIOUS ANEMIA		HASHIMOTO MYXEDEMA		HOSPITAL CONTROLS
	PTS.	RELS.	PTS.	RELS.	
Gastric parietal cytoplasm	89	36	32	20	2–16*
Thyroid acinar cytoplasm	55	50	87	46	0–15*

*Incidence increases with age; F > M
Source: Doniach D, Roitt IM, Taylor KB: *Br Med J* I: 1374–1379, 1963.

dental clinical association of thyroid atrophy and pernicious anemia was the finding of W. J. Irvine et al.[116] in 1962 and of Doniach's group[117] the following year that in pernicious anemia, about 30 percent of the patients have such an antibody in their serum and that a similar percentage of thyroiditis patients have an antibody that is directed against the parietal cells of their stomachs. The serum of 90 percent of the pernicious anemia patients contains the antiparietal cell antibody, and it is also found in 10 percent of normal elderly subjects and in somewhat greater numbers in patients with gastritis and iron deficiency as well as in Addison's other disease, adrenocortical atrophy.

Nevertheless, it is not easy to show that such serum antibodies, anti-intrinsic factor or antiparietal cell, although they combine with their target antigens, are injurious to the cells that contain them. Indeed, it is possible that the antibodies are the *result* rather than the *cause* of the gastritic process. However, in the course of experimental work during the past 10 years, an interest in so-called cellular as well as humoral immunity has grown, as will be discussed in Chapter 14. In the gastric mucosa, many antibody-producing lymphoid cells and macrophages are in close proximity to the parietal cells that are, in some way, injured. Perhaps this is a deceptive appearance of guilt by association, but it does resemble experimental examples of *delayed cellular immunity* in animals or humans. In this reaction, certain lymphocytes with a thymic gland origin or developmental influence are *transformed* in the test tube by antigens with which they have had a previous passing acquaintance. Again in vitro, in the presence of antigens to which they have previously been introduced, such lymphocytes produce not specific antibodies but, instead, molecules of a much smaller size collectively called *lymphokines.* Such molecules individually, or as a group, exhibit toxicity for tissue cells in vitro, activate other lymphocytes, or inhibit the normal amoeboid motion of macrophages, which are "helper" blood or tissue cells found in immune responses. The last of these effects is the easiest to measure. The measured quantity is the so-called migration inhibition factor, which is determined by the effect on guinea pig peritoneal macrophages.

An early indication of the possible importance of cellular immunity was reported by Tai and McGuigan[118] in 1969, when they found that the circulating lymphocytes of some patients with pernicious anemia became specifically transformed when exposed to gastric juice. In 1974, Chanarin and James,[119] of London University, found by one or the other of the tests just mentioned that all but 1 of 25 pernicious anemia patients exhibited cell-mediated immunity to human intrinsic factor. Especially suggestive of the possible role of cellular immunity was the occurrence of gastritis and pernicious anemia in an unusually young group of patients who lacked the ability to produce antibodies but retained their cell-mediated immunity intact. Ten such individuals were reported by J. J. Twomey and associates[120] in 1969. It has been proposed that, because of some undefined lack of resistance, a primary viral infection is not eliminated and that seemingly normal body cells are antigenically altered by its persistence. In theory, this would account for the gastritis by the misuse of a normally protective response in the form of a prolonged and perverted cellular immune reaction, a kind of biologic *auto-da-fé* for such presumed cellular heretics.

A Summing Up

The study of pernicious anemia over the past century and a quarter by men and women in many parts of the world has provided insight into much previously unknown. First, by shrewd clinical observation, physicians identified the problems, and later, with tools borrowed from microscopic anatomy, physiology, and biochemistry, they opened challenging new vistas to further exploration by many workers from those fields. It was fortunate that relief from the dreadful urgency of finding a cure came over 50 years ago. That dramatic discovery helped to convert hematology from a largely descriptive science to a dynamic one by providing impetus and initial guidance toward later achievements in clinic and laboratory. Eventually came the discovery of the two new vitamins—folic acid and vitamin B_{12}—of fundamental importance to cellular proliferation and metabolism. Their ready availability has greatly facilitated the prevention and treatment of the megaloblastic anemias, due to their respective deficiencies. Knowledge of the structure of folic acid has permitted chemists to synthesize the molecular modifications that are the inhibitors of the leukemic process (Chapter 15). The discovery of cobalt in the vitamin B_{12} molecule explained its essential role as a trace element in animal nutrition. The study of the clinical association between achylia gastrica and pernicious anemia has shown how and why the so-called intrinsic factor of normal gastric juice is essential to the efficient assimilation of vitamin B_{12} from the small amounts present in the normal diet. An analysis of the sequential steps concerned has stimulated further interest in other aspects of alimentary assimilation and has converted the theory of intestinal intoxication by parasites to the reality of their competition for nutrients in humans. The gastritis resulting in the failure of intrinsic factor secretion in pernicious anemia is now being considered as a manifestation of a chronic, cell-mediated, autoimmune reaction. The peculiar morphologic and staining characteristics of the red cell precursors in the bone marrow were involved in early histochemical studies concerning the cellular functions of the deoxyribo- and ribonucleic acids, the DNA and RNA, respectively, of nucleus and cytoplasm. These master molecules are of fundamental importance to modern molecular biology and its concern with the operations of genes, the chemistry of viruses, and the origins of cancer. Over the years, mistaken interpretations sometimes placed obstacles in the path of progress, but wherever the way was paved with reproducible experiments, confirmation or correction of their meaning again guided onward the advance of knowledge.

Bibliography

Castle WB: A century of curiosity about pernicious anemia. The Gordon Wilson Lecture. *Trans Am Clin Climatol Assoc* 73:54–80, 1961.

Babior BM (ed): *Cobalamin: Biochemistry and Pathophysiology.* New York, Wiley, 1975, 477 pp (Brief historical introduction).

Cornell BS: The etiology of pernicious anaemia: historical etiological conceptions. *Medicine* (Baltimore) 6:375–417, 1927.

Hunter W: *Severest Anaemias.* London, MacMillan, 1909, vol I, 226 pp (Bibliography 1822–1902).

Kass L: *Pernicious Anemia,* vol VII in Smith LH Jr (ed): *Major Problems in Internal Medicine.* Philadelphia, Saunders, 1976, 247 pp (Historical aspects, portraits, and personal communications).

Robb-Smith AHT: The advantages of false assumptions. Part III. *Oxford Med Sch Gaz* 2:53–75, 1950 (History of pernicious anemia).

Smith EL: *Vitamin B₁₂,* 3d ed. London, Methuen, 1965, 180 pp (Discovery of vitamin B_{12} and its biochemistry).

References

1 Cabot RC: Pernicious and secondary anaemia, chlorosis and leukemia, chap 15 in Osler W, McCrae T (eds): *Modern Medicine: Its Theory and Practice.* Philadelphia, Lea and Febiger, 1908, vol 4, 865 pp, pp 612–618, 636.

2 Minot GR, Murphy WP: Observations on patients with pernicious anemia partaking of a special diet. A. Clinical aspects. *Trans Assoc Am Physicians* 41:72–75, 1926.

3 Addison T: *On the Constitutional and Local Effects of Disease of the Suprarenal Capsules.* London, Samuel Highley, 1855, 43 pp.

4 Barclay AW: Death from anaemia. *Med Times Gaz (Lond)* 23:480–482, 1851.

5 Hunter W: *Pernicious Anaemia.* London, Charles Griffin, 1901, 464 pp.

6 Osler W, Gardner W: A case of progressive pernicious anemia (idiopathic of Addison). *Can Med Surg J* 5:385–404, 1876–1877.

7 Leichtenstern O: Ueber "progressive perniciöse Anämie bei Tabeskranken." *Dtsch Med Wochenschr* 10:849, 1884.

8 Lichtheim L: Zur Kenntniss der perniciösen Anämie. *Munch Med Wochenschr* 34:300, 1887.
9 Russell JSR, Batten FE, Collier J: Subacute combined degeneration of the spinal cord. *Brain* 23:39–110, 1900.
10 Hurst AF, Bell JR: The pathogenesis of subacute combined degeneration of the spinal cord, with special reference to its connection with Addison's (pernicious) anaemia, achlorhydria and intestinal infection. *Brain* 45:266–281, 1922.
11 Sörensen ST: Taellinger af Blodlegemer i 3 Tilfaelde af excessiv Oligocythaemi. *Hospitals Tidende* 1:513–21, 1874.
12 Quincke H: Weiterer Beobachtungen über perniciöse Anämie. *Dtsch Arch Klin Med* 20:1–31, 1877.
13 Eichhorst H: *Die Progresive Perniciöse Anämie.* Leipzig, von Veit, 1878, 386 pp.
14 Laache S: *Die Anämie.* Christiana (Oslo), Malling, 1883, 276 pp.
15 Hayem G: Des alterations anatomique du sang dans l'anémie, in *Congrés Périodiques Internat Sciences Med,* 5'me Session. Genève, M.M. Prévost et al., 1877, 895 pp, pp 211–217.
16 Ehrlich P: Üeber Regeneration und Degeneration rother Blutscheiben bei Anämien. *Berl Klin Wochenschr* 17:405, 1880.
17 Ehrlich P: Zur Physiologie und Pathologie der Blutscheiben. *Charité Ann* 10:136–146, 1885.
18 Smith T: On changes in the red blood corpuscles in the pernicious anaemia of Texas cattle fever. *Trans Assoc Am Physicians* 6:263–78, 1891.
19 Krumbhaar EB: Reticulosis—increased percentage of reticulated erythrocytes in the peripheral blood. *J Lab Clin Med* 8:11–18, 1922.
20 Vogel KM, McCurdy UF: Blood transfusion and regeneration in pernicious anemia. *Arch Intern Med* 12:707–722, 1913.
21 Lee RI, Minot GR, Vincent B: Splenectomy in pernicious anemia: studies on bone marrow stimulation. *JAMA* 67:719–723, 1916.
22 Huser H-J: A note on Biermer's anemia. *Med Clin North Am* 50:1611–1626, 1966.
23 Pernicious anaemia. A new disease. *Med Times Gaz (Lond)* 2:581–582, 1874.
24 Wilks S: Idiopathic anaemia. *Br Med J* 2:680, 1874.
25 Arneth J: *Diagnose und Therapie der Anämien.* Wurzburg, Stuber, 1907, 208 pp.
26 Pepper W: Progressive pernicious anemia or anematosis. *Am J Med Sci* 70:313–317, 1875.
27 Cohnheim J: Erkrankung des Knochenmarkes bei perniciöser Anämie. *Arch Pathol Anat Physiol Klin Med* 68:291–293, 1876.
28 Neumann E: Ueber das Verhalten des knochen markes bei progressiver perniciöser Anämie. *Berl Klin Wochenschr* 17:685–686, 1877.
29 Ehrlich P: Ueber einige Beobachtungen am anämishen Blut. *Berl Klin Wochenschr* 18:43, 1881.
30 Birkeland IW: "Bothriocephalus anemia," *Diphyllobothrium latum* and pernicious anemia. *Medicine* (Baltimore) 11:72, 87, 1932.
31 Peabody FW: The pathology of the bone marrow in pernicious anemia. *Am J Pathol* 3:179–202, 1927.
32 Arinkin MA: Die intravitale Untersuchungsmethodik des Knochenmarks. *Folia Haematol (Leipz)* 38:233–240, 1929.
33 Finch CA et al: Erythrokinetics in pernicious anemia. *Blood* 11:807–820, 1956.

34   Jedlicka V: Über die Lebertherapie und das Wesen der perniciöser Anämie. *Folia Haematol (Leipz)* 42:359–396, 1930.

35   Whipple GH: Pigment metabolism and regeneration of hemoglobin in the body. *Arch Intern Med* 29:711–731, 1922.

36   Eijkmann C: Eine Beri-Beri ähnliche Krankheit der Hühner. *Arch Pathol Anat* 148:523–532, 1897.

37   Grijns G: Over polyneuritis gallinarum. *Geneesk Tidjschr Ned-Ind* 41:3–110, 1901.

38   Funk C: The etiology of the deficiency diseases. *J State Med* 20:341–368, 1912.

39   Whipple GH, Robscheit-Robbins FS: Blood regeneration in severe anemia. II. Favorable influence of liver, heart and skeletal muscle in diet. *Am J Physiol* 72:408–418, 1925.

40   Fraser TR: Bone marrow in the treatment of pernicious anemia. *Br Med J* 1:1172–1174, 1894.

41   Barker LF, Sprunt TP: The treatment of some cases of so-called "pernicious anemia," a regimen that has been found helpful. *JAMA* 69:1919–1927, 1917.

42   Gibson RB, Howard CP: Metabolic studies in pernicious anemia. *Arch Intern Med* 32:1–16, 1923.

43   Rackemann FM: *The Inquisitive Physician. The Life and Times of George Richards Minot, AB, MD, DSc.* Cambridge, Harvard University Press, 1956, 288 pp.

44   Minot GR: The development of liver therapy in pernicious anaemia: a Nobel Lecture. *Lancet* 1:361–364, 1935.

45   Whipple GH, Robscheit-Robbins FS: I. Iron and its utilization in experimental anemia. *Am J Med Sci* 191:11–24, 1936.

46   Castle WB: Award of the Nobel Prize for the treatment of anemia. *Sci Month* 40:194–196, 1935.

47   Minot GR, Murphy WP: Treatment of pernicious anemia by a special diet. *JAMA* 87:470–476, 1926.

48   Minot GR, Cohn EJ, Murphy WP, Lawson HA: Treatment of pernicious anemia with liver extract: effects upon the production of immature and mature red cells. *Am J Med Sci* 175:599–622, 1928.

49   Gänsslen M: Ein hochwirksamer injizierbarer Leberextrakt. *Klin Wochenschr* 9:2099–2103, 1930.

50   Strauss MB, Taylor FHL, Castle WB: Intramuscular use of liver extract. Maximal responses of reticulocytes from daily intramuscular injection of extract derived from ten grams of liver. Preliminary communication. *JAMA* 97:313–314, 1931.

51   Ungley CC, Davidson LSP, Wayne EJ: The treatment of pernicious anaemia with Dakin and West's liver fraction (anahaemin). *Lancet* 1:349–354, 1936.

52   Wills L, Evans BDF: Tropical macrocytic anaemia: its relation to pernicious anaemia. *Lancet* 2:416–421, 1938.

53   Snell EE, Peterson WH: Growth factors for bacteria. X. Additional factors required by certain lactic acid bacteria. *J Bacteriol* 39:273–285, 1940.

54   Pfiffner JJ et al: Isolation of the antianemia factor (vitamin B_c) in crystalline form from liver. *Science* 97:404–405, 1943.

55   Stokstad ELR: Some properties of a growth factor for *Lactobacillus casei. J Biol Chem* 149:573–574, 1943.

56   Shorb MS: Unidentified growth factors for *Lactobacillus lactis* in refined liver extracts. *J Biol Chem* 169:455–456, 1947.

57 Rickes EL et al: Crystalline vitamin B_{12}. *Science* 107:396–397, 1948.
58 West R: Activity of vitamin B_{12} in Addisonian pernicious anemia. *Science* 107:398, 1948.
59 Smith EL, Parker LFJ: Purification of antipernicious anaemia factor. *Biochem J* 43:viii, 1948.
60 Marston HR: The cobalt story. *Med J Aust* 46:105–113, 1959.
61 Hodgkin DC et al: Structure of vitamin B_{12}. *Nature* 178:64–66, 1956.
62 Woodward RB: The total synthesis of vitamin B_{12}. *Pure Appl Chem* 33:145–177, 1973.
63 Chaiet L, Rosenblum C, Woodbury DL: Biosynthesis of radioactive vitamin B_{12} containing cobalt.[60] *Science* 111:601–602, 1950.
64 Barker HA, Weissbach H, Smyth DD: A coenzyme containing pseudovitamin B_{12}. *Proc Natl Acad Sci USA* 44:1093–1097, 1958.
65 Kisliuk RL, Woods DD: Interrelationships between folic acid and cobalamin in the synthesis of methionine by extracts of *Escherichia coli*. *Biochem J* 75:467–477, 1960.
66 Larrabee AR et al: A methylated derivative of tetrahydrofolate as an intermediate of methionine biosynthesis. *J Am Chem Soc* 83:4094–4095, 1961.
67 Herbert V, Zalusky R: Interrelations of vitamin B_{12} and folic acid metabolism: folic acid clearance studies. *J Clin Invest* 41:1263–1267, 1962.
68 Foster MA, Dilworth MJ, Woods DD: Cobalamin and the synthesis of methionine by *Escherichia coli*. *Nature* 201:39–42, 1964.
69 Killmann SA: Effect of deoxyuridine on incorporation of tritiated thymidine: difference between normoblasts and megaloblasts. *Acta Med Scand* 175:483–488, 1964.
70 Foroozan R, Trier JS: Mucosa of the small intestine in pernicious anemia. *N Engl J Med* 277:553–559, 1967.
71 Spies TD et al: Observations of the anti-anemic properties of synthetic folic acid. *South Med J* 38:707–709, 1945.
72 Vilter RW, Vilter CF, Hawkins R: Combined system disease and hematologic relapse occurring in persons with pernicious anemia treated with synthetic folic (pteroylglutamic) acid for a period of two years. *J Lab Clin Med* 32:1426–1427, 1947 (abstract).
73 Marshall RA, Jandl JH: Responses to "physiologic" doses of folic acid in the megaloblastic anemias. *Arch Intern Med* 105:352–360, 1960.
74 Wintrobe MM: The antianemic effect of yeast in pernicious anemia. *Am J Med Sci* 197:286–310, 1939.
75 Frankel EP: Abnormal fatty acid metabolism in peripheral nerves of patients with pernicious anemia. *J Clin Invest* 52:1237–1245, 1973.
76 Combe JS: History of a case of anaemia. *Trans Med Chir Soc Edinburgh* 1:194–203, 1824.
77 Flint A: A clinical lecture on anaemia. *Am Med Times* 1:181–186, 1860.
78 Jones EH: Observations of morbid changes in the mucous membrane of the stomach. *Trans Med Chir Soc Lond* 19:86–151, 1854.
79 Fenwick S: On atrophy of the stomach. *Lancet* 2:78–80, 1870.
80 Cahn A, Mering, J von: Die Säuren des gésunden und kranken Magens. *Dtsch Arch Klin Med* 39:233–253, 1886.
81 Faber K, Bloch CE: Ueber die pathologishen Veränderung am Digestionstractus bei der perniciösen Anämie und über die sogennante Darmatrophie. *Z Klin Med* 40:98–136, 1900.

82 Levine SA, Ladd WS: Pernicious anemia: a clinical study of one hundred and fifty consecutive cases with special reference to gastric acidity. *Bull Johns Hopkins Hosp* 32:254–266, 1921.

83 Hurst AF: Addison's (pernicious) anaemia and subacute combined degeneration of the spinal cord. *Br Med J* 1:93–100, 1924.

84 Castle WB: I. The effect of the administration to patients with pernicious anaemia of the contents of the normal human stomach after ingestion of beef muscle. *Am J Med Sci* 178:748–763, 1929.

85 Elders C: Tropical sprue and pernicious anaemia: aetiology and treatment. *Lancet* 1:75–77, 1925.

86 Sturgis CC, Isaacs R: Desiccated hog stomach in the treatment of pernicious anemia. *JAMA* 93:747–749, 1929.

87 Castle WB, Townsend WC, Heath CW: III. The nature of the reaction between normal human gastric juice and beef muscle leading to clinical improvement and increased blood formation similar to the effect of liver feeding. *Am J Med Sci* 180:305–335, 1930.

88 Helmer OM, Fouts PJ, Zerfas LG: Increased potency of liver extract by incubation with human gastric juice. *Proc Soc Exp Biol Med* 30:775–778, 1933.

89 Helmer OM, Fouts PJ: Fractionation studies on intrinsic factor in normal human gastric juice. *Am J Med Sci* 194:399–410, 1937.

90 Formijne P: Experiments on properties of extrinsic factor and on reaction of Castle. *Arch Intern Med* 66:1191–1214, 1940.

91 Berk L et al: X. Activity of vitamin B_{12} as food (extrinsic) factor. *N Engl J Med* 239:911–913, 1948.

92 Ternberg JL, Eakin RE: Erythein and apoerythein and their relation to the anti-pernicious anemia principle. *J Am Chem Soc* 71:3858, 1949.

93 Gräsbeck R: Studies on the vitamin B_{12} binding principle and other biocolloids of human gastric juice. *Acta Med Scand* 154(suppl. 314):1–87, 1956.

94 Gräsbeck R, Simons K, Sinkkonnen I: Isolation of intrinsic factor and its probable degradation product as their vitamin B_{12} complexes from human gastric juice. *Biochem Biophys Acta* 127:47–58, 1966.

95 Hoedemaeker PJ et al: Investigations about the site of production of Castle's gastric intrinsic factor. *Lab Invest* 13:1394–1399, 1964.

96 Heinle RW et al: Studies of excretion (and absorption) of Co^{60}-labelled vitamin B_{12} in pernicious anemia. *Trans Assoc Am Physicians* 65:214–222, 1952.

97 Schilling RF: II. The effect of gastric juice on the urinary excretion of radioactivity after the oral administration of radioactive vitamin B_{12}. *J Lab Clin Med* 42:860–866, 1953.

98 Doscherholmen A, Hagen PS: A dual mechanism of vitamin B_{12} plasma absorption. *J Clin Invest* 36:1551–1557, 1957.

99 Watson GM, Florey HW: The absorption of vitamin B_{12} in gastrectomized rats. *Br J Exp Pathol* 36:479–486, 1955.

100 Nieweg HO, Shen SC, Castle WB: Mechanism of intrinsic factor action in gastrectomized rat. *Proc Soc Exp Biol Med* 94:223–230, 1957.

101 Hines JD, Rosenberg A, Harris JW: Intrinsic factor-mediated radio-B_{12} uptake in sequential incubation studies using everted sacs of guinea pig small intestine. Evidence that IF is not absorbed into the intestinal cell. *Proc Soc Exp Biol Med* 129:653–658, 1968.

102 Herbert V, Castle WB: Divalent cation and pH dependence of rat intrinsic factor action in everted sacs and mucosal homogenates of rat small intestine. *J Clin Invest* 40:1978–1983, 1961.
103 Booth CC, Mollin DL: The site of absorption of vitamin B$_{12}$ in man. *Lancet* 1:18–21, 1959.
104 Toskes PP et al: Vitamin B$_{12}$ malabsorption in chronic pancreatic insufficiency. Studies suggesting the presence of a pancreatic intrinsic factor. *N Engl J Med* 284:627–632, 1971.
105 Bonsdorff B von: "Castle's test" in pernicious tapeworm anemia. *Acta Med Scand* 128(suppl 194):456–477, 1947.
106 Nyberg W: The influence of *Diphyllobothrium latum* on the vitamin B$_{12}$-intrinsic factor complex. I. *In vivo* studies with Schilling test technique. *Acta Med Scand* 167:185–187, 1960.
107 Halstead JA, Lewis PM, Gasster M: Absorption of radioactive vitamin B$_{12}$ in the syndrome of megaloblastic anemia associated with intestinal stricture or anastomosis. *Am J Med* 20:42–52, 1956.
108 Donaldson RM: Malabsorption of ^{60}Co-labelled cyanocobalamin in rats with intestinal diverticula. *Gastroenterology* 43:271–281, 1962.
109 Mollin DL, Booth CC, Baker SJ: The absorption of vitamin B$_{12}$ in control subjects, in Addisonian pernicious anaemia and in the malabsorption syndrome. *Br J Haematol* 3:412–428, 1957.
110 Magnus HA, Ungley CC: The gastric lesions in pernicious anaemia. *Lancet* 1:420–421, 1938.
111 Wood IJ: Gastric biopsy: report on fifty-five biopsies using a new flexible gastric biopsy tube. *Lancet* 1:18–21, 1949.
112 Schwartz M: Intrinsic factor-inhibiting substance in serum of orally treated patients with pernicious anaemia. *Lancet* 2:61–62, 1958.
113 Taylor KB: Inhibition of intrinsic factor by pernicious anaemia sera. *Lancet* 2:106–108, 1959.
114 Roitt IM, Doniach D, Shapland C: Intrinsic factor autoantibodies. *Lancet* 2:469–470, 1964.
115 Kaplan ME et al: Immunologic studies with intrinsic factor in man. *J Clin Invest* 42:368–382, 1963.
116 Irvine WJ et al: Immunological relationship between pernicious anaemia and thyroid diseases. *Br Med J* 2:454–456, 1962.
117 Doniach D, Roitt IM, Taylor KB: Autoimmune phenomena in pernicious anaemia. Serologic overlap with thyroiditis, thyrotoxicosis and systemic lupus erythematosus. *Br Med J* 1:1374–1379, 1963.
118 Tai C, McGuigan JE: Immunologic studies in pernicious anemia. *Blood* 34:63–71, 1969.
119 Chanarin I, James D: Humoral and cell-mediated intrinsic factor antibody in pernicious anaemia. *Lancet* 1:1078–1080, 1974.
120 Twomey JJ et al: The syndrome of immunoglobulin deficiency and pernicious anemia. *Am J Med* 47:340–350, 1969.

CHAPTER 11

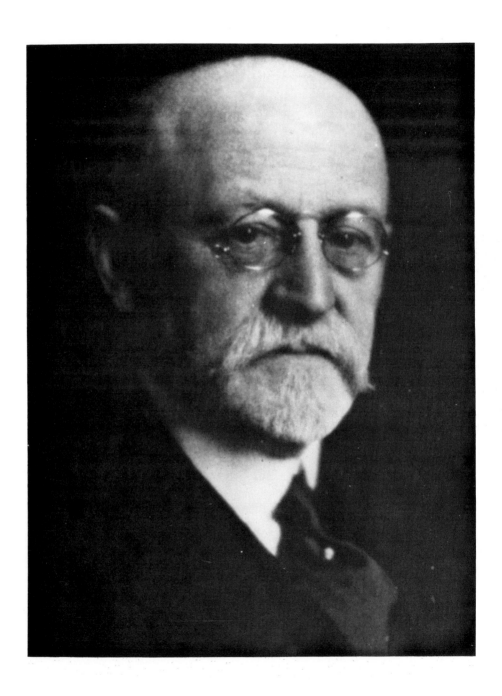

SICKLE-CELL ANEMIA—THE FIRST MOLECULAR DISEASE

C. Lockard Conley

Sickle-cell anemia is an inherited disease which occurs predominantly but not exclusively in black populations. Affected persons have unrelenting severe anemia with varying numbers of sickle-shaped red cells in the blood. Anemia often is well tolerated, although ability to engage in physical activity is limited. Pallor may be overlooked because of pigmentation of the skin, but the eyes usually appear yellow as a result of chronic jaundice. Large ulcers tend to occur on the lower legs and may recur or persist. Growth and development are retarded, and fertility is reduced. Victims of the illness are inordinately susceptible to serious infections, particularly during infancy. The "crises" that characterize the clinical course are manifested by recurrent episodes of agonizing pain in the extremities, the back, or the abdomen. Irreversible tissue damage in vital organs may lead to progressive disability and to premature death. Nevertheless, some patients are remarkably well between crises and during these times may be able to live in a virtually normal way. Almost all patients with sickle-cell anemia have a greatly shortened life span, many dying in infancy or childhood.

Much more frequent than sickle-cell anemia is the benign and clinically inapparent sickle-cell trait. Persons with that anomaly are perfectly well, without anemia or any of the manifestations of sickle-cell disease. However, their red cells can be made to assume the sickle shape under certain conditions in the laboratory. Sickle-cell trait invariably occurs in some members of the families of patients with sickle-cell anemia. It can be detected also in many persons not known to be related to patients with the disease.

Sickle cells have existed in human populations for perhaps thousands of years, often causing dramatic clinical symptoms and premature death. Felix I.D. Konotey-Ahulu, a Ghanian physician, reports that among West African tribes, specific vernacular names were assigned to clinical syndromes now identifiable as the sickle-cell diseases.[1] However, a written description of these disorders did not appear until 1910. Physicians who staffed clinics in Africa did not recognize sickle cells or sickle-cell anemia. The distorted cells went unnoticed in those hospitals in the United States in which numerous black patients were seen.

That the striking abnormality of the erythrocytes was undiscovered for so many years may seem surprising. "Crescentic" red cells had been described in the blood of several species of deer in 1840 by George Gulliver, Assistant Surgeon to the Royal Regiment of Horse Guards.[2] The misshapen erythrocytes

Chapter Opening Photo   James B. Herrick (1861–1954) in 1925.

319

are well illustrated in a woodcut in his initial report. Gulliver, who studied the blood in a number of species of animals in the London Zoological Gardens, observed that the crescent-shaped forms in the blood of deer increased in number after the blood was drawn and that the cells reverted to an oval or disc shape when a small amount of water was added. The eminent French hematologist Georges Hayem described many real and artifactual distortions of red cell shape.[3] His illustrations depict reniform and lunate erythrocytes; however, it is clear that he did not observe sickle cells. "Demi-lune" cells were observed in blood films of patients with malaria by Sergent and Sergent,[4] but the illustrations and descriptions of the cells and the conditions in which they were encountered indicate that they were artifacts. The long delay in recognizing sickle-cell anemia was largely the result of the primitive conditions of life, the prevalence of anemia caused by rampaging infectious and nutritional diseases, the inadequacy of medical care, and the premature deaths of affected persons in black populations, in which the disease occurs most frequently.[5] The varied manifestations of sickle-cell anemia, which often simulates other disorders, added to the difficulty of identification.[6]

Discovery of Sickle-cell Anemia

The discovery of human sickle cells and of sickle-cell anemia was announced in the form of a case report presented at the twenty-fifth annual meeting of the Association of American Physicians at the New Willard Hotel in Washington, D.C., on the morning of May 5, 1910.[7] The essayist was James B. Herrick, of Chicago (Chapter Opening Figure). The roster of physicians in attendance was a "who's who" of the eminent internists of that era, but there was no discussion of Herrick's paper. None of his distinguished colleagues recognized the unique disorder that he described. The full report, published in the *Archives of Internal Medicine* in 1910, provides a splendid account of many of the now well-known features of the disease.[8]

Actually the story had begun 6 years earlier, when Herrick examined a young black student from Granada, West Indies, who had entered one of the professional schools in Chicago. Herrick noted that the patient was anemic and observed in the blood film elongated and sickle-shaped red cells (Figure 11-1). After some simple tests, he suggested "that some change in the composition of the corpuscle itself may be the determining factor." The patient was seen on several occasions during the subsequent 3 years by Herrick and by Dr. E.E. Irons; their cumulative observations formed the basis for the report. Herrick could only speculate on the relationship between the abnormal red cells and the clinical disorder. As additional case reports slowly appeared over the following decades, the clinical pattern of sickle-cell anemia was firmly established.

What kind of person was Herrick, who saw what many others had failed

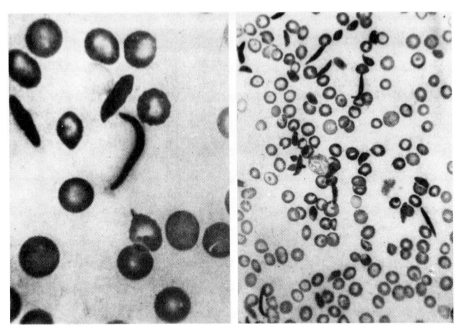

Figure 11-1 Blood films showing "peculiar elongated forms of the red corpuscles" in a case of severe anemia. (*Herrick JB: Arch Intern Med 6:517–521, 1910.*)

to see? A graduate of the University of Michigan, he had been a high school teacher of English before attending Rush Medical College. After internship, he engaged in general practice for 10 years before assuming the role of a consultant. Always a clinical teacher, he became a professor of medicine at his alma mater. He keenly felt the impact of advancing biological science and recognized the important role that chemistry was to have in medicine. In 1904, when he was 43 years old and a busy practitioner, he took courses in physical and organic chemistry at the University of Chicago. He traveled abroad to the laboratory of the Nobel Prize–winning chemist Emil Fischer, where he undertook a project and published a paper with Abderhalden.[9] Fischer's laboratory was humming with activity, and Herrick learned about proteins, polypeptides, and amino acids. He did not, thereafter, undertake laboratory research but was a scholarly and perceptive clinical observer, best known as the first to recognize and describe the clinical features of coronary thrombosis.[10] In 1930, the Association of American Physicians awarded Herrick the Kober Medal, one of the greatest honors that a physician can receive. In his statement of acceptance, Herrick said, "I am sure when the Council awarded me this medal they did it largely because they felt that I, in some way, represented the clinical side of medicine and they wished to put the stamp of approval on creditable work done by clinicians."[11] Herrick's last address before the Association of American Physicians, an after dinner talk at the annual meeting in 1931, was entitled, "Why I Read Chaucer at Seventy." Reflecting the literary interest that he had developed in his premedical days, he read Chaucer at seventy "because I read him at nineteen."[12] Herrick died in 1954. He lived long enough to witness some of the extraordinary developments that had evolved from the study of sickle-cell anemia, but he minimized his own contribution. In his autobiography, written in 1949, there is barely a passing reference to the disease.[13]

Herrick's report appeared in the November 1910 issue of the *Archives of Internal Medicine*.[8] At that time a 25-year-old black woman with anemia and abdominal pain was under observation in the medical ward of the University of Virginia Hospital. She had been admitted on prior occasions since 1907 for pain, leg ulcers, gall stones, and anemia. Blood films in 1909 had been described as containing "poikilocytes in a variety of shapes, the most common variety being of a crescent shape." Russell L. Haden, a student who later became an eminent hematologist, is reported to have taken a sample of the patient's blood to the Johns Hopkins Hospital, where an unusual type of pernicious anemia was suggested.[14] On reading the report of Herrick's case, R.E. Washburn, of the University of Virginia, recognized that the two patients had strikingly similar clinical manifestations and blood abnormalities. In an article in *The Virginia Medical Semi-monthly* in 1911, Washburn described the second case of sickle-cell anemia to be reported.[15]

Early Studies

Studies of sickle-cell anemia have had an enormous impact, initially more on biological science than on clinical medicine. It was the first disease in which every manifestation could be traced to a precisely identified submolecular abnormality, an abnormality that by inference could be explained by a specific alteration in the DNA itself. How was this incredible body of knowledge amassed? Who were the people who made the great discoveries?

The first experimental studies of sickle cells were performed by Victor E. Emmel, a Kansas farmer who became an anatomist.[16] Until he was 20 years old, Emmel toiled with his father on the land and had received virtually no formal schooling. Subsequently, making up for the deficiencies in his education, he obtained a Ph.D. degree in biology at Brown University. During a year at the Harvard Medical School as Austin Teaching Fellow in Anatomy, he came under the spell of Professor Charles Sedgwick Minot, who at that time was involved in a study of the genetic history of the blood. Professor Minot, a member of the distinguished Boston family that included George Richards Minot, of pernicious anemia fame, turned Emmel's interest to hematology. Emmel became a member of the faculty in anatomy at Washington University in St. Louis and was on the scene in 1915 when the first patient with sickle-cell anemia was recognized at that institution.[17]

The second decade of the twentieth century was the heyday of the pioneers of tissue culture. Given the blood of the patient with sickle-cell anemia, Emmel did what came naturally to an anatomist of that period.[18] He prepared a cell "culture." His technique was to seal a drop of blood between a sterile slide and cover slip using petrolatum. In his cultures, Emmel observed that sickling occurred in cells that previously had appeared to be normal (Figure 11-2). Using his method, the red cells of the patient's nonanemic father could be made to sickle, although sickle cells were not seen in the blood smear. Emmel had no idea why the erythrocytes sickled under the conditions of his experiments, but his technique became standard for detecting the sickling abnormality for many years thereafter. The sealed wet preparation was indispensable for the clinical investigations, population surveys, and genetic studies that were to be carried out by succeeding investigators. Emmel's method was used without modification for almost 30 years, when its reliability was improved by adding bacterial cultures or chemical reducing agents to blood to accelerate and enhance sickling.[19–21]

Interest in sickle-cell anemia was aroused slowly. Only three cases had been reported by 1922, when Verne R. Mason, resident physician at the Johns Hopkins Hospital, described the first patient recognized to have the disease at that institution.[22] Mason entitled his report "Sickle Cell Anemia," thus introducing the term that was to become the standard designation for the disorder. Attaching a name to a newly described disease is important in enhancing its recognition. Mason became an outstanding internist in Los Angeles, the personal physician of Howard Hughes, and a founder of the Howard Hughes Institute for Medical Research.

The first genetic study of sickling was reported by Guthrie and Huck in 1923.[23] They investigated the family of a patient with newly discovered sickle-cell anemia and found that the red cells of both parents and of a number

Figure 11-2 Film of the patient's fresh blood (left) compared with an 8-day culture prepared at the same time (right). (*Emmel VE: Arch Intern Med 20:586–589, 1917.*)

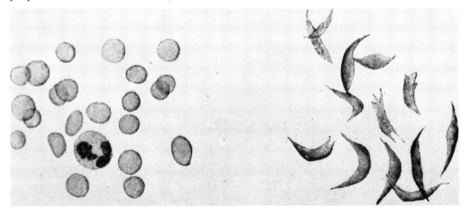

of other relatives could be made to sickle (Figure 11-3). Observations by Huck on that family and on another in which sickling occurred in three generations led to the conclusion that the sickle-cell condition is transmitted according to the Mendelian law for inheritance of a single factor, is dominant, and occurs in both sexes with equal frequency.[24,25] Huck did not differentiate sickle-cell anemia from the sickling that occurred in nonanemic persons, considering that the spectrum of the disease included severe, mild, and symptomless cases. He recognized that sickling was an intrinsic property of the red cells and not of the plasma and concluded that persons with sickle cells were heterozygous for the abnormal condition. Using Emmel's technique, he examined the blood of 100 blacks but found no sickling, although the preparations were observed for a week.

John Huck, a noted athlete during his college days, graduated from the Johns Hopkins University School of Medicine in 1918. His studies of sickle-cell anemia were performed while he was an instructor in medicine participating in the teaching of what was termed clinical microscopy. Later he served as

Figure 11-3   Distribution of sickle cells in the family of C.T., a patient with sickle-cell anemia. Blood groups are designated according to the Moss system. (*Guthrie CG, Huck JG: Bull Johns Hopkins Hosp 34:37–48, 1923.*)

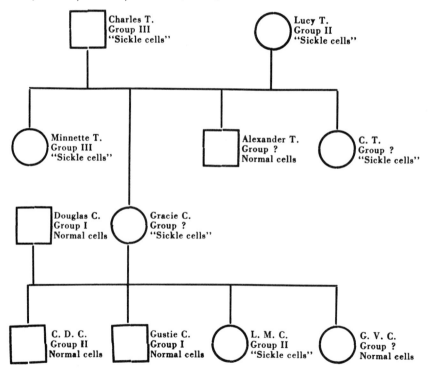

assistant professor at the University of Maryland School of Medicine and as physician to Hutzler Brothers Department Store in Baltimore.

The first student of sickle-cell anemia who had more than an ephemeral interest in the disease was Virgil P. Sydenstricker of Georgia. In the same year that Huck described his genetic studies, Sydenstricker and his associates reported a case of sickle-cell anemia in which both parents were observed to have "latent" sickling.[26] In an unrelated family, two brothers of a patient with sickle-cell anemia were found to have the disease. Later he wrote: "From personal observations it seems probable that children born of parents, both of whom show meniscocytosis,* develop sickle cell anemia more frequently than those born of one normal and one affected parent."[28] Sydenstricker carefully observed and recorded many of the clinical and hematologic features of the disorder.[26,29] He introduced the term *crisis* and was the first to suggest that the anemia is hemolytic. He reported the first autopsy, describing many of the typical lesions, including the scarred and atrophic spleen. He was the first to describe sickle-cell anemia in childhood, noting the peculiar susceptibility to infection and the high mortality. In a population survey of about 300 black persons, he discovered latent sickling in 13 but found none in a similar number of Caucasians. He reported that sickling of red cells is temperature dependent and inhibited by cold, an observation later to have importance in elucidating the nature of the sickling phenomenon.[30] His comments on treatment were astute. Observing that iron, arsenic, transfusions, and liver therapy had little effect on the blood, he pointed out, "In evaluating any method of treatment it must be borne in mind that the disease is characterized by remissions and relapses, and that patients without treatment have been observed to pass from a severe anemic state into one of relatively good health with disappearance of sickle cells from the blood."[28]

Sydenstricker received B.A. and M.A. degrees from Washington and Lee University and graduated from the Johns Hopkins University School of Medicine in 1915. He and his classmate Verne Mason helped to organize the Hopkins military medical unit that participated in World War I. His first paper, published when he was a medical student, was written with George Hoyt Whipple, who later was awarded the Nobel Prize for his contribution to the successful use of liver therapy in pernicious anemia.[31] Sydenstricker went to Georgia in 1919 as resident physician at the University Hospital in Augusta and in 1922, was appointed professor of medicine in the Medical College of Georgia, a position he held until his retirement in 1957. A persistent clinical investigator, he played a major role in the elimination of pellagra from the southern United States and received many distinguished awards. Sydenstricker maintained his interest in sickle-cell anemia throughout his life. In 1932, he noted that sickle-cell anemia had never been reported in a patient

*"Meniscocytosis"—a term proposed as a synonym for sickling by Graham and McCarty.[27]

over the age of 30, although sickling had been found in persons of all ages up to 78. His last paper on the subject, published in 1962, included a description of 10 patients with sickle-cell anemia who had lived past the age of 30, one of whom was still living at 59.[32] The outlook for patients with sickle-cell anemia had improved during his professional lifetime.

Mode of Inheritance

By 1923, tests for sickling had been performed on the blood of the parents of four patients who had sickle-cell anemia.[18,24,26] Six parents were tested, and all except one of them were positive, a remarkable observation since sickling was then thought to be a rare phenomenon. These and other genetic data available at the time might have suggested that sickle-cell anemia is the expression of the homozygous state of a gene that in the heterozygous state produces "latent" sickling. But Huck and Sydenstricker were not geneticists; in their era, heterozygous carriers of recessively transmitted diseases were thought to be phenotypically normal. More than 25 years passed before Neel[33] and Beet[34] independently concluded that sickle-cell anemia does represent homozygosity for the mutant gene. During the long interim, there was much confusion about the relationship between the anemia and the latent disorder. Sydenstricker, like Huck, believed that the "active" and the "latent" disease were merely different phases of a single process.

That the asymptomatic carriers of a serious blood disease may be detected by laboratory tests was reported in 1938 by Caminopetros, who examined members of the families of patients with Cooley's anemia.[35] Concluding that Cooley's anemia (thalassemia in later terminology) is a hereditary disease, probably transmitted as a recessive trait, he suggested that examination of the red cells for resistance to osmotic lysis could be used as a method to identify asymptomatic carriers within families. Indeed, thalassemia (Chapter 12) was the first inherited condition of any importance in which it seemed possible to detect carriers with a high degree of accuracy.[36] In 1946, Silvestroni and Bianco recognized that a person could derive the sickling abnormality from one parent and "constitutional microcytic anemia" from the other and, as a result, have a unique disease (sickle-thalassemia).[37] Neither they nor others who preceded them seem to have considered what condition would be produced if a person derived the gene for sickling from both parents. Neel apparently was the first to suggest the possibility that patients with sickle-cell anemia might be homozygous for the mutant gene, but in 1947, he was unable to establish the mode of inheritance of the disease even using the large volume of genetic data that had become available by that time.[38] We know now that the published data were replete with errors primarily because of the inaccuracy of the methods employed to detect sickling in many of the reported studies.

James V. Neel of the University of Michigan, a pioneer in the study of human genetics, was a zoologist before he became a physician. His sophisticated studies of heredity earned him numerous honors, including the Lasker Award and the National Medal of Science. In 1949, he reported that he had examined 42 parents of 29 patients with sickle-cell anemia using several methods with meticulous care to detect sickling. The red cells could be made to sickle in every parent tested![38] E.A. Beet, a medical officer of the Colonial Medical Service in Northern Rhodesia, had obtained and collated data on the frequency of sickling in several areas of Africa. His conclusion pertaining to the mode of inheritance of sickle-cell anemia was based on a single case—both parents of a patient with the disease had positive tests for sickling.[34] Beet had no more data than were available to Guthrie and Huck in 1923, but he was more knowledgeable in interpreting the facts. The mode of inheritance of sickle-cell anemia proposed by Neel and by Beet was confirmed almost simultaneously by the impressive studies of Pauling and his associates.[39]

Sickle-cell Anemia in Africa

The first case of sickle-cell anemia to be reported from Africa was described in 1925. The patient, a 10-year-old Arab boy, was admitted to the CMS Hospital in Omdurman with a febrile illness. On examination of the blood film for malarial parasites, Dr. Gwyndolen Hunton observed a remarkable and unfamiliar abnormality of the red cells; Dr. R.G. Archibald, director of the Wellcome Tropical Research Laboratory in Khartoum, was consulted. Neither Hunton nor Archibald had heard of sickle cells or sickle-cell anemia, but they subsequently discovered the published reports from the United States. After a year of observation, Archibald described the typical features of the disease in the patient.[40] Sickle-cell anemia in a black African was first reported from Ghana by Russell and Taylor in 1932.[41] At the African Hospital in Lagos, Smith recognized three cases at autopsy by the splenic and other characteristic lesions, although blood examinations had not been performed during life.[42] In 1934, he reported the autopsy findings on a patient with sickle-cell anemia in whom the diagnosis had been made before death.[43]

A survey to determine the frequency of sickle-cell trait in an African population was described in 1944 by R. Winston Evans, pathologist at the West African Military Hospital.[44] In a study of almost 600 native men of Gambia, the Gold Coast, Nigeria, and the Cameroons, he found approximately 20 percent to be affected. The sickling rate was about three times that reported from the United States. In East Africa, Beet obtained positive tests for sickling in 12.9 percent of 815 consecutive inpatients in the Balovale District of Northern Rhodesia. He reported a striking tribal difference in the prevalence of sickle-cell trait, the high frequencies being found on the east side of the Zambesi River.[45] By 1945, Trowell considered that sickle-cell anemia was probably one of the most common and least frequently diagnosed diseases in Africa.[46] In his own clinic in Uganda, no cases had been recognized before 1940, but 21 cases were seen within the first 6 months of 1944, when routine testing for sickling began.

The impression that sickle-cell anemia was rare in Africa, in contrast with its apparently greater prevalence in America, nevertheless persisted. The enigma was unresolved for years. Raper in 1950, again noting that sickle-cell trait was nearly three times as frequent in blacks in Central and West Africa as in those in America, cited evidence that sickle-cell *anemia* in Africa was much less common than in the United States.[47] To explain this discrepancy he suggested that "some factor, imported by marriage with white persons is especially liable to bring out the haemolytic aspect of the disease, while the anomaly remains a harmless one in the communities in which it originated." His concept that race crossing has untoward biologic effects has only recently been discarded.[48] In 1952, the apparent rarity of sickle-cell anemia in Africa led Lehmann to write: "I do not believe that in Uganda we could have overlooked sickle-cell anaemia present in all homozygous carriers of the trait. Even if they had died in early infancy, it would have been such a 'slaughter of the innocents' that it could not have escaped our attention."[49] But the paucity of recognized cases was indeed the result of the high infant mortality rate, as was shown in a remarkable study in Leopoldville by J. and C. Lambotte-Legrand.[50,51] They noted that by 1955, only two cases of sickle-cell anemia had been reported among adults in the Belgian Congo, although sickling occurred in about 25 percent of the black population. Identifying 300 infants with sickle-cell anemia, they demonstrated that of the 297 mothers tested, 294 gave positive tests for sickling (99 percent); of 277 fathers tested, 259 were positive (93.4 percent). Seventy-two of the 300 infants were known to be dead before the age of 1 year, 120 by the second year, and 144 or almost half by age 5. The rarity of adults with sickle-cell anemia in Africa was extensively documented by several groups of investigators.[52]

As late as 1970, probably half of all children with sickle-cell anemia in Zambia died before age 3,[53] and in Rhodesia, only 3 of 31 patients known to have the disease were over the age of 10.[54] Trowell and his associates in Uganda observed that patients who survived to adolescence came from the higher social groups and suggested that general infantile mortality in different countries might, in part, explain differences in the lethality of sickle-cell anemia.[6] The standard of living, the prevalence of infection, nutritional deficiency, and the level of general health care appear to be the principal factors affecting the virulence of sickle-cell anemia in young children. Folate deficiency was shown to be relatively common among patients with sickle-cell anemia in Africa, contributing to the morbidity and the mortality of the disease.[55] Where improved health care became available, the course of the disease was altered. By 1971, at the Sickle Cell-Haemoglobinopathy Clinic of the University of Ghana, 50 percent of the patients with sickle-cell anemia lived past the age of 10.[56]

Geographic Distribution and Gene Frequency

By 1950, the prevalence of sickling in black populations in various parts of the United States had been well established.[14] Numerous surveys in Central and South America revealed that the frequency of sickling varied, but the occurrence of the gene could be accounted for by the influx of blacks from Africa.[57]

In Africa, surveys to ascertain the distribution and frequency of sickling were performed by many investigators after World War II.[14,52,57–61] More than 20 percent of the individuals in certain populations across a broad belt of tropical Africa were found to be carriers of the sickle-cell trait. High frequencies were discovered in some areas of Sicily, southern Italy, Greece, Turkey, Arabia, and South India. In contrast, sickling was virtually absent in a large segment of the world extending from Northern Europe to Australia. These observations led to speculations on where the mutant gene had had its origin and how such high frequencies of a deleterious gene were maintained.

Spread of the gene appears to have occurred in contiguous populations. Whether the mutation appeared on multiple occasions is unknown, but the present day distribution of sickling throughout the world can be explained on the basis of a single event. H. Lehmann, who became deeply interested in the implications of the accumulating data, presented evidence that sickling may have had its origin in neolithic times in Arabia, the gene then being distributed by migrations eastward to India and westward to Africa. The archaeologic and anthropologic evidence to support his belief is summarized in a colorful fashion in a book entitled *Man's Hemoglobins*.[62]

Hermann Lehmann was born in Germany in 1910 and received his early education in Dresden. In his youth, he won a prize for accomplishment in the study of ancient history, an interest that influenced his later career. After studies in several German universities, he attended the University of Basel, where he was awarded the M.B. degree. His scientific training began in the department of Otto Meyerhof, where he studied phosphorylating enzymes. Because of difficulties under the Nazi regime, he moved to Cambridge, where he received the Ph.D. degree in 1938. He maintained his interest in phosphorylation and glucose metabolism but, in addition, he worked for a time with Robert Hill on the metabolism of chlorophyll and the association in plants between chlorophyll and iron concentration. After joining the British Army, he was sent to India as a general duty officer. Because of his experience in the measurement of iron, he was assigned to a study of iron-deficiency anemia, his introduction to hematology. After the war, he was transferred to Uganda to investigate hypochromic anemia caused by hookworm infestation. While there, he became acquainted with the sickling phenomenon, established that the sickle-cell trait was widely distributed, and observed a differing frequency of sickling among tribes. Those observations led to a broad search for sickling in eastern Africa and to the recognition of a tribal association of the sickle-cell trait.[63] During all of these studies he encountered only two children with sickle-cell anemia in Africa.

Later, Lehmann joined the department of pathology at St. Bartholomew's Hospital in London as a chemical pathologist. In a very small section of the laboratory, he performed electrophoretic and other studies of hemoglobin, soon becoming a prolific investigator in the rapidly developing field of abnormal hemoglobins. He established and maintained contacts with physicians and investigators in many parts of the world, collaborating in the discovery and descriptions of new hemoglobins and acquiring unparalleled expertise. He headed the Medical Research Council Abnormal Hemoglobin Research Unit at St. Bartholomew's Hospital and, in 1963, transferred the Unit to Cambridge, where his prodigious research output continued past his retirement in 1977. In 1963, the Royal Anthropological Institute awarded Lehmann the Rivers Medal for his contributions to anthropology. He had received the Sc.D. degree from the University of Cambridge in 1957. A tireless and scholarly student of hemoglobin, he maintained his broad interests and his far-flung contacts. He taught and assisted many who initiated studies of hemoglobin in the underdeveloped areas of the world. In Cambridge, his proximity to M.F. Perutz fostered productive collaboration, especially in the study of the "molecular pathology" of hemoglobin.[64] By his many original papers and reviews, Lehmann made it possible for other investigators to keep abreast of a rapidly expanding field, one in which he was able to maintain a remarkable degree of virtuosity.

Sickle-cell Trait—A Balanced Polymorphism

Much interest centered on the cause of the high frequency of the sickle gene in some areas of Africa. In his report on sickling in hospitalized patients in Northern Rhodesia in 1946, Beet noted without comment that only 9.8 percent of the sicklers had malaria, whereas 15.3 percent of the nonsicklers were affected.[45] P. Brain, of Southern Rhodesia, wrote a brief letter to the *British Medical Journal* in 1952, in which he suggested that "red cells in sicklers offer a less favourable environment for malarial parasites."[65] J.P. Mackey and F. Vivarelli, of Dar es Salaam, in another letter to the *British Medical Journal* in 1954, considered that "the survival value may lie in there being some advantage to the heterozygous sickle-cell trait individual in respect of decreased susceptibility of a proportion of his red cells to parasitization by *P. falciparum*." They further suggested that sickle-cell hemoglobin may not be suitable for the parasite or that the life cycle of the parasite may be interrupted by sickling and by the premature destruction of the parasitized red cell.[66]

A thorough study of the relationship between the sickle-cell trait and falciparum malaria was reported by A.C. Allison in 1954.[59,67] He noted that the heterozygote (sickle-cell trait) frequency was as high as 40 percent in some African tribes and, therefore, a high homozygote (sickle-cell anemia) frequency would be expected. If there were no selective advantage of the sickling gene, elimination of the gene should be remarkably rapid since most homozygotes die without reproducing. To balance that loss, a mutation rate in some tribes would be required that is about 1000 times other estimations of mutation rates in humans. Deciding that an increased mutation rate could not account for the high but varying frequencies of the sickle-cell trait in Africa, he proposed that the occurrence of sickle-cell trait is a true polymorphism, maintained by a selective advantage conferred upon the heterozygote. On comparing the distribution of falciparum malaria and sickling, he found that high frequencies of the sickle-cell trait were invariably found in those populations who suffered from hyperendemic malaria. He presented evidence that individuals with the sickle-cell trait suffer from malaria less frequently and less severely than other persons. Allison concluded that in areas where malaria is hyperendemic, children with sickle-cell trait have an advantage in survival.[68] How protection is conferred by the sickle-cell trait has not been fully established. Some of the possibilities have been discussed by Power.[69] Malaria has increased where agriculture has been developed, and the interplay of malaria, agriculture, and sickling on the destiny of populations is of considerable anthropologic interest.[70]

Anthony C. Allison, an astute scientist with broad biological interests, was born in 1925 and received medical and D. Phil. degrees from the University of Oxford. His scientific training was in biochemistry and genetics, and the subject of his predoctoral research was polymorphisms in animals. In that work, he was closely associated with E.B. Ford, whose definition of polymorphism has become a genetic byword: "Polymorphism may be defined as the occurrence together in the same habitat of two or more discontinuous forms of a species in such proportions that the rarest of them cannot be maintained merely by recurrent mutation.[70a] Allison began his studies of sickling when he was Staines Research Fellow of Exeter College in the clinical pathology laboratory of the Radcliffe Infirmary at Oxford. He traveled to Kenya to determine the prevalence of sickling and found that rates were high near the sea and around Lake Victoria, where malaria was hyperendemic, and much lower in the highlands. He then proceeded to compare the rates of sickling and of falciparum malaria in other parts of Africa, thereby providing the evidence for their close association. Allison also performed important studies of the sickling phenomenon, describing factors that inhibit or enhance the reaction.[71] Later, he became Head, Cell Pathology Division, Clinical Research Center of the Medical Research Council in London.

Dependence of Sickling
on the State of Oxygenation
of the Hemoglobin

One of the great milestones in the evolution of knowledge about sickle-cell anemia was the key discovery by Hahn and Gillespie, reported in 1927, that sickling of the red cells occurs when the hemoglobin is deoxygenated.[72] Observing a suspension of red cells from a patient with sickle-cell anemia, Hahn fortuitously noted that many sickled forms appeared at the bottom of the tube. After agitation of the suspension, sickled cells were no longer seen. That simple observation suggested a possible role for oxygen in the sickling phenomenon. Hahn and Gillespie then performed beautifully designed experiments that clearly showed that the sickling deformation is related to the state of oxygenation of the hemoglobin, determined by oxygen tension and pH. Under the conditions of their experiments, red cells sickled when oxygen tension was reduced to about 45 mmHg. Carbon monoxide was as effective as oxygen in restoring the discoid form. They found that red cell ghosts (red cells devoid of hemoglobin) do not sickle, an observation consistent with their hypothesis that the change of shape is concerned with the hemoglobin. Thus, the hemoglobin was implicated in sickle-cell anemia 22 years before Pauling and his associates established its role beyond question. Hahn and Gillespie concluded, "It is reasonable to suppose that sickle cells are formed in the body of an affected person wherever the oxygen tension and hydrogen ion concentration are such as to render the distorted form of the corpuscles stable. It is also probable that a condition of general anoxemia would induce the formation of sickle cells in vivo." They preferred the term *sickle-cell trait* to *latent sickle-cell anemia* because some individuals live long lives without ever developing anemia. Hahn observed an important difference between persons with the sickle-cell trait and patients with sickle-cell anemia when he noted that ". . . in the non-anemic, sickle cells in considerable numbers do not occur preformed in the circulating blood, whereas in the anemic they do."[73] But using his relatively crude method, he was unable to demonstrate a difference between the cells in vitro.

E. Vernon Hahn, a graduate of the University of Indiana School of Medicine, was a young surgeon at the time of his study. His experiments were performed with homemade equipment (Figure 11-4) in the laboratory of surgical pathology of the medical school in Indianapolis, where a 4-year-old child with sickle-cell anemia was under observation. A huge spleen was removed after the diagnosis had been established, the first reported instance of splenectomy for sickle-cell anemia. Dr. Elizabeth B. Gillespie, later a general practitioner in Cincinnati, was an intern at the time and assisted in the laboratory work. Hahn subsequently became a neurosurgeon and psychiatrist. He was chief of neurological surgery at Indianapolis General Hospital, clinical

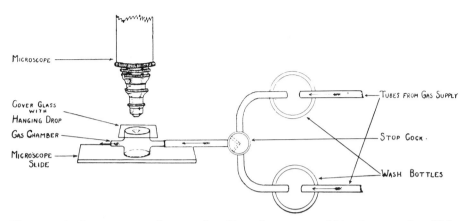

Figure 11-4 Apparatus used to test the effect of gases on red blood corpuscles. (*Hahn EV, Gillespie EB: Arch Intern Med 39:233–254, 1927.*)

professor of psychiatry at the University of Indiana, president of the local medical society, and a leader in the medical community. None of his other accomplishments are likely to have the lasting significance of his brief exploration of sickle-cell anemia.

Significant new observations were described in 1930 by Scriver and Waugh, of McGill University, following the study of a 7-year-old black girl, the first case of sickle-cell anemia to be reported from Canada.[74] Confirming the report of Hahn and Gillespie, they found that the patient's red cells showed a definite increase in sickling when oxygen tension was reduced to 40 to 45 mmHg. Increased sickling occurred in venous blood in vivo when anoxemia was produced by application of a tourniquet to the arm. The oxygen dissociation curve of the blood of their patient was shifted to the right, "as seen in other anemias," an aberration that they thought was probably dependent on pH. They recognized that the result was greater ease of release of oxygen to the tissues. That the oxygen affinity of the blood is low in sickle-cell anemia was later confirmed by other investigators and has been attributed in part to elevated levels of 2,3-diphosphoglycerate and to aggregation of sickle hemoglobin molecules at the high concentration in which they occur in red cells.[75,76] Scriver and Waugh attempted to make dry smears from sealed wet preparations of blood but found that there was immediate unsickling of most of the cells. Some erythrocytes retained the sickle shape, suggesting that "they represent the original sickle cells and are of a more resistant character." "Irreversibly sickled cells" were later observed by Diggs and Bibb[77] and were extensively studied by subsequent investigators, who showed that permanently deformed cells could be produced in sickle cell blood in vitro by prolonged deoxygenation,[78] that they are formed preferentially in red cells containing low concentrations of fetal hemoglobin,[79] and that they are associated with permanent membrane damage[80] with an excessive accumulation of membrane calcium probably "fixing" the membrane in the sickled shape.[81]

Pathology and Pathophysiology

The discovery of the conditions that cause red cells to assume the sickle form was an indispensable step in the comprehension of sickle-cell disease, but there was no possibility of understanding the mechanisms involved until the clinical disorder had been delineated and the pathologic lesions adequately described and interpreted. In that area, L.W. Diggs, of Memphis, was the uncontested leader. In 1932, he performed a large number of sickling tests on blood obtained from patients with sickle-cell anemia and from apparently healthy persons with *sicklemia* (sickle-cell trait).[82] The rate of sickling was variable and the results of a single test unreliable. On the average, however, sickling occurred more rapidly and in a higher proportion of the red cells in blood from anemic patients. In the following year, Diggs and his associates reported on a meticulous study of sickling in over 3000 blacks.[83] The sickle-cell trait was demonstrated in 8.3 percent of the 2539 individuals tested in Memphis, a higher prevalence than had been reported by earlier investigators but very similar to that obtained years later by others using more reliable methods. A low frequency of sickling was encountered in newborn infants, in whose blood sickling was less marked and less rapid than in that of older persons. After the newborn period, the incidence of sickling was not significantly related to age or state of health. Diggs and his coworkers observed that the sickle-cell trait was compatible with long life and was not associated with an increased frequency of leg ulcers or other abnormalities. They showed that the distribution of hemoglobin levels of the blood of children with the trait was virtually identical with that of children whose red cells did not sickle. Their mathematically precise comparisons established beyond doubt that the sickle-cell trait is benign and quite distinct from sickle-cell anemia. On the basis of their experience, they computed the ratio of sickle-cell anemia patients to sickle trait carriers to be 1:40. Had their knowledge of genetics been more sophisticated, they would have recognized how close this figure approximates the expected homozygote/heterozygote ratio.

At a meeting of the Southern Medical Association in 1933, Diggs presented a remarkably complete description of the lesions seen at autopsy in a large group of patients with sickle-cell anemia.[84] The report reveals the clarity and accuracy of his observations and interpretations and his concern with pathophysiologic mechanisms. He stated:

> A possible explanation of the capillary engorgement is that the elongated and spiked cells interlock and pass with more difficulty through narrow spaces than do normal cells. . . . Experimental confirmation of this tendency to mat together is

found in the test tube, where difficulty of resuspension of centrifugalized blood is encountered. . . . Since the distortion is increased under conditions of anoxemia, it is reasonable to assume that it will be greatest in tissue where there is stasis. . . . The sudden pains experienced by patients with sickle cell anemia, which often disappear as mysteriously as they come, may in part be explained by this capillary blockade.

These concepts were further developed in a report in 1939 dealing with the character of the erythrocytes in sickle-cell anemia.[77] His hand-drawn illustrations of the sickling process (Figure 11-5) showed a spicular arrangement of the hemoglobin in what he called "foci of hemoglobin condensation." By agitating blood with glass beads, he demonstrated the increased mechanical fragility of sickled red cells, a property believed by subsequent investigators[85] to account for the intravascular destruction of some erythrocytes in patients with sickle-cell anemia. Again he wrote: "It is possible that the abnormal shape of the cells and their great length interfere with the free circulation of blood and is a factor

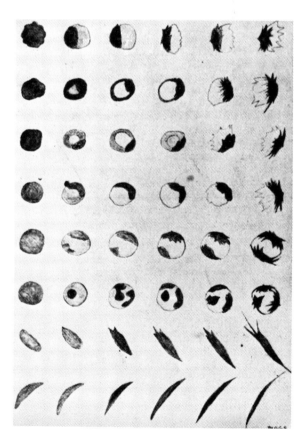

Figure 11-5 Hand-drawn illustrations of the sickling phenomenon. (*Diggs LW, Bibb J: JAMA 112:695–701, 1939.*)

in the production of thrombosis, which is a common feature of this disease." In a series of reports during a lengthy professional lifetime, Diggs described in detail many of the clinical, hematologic, and pathologic features of the sickling disorders.

Lemuel Whitley Diggs (1900–) earned an M.A. at Randolph Macon College, where he was an instructor in English for a short time, and graduated from the Johns Hopkins University School of Medicine in 1926. Always interested in art, he studied briefly with Max Broedel. During the medical school course in clinical microscopy, he learned about sickle-cell anemia from John Huck, an inspiring teacher. At that time, Diggs made his first drawings of sickle cells. He went on to the University of Rochester for internship and residency training in internal medicine, a member of the first group of house officers in that newly established institution. There he came under the influence of George Hoyt Whipple, participated in the ongoing studies of thalassemia and pernicious anemia, and taught the first course in clinical pathology at the medical school. In 1929, Diggs moved to the department of pathology of the University of Tennessee in Memphis. He served as director of the clinical laboratories and again taught clinical pathology to medical students. His intention had been to investigate the effects of nutritional deficiencies on the blood, but, almost immediately, he encountered patients with sickle-cell anemia; he examined their blood and studied the lesions at autopsy. He was so fascinated by the disease that it became his principal interest during the next five decades. Diggs joined the department of medicine in 1936 as the only full-time member of the clinical staff and subsequently rose to the rank of professor. His dual expertise as clinician and pathologist facilitated his many contributions to our understanding of sickle-cell anemia. As director of the Sickle Cell Center at the University of Tennessee, he extended his vigorous academic career long past the usual retirement age. At the time that Diggs began his studies of sickle-cell anemia, little research was being conducted in Memphis, and facilities and resources were limited. That he accomplished so much is a reflection of his enthusiasm and energy combined with imagination, independence, and determination.

Many of the links in the chain of developing knowledge about sickle-cell anemia were contributed by persons who had only a passing interest in the disease. Such is the case with Irving J. Sherman, whose single published report on the subject appeared in 1940.[86] Sherman, attempting to determine whether red cells are sickled in the blood stream, drew blood in such a way as to preclude exposure to air and introduced it immediately into a solution of formalin-saline. Beck and Hertz,[87] modifying a technique of Hahn,[73] had demonstrated that a solution of 10% formalin made isotonic with sodium chloride fixes cells in the shape in which they exist at the time. Sherman observed that between 30 and 60 percent of the red cells were sickled in the venous blood of patients with sickle-cell anemia, but virtually none in the blood of persons with the sickle-cell trait. He concluded, "This method thus provides a quick and simple diagnostic test for sickle cell anemia, differentiating it from sickle cell trait, which has no apparent clinical significance."[86] Arterial blood from patients with sickle-cell anemia contained only 5 to 20 percent sickle cells, and even these appeared "incompletely sickled." Interpreting this observation, Sherman wrote: "In sickle cell anemia the finding of much less extensive sickling in the arterial circulation than in the venous circulation indicates that a cyclic morphologic change occurs in a large percentage of the erythrocytes with each passage through the systemic and pulmonary circulation. If this constantly changing morphology decreases the life span of the erythrocytes it could of itself cause a hemolytic anemia such as we find in these patients." That the sickling-unsickling cycle does, in fact, damage red cells was demonstrated years later.[88] Sherman confirmed the role of deoxygenation in the sickling process, and he was able to show convincingly for the first time that the red cells of patients with sickle-cell anemia differ from those of persons with sickle-cell trait. Using a vacuum apparatus, he demonstrated that a much lower pressure is required to produce sickling in sickle trait cells than in sickle-cell anemia cells. At an air pressure of 50 mmHg, sickling appeared regularly in the blood of patients with the anemia but did not occur in the blood of persons with the trait (Figure 11-6). He emphasized the significance of his observations, which "probably explain why sickling occurs in vivo in patients with sickle cell anemia but not in patients with sickle cell trait." That there is a difference between the red cells of persons with sickle-cell trait and sickle-cell anemia was abundantly confirmed by others.[89] The survival time of transfused cells was shown to be normal for sickle-cell

Figure 11-6 Production of sickling by reduced atmospheric pressure. (*Sherman IJ: Bull Johns Hopkins Hosp 67:309–324, 1940.*)

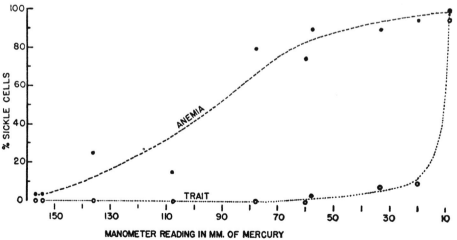

trait cells and greatly shortened in the case of sickle-cell anemia cells.[90,91] The revelations of Pauling and his associates defined the nature of the difference.[39] In the course of his studies, Sherman observed that "under the polarizing microscope characteristic sickle cells exhibit a definite birefringence which disappears after aeration of the cells and the consequent return to the normal discoid form." As it turned out, that discovery was of seminal importance; it was the bit of evidence that led Pauling and his associates to identify sickle-cell anemia as a "molecular disease."

Sherman initiated his studies of sickle-cell anemia when he undertook a project in genetics as an undergraduate college student at the Johns Hopkins University. He continued his investigations in the clinical microscopy laboratory, which was headed by Maxwell M. Wintrobe, and was a senior medical student at Johns Hopkins at the time of his report. After graduation from medical school, Sherman received his surgical training under Walter Dandy, later becoming a practicing neurosurgeon in Bridgeport, Connecticut. Sherman recalled that in the course of his experiments, he had tried to demonstrate without success antigenic differences among the preparations of hemoglobin obtained from normal individuals, from persons with the sickle-cell trait, and from patients with sickle-cell anemia. He did not understand why sickled cells are birefringent in polarized light and did not intend to mention the observation in his manuscript, but he was urged to do so by Wintrobe. Four years later, Murphy and Shapiro, of St. Luke's Hospital in New York City, interpreted Sherman's description of birefringence as suggesting "that certain molecules of the cell become orientated when the cell undergoes sickling."[92]

Sickle Hemoglobin

The implication of the birefringence of sickled cells was recognized by William B. Castle, professor of medicine in the Harvard Medical School. Castle, the ingenious clinical investigator who had elucidated the pathogenesis of pernicious anemia, became entranced by the sickling phenomenon in 1938 when a white woman with sickle-cell disease was admitted to the Boston City Hospital. The patient was a member of an Italian family in Cleveland and had been described by Haden and Evans in a report on sickle-cell anemia in the white race.[93] She later was found to have sickle-cell-thalassemia disease.[94] When her blood was exposed to a gas mixture that was made up of 90% nitrogen and 10% carbon dioxide, the sickled cells that resulted did not pack normally on centrifugation in a hematocrit tube, but packing was complete when the blood was oxygenated. Castle postulated that the sickled forms were like "hay wire" and, therefore, should show increased viscosity of flow in a capillary tube. Ham and Castle then demonstrated that deoxygenated blood from patients with sickle-cell anemia passed through an Ostwald viscometer at a retarded rate.[95] They concluded that increased cell destruction in sickle-cell anemia is the result of erythrostasis in the spleen and other organs and proposed that a "vicious cycle of erythrostasis" is established because the critical oxygen tension for a marked increase in sickling is relatively close to that of normal venous blood.

Castle recalled that he described this work to Linus Pauling, the eminent chemist and Nobel laureate, in a chance conversation:

> He and I were both members of a committee that eventuated in the publication of the book by Vannevar Bush, *Science, the Endless Frontier,* which among other places, met in Denver I think in 1945. On the overnight train between Denver and Chicago, not long after leaving Denver, I had a conversation with Doctor Pauling about the molecular relation of antibody to antigen, etc., which was very informative to me. I then sketched a little bit of the work that Doctor Ham and I had been doing since 1940 on sickle cell disease and mentioned that, as stated by Doctor I.J. Sherman in 1940, when the cells were deoxygenated and sickled they showed birefringence in polarized light. This, I stated, meant to me some type of molecular alignment or orientation, and ventured to suggest that this might be 'the kind of thing in which he would be interested'. I am equally clear that I did not make the further generalization that it was orientation of the hemoglobin that might be doing this.[96]

Pauling's recollection of the meeting differs only slightly from Castle's account. In the course of their discussion he had

> pointed out that the relation of sickling to the presence of oxygen clearly indicated that the hemoglobin molecules in the red cell are involved in the phenomenon of sickling, and that the difference between sickle-cell anemia red corpuscles and normal red corpuscles could be explained by postulating that the former contain an abnormal kind of hemoglobin, which when deoxygenated has the power of combining with itself into long rigid rods, which then twist the red cell out of shape.[97]

At the time, Pauling already had a considerable familiarity with hemoglobin. For years, he had been interested in the structural basis of the sigmoidal oxygen dissociation curve, and he had studied the nature of the bonds formed by the iron atoms with the neighboring atoms of the porphyrin ring, the globin, and the oxygen. He did not forget the casual conversation about sickle-cell anemia that took place in the spring of 1945, and the developments that resulted from the discussion had an unforeseen impact on biomedical science. In September 1955, Castle wrote to Pauling, "Never has a chance remark of mine turned out so well as my mention to you some years ago during our railroad journey from Denver to Chicago of the phenomenon of birefringence when sickle cells are deoxygenated that had been observed by Sherman!"[98]

Early in 1946, Dr. Harvey A. Itano, a rotating intern at the Detroit Receiving Hospital, decided that he preferred a research career in chemistry to the practice of medicine. An American citizen born in California of Japanese heritage, Itano was one of the Nisei temporarily incarcerated after the onset of World War II. Although he had the highest scholastic record for the University of California class of 1942 in Berkeley, he was unable to attend the ceremonies to receive his degree in chemistry because, as President Robert Gordon Sproul said at the graduation, "His country has called him elsewhere."[99] After his liberation, he attended the St. Louis University School of Medicine, receiving his M.D. degree in 1945. He had read Karl Landsteiner's book *The Specificity of Serological Reactions* and was stimulated by Pauling's chapter.[100] Seeking advice from a former teacher, he wrote to Edward A. Doisy about his interest in applying physical chemistry to biological problems. Doisy replied, "I regard Pauling as one of the greatest scientists of the world. Since he is interested in using physical chemistry in solving some of the difficult problems related to medicine, you might enjoy working with him; if so, I suggest that you write directly to Pauling."[98] In a letter in which Itano was accepted as a graduate student, Pauling wrote, "I think that we can postpone the discussion of the research problem in which you might work until your arrival here. I am very much interested in having a study carried out of the relation of the sickling of red cells in sickle-cell anemia to the chemical nature of hemoglobin in the cells, and perhaps this would be a suitable problem."[98]

Itano accepted a predoctoral fellowship in chemistry of the American Chemical Society and, in the fall of 1946, went to the California Institute of Technology, in Pasadena. He took the required predoctoral courses but started early on a study of the hemoglobin of patients with sickle-cell anemia. The properties of the heme group were first investigated. Cells containing methemoglobin did not sickle, and the idea evolved that sodium nitrite might be tried in the treatment of sickle-cell anemia. At the suggestion of Pauling, a brief trial was carried out by George Burch and his associates in New Orleans but without success, and the results were not published. Years later, Beutler and Mikus reported a similar study in which the administration of sodium nitrite led to some degree of lengthening of the life span of the red cells in patients with the disease.[101] S.J. Singer and I.C. Wells also joined Pauling's group of postdoctoral students. After an electrophoresis apparatus modified from that of Tiselius was constructed, Itano and Singer compared the electrophoretic mobility of normal hemoglobin with that of persons with sickle cells. The crucial experiments, performed in the summer of 1948, demonstrated the aberrant mobility of sickle hemoglobin. Wells showed that the heme groups of the two hemoglobins are identical.

The results of the studies were presented in the spring of 1949 to the American Society of Biological Chemists and to the National Academy of Sciences. The report, published in *Science* in November 1949,[39] described the altered electrophoretic mobility of the hemoglobin of patients with sickle-cell anemia and ascribed the abnormality to a change in the globin. The red cells of the patients contained the abnormal hemoglobin almost exclusively, while those of persons with sickle-cell trait contained both the normal and abnormal components (Figure 11-7). Interpreting their observations, Pauling and his associates wrote:

> Let us propose that there is a surface region on the globin of the sickle cell anemia hemoglobin molecule which is absent in the normal molecule and which has a configuration complementary to a different region of the surface of the hemoglobin molecule. This situation would be somewhat analogous to that which very probably exists in antigen-antibody reactions. The fact that sickling occurs only when the partial pressures of oxygen and carbon monoxide are low suggests that one of these sites is very near to the iron atom of one or more of the hemes, and that when the iron atom is combined with either one of these gases, the complementariness of the two structures is considerably diminished. Under the appropriate conditions, then, the sickle cell anemia hemoglobin molecules might be capable of interacting with one another at these sites sufficiently to cause at least a partial alignment of the molecules within the cell, resulting in the erythrocyte's becoming birefringent, and the cell membrane's being distorted to accommodate the now relatively rigid structures within its confines.

That each red cell in sickle-cell trait contained the products of both the normal and the mutant gene beautifully supported the genetic basis of sickle-cell anemia proposed by Neel,[33] namely that the person with sickle-cell trait is a heterozygous carrier of the sickling gene. The study supplied a direct link between defective hemoglobin molecules and their pathological consequences, providing a firm basis for the concept of "molecular disease." A result of these discoveries was to shift the direction of much of the research on sickle-cell anemia. Scientists, some far removed from clinical medicine, became involved and produced many of the subsequent advances. The clinicians

Figure 11-7 Longsworth scanning diagrams of carboxyhemoglobins in phosphate buffer of 0.1 ionic strength and pH 6.90 taken after 20 hours' electrophoresis at a potential gradient of 4.73 volts per centimeter. (*Pauling L, Itano HA, Singer SJ, Wells IC: Science 110:543–548, 1949.*)

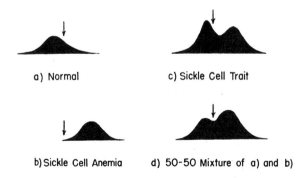

a) Normal

c) Sickle Cell Trait

b) Sickle Cell Anemia

d) 50-50 Mixture of a) and b)

who had made the earlier observations could barely comprehend the work of some of the succeeding investigators.

Earlier Observations on Hemoglobin Variants

Actually, the concept of a structural variant of the human hemoglobin molecule was not new. The first abnormal hemoglobin to be discovered was described by H. Hörlein, a young physician, and G. Weber, his medical student associate, in a remarkable paper presented at a meeting of the Westphalian Society for Internal Medicine in 1947.[102–104] They clearly demonstrated that the methemoglobinemia with cyanosis occurring in four generations of a German family was attributable to a variant of the globin fraction of hemoglobin. Their important study, which preceded by 2 years the report of Pauling and his associates, was overlooked by subsequent investigators and was not even mentioned in the numerous reviews of abnormal hemoglobins, which appeared as late as 1956.[97,105–108] Karl Singer, in a seminar published in 1955, mentioned the methemoglobinemia described by Hörlein and Weber and proposed the designation *HbM*.[109] But it was not until other families with a similar disorder were encountered that the hemoglobins M were generally recognized.[110] The methemoglobin in the report of Hörlein and Weber subsequently was found to be similar to hemoglobin M Saskatoon.[111]

Fetal hemoglobin, the predominant hemoglobin of the fetus and newborn, had been known since 1866 to differ from adult hemoglobin. Disparate chemical and immunologic properties were recognized, and by 1944, the electrophoretic mobility of the two normal hemoglobins had been reported to differ.[112,113] In 1948, Janet Watson, hematologist at Long Island College of Medicine in Brooklyn, New York confirmed the observation of Diggs that erythrocytes of newborn infants sickle slowly and in small numbers. She attributed the impaired sickling to the high concentration of fetal hemoglobin in the red cells of newborns. In normal infants, fetal hemoglobin is replaced by adult hemoglobin during the early months of life. Watson concluded that "the sickling trait progressively becomes 100 percent with the gradual formation of the new red cells containing the adult type of hemoglobin which possesses the sickling property."[114] Her interest in the hemoglobin of sickle cells led her to consult F. Eirich, a physical chemist in the Polymer Institute of the Polytechnic Institute of Brooklyn, who had been interested in abnormal proteins. Their discussions stimulated Eirich and his colleagues to undertake studies of the hemoglobin of patients with sickle-cell anemia.[115] It was Eirich, a lifelong friend of M.F. Perutz, who later provided hemoglobin from Janet Watson's patients for the solubility studies reported by Perutz and Mitchison.[116] A.M. Liquori, a visiting scientist in Eirich's institute, became involved in the research and, on moving to Cambridge, collaborated with Perutz and Eirich in a further report on the properties of sickle hemoglobin.[117]

Heterogeneity of Sickling Disorders— Discovery of Other Abnormal Hemoglobins

Following the initial success in Pauling's laboratory, Itano employed the electrophoretic method in a further search for abnormalities of hemoglobin. In collaboration with Philip Sturgeon, he examined the hemoglobin of a number of anemic children but found no abnormality. Neel, continuing his studies of the inheritance of the sickling phenomenon, encountered two families in which one or more children had a disorder resembling sickle-cell disease but of less severity; in each family the red cells of only one parent could be made to sickle. Itano showed that in these families, an unknown abnormal hemoglobin had been transmitted by the nonsickling parent to the affected children, who had both sickle hemoglobin and the new component.[118] The newly discovered hemoglobin was later designated *hemoglobin C*, and these were the first cases of sickle-cell-hemoglobin C disease to be recognized.[119] A new hemoglobin, subsequently known as hemoglobin D Los Angeles, was discovered by Itano and his associates[120] in a family in which hemoglobin S coexisted with hemoglobin D.[121] The propositus, who was found to have sickle-cell-hemoglobin D disease, was a Caucasian man whose case had been reported earlier as an instance of sickle-cell anemia in the white race.[122] In addition to the discovery of new hemoglobins, Itano demonstrated that the electrophoretic pattern in cases of sickle-cell-thalassemia disease differs from that of the sickle-cell trait—the fraction of sickle hemoglobin is larger.[123]

Various designations were applied to normal and fetal hemoglobin and to the first abnormal hemoglobins that were recognized. In January 1953, the Hematology Study Section of the National Institutes of Health sponsored a symposium at which a standard nomenclature was recommended.[124] Normal adult hemoglobin became *hemoglobin A*, fetal hemoglobin was designated *hemoglobin F*, and sickle hemoglobin, *hemoglobin S*. The letters *C* and *D* were employed to designate the abnormal hemoglobins that had been discovered at that time. New hemoglobins thereafter were to be named in the order of their discovery by successive letters of the alphabet. The designation hemoglobin *b* had been proposed earlier for sickle hemoglobin; because that term was discarded, there is no hemoglobin B. The immediate result of the recommendation was advantageous, but the proposed convention was not accepted by everyone when new hemoglobins were discovered. Furthermore, the number of abnormal hemoglobins soon far exceeded the number of letters in the alphabet.

The electrophoretic method used in Pauling's laboratory employed a modification of the Tiselius apparatus, equipment not generally available in clinical research units. Consequently, the new discovery could not readily be exploited by clinicians. In 1953, Spaet[125] and Smith and Conley[126] demonstrated that separation of hemoglobin components could be achieved by electrophoresis on filter paper using inexpensive homemade equipment modeled after that of Durrum[127] or of Kunkel and Tiselius.[128] A previously complex technique was thus rendered so simple that it could be employed by inexperienced technicians anywhere in the world. The first population survey employing the method included 1000 subjects in Baltimore. An abnormal hemoglobin was not encountered among 500 white persons, but 7.2 percent of the black subjects were found to be heterozygous for hemoglobin S and 2 percent, for hemoglobin C.[126]

The Abnormality of the Sickle Hemoglobin Molecule

Following the demonstration by Pauling's group that the hemoglobin of patients with sickle-cell anemia has an electrical charge different from that of normal hemoglobin, efforts were made in several laboratories to account for the abnormality. Most of the properties of the two hemoglobins appeared to be virtually identical. With the methods then available, a specific difference in amino acid composition could not be demonstrated, and speculations included the possibility that the molecule was folded in an aberrant fashion.[129] The similarity in structure of sickle hemoglobin was further shown by the barely detectable difference in antigenic properties, in contrast to the major differences between sickle and fetal hemoglobins.[130] In 1956, V.M. Ingram reported a discovery of profound significance—that sickle hemoglobin differs from the normal in only one tiny part of the molecule.[131] Soon thereafter, he identified the alteration as a replacement of a single amino acid among the approximately 300 residues that constitute the symmetrical half-molecule.[132] For the first time, the one gene–one enzyme hypothesis of Beadle and Tatum[133] (modified to one gene–one polypeptide) had not only been confirmed but had been explained in chemical terms. The implications of Ingram's discovery for molecular biology, genetics, and protein chemistry were immense.

Vernon M. Ingram was born in 1924 in Breslau. By the age of 12, he was sure that he wanted to study chemistry, but soon thereafter, as a member of a Jewish family, he was barred from attending school. Moving to London with his family, he later became a part-time student at Birkbeck College, the University of London, and earned a B.S. degree in chemistry. At the same time, he held a full-time position as a chemist. Despite fire bombs and other wartime interruptions, he continued postgraduate studies in chemistry and received a Ph.D. in 1949. On the advice of J.D. Bernal, Ingram spent a postdoctoral year at the Rockefeller Institute in New York, where he worked with Moses Kunitz and learned to prepare crystals of protein for x-ray studies. During a second postdoctoral year at Yale, he worked with J.S. Fruton in the study of peptide chemistry. While there, Ingram fortuitously came to the attention of M.F. Perutz, who was seeking a protein chemist to aid in the preparation of protein crystals suitable for x-ray crystallography. In Perutz' laboratory in the MRC unit at Cambridge, Ingram assisted in introducing a mercury atom into molecules of hemoglobin and myoglobin, thus facilitating the crystallographic studies by Perutz and J.C. Kendrew. He became interested in the chemistry of hemoglobin and myoglobin, and particularly in the portion of the peptide chain that is adjacent to the heme group. He was quite aware of the work of F. Sanger in the nearby biochemistry department. Sanger was elucidating the structure of insulin. The techniques of paper electrophoresis and paper chromatography that Ingram was using had been perfected by Sanger. At the same time, F.H.C. Crick was attempting to identify a chemical alteration in a protein produced by a mutant gene. Ingram assisted Crick in those studies, but they were unable to demonstrate amino acid differences among egg-white lysozymes from different strains of hens, or among lysozymes obtained from human tears collected with the aid of onion slices.

Ingram was having little success with his heme peptide when A.C. Allison came to perform some x-ray diffraction studies of sickle hemoglobin. The effort was not successful, and Allison left his samples of sickle hemoglobin at the laboratory. Perutz was interested in sickle hemoglobin, having reported earlier its insolubility when deoxygenated.[116] Members of the laboratory group suggested that it would be interesting to look at the tryptic peptides of the abnormal hemoglobin. Using electrophoresis and chromatography alone, Ingram was unable to demonstrate an abnormality. Only when the two methods were combined, probably for the first time, was an abnormal "fingerprint" obtained (Figure 11-8). The discovery that a single peptide was abnormal led immediately to intense interest and excitement, but it was necessary to confirm the observation with hemoglobin from other patients with sickle-cell anemia. Four additional samples ultimately were obtained; all gave the same result.

Ingram first presented his observations at a subsession of the annual meeting of the British Association for the Advancement of Science in the summer of 1956. He anticipated the meeting with great enthusiasm but was distressed when only about six people attended, none of whom asked questions or displayed any reaction at all. Returning to Cambridge, he proceeded with the tedious task of isolating the aberrant peptide and determining its composition and sequence.[134] The results were ready in time for the important Conference on Hemoglobin held in Washington in May 1957; he reported that sickle hemoglobin differs from normal hemoglobin in that one glutamic acid residue is replaced by valine in each half-molecule.[135] We now know that all of the manifestations of sickle-cell anemia are the result of that single change.

The first abnormal hemoglobins to be discovered by the electrophoretic method were inherited as if transmitted by allelic genes at a single locus. But Rhinesmith, Schroeder, and Pauling, in the United States, and Braunitzer, in Germany, reported chemical evidence that there are two kinds of polypeptide

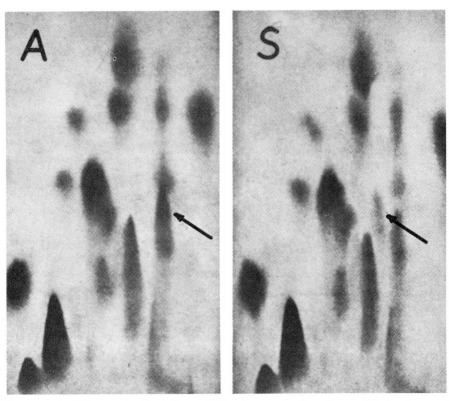

Figure 11-8 "Fingerprints" of hemoglobin fragments (tryptic peptides) of normal hemoglobin (A) and sickle hemoglobin (S) obtained by a combination of electrophoresis and chromatography. The arrows indicate the significant difference. (*Ingram VM: Scientific American 198:68–74, 1958.*)

chains in normal globin,[136,137] subsequently designated alpha and beta chains.[138] Almost simultaneously, Smith and Torbert described a new abnormal hemoglobin (hemoglobin Hopkins 2) in a family in which hemoglobin S was also present.[139] The distribution of abnormal hemoglobins in the family established that they were determined by nonlinked genes; a carrier of both abnormal hemoglobins also had hemoglobin A in his red cells and was able to transmit one, both, or neither of the abnormalities to an offspring. That there are two independent loci for hemoglobin formation was clearly established.* Through the efforts of several groups of investigators, the amino acid sequences of normal alpha and beta chains were soon determined,[140-142] and the entire primary structure of hemoglobin A was elucidated. The site of the amino acid replacement in sickle hemoglobin is at the sixth residue of the beta chain.[143]

*The genetic control of hemoglobin synthesis is discussed fully in Chapter 12.

The Sickling Phenomenon

Identification of the molecular lesion in sickle hemoglobin provided no clue to why the red cells sickle. Understanding of the effects of the amino acid substitution was acquired in other ways. Diggs had described "foci of hemoglobin condensation" in cells undergoing the sickling deformation, and his drawings showed a distortion of the cell membrane by a spicular arrangement of hemoglobin.[77] Years later, the same phenomenon was interpreted as "incipient intracellular crystallization" of hemoglobin by Rebuck and his associates, who employed an electron microscope at low resolution.[144] Murphy and Shapiro in 1944 had observed, "The moment a cell becomes sickled its flexibility is lost and it appears as fixed and rigid as a crystal of ice."[92] Eric Ponder, a sophisticated student of red cell structure, considered the forces that determine red cell shape and suggested that asymmetric hemoglobin molecules are close to one another and may be preferentially oriented. He was aware that sickled erythrocytes are birefringent in polarized light and concluded that sickle cells are probably paracrystalline structures.[145]

The crucial observations were reported in 1950 by John W. Harris, who studied concentrated solutions of sickle hemoglobin. When the solutions were progressively deoxygenated, marked increases in viscosity occurred in the lower range of oxygen saturations, and the more concentrated hemoglobin preparations actually formed a semisolid gel. The increase in viscosity, which occurred only in solutions containing more than 10 g of sickle hemoglobin per 100 ml, was readily reversed by reoxygenation. When the deoxygenated preparations were observed under the phase microscope, spindle-shaped bodies resembling sickled cells were observed and were found to be birefringent in polarized light (Figure 11-9). These structures were identified as tactoids, which contain more water than true crystals. They were taken as evidence of a specific arrangement of the individual molecules with formation of long chains and subsequent alignment of hemoglobin elements (Figure 11-10). Harris concluded:

> The following sequence of events would be adequate to explain the major aspects of the pathologic physiology of sickle cell disease. The alignment and parallel aggregation of the molecules of deoxygenated hemoglobin derived from the red cells of patients with sickle cell disease are manifested as increased viscosity of hemoglobin solutions and the formation of hemoglobin tactoids. These effects take place in solutions at concentrations comparable to those of the intracellular hemoglobin. The resemblance of tactoids to sickled erythrocytes is so striking that the sickled red cell in all probability is essentially a membrane-covered hemoglobin tactoid. Due entirely to the sickled form of the erythrocytes, the viscosity of the whole blood and the mechanical fragility of sickled cells are significantly increased at low oxygen tensions. The increase in viscosity appears to explain the multiple venous thromboses, and the increase in mechanical fragility may largely explain the hemolytic anemia—phenomena which are characteristic of the active disease.[146]

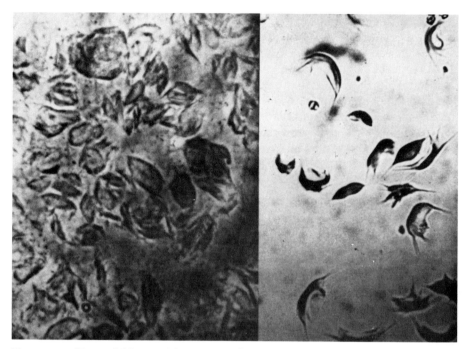

Figure 11-9 Hemoglobin tactoids in stroma-free solutions of deoxygenated hemoglobin S, compared with sickled red cells photographed at the same magnification (phase microphotography). (*Harris JW: Proc Soc Exp Biol Med 75:197–201, 1950.*)

Harris, a graduate of Harvard Medical School, began his research training in 1948 at the Thorndike Memorial Laboratory of the Boston City Hospital, then headed by William B. Castle. At first involved with ongoing studies of pernicious anemia, Harris became intrigued by sickle-cell anemia while caring for a patient with that disease. He was aware of the studies of blood viscosity that had been reported by Ham and Castle, and he read the report by Pauling and his associates about the molecular abnormality of sickle hemoglobin. In the course of a teaching session with Harvard medical students, the idea came to him to look for viscosity changes in solutions of sickle hemoglobin during progressive deoxygenation. In his first experiments, done with a crude he-molysate at a hemoglobin concentration approaching that of the intact cell, there were obvious increases in viscosity. The preparation plugged the transfer pipettes and was impossible to manage in the capillary tube of the Ostwald viscometer, changes that were reversed by reoxygenation. Under the micro-scope, the structures later identified as tactoids were seen and were observed to crumble and fade from view when oxygen was permitted to diffuse into the preparation. Castle made arrangements for Harris to visit David F. Waugh, then associate professor of physical biology at the Massachusetts Institute of

Technology. Accompanied by the technician who subsequently became his wife, Harris demonstrated the reversible sol-gel transformation and the microscopic appearance of the gel to Waugh, who immediately identified the structures as tactoids. Returning later with a preparation of intact sickle cells and a gel of deoxygenated sickle hemoglobin, Harris was given access to the excellent polarizing microscope at the Massachusetts Institute of Technology. He was able to show that tactoids polarize light in the same way that sickle cells do and that the polarization is lost with reoxygenation. After the experiments were repeated in a more quantitative way, a manuscript was prepared and submitted. Rejected by one prestigious journal, it was published promptly by another.[146]

In the same month in which the paper by Harris appeared, an article entitled "State of haemoglobin in sickle-cell anaemia" by Perutz and Mitchison was published in a British journal.[116] The birefringence of sickle cells in polarized light was again confirmed. Isolated crystals of deoxygenated sickle

Figure 11-10 Diagrammatic illustration showing how tactoids are formed. Deoxygenated hemoglobin S molecules form elongated filaments that associate laterally, deforming the red cell as outlined. The filaments later were shown to be produced by a helical arrangement of the individual molecules. (*Drawing by S. Charache.*)

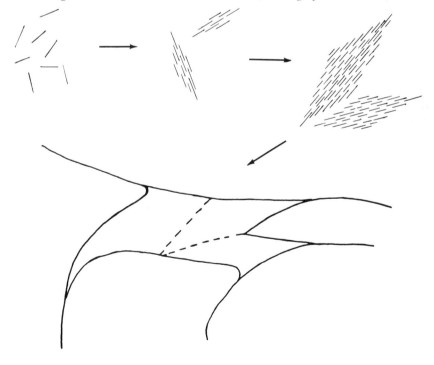

hemoglobin also were birefringent, and some of the hemoglobin crystallized in the form of sickles. Deoxygenated sickle hemoglobin was demonstrated to be markedly insoluble, its solubility no more than one-hundredth that of oxyhemoglobin. These investigators had not observed tactoids and concluded that the hemoglobin in deoxygenated sickle cells is in a crystalline state, going into solution when the hemoglobin is reoxygenated. Perutz had learned about sickle-cell anemia from F. Eirich, who had submitted the sickle-cell-hemoglobin solution that he used. The idea that the sickling process bore some resemblance to crystallization had been suggested to Perutz by Chandler A. Stetson, Jr., who provided the sickle cells for the study. When Perutz and his associates became interested in sickle cells, two elongating paths of scientific development converged in a manner that was to be incredibly profitable.

Max F. Perutz (1914–) began graduate study at Cambridge University in 1936, soon after moving to England from his native Austria.[147,148] His research supervisor was J.D. Bernal, the noted x-ray crystallographer. Only a short time before Perutz arrived, Bernal and Dorothy Crowfoot Hodgkin had taken the first x-ray diffraction pictures of crystals of protein, demonstrating that protein molecules, in spite of their large size, have highly ordered structures. In 1937, Perutz went to Prague to visit Felix Haurowitz, who first interested him in hemoglobin. He chose the x-ray analysis of hemoglobin as a subject for his research. Hemoglobin was one of the very few crystalline proteins then available, it had unique physiological importance, and it was abundant. But it contained about 10,000 atoms. When Perutz began his work, the largest organic molecule whose structure had been determined by x-ray analysis contained only 58 atoms. Through many years of tedious effort, Perutz established the structure of the hemoglobin molecule at high resolution, an accomplishment for which he was awarded the Nobel Prize in 1962. But his studies could not have been completed if the amino acid sequences of the hemoglobin chains had not already been determined, an achievement that had its beginning in his own laboratory with the study of sickle hemoglobin by Vernon Ingram. The molecular model constructed by Perutz revealed the location of the amino acids in three-dimensional space. The substituted amino acid in hemoglobin S is on the surface of the molecule and does not distort its configuration.[117]

Sickle hemoglobin transports oxygen in a normal fashion[30] and is harmful only because of its tendency to form molecular aggregates when deoxygenated in high concentration. The nature of the aggregates and the intermolecular bonds involved became a subject of primary interest. Sydenstricker had observed that sickling is inhibited by low temperatures, and in 1954, Allen and Wyman found that gels of deoxygenated hemoglobin S liquefy when cooled.[30] Confirming that observation, Allison measured quantitatively the dependence of gelation on hemoglobin concentration and also showed that gelation is inhibited by high concentrations of urea.[71] These and other studies led him to conclude that hydrogen bonding plays an important part in the sickling phenomenon and that sulfhydryl groups probably are not involved. He suggested that asymmetric molecules polymerize in a helical arrangement.

The molecular alignment implied by the tactoids described by Harris was confirmed by other methods. Makio Murayama, working at the National Institutes of Health, showed that sickled erythrocytes in a magnetic field become oriented with their long axes perpendicular to the magnetic lines of force, an observation that could be explained by stacking of hemoglobin S molecules with the heme groups parallel to the long axis of the cells.[149] Early attempts to demonstrate an organized internal structure of sickled red cells with the electron microscope revealed intracellular fibers.[150] In 1966, Chandler A. Stetson, Jr., of New York University School of Medicine, demonstrated that sickled cells, when fixed with glutaraldehyde and examined by electron microscopy, show regularly spaced lines parallel to the long axis of the sickled erythrocyte. In cross section, these structures appeared as hexagonal configurations (Figure 11-11).[151] A few months later, Murayama described electron micrographs of threads of deoxygenated sickle hemoglobin, which he inter-

Figure 11-11 Electron micrograph of a sickled cell sectioned in a plane perpendicular to the long axis of the cell, showing close packing of hexagonal units, each measuring approximately 150 Å between opposite sides. (*Stetson CA Jr: J Exp Med 123:341–346, 1966.*)

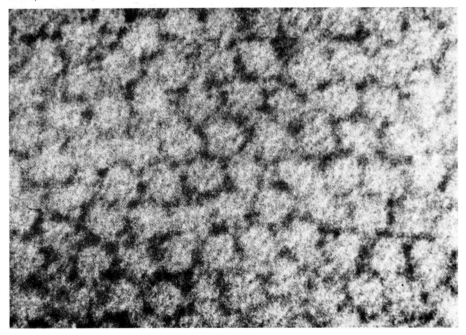

preted as containing microtubules composed of six strands of hemoglobin S monofilaments that were twisted together to form a hollow cable.[152] Thereafter, several groups of scientists employed electron microscopy and x-ray diffraction to ascertain in more detail the way the hemoglobin molecules are arranged in the filamentous structures.[153-159] Linear monomolecular strands containing many molecules become laterally associated in a spiral arrangement to form microtubular fibers with the fibers generally parallel to the long axis of the cell. Several models have been proposed to explain the properties of these aggregates. Studies of crystals of deoxygenated hemoglobin S by x-ray diffraction have made possible the discovery of the sites of intermolecular contacts; these involve residues 6, 73, and 121 of the beta chain and residue 23 of the alpha chain.[160] It is clear that polymerization is a complex phenomenon highly dependent on hemoglobin concentration and involving multiple intermolecular contacts.[159,161]

There is no doubt that the primary reaction in sickling is the polymerization of hemoglobin, but the cell membrane is secondarily involved. The suggestion of Sherman[86] that the sickling cycle damages the cell membrane was confirmed in 1955 by Tosteson and his associates, who demonstrated abnormalities of ion transport.[162] Jensen and his colleagues observed the loss of fragments of membrane during the sickle-unsickle process.[163] Studies of the irreversibly sickled cell have led to greater interest in the cell membrane. In these permanently deformed and rigid cells, the parallel fibrillar structures usually seen in sickled erythrocytes often cannot be demonstrated by electron microscopy.[80] Ghosts of these cells produced by hypotonic hemolysis tend to retain their shape, suggesting that the membrane may have special importance in their formation.[164] The mechanism by which the changes are produced is a subject of current investigation by many scientists, and there is evidence that the interaction of membrane proteins and calcium may play a role in fixing the sickle cell in the irreversible form.[165]

Pathogenesis of the Clinical Disease: The Hybrid Sickling Disorders

Persons with the sickle-cell trait have less than 50 percent hemoglobin S in their red cells and are as well as normal persons. Their erythrocytes do not sickle under physiologic conditions, and, with rare exceptions, they show no manifestations of disease. But patients with sickle-cell-hemoglobin C disease are often ill, although their red cells also contain less than 50 percent hemoglobin S. To explain these phenomena, Karl Singer and his wife, in Chicago, and A.C. Allison independently made use of the earlier observations of Harris that concentrated solutions of hemoglobin S gel when deoxygenated.[71,166] Measuring the minimum concentration of hemoglobin required for gelation, they found that the kind and quantity of non-S hemoglobin had a marked influence. Hemoglobin C was more effective than hemoglobin A in reducing minimum gelling concentration while hemoglobin F was almost inert. Later, Harris and his associates measured the degree of sickling of defibrinated blood at a fixed hematocrit level and at varying oxygen tensions and found that there was a good correlation among sickling disorders between clinical severity and increase in sickling in blood on partial deoxygenation.[167,168] The techniques of Singer and Harris have since been modified and exploited by many subsequent investigators to study hemoglobin interactions. The results of some of these procedures have been useful in identifying the points of contact between the hemoglobin molecules during the sickling process. Both hemoglobin D Punjab and hemoglobin O Arab have amino acids that replace the glutamic acid residue in position 121 of the beta chain, and both interact strongly with hemoglobin S.[169] Patients with hemoglobin S-D Punjab disease and hemoglobin S-O Arab disease are severely affected. In contrast, hemoglobin C Harlem and hemoglobin Korle-Bu have amino acid substitutions at residue 73 of the beta chain, and both react less readily with hemoglobin S.[170] Of intense interest is the discovery that the beta-121 and beta-73 sites have been identified as points of contact between sickle hemoglobin molecules in the crystals examined by x-ray diffraction.[160] That hemoglobin F interacts so weakly with hemoglobin S is especially noteworthy. As pointed out by Watson, young infants are protected against the manifestations of sickle-cell anemia by the high concentration of hemoglobin F in their red cells. Adults with as much as 70 percent hemoglobin S in the erythrocytes are virtually without evidence of disease when the remaining hemoglobin in each red cell is hemoglobin F.[171]

Whether intracellular polymerization of the hemoglobin molecules occurs is dependent upon several variables, most important of which are the concentration of hemoglobin S within the red cell, the intracellular oxygen tension and pH, and the kind and quantity of other hemoglobins in the cell. Each red cell is an independent unit, and all are not equally susceptible. Fetal hemoglobin tends to be increased in the erythrocytes of patients with sickle-cell anemia[172] but is not uniformly distributed among the red cells. As shown by Singer and Fisher,[173] those cells containing the larger amounts of hemoglobin F survive longer. The rate at which sickling occurs as blood flows through capillaries and veins is of undoubted physiologic significance.[174] Sickling is not instantaneous, and the length of time that a red cell is exposed to low oxygen tension and to low pH is a factor in determining the effect. The rate of sickling in vitro varies according to the experimental conditions, but it can be very rapid and is accompanied with increasing rigidity of the cell preceding deformation.[175] Rigid sickled cells may have difficulty traversing the minute vascular passages. Jandl and his associates observed that as blood is deoxygenated, sickle cells are unable to pass through a millipore filter that permits passage of normal cells.[176] In patients with sickle-cell anemia, red cells are not destroyed as a function of age but randomly, presumably as a result of the sickling phenomenon and its consequences.[177] The specific sites of clinical involvement probably are influenced by the character of the circulation, rates of blood flow, degree of deoxygenation, and pH changes.

Natural History of the Disease

The natural history of sickle-cell anemia as it occurs in the United States has been defined by a huge number of clinical reports published since Herrick's first paper.[14,178-180] There are many descriptions of the clinical disease as it is seen in Africa.[6,52,181-183] Certain features, for example overgrowth and distortion of the jaw ("gnathopathy"), which results from expansion of the bone marrow, are relatively common in Africa but rare in the United States. Differences most likely are principally the result of environmental rather than genetic factors. The disease is characterized by an erratic course, with dramatic "crises" recurrently and unpredictably interrupting periods of reasonably good health. Anemia often is remarkably well tolerated but may be fatal at times of the rare "sequestration crises" or "aplastic crises," when extremely severe anemia may appear abruptly. Much of the havoc of the disease is the result of the recurrent and painful "vascular occlusive crises," well described by Diggs; these usually are not associated with increased anemia.[184] However, permanent organ damage results from ischemia and infarction. The medical literature abounds with detailed descriptions of every aspect of sickle-cell disease, which has attracted the attention of diverse medical specialists. Full accounts document individually the affections of the heart, lungs, liver, kidneys, bones, eyes, skin, endocrine glands, reproductive organs, nervous system, and immunologic mechanisms.

There is no question that as living conditions have improved in North America, the course of the disease has been ameliorated. The "meat, meal, and molasses" diet; the primitive living conditions; and the prevalence of infections on the plantations of the old South must have been disastrous to patients with sickle-cell anemia. Greatly improved nutrition and sanitation and more adequate prevention and treatment of infections have had a salutary effect. As a result, the outlook has improved, even though specific therapeutic measures have not become available. Many patients with sickle-cell anemia now live to middle life or beyond, and increasing numbers are gainfully employed. Nevertheless, the disease remains serious, and recurrent or chronic invalidism and premature death persist as typical features.

To a large extent, concepts about the character of the disease have been derived from patients who seek care in hospitals, often at times of severe illness, while less severely affected patients may have gone unnoticed. An informative study of the natural history of sickle-cell anemia in a confined population was conducted on the island of Jamaica by Graham R. Serjeant at the University of the West Indies.[185] Using a minibus as a mobile unit, he visited the families of clinic patients and identified and examined many individuals with sickle-cell disease who had never sought medical care. The exploration revealed that the spectrum of the illness is broader than had been realized and that some patients are relatively mildly affected even though homozygous for sickling. Serjeant found that the less severely affected persons tended to have somewhat higher levels of hemoglobin F in their red cells, but he was unable to identify any other specific factors that might account for the clinical differences. In Jamaica, where there were extremes of social conditions, the environmental effect was notable. Mild sickle-cell anemia has been recognized with increasing frequency in the United States, where the features do not appear to differ from those encountered in Jamaica.[186,187] But even now, full knowledge of the natural course of the disease is not available.[188]

Sickle-cell anemia in certain Arabs of the Middle East has attracted special notice because of its relatively benign character.[189–192] There is no doubt that the severe manifestations of the disease seen in blacks are less frequent among Arabs. Thus, among 270 Saudi Arabs with homozygous sickle-cell anemia, not one had leg ulcers, lesions that are quite common in black patients.[192] A striking feature of the disease in Arabs is the high level of hemoglobin F in the blood, values sometimes exceeding 25 percent, but the explanation of these high values is unknown. The amino acid sequence of the beta chain has been examined in some and shows only the expected substitution.[191] Alpha thalassemia (Chapter 12) has a high frequency in Saudi Arabia[193] and has been encountered in persons homozygous for hemoglobin S.[189] But there is no evidence that thalassemia can account for the mild disease in the majority of patients.

Treatment of Sickle-cell Anemia

Empirical measures were used in early attempts to treat sickle-cell anemia. The patients of Herrick and of Washburn were reported to show gratifying improvement after rest, nourishing food, the administration of iodide, arsenic, and thymol, and the application of boric ointment to the leg ulcers.[8,15] Splenectomy was suggested by Sydenstricker but was first performed in the case reported by Hahn and Gillespie in 1927.[72] The results of the operative procedure seemed favorable, but enthusiasm soon waned. In 1930 the "outstanding methods of treatment" of sickle-cell anemia were considered to be splenectomy, liver diet, and blood transfusion.[178] By 1932, Sydenstricker, who was familiar with the vagaries of the disease and the long asymptomatic intervals, recognized that iron, arsenic, liver diet, and transfusion had little beneficial effect and that splenectomy was useful only when the spleen became enlarged.[28] His experience and wisdom were not shared by many other physicians, who enthusiastically reported favorable results with one or another of an array of measures, few of which had more than ephemeral use.[194]

As understanding of the pathogenesis of the disease evolved, treatment was based on seemingly rational concepts. Vascular occlusive lesions were regarded by some physicians as having a major thrombotic component, and anticoagulant and other drugs thought to be useful in preventing or treating thromboses were recommended. But clinical experience was disappointing,[195] and in controlled trials, therapeutic benefits could not be demonstrated.[196] When evidence developed that the clinical manifestations of sickle-cell disease are caused by intravascular sickling, efforts were then directed at preventing the sickling phenomenon—if the patient's red cells could be replaced by normal cells, perhaps the crises could be prevented. In fact, Anderson and his associates and others provided evidence that sickle-cell crises rarely occur when about half of the patient's erythrocytes have been replaced.[197] Thus, partial exchange transfusions have acquired a place in the management of the disease, in particular for the prevention of crises at times of surgical procedures or in other stressful situations.[194] Sickling can be inhibited by methemoglobin and carboxyhemoglobin. Agents that produce these modified hemoglobins, e.g., nitrites and carbon monoxide, have had only brief experimental trials in patients.[101,198] Their clinical use has not been feasible because of the difficulty of safe administration.

Effective antisickling agents would be expected to prevent the manifestations of sickle-cell disease. Whether they would be effective in terminating crises is more speculative. Diggs and Ching suggested that the pain associated with crises is the result of local anoxia caused by blockade of blood vessels.[84] A general assumption seems to have been made that pain can be relieved by causing the red cells to unsickle. Proof of that assumption is lacking. In at least some instances, pain is the result of infarction. Charache and Page demonstrated that necrotic marrow can be aspirated from some painful areas of bone, a lesion not likely to be benefited by unsickling agents.[199] Sodium bicarbonate and sodium citrate, which tend to lessen sickling by increasing pH, were reported to be useful in the treatment as well as the prevention of crises.[200,201] Controlled trials, however, to the extent that they have been performed, have failed to demonstrate efficacy for either prophylaxis or therapy.[202–204]

The effects of breathing pure oxygen were evaluated by Reinhard and his associates at Washington University in St. Louis.[205] Four patients with sickle-cell anemia were fitted with masks that permitted them to breathe oxygen without interruption over periods of 8 to 20 days. The venous oxygen saturation was substantially increased, and the number of sickled cells in the blood lessened, but the rate of red cell destruction was not greatly reduced. Reticulocytosis was inhibited, and anemia became more severe, undoubtedly because the production of erythropoietin was suppressed by the high oxygen tension of the blood. Other investigators who have employed brief exposure to hyperbaric oxygen in the treatment of sickle-cell crises have not often been rewarded with favorable results.[206,207]

Two attempts to treat sickle-cell anemia with chemical antisickling agents attracted unusually intense interest and excitement. The background of the introduction of these substances, urea and cyanate, and the rise and fall of enthusiasm for their use are noteworthy—all the more because they appeared at a time of unprecedented public concern about sickle-cell disease. In a long series of publications beginning in 1970, Robert M. Nalbandian, a pathologist of Grand Rapids, Michigan, reported that a solution of urea in invert sugar was effective in blocking and reversing sickling in vitro and in preventing and ameliorating sickle-cell crises in vivo.[208,209] The apparent virtue of urea was attributed to its action in disrupting nonpolar bonds, which were considered by Murayama at that time to be of primary importance in the sickling phenomenon.[152] In 1957, Allison had reported that urea in molar concentration inhibits gelation of deoxygenated sickle hemoglobin, but he found that lower concentrations were ineffective.[71] In Nalbandian's articles, dramatic clinical effects were described in patients whose blood urea concentrations were relatively low. His method of treatment was given wide publicity, and many patients received urea with varying results. Some investigators observed seemingly beneficial effects.[210] As experience and skepticism increased, however, an urgent need for controlled clinical trials became apparent. When these were performed, a significant difference could not be demonstrated between the effects of solutions containing urea and of those with sugar alone in patients in sickle-cell crises.[204,211,212] Urea therapy was soon discarded.

Introduction of cyanate as a potential treatment of sickle-cell anemia followed directly from the use of urea. Anthony Cerami, a biochemist, and James M. Manning, of the Rockefeller University, read the optimistic reports of the benefits of urea in sickle-cell disease. They recognized that the proposed mechanism for its action, the disruption of the nonpolar bonds of the hemoglobin molecules, was untenable because the blood concentrations of urea achieved were too low to produce that effect. Believing at the time that urea had therapeutic value, they conceived another mechanism based on earlier observations of distinguished colleagues. William H. Stein and Stanford Moore, of the Rockefeller Institute, had won Nobel prizes for their work on ribonuclease. In 1960, George R. Stark along with Stein and Moore sought an explanation for the loss of activity of ribonuclease when it is incubated in 8-molar urea. They showed that the protein reacts with cyanate, which exists in equilibrium with urea in solution. They warned that when urea is employed to bring about physical changes in a protein, the possibility of carbamylation by coexisting cyanate must be kept in mind.[213] Kilmartin and Rossi-Bernardi in 1969 used cyanate to block the alpha amino groups of the polypeptide chains of horse hemoglobin, a reaction that impaired the binding of carbon dioxide and altered the Bohr effect.[214] Cerami and Manning thought that the reported effects of urea in patients with sickle-cell anemia might be due to the presence of cyanate in the urea solutions. They demonstrated that cyanate irreversibly inhibited sickling in concentrations much lower than the concentration of urea required for reversible inhibition.[215] Cyanate was found to exert its antisickling effect principally by increasing the oxygen affinity of the hemoglobin.[216,217] After extended animal experiments indicated a lack of toxic effects, clinical trials with cyanate were begun. The early experience was encouraging— patients with sickle-cell anemia responded with higher hemoglobin levels and fewer crises.[218] The life span of the red cells of treated patients was pro- longed.[219] Enthusiasm reached a high pitch, and many investigators became involved in related research. Large scale clinical trials were contemplated. But in 1973, a severe peripheral neuropathy was observed in a few patients receiving cyanate. Study of other patients showed nerve conduction abnor- malities in many more.[220] Then, cataracts began to appear in the eyes of some recipients. Clinical trials with orally administered cyanate abruptly came to an end. In the one double-blind clinical evaluation, performed by Harkness and Roth in a small group of patients, there was no demonstrable symptomatic benefit.[221]

Until 1970, the extraordinary scientific advances that had evolved from the study of sickle-cell anemia were unfamiliar to the general public; the disease was unknown, and the patients were largely neglected. In November 1970, Leonard J. Patricelli, president of a television station in Hartford, Connecticut, delivered the first of four prime-time editorials on sickle-cell anemia, the beginning of a series of events that made sickle-cell disease an issue of national and international importance.[222] Patricelli had learned about sickle-cell anemia indirectly from a staff member of the United States Department of Health, Education, and Welfare, where information on the disease was being assem- bled. The response to the broadcasts was amazing, one result being the receipt of substantial gifts to establish a sickle-cell center at Howard University in Washington, D.C. In 1971, President Richard M. Nixon gave special attention to sickle-cell anemia in his health message: "It is a sad and shameful fact that the causes of this disease have been largely neglected throughout our history. We cannot rewrite this record of neglect, but we can reverse it." Almost instantly, there was a burst of interest in sickle-cell anemia throughout the United States. The Congress enacted the National Sickle Cell Control Act, and funds were made available for research and for community service and education.

The public attention given to sickle-cell disease coincided in time with enthusiastic reports of the therapeutic benefits of urea and of cyanate. Scien- tists, some previously unfamiliar with the disease, were fascinated by the theoretical simplicity of an approach to effective treatment—some small modification of the hemoglobin molecule that would prevent polymerization should eliminate manifestations of the disease. The disappointment engen- dered by the failure of urea and cyanate spurred efforts to find more satisfac- tory agents. Several chemical compounds were identified that inhibit sickling in vitro.[223–226] The search goes on, but an antisickling agent suitable for clinical use has not yet been developed.

Even though specific treatment of sickle-cell anemia is not available, much has been done to improve the life span and quality of life of affected persons. Infections, particularly malaria and pneumococcal sepsis, have been common causes of death of children with sickle-cell anemia. Such nonspecific measures as malaria control and the use of polyvalent pneumococcal polysaccharide immunization may reduce mortality.[227] Many useful procedures are available to deal with the lesions and complications of the disease.[194]

The Explosion of Knowledge

Within little more than half a century after the discovery of sickle-cell anemia, fundamental knowledge derived from investigations of the disease probably exceeded that obtained by study of any other clinical disorder. Identification of the first "molecular disease" led directly to the recognition of hundreds of other abnormalities of hemoglobin synthesis, some of which produce diseases that previously were unknown.[161] During the numerous population surveys that were conducted, new abnormal hemoglobins were encountered in almost every part of the world, some with surprising frequency. Hemoglobin C, discovered in Detroit,[118] was found to have a focal distribution in West Africa, where more than 25 percent of the population are carriers in some local areas.[228] Hemoglobin D, first identified in Los Angeles,[120] is identical with hemoglobin D Punjab, which has a relatively high frequency in certain parts of India.[229] Hemoglobin E, initially described in California,[230] is prevalent in Southeast Asia, where the carrier rate exceeds 30 percent in some areas.[231] Several types of hemoglobin M were recognized in scattered Caucasian families,[232] but that form of methemoglobinemia turned out to be the cause of a strange disease known for more than a century as "kuchikuru" (black mouth) or "hereditary nigremia" in a restricted area of Northern Japan.[233] Various forms of thalassemia were found to be widely distributed throughout the world and not restricted to Mediterranean populations as originally thought (Chapter 12). Most of the new abnormal hemoglobins appeared to be harmless, at least in the heterozygous carriers in whom they were discovered. But some were discovered that were chemically unstable, precipitating within the red cells and causing hemolytic anemia,[234] as more fully discussed in Chapter 8. In a few instances, the instability of the abnormal molecules was enhanced by certain drugs, notably the sulfonamides, accounting for a previously unrecognized type of drug reaction.[235] Still other variant hemoglobins were found to bind oxygen in an abnormal fashion, causing an increase in the number of red cells in the blood (polycythemia), or a bluish discoloration of the skin (cyanosis), or anemia.[236] The electrophoretic method, used in initial surveys, proved to be inadequate; some abnormal hemoglobins have normal electrophoretic mobility, and several hemoglobin variants have the same abnormal mobility. Increasingly sophisticated methods were devised to study the properties of hemoglobin and to analyze its structure. The specific abnormality of the amino acid sequences has been precisely identified in many of the several hundred variants that have been recognized. Knowledge of the three-dimensional structure of the hemoglobin molecule has made possible a remarkably clear delineation of the relation of structure to function and the development of a "molecular pathology" of hemoglobin.[64]

Sickle-cell anemia provided the first demonstration of one mechanism of gene action, and study of other hemoglobinopathies revealed how other mutational events produce their effects.[161] The numerous ways in which a gene product may be altered by mutation have been elucidated magnificently by exploration of the heritable disorders of hemoglobin production. The hemoglobinopathies now serve as the prototype for an understanding of the mechanisms of inheritance, clarifying in specific chemical detail such abstract genetic concepts as interaction between heredity and environment, gene interaction, dominance, penetrance, and pleiotropy. The distribution of mutant hemoglobin genes in populations has been of importance to anthropologists,[62] and comparison of amino acid sequences of the hemoglobin polypeptides of various animal species has become a valuable tool in the study of evolution.[237,238]

In 1948, a discovery of singular importance was announced—the red cells of patients with sickle-cell anemia, in contrast with those of normal persons, are capable of synthesizing heme, a portion of the hemoglobin molecule.[239] That observation was followed quickly by recognition that reticulocytes synthesize hemoglobin even after removal from the body.[240,241] Reticulocytes are young red cells, released into the circulation at an accelerated rate in sickle-cell anemia as a compensatory mechanism for the rapid destruction of the abnormal cells. The reticulocyte-rich blood of humans and animals became a readily available and invaluable laboratory tool for the study of many aspects of hemoglobin synthesis. As a result, much has been learned about the manner in which the molecule is assembled and about the genetic control of hemoglobin synthesis.[242] Many of the principles derived from these studies are of broad biologic importance since they apply to protein synthesis in general.

Contributions to the development of knowledge about sickle-cell anemia have come from a remarkably heterogeneous group of physicians and scientists. Fortunately a much larger and more heterogeneous group has profited from the results of the studies.

References

1 Konotey-Ahulu FID: Hereditary qualitative and quantitative erythrocyte defects in Ghana: An historical and geographical survey. *Ghana Med J* 7:118–119, 1968.

2   Gulliver G: Observations on the blood corpuscles of certain species of the genus Cervus. *Lond Edinburgh Dublin Philos Mag J Sci* 17:327–331, 1840.

3   Hayem G: *Du Sang et ses Alterations Anatomique.* Paris, Masson, 1889, 1023 pp.

4   Sergent E, Sergent É: Sur des corps particuliers du sang des paludéens. *C R Soc Biol (Paris)* 58:51–53, 1905.

5   Jelliffe DB: The African child. *Trans R Soc Trop Med Hyg* 46:13–46, 1952.

6   Trowell HC, Raper AB, Welbourn HF: The natural history of homozygous sickle-cell anaemia in Central Africa. *Q J Med* 26:401–423, 1957.

7   Herrick JB: Peculiar elongated and sickle-shaped red blood corpuscles in a case of severe anemia. *Trans Assoc Am Physicians* 25:553–561, 1910.

8   Herrick JB: Peculiar elongated and sickle-shaped red blood corpuscles in a case of severe anemia. *Arch Intern Med* 6:517–521, 1910.

9   Abderhalden E, Herrick JB: Beitrag zur Kenntnis der Zusammensetzung des Conglutins aus Samen von Lupinus. *Z Physiol Chem* 45:479–485, 1905.

10 Herrick JB: Certain clinical features of sudden obstruction of the coronary arteries. *Trans Assoc Am Physicians* 27:100–116, 1912.

11 Herrick JB: Presentation of the Kober Medal to James B. Herrick, M.D. for research in scientific medicine. Remarks by James B. Herrick, M.D. *Trans Assoc Am Physicians* 45:10–11, 1930.

12 Herrick JB: Why I read Chaucer at seventy. *Trans Assoc Am Physicians* 46:13–28, 1931.

13 Herrick JB: *Memories of Eighty Years.* Chicago, University of Chicago Press, 1949, 270 pp.

14 Margolies WP: Sickle cell anemia. A composite study and survey. *Medicine (Baltimore)* 30:357–443, 1951.

15 Washburn RE: Peculiar elongated and sickle-shaped red blood corpuscles in a case of severe anemia. *Va Med Semimonthly* 15:490–493, 1911.

16 Kampmeier OF: Victor Emanuel Emmel. *Anat Rec* 42:75–89, 1929.

17 Cook JE, Meyer J: Severe anemia with remarkable elongated and sickle-shaped red blood cells and chronic leg ulcer. *Arch Intern Med* 16:644–651, 1915.

18 Emmel VE: A study of the erythrocytes in a case of severe anemia with elongated and sickle-shaped red blood corpuscles. *Arch Intern Med* 20:586–598, 1917.

19 Neuda PM, Rosen MS: Preliminary report on a rapid method for the diagnosis of sickle cell disease. *J Lab Clin Med* 30:456–461, 1945.

20 Thomas L, Stetson CA Jr: Sulfhydryl compounds and the sickling phenomenon. A preliminary report. *Bull Johns Hopkins Hosp* 83:176–180, 1948.

21 Castle WB, Daland GA: A simple and rapid method for demonstrating sickling of the red blood cells: the use of reducing agents. *J Lab Clin Med* 33:1082–1088, 1948.

22 Mason VR: Sickle cell anemia. *JAMA* 79:1318–1320, 1922.

23 Guthrie CG, Huck JG: On the existence of more than four isoagglutinin groups in human blood. *Bull Johns Hopkins Hosp* 34:37–48, 1923.

24 Huck JG: Sickle cell anemia. *Bull Johns Hopkins Hosp* 34:335–344, 1923.

25 Taliaferro WH, Huck JG: The inheritance of sickle-cell anaemia in man. *Genetics* 8:594–598, 1923.

26 Sydenstricker VP, Mulherin WA, Houseal RW: Sickle cell anemia. Report of 2 cases in children, with necropsy in one case. *Am J Dis Child* 26:132–154, 1923.

27 Graham GS, McCarty SH: Notes on sickle cell anemia. *J Lab Clin Med* 12:536–547, 1927.

28 Sydenstricker VP: Sickle cell anemia (Herrick's syndrome), in Christian HA (ed): *Oxford Medicine*. New York, Oxford Univ Press, 1932, vol II, pp 849–860.

29 Sydenstricker VP: Sickle cell anemia. *South Med J* 17:177–183, 1924.

30 Allen DW, Wyman J Jr: Équilibre de l'hémoglobine de drépanocytose avec l'oxygène. *Rev Hematol* 9:155–157, 1954.

31 Sydenstricker VP, Delatour BJ, Whipple GH: The adrenalin index of the suprarenal glands in health and disease. *J Exp Med* 19:536–551, 1914.

32 Sydenstricker VP, Kemp JA, Metts JC: Prolonged survival in sickle cell disease. *Am Practitioner* 13:584–590, 1962.

33 Neel JV: The inheritance of sickle cell anemia. *Science* 110:64–66, 1949.

34 Beet EA: The genetics of the sickle-cell trait in a Bantu tribe. *Ann Eugenics* 14:279–284, 1949.

35 Caminopetros J: Recherches sur l'anémie érythroblastique infantile des peuples de la Méditerranée orientale. Étude anthropologique étiologique et pathogénique. La transmission héréditaire de la maladie. *Ann Med* 43:104–125, 1938.

36 Valentine WN, Neel JV: Hematologic and genetic study of the transmission of thalassemia (Cooley's anemia; Mediterranean anemia). *Arch Intern Med* 74:185–196, 1944.

37 Silvestroni E, Bianco I: Una nuova entità nosologica: "La malattia microdrepanocitica." *Haematologica* (Pavia) 29:455–488, 1946.

38 Neel JV: The clinical detection of the genetic carriers of inherited disease. *Medicine* (*Baltimore*) 26:115–153, 1947.

39 Pauling L, Itano HA, Singer SJ, Wells IC: Sickle cell anemia, a molecular disease. *Science* 110:543–548, 1949.

40 Archibald RG: A case of sickle cell anaemia in the Sudan. *Trans R Soc Trop Med Hyg* 19:389–393, 1925–1926.

41 Russell H, Taylor CJSO: A case of sickle cell anaemia. *West Afr Med J* 5:68–69, 1932.

42 Smith EC: Sickle-cell anaemia. A report on three cases diagnosed from microscopic sections of the spleen. *Trans R Soc Trop Med Hyg* 27:201–206, 1933–1934.

43 Smith EC: Postmortem report on a case of sickle-cell anaemia. *Trans R Soc Trop Med Hyg* 28:209–214, 1934–1935.

44 Evans RW: The sickling phenomenon in the blood of West African natives. *Trans R Soc Trop Med Hyg* 37:281–286, 1943–1944.

45 Beet EA: Sickle cell disease in the Balovale District of Northern Rhodesia. *East Afr Med J* 23:75–86, 1946.

46 Trowell HC: Sickle cell anaemia. *East Afr Med J* 22:34–45, 1945.

47 Raper AB: Sickle-cell disease in Africa and America—a comparison. *J Trop Med Hyg* 53:49–53, 1950.

48 Provine WB: Geneticists and the biology of race crossing. *Science* 182:790–796, 1973.

49 Lehmann H: Discussion of Jelliffe DB: The African child. *Trans R Soc Trop Med Hyg* 46:42–43, 1952.

50 Lambotte-Legrand J, Lambotte-Legrand C: Anémie drépanocytaire et homozygotisme (À propos de 300 cas). *Ann Soc Belg Med Trop* 35:47–51, 1955.

51 Lambotte-Legrand J, Lambotte-Legrand C: Le prognostic de l'anémie drépanocytaire au Congo Belge (À propos de cas de 150 décès). *Ann Soc Belg Med Trop* 35:53–57, 1955.

52 Jonxis JHP (ed): *Abnormal Haemoglobins in Africa*. Oxford, Blackwell Scientific, 1965, 477 pp.
53 Barclay GPT, Huntsman RG, Robb A: Population screening of young children for sickle cell anaemia in Zambia. *Trans R Soc Trop Med Hyg* 64:733–739, 1970.
54 Bell RMS, Gelfand M: Sickle cell disease in Rhodesia. *J Trop Med Hyg* 74:148–153, 1971.
55 Watson-Williams EJ: Folic acid deficiency in sickle-cell anaemia. *East Afr Med J* 39:213–221, 1962.
56 Konotey-Ahulu FID: Computer assisted analysis of data on 1,697 patients attending the Sickle Cell/Haemoglobinopathy Clinic of Korle-Bu Teaching Hospital, Accra, Ghana. Clinical features. I. Sex, genotype, age, rheumatism and dactylitis frequencies. *Ghana Med J* 10:241–260, 1971.
57 Livingstone FB: *Abnormal hemoglobins in human populations*. Chicago, Aldine, 1967, 470 pp.
58 Lehmann H: Distribution of the sickle cell gene. A new light on the origin of the East Africans. *Eugenics Rev* 46:3–23, 1954.
59 Allison AC: Notes on sickle-cell polymorphism. *Ann Hum Genet* 19:39–57, 1954.
60 Livingstone FB: Anthropological implications of sickle cell gene distribution in West Africa. *Am Anthropologist* 60:533–562, 1958.
61 Singer R: The origin of the sickle cell. *S Afr J Sci* 50:287–291, 1954.
62 Lehmann H, Huntsman RG: *Man's Haemoglobins*. Oxford, North-Holland, 1974, 478 pp.
63 Lehmann H, Raper AB: Distribution of the sickle-cell trait in Uganda and its ethnological significance. *Nature* 164:494–495, 1949.
64 Perutz MF, Lehmann H: Molecular pathology of human haemoglobin. *Nature* 219:902–909, 1968.
65 Brain P: Sickle-cell anaemia in Africa. *Br Med J* 2:880, 1952.
66 Mackey JP, Vivarelli F: Sickle-cell anaemia. *Br Med J* 1:276, 1954.
67 Allison AC: Protection afforded by sickle-cell trait against subtertian malarial infection. *Br Med J* 1:290–294, 1954.
68 Allison AC: Population genetics of abnormal haemoglobins and glucose-6-phosphate dehydrogenase deficiency, in Jonxis JHP (ed): *Abnormal Haemoglobins in Africa*. Oxford, Blackwell Scientific, 1965, 477 pp, pp 365–391.
69 Power HW: A model of how the sickle-cell gene produces malaria resistance. *J Theor Biol* 50:121–127, 1975.
70 Wiesenfeld SL: Sickle-cell trait in human biological and cultural evolution. *Science* 157:1134–1140, 1967.
70a Ford EB: Polymorphism and taxonomy, in Huxley J (ed): *The New Systematics*. Oxford, Clarendon Press, 1940, 583 pp, pp 493–513.
71 Allison AC: Properties of sickle-cell haemoglobin. *Biochem J* 65:212–219, 1957.
72 Hahn EV, Gillespie EB: Sickle cell anemia. Report of a case greatly improved by splenectomy. Experimental study of sickle cell formation. *Arch Intern Med* 39:233–254, 1927.
73 Hahn EV: Sickle-cell (drepanocytic) anemia. With report of a second case successfully treated by splenectomy and further observations on the mechanism of sickle-cell formation. *Am J Med Sci* 175:206–217, 1928.
74 Scriver JB, Waugh TR: Studies on a case of sickle-cell anemia. *Can Med Assoc J* 23:375–380, 1930.

75 Charache S, Grisolia S, Fiedler AJ, Hellegers AE: Effect of 2,3-diphosphoglycerate on oxygen affinity of blood in sickle cell anemia. *J Clin Invest* 49:806–812, 1970.

76 Seakins M, Gibbs WN, Milner PF, Bertles JF: Erythrocyte Hb-S concentration. An important factor in the low oxygen affinity of blood in sickle cell anemia. *J Clin Invest* 52:422–432, 1973.

77 Diggs LW, Bibb J: The erythrocyte in sickle cell anemia. Morphology, size, hemoglobin content, fragility and sedimentation rate. *JAMA* 112:695–701, 1939.

78 Shen SC, Fleming EM, Castle WB: Studies on the destruction of red blood cells. V. Irreversibly sickled erythrocytes: their experimental production in vitro. *Blood* 4:498–504, 1949.

79 Bertles JF, Milner PFA: Irreversibly sickled erythrocytes: a consequence of the heterogeneous distribution of hemoglobin types in sickle-cell anemia. *J Clin Invest* 47:1731–1741, 1968.

80 Bertles JF, Döbler J: Reversible and irreversible sickling: a distinction by electron microscopy. *Blood* 33:884–898, 1969.

81 Eaton JW, Skelton TD, Swofford HS, Kolpin CE, Jacob HS: Elevated erythrocyte calcium in sickle cell disease. *Nature* 246:105–106, 1973.

82 Diggs LW: The sickle cell phenomenon. I. The rate of sickling in moist preparations. *J Lab Clin Med* 17:913–920, 1932.

83 Diggs LW, Ahmann CF, Bibb J: The incidence and significance of the sickle cell trait. *Ann Intern Med* 7:769–778, 1933.

84 Diggs LW, Ching RE: Pathology of sickle cell anemia. *South Med J* 27:839–845, 1934.

85 Crosby WH, Dameshek W: The significance of hemoglobinemia and associated hemosiderinuria, with particular reference to various types of hemolytic anemia. *J Lab Clin Med* 38:829–841, 1951.

86 Sherman IJ: The sickling phenomenon, with special reference to the differentiation of sickle cell anemia from the sickle cell trait. *Bull Johns Hopkins Hosp* 67:309–324, 1940.

87 Beck JSP, Hertz CS: Standardizing sickle cell method and evidence of sickle cell trait. *Am J Clin Pathol* 5:325–332, 1935.

88 Padilla F, Bromberg PA, Jensen WN: The sickle-unsickle cycle: a cause of cell fragmentation leading to permanently deformed cells. *Blood* 41:653–660, 1973.

89 Lange RD, Minnich V, Moore CV: Effect of oxygen tension and of pH on the sickling and mechanical fragility of erythrocytes from patients with sickle cell anemia and the sickle cell trait. *J Lab Clin Med* 37:789–802, 1951.

90 Singer K, Robin S, King JC, Jefferson RN: The life span of the sickle cell and the pathogenesis of sickle cell anemia. *J Lab Clin Med* 33:975–984, 1948.

91 Callender STE, Nickel JF, Moore CV, Powell EO: Sickle cell disease: studied by measuring the survival of transfused red blood cells. *J Lab Clin Med* 34:90–104, 1949.

92 Murphy RC Jr, Shapiro S: Sickle cell disease. I. Observations on behavior of erythrocytes in sickle cell disease. *Arch Intern Med* 74:28–35, 1944.

93 Haden RL, Evans FD: Sickle cell anemia in the white race. *Arch Intern Med* 60:133–142, 1937.

94 Ham TH, Battle JD Jr: Viscosity of sickle cells. A 34 year study of an Italian family with sickle cell and thalassemia traits: splenectomy in two members. *Trans Am Clin Climatol Assoc* 68:146–154, 1956.

95 Ham TH, Castle WB: Relation of increased hypotonic fragility and of erythrostasis to the mechanism of hemolysis in certain anemias. *Trans Assoc Am Physicians* 55:127–132, 1940.

96 Castle WB, quoted by Strauss MB: Of medicine, men and molecules: wedlock or divorce? *Medicine (Baltimore)* 43:619–624, 1964.

97 Pauling L: Abnormality of hemoglobin molecules in hereditary hemolytic anemias. In Harvey Lect, 1953–1954, series 49. New York, Academic Press, 1955, pp 216–241.

98 Itano HA: Personal communication. From letter in Dr. Itano's possession.

99 Hosokawa WK: *Nisei. The Quiet Americans.* New York, William Morrow, 1969, 522 pp, p 354.

100 Landsteiner K: *The Specificity of Serological Reactions,* with a chapter on Molecular Structure and Intermolecular Forces by Linus Pauling. Cambridge, Mass., Harvard University Press, 1945, 310 pp.

101 Beutler E, Mikus BJ: The effect of methemoglobin formation in sickle cell disease. *J Clin Invest* 40:1856–1870, 1961.

102 Hörlein H, Weber G: Über chronische familiäre Methämoglobinämie und eine neue Modifikation des Methämoglobins. *Dtsch Med Wochenschr* 73:476–478, 1948.

103 Hörlein H, Weber G: Chronische familiäre methämoglobinämie. *Z Gesamte Inn Med* 6:197–201, 1951.

104 Heller P: Hemoglobin M—an early chapter in the saga of molecular pathology. *Ann Intern Med* 70:1038–1041, 1969.

105 White JC, Beaven GH: A review of the varieties of human haemoglobin in health and disease. *J Clin Pathol* 7:175–200, 1954.

106 Itano HA: Clinical states associated with alterations of the hemoglobin molecule. *Arch Intern Med* 96:287–297, 1955.

107 Chernoff AI: The human hemoglobins in health and disease. *N Engl J Med* 253:322–331, 365–374, 416–423, 1955.

108 Zuelzer WW, Neel JV, Robinson AR: Abnormal hemoglobins, in Brown EB (ed): *Progress in Hematology.* New York, Grune and Stratton, 1956, vol 1, pp 91–137.

109 Singer K: Hereditary hemolytic disorders associated with abnormal hemoglobins. *Am J Med* 18:633–652, 1955.

110 Gerald PS, Cook CD, Diamond LK: Hemoglobin M. *Science* 126:300–301, 1957.

111 Betke K: Hämoglobin M: Typen und ihre differenzierung (Übersicht), in Lehmann H, Betke K (eds): *Haemoglobin-Colloquium.* Stuttgart, Georg Thieme Verlag, 1962, 113 pp, pp 39–47.

112 Andersch MA, Wilson DA, Menten ML: Sedimentation constants and electrophoretic mobilities of adult and fetal carbonylhemoglobin. *J Biol Chem* 153:301–305, 1944.

113 Jope HM, O'Brien JRP: Crystallization and solubility studies on human adult and foetal haemoglobins, in Roughton FJW, Kendrew JC (eds): *Haemoglobin.* London, Butterworths Scientific, 1949, 317 pp, pp 269–278.

114 Watson J, Stahman AW, Bilello FP: The significance of the paucity of sickle cells in newborn Negro infants. *Am J Med Sci* 215:419–423, 1948.

115 Eirich F: Personal communication.

116 Perutz MF, Mitchison JM: State of haemoglobin in sickle-cell anaemia. *Nature* 166:677–679, 1950.

117 Perutz MF, Liquori AM, Eirich F: X-ray and solubility studies of the haemoglobin of sickle-cell anaemia patients. *Nature* 167:929–931, 1951.

118 Itano HA, Neel JV: A new inherited abnormality of human hemoglobin. *Proc Natl Acad Sci USA* 36:613–617, 1950.

119 Kaplan E, Zuelzer WW, Neel JV: A new inherited abnormality of hemoglobin and its interaction with sickle hemoglobin. *Blood* 6:1240–1259, 1951.

120 Itano HA: A third abnormal hemoglobin associated with hereditary hemolytic anemia. *Proc Natl Acad Sci USA* 37:775–784, 1951.

121 Sturgeon P, Itano HA, Bergren WR: Clinical manifestations of hemoglobin-S with hemoglobin-D. The interaction of hemoglobin-S with hemoglobin-D. *Blood* 10:389–404, 1955.

122 Cooke JV, Mack JK: Sickle-cell anemia in a white American family. *J Pediatr* 5:601–607, 1934.

123 Itano HA: Abnormal hemoglobins in hemolytic anemias. *Fed Proc* 11:235–236, 1952.

124 Hematology Study Section, National Institutes of Health: Statement concerning a system of nomenclature for the varieties of human hemoglobin. *Blood* 8:386–387, 1953.

125 Spaet TH: Identification of abnormal hemoglobins by means of paper electrophoresis. *J Lab Clin Med* 41:161–165, 1953.

126 Smith EW, Conley CL: Filter paper electrophoresis of human hemoglobins with special reference to the incidence and clinical significance of hemoglobin C. *Bull Johns Hopkins Hosp* 93:94–106, 1953.

127 Durrum EL: A microelectrophoretic and microiontophoretic technique. *J Am Chem Soc* 72:2943–2948, 1950.

128 Kunkel HG, Tiselius A: Electrophoresis of proteins on filter paper. *J Gen Physiol* 35:89–118, 1951.

129 Pauling L, Itano HA, Wells IC, Schroeder WA, Kay LM, Singer SJ, Corey RB: Sickle cell anemia hemoglobin. *Science* 111:459, 1950.

130 Goodman M, Campbell DH: Differences in antigenic specificity of human normal adult, fetal, and sickle cell anemia hemoglobin. *Blood* 8:422–433, 1953.

131 Ingram VM: A specific chemical difference between the globins of normal human and sickle-cell anaemia haemoglobin. *Nature* 178:792–794, 1956.

132 Ingram VM: Gene mutations in human haemoglobin: the chemical difference between normal and sickle cell haemoglobin. *Nature* 180:326–328, 1957.

133 Beadle GW, Tatum EL: Genetic control of biochemical reactions in Neurospora. *Proc Natl Acad Sci USA* 27:499–506, 1941.

134 Ingram VM: How do genes act? *Sci Am* 198:68–74, 1958.

135 Ingram VM: The chemical difference between normal human and sickle cell anaemia haemoglobins. *Conference on Hemoglobin.* Publication 557 National Academy of Sciences—National Research Council, 1958, pp 233–238.

136 Rhinesmith HS, Schroeder WA, Pauling L: A quantitative study of the hydrolysis of human dinitrophenyl (DNP) globin: the number and kind of polypeptide chains in normal adult human hemoglobin. *J Am Chem Soc* 79:4682–4686, 1957.

137 Braunitzer G: Vergleichende Untersuchungen zur Primärstruktur der Proteinkomponente Einiger Hämoglobine. *Z Physiol Chem* 312:72–84, 1958.

138 Rhinesmith HS, Schroeder WA, Martin N: The N-terminal sequence of the β chains of normal adult human hemoglobin. *J Am Chem Soc* 80:3358–3361, 1958.

139 Smith EW, Torbert JV: Study of two abnormal hemoglobins with evidence for a new genetic locus for hemoglobin formation. *Bull Johns Hopkins Hosp* 102:38–45, 1958.

140 Braunitzer G, Gehring-Müller R, Hilschmann N, Hilse KK, Hobom G, Rudloff V, Wittman-Liebold B: Die Konstitution des normalen adulten Humanhämoglobins. *Z Physiol Chem* 325:283–286, 1961.

141 Konigsberg W, Guidotti G, Hill RJ: The amino acid sequence of the α chain of human hemoglobin. *J Biol Chem* 236:PC55–56, 1961.

142 Goldstein J, Konigsberg W, Hill RJ: The structure of human hemoglobin. VI. The sequence of amino acids in the tryptic peptides of the β chain. *J Biol Chem* 238:2016–2027, 1963.

143 Ingram VM: *Hemoglobin and Its Abnormalities*. Springfield, Charles C Thomas, 1961, 153 pp.

144 Rebuck JW, Sturrock RM, Monaghan EA: Sickling processes in anemia and trait erythrocytes with the electron microscopy of their incipient crystallization. *Fed Proc* 9:340, 1950.

145 Ponder E: *Hemolysis and Related Phenomena*. New York, Grune and Stratton, 1948, 398 pp, pp 145, 153, 342–343.

146 Harris JW: Studies on the destruction of red blood cells. VIII. Molecular orientation in sickle cell hemoglobin solutions. *Proc Soc Exp Biol Med* 75:197–201, 1950.

147 Perutz MF: The hemoglobin molecule. *Sci Am* 211:64–76, 1964.

148 Perutz M: Life with living molecules. *New Scientist* 71:144–147, 1976.

149 Murayama M: Orientation of sickled erythrocytes in a magnetic field. *Nature* 206:420–422, 1965.

150 Bessis M, Nomarski G, Thíery JP, Breton-Gorius J: Etudes sur la falciformation des globules rouges au microscope polarisant et au microscope électronic. II. L'intérieur du globule. Comparison avec les cristaux intraglobulaires. *Rev Hematol* 13:249–270, 1958.

151 Stetson CA Jr: The state of hemoglobin in sickled erythrocytes. *J Exp Med* 123:341–346, 1966.

152 Murayama M: Molecular mechanism of red cell "sickling." *Science* 153:145–149, 1966.

153 Döbler J, Bertles JF: The physical state of hemoglobin in sickle-cell anemia erythrocytes in vivo. *J Exp Med* 127:711–716, 1968.

154 White JG, Heagan B: Gels of normal and sickled hemoglobin. Comparative study. *J Exp Med* 131:1079–1092, 1970.

155 Edelstein SJ, Telford JN, Crepeau RH: Structure of fibers of sickle cell hemoglobin. *Proc Natl Acad Sci USA* 70:1104–1107, 1973.

156 Finch JT, Perutz MF, Bertles JF, Döbler J: Structure of sickled erythrocytes and of sickle-cell hemoglobin fibers. *Proc Natl Acad Sci USA* 70:718–722, 1973.

157 Hofrichter J, Hendricker DG, Eaton WA: Structure of hemoglobin S fibers: optical determination of the molecular orientation in sickled erythrocytes. *Proc Natl Acad Sci USA* 70:3604–3608, 1973.

158 Josephs R, Jarosch HS, Edelstein SJ: Polymorphism of sickle cell hemoglobin fibers. *J Mol Biol* 102:409–426, 1976.

159 May A, Huehns ER: The mechanism and prevention of sickling. *Br Med Bull* 32:223–233, 1976.

160 Wishner BC, Ward KB, Lattman EE, Love WE: Crystal structure of sickle-cell deoxyhemoglobin at 5 Å resolution. *J Mol Biol* 98:179–194, 1975.

161 Bunn HF, Forget BG, Ranney HM: *Human Hemoglobins*. Philadelphia, Saunders, 1977, 432 pp, pp 228–245.

162 Tosteson DC, Shea E, Darling RC: Potassium and sodium of red blood cells in sickle cell anemia. *J Clin Invest* 31:406–411, 1952.

163 Jensen WN, Lessin LS: Membrane alterations associated with hemoglobinopathies. *Semin Hematol* 7:409–426, 1970.

164 Jensen W, Bromberg P, Barefield K: Membrane deformation: a cause of the irreversibly sickled cell (ISC). *Clin Research* 17:464, 1969.

165 Palek J: Red cell membrane injury in sickle cell anaemia. *Br J Haematol* 35:1–9, 1977.

166 Singer K, Singer L: Studies on abnormal hemoglobins. VIII. The gelling phenomenon of sickle cell hemoglobin: its biologic and diagnostic significance. *Blood* 8:1008–1023, 1953.

167 Harris JW, Brewster HH, Ham TH, Castle WB: Studies on the destruction of red blood cells. X. The biophysics and biology of sickle-cell disease. *Arch Intern Med* 97:145–168, 1956.

168 Griggs RC, Harris JW: The biophysics of the variants of sickle-cell disease. *Arch Intern Med* 97:315–326, 1956.

169 Milner PF, Miller C, Grey R, Seakins M, DeJong WW, Went LN: Hemoglobin O Arab in four negro families and its interaction with hemoglobin S and hemoglobin C. *N Engl J Med* 283:1417–1425, 1970.

170 Bookchin RM, Nagel RL, Ranney HM: The effect of β^{73Asn} on the interactions of sickling hemoglobins. *Biochim Biophys Acta* 221:373–375, 1970.

171 Conley CL, Weatherall DJ, Richardson SN, Shepard MK, Charache S: Hereditary persistence of fetal hemoglobin: a study of 79 affected persons in 15 negro families in Baltimore. *Blood* 21:261–281, 1963.

172 Singer K, Chernoff AI, Singer L: Studies on abnormal hemoglobins: I. Their demonstration in sickle cell anemia and other hematologic disorders by a means of alkali denaturation. *Blood* 6:413–428, 1951.

173 Singer K, Fisher B: Studies on abnormal hemoglobins. V. The distribution of type S (sickle cell) hemoglobin and type F (alkali resistant) hemoglobin within the red cell population in sickle cell anemia. *Blood* 7:1216–1226, 1952.

174 Charache S, Conley CL: Rate of sickling of red cells during deoxygenation of blood from persons with various sickling disorders. *Blood* 24:25–48, 1964.

175 Messer MJ, Harris JW: Filtration characteristics of sickle cells: rates of alteration of filterability after deoxygenation and reoxygenation, and correlations with sickling and unsickling. *J Lab Clin Med* 76:537–547, 1970.

176 Jandl JH, Simmons RL, Castle WB: Red cell filtration and the pathogenesis of certain hemolytic anemias. *Blood* 18:133–148, 1961.

177 London IM, Shemin D, West R, Rittenberg D: Heme synthesis and red blood cell dynamics in normal humans and in subjects with polycythemia vera, sickle-cell anemia, and pernicious anemia. *J Biol Chem* 179:463–484, 1949.

178   Steinberg B: Sickle cell anemia. *Arch Pathol* 9:876–897, 1930.

179   Henderson AB: Sickle cell anemia. Clinical study of fifty-four cases. *Am J Med* 19:757–765, 1950.

180   Powars DR: Natural history of sickle cell disease—the first ten years. *Semin Hematol* 12:267–285, 1975.

181   Lewis RA: *Sickle States: Clinical Features in West Africans.* Accra, Ghana Universities Press, 1970, 138 pp.

182   Konotey-Ahulu FID: The sickle cell diseases. Clinical manifestations including the "sickle crisis." *Arch Intern Med* 133:611–619, 1974.

183   Cabannes R (ed): *La Drepanocytose (Sickle-Cell Anemia)*. Paris, Editions Inserm, 1976, 435 pp.

184   Diggs LW: Sickle cell crisis. *Am J Clin Pathol* 44:1–19, 1965.

185   Serjeant GR: *The Clinical Features of Sickle Cell Disease.* Amsterdam, North-Holland, 1974, 375 pp.

186   Charache S, Richardson SN: Prolonged survival of a patient with sickle cell anemia. *Arch Intern Med* 113:844–849, 1964.

187   Steinberg MH, Dreiling BJ, Morrison FS, Necheles TF: Mild sickle cell disease. Clinical and laboratory studies. *JAMA* 224:317–321, 1973.

188   Charache S: Sickle-cell anemia: the known and the unknown. *Ann Intern Med* 77:148–149, 1972.

189   Weatherall DJ, Clegg JB, Blankson J, McNeil JR: A new sickling disorder resulting from interaction of the genes for haemoglobin S and α-thalassemia. *Br J Haematol* 17:517–526, 1969.

190   Ali SA: Milder variant of sickle-cell disease in Arabs in Kuwait associated with unusually high levels of foetal haemoglobin. *Br J Haematol* 19:613–619, 1970.

191   Perrine RP, Brown MJ, Clegg JB, Weatherall DJ, May A: Benign sickle-cell anaemia. *Lancet* 2:1163–1167, 1972.

192   Perrine RP, Pembrey ME, John P, Perrine S, Shoup F: Natural history of sickle cell anemia in Saudi Arabs. A Study of 270 subjects. *Ann Intern Med* 88:1–6, 1978.

193   Pembrey ME, Weatherall DJ, Clegg JB, Bunch C, Perrine RP: Haemoglobin Bart's in Saudi Arabia. *Br J Haematol* 29:221–234, 1975.

194   Charache S: The treatment of sickle cell anemia. *Arch Intern Med* 133:698–705, 1974.

195   Salvaggio JE, Arnold CA, Banov CH: Long-term anticoagulation in sickle-cell disease. A clinical study. *N Engl J Med* 269:182–186, 1963.

196   Mann JR, Deeble TJ, Breeze GR, Stuart J: Ancrod in sickle-cell crisis. *Lancet* 1:934–937, 1972.

197   Anderson R, Cassell M, Mullinax GL, Chaplin H Jr: Effect of normal cells on viscosity of sickle-cell blood. *Arch Intern Med* 111:286–294, 1963.

198   Sirs JA: The use of carbon monoxide to prevent sickle cell formation. *Lancet* 1:971–972, 1963.

199   Charache S, Page DL: Infarction of bone marrow in the sickle cell disorders. *Ann Intern Med* 67:1195–1200, 1967.

200   Greenberg MS, Kass EH: Studies on the destruction of red blood cells. XIII. Observations on the role of pH in the pathogenesis and treatment of painful crisis in sickle cell disease. *Arch Intern Med* 101:355–363, 1958.

201   Barreras L, Diggs LW: Sodium citrate orally for painful sickle cell crises. *JAMA* 215:762–768, 1971.

202 Schwartz E, McElfresh AE: Treatment of painful crises of sickle cell disease. A double-blind study. *J Pediatr* 64:132–133, 1964.

203 Mann JR, Stuart J: Sodium bicarbonate prophylaxis of sickle cell crisis. *Pediatrics* 53:414–416, 1974.

204 Kraus AP, representing Cooperative Urea Clinical Trials Group: Clinical trials of therapy for sickle cell vaso-occlusive crises. *JAMA* 228:1120–1124, 1974.

205 Reinhard EH, Moore CV, Dubach R, Wade LJ: Depressant effects of high concentrations of inspired oxygen on erythrocytogenesis. Observations on patients with sickle cell anemia with a description of the observed toxic manifestations of oxygen. *J Clin Invest* 23:682–698, 1944.

206 Laszlo J, Obenour W Jr, Saltzman HA: Effects of hyperbaric oxygenation on sickle syndromes. *South Med J* 62:453–456, 1969.

207 Reynolds JDH: Painful sickle cell crisis. Successful treatment with hyperbaric oxygen therapy. *JAMA* 216:1977–1978, 1971.

208 Nalbandian RM, Shultz G, Lusher JM, Anderson JW, Henry RL: Sickle cell crisis terminated by intravenous urea in sugar solutions—a preliminary report. *Am J Med Sci* 261:309–324, 1971.

209 Nalbandian RM, Anderson JW, Lusher JM, Agustsson A, Henry RL: Oral urea and the prophylactic treatment of sickle cell disease—a preliminary report. *Am J Med Sci* 261:325–334, 1971.

210 McCurdy PR, Mahmood L: Intravenous urea treatment of the painful crisis of sickle-cell disease. A preliminary report. *N Engl J Med* 285:992–994, 1971.

211 Opio E, Barnes PM: Intravenous urea in treatment of bone-pain crises of sickle-cell disease. A double-blind trial. *Lancet* 2:160–162, 1972.

212 McCurdy PR, representing Cooperative Urea Trials Group: Treatment of sickle cell crisis with urea in invert sugar. A controlled trial. *JAMA* 228:1125–1128, 1974.

213 Stark GR, Stein WH, Moore S: Reactions of the cyanate present in aqueous urea with amino acids and proteins. *J Biol Chem* 235:3177–3181, 1960.

214 Kilmartin JV, Rossi-Bernardi L: Inhibition of CO_2 combination and reduction of the Bohr effect in haemoglobin chemically modified at its α-amino groups. *Nature* 222:1243–1246, 1969.

215 Cerami A, Manning JM: Potassium cyanate as an inhibitor of the sickling of erythrocytes *in vitro*. *Proc Natl Acad Sci USA* 68:1180–1183, 1971.

216 de Furia FG, Miller DR, Cerami A, Manning JM: The effects of cyanate in vitro on red blood cell metabolism and function in sickle cell anemia. *J Clin Invest* 51:566–574, 1972.

217 May A, Bellingham AJ, Huehns ER, Beavan GH: Effect of cyanate on sickling. *Lancet* 1:658–661, 1972.

218 Gillette PN, Peterson CM, Lu YS, Cerami A: Sodium cyanate as a potential treatment for sickle-cell disease. *N Engl J Med* 290:654–660, 1974.

219 Milner PF, Charache S: Life span of carbamylated red cells in sickle cell anemia. *J Clin Invest* 52:3161–3171, 1973.

220 Peterson CM, Tsairis P, Ohnishi A, Lu YS, Grady R, Cerami A, Dyck PJ: Sodium cyanate induced polyneuropathy in patients with sickle cell disease. *Ann Intern Med* 81:152–158, 1974.

221 Harkness DR, Roth S: Clinical evaluation of cyanate in sickle cell anemia, in Brown EB (ed): *Progress in Hematology*. New York, Grune and Stratton, 1975, vol 9, pp 157–184.

222 Culliton BJ: Sickle cell anemia: The route from obscurity to prominence. *Science* 178:138–142, 1972.

223 Roth EF Jr, Nagel RL, Bookchin RM, Grayzel AL: Nitrogen mustard: an "in vitro" inhibitor of erythrocyte sickling. *Biochem Biophys Res Commun* 48:612–618, 1972.

224 Benesch R, Benesch RE, Yung S: Chemical modifications that inhibit gelation of sickle hemoglobin. *Proc Natl Acad Sci USA* 71:1504–1505, 1974.

225 Lubin BH, Pena V, Mentzer WC, Bymun E, Bradley TB, Packer L: Dimethyl adipimidate: a new antisickling agent. *Proc Natl Acad Sci USA* 72:43–46, 1975.

226 Milosz A, Settle W: A new approach to the treatment of sickle cell anemia. *Res Commun Chem Pathol Pharmacol* 12:137–146, 1975.

227 Ammann AJ, Addiego J, Wara DW, Lubin B, Smith WB, Mentzer WC: Polyvalent pneumococcal-polysaccharide immunization of patients with sickle-cell anemia and patients with splenectomy. *N Engl J Med* 297:897–900, 1977.

228 Edington GM, Lehmann H: The distribution of haemoglobin C in West Africa. *Man* 36:1–3, 1956.

229 Bird GWG, Lehmann H: Haemoglobin D in India. *Br Med J* 1:514, 1956.

230 Itano HA, Bergren WR, Sturgeon P: Identification of a fourth abnormal human hemoglobin. *J Am Chem Soc* 76:2278, 1954.

231 Lie-Injo LE: Distribution of genetic red cell defects in South-East Asia. *Trans R Soc Trop Med Hyg* 63:664–674, 1969.

232 Jaffe ER, Heller P: Methemoglobinemia in man. *Prog Hematol* 4:48–71, 1964.

233 Shibata S, Miyaji T, Iuchi I, Ohba Y, Yamamoto K: Hemoglobin M's of the Japanese. *Bull Yamaguchi Medical School* 14:141–179, 1967.

234 White JM: The unstable haemoglobin disorders. *Clin Haematol* 3:333–356, 1974.

235 Frick PG, Hitzig WH, Betke K: Hemoglobin Zürich. I. A new hemoglobin anomaly associated with acute hemolytic episodes with inclusion bodies after sulfonamide therapy. *Blood* 20:261–271, 1962.

236 Nagel RL, Bookchin RM: Human hemoglobin mutants with abnormal oxygen binding. *Semin Hematol* 11:385–403, 1974.

237 Hill RL, Buettner-Janusch J: Evolution of hemoglobin. *Fed Proc* 23:1236–1242, 1964.

238 Boyer SH, Noyes AN, Timmons CF, Young RA: Primate hemoglobins: Polymorphisms and evolutionary patterns. *J Hum Evolution* 1:515–543, 1972.

239 London IM, Shemin D, Rittenberg D: The *in vitro* synthesis of heme in the human red blood cell of sickle cell anemia. *J Biol Chem* 173:797–798, 1948.

240 London IM, Shemin D, Rittenberg D: Synthesis of heme in vitro by the immature non-nucleated mammalian erythrocyte. *J Biol Chem* 183:749–755, 1950.

241 Borsook H, Deasy CL, Haagen-Smit AJ, Keighley G, Lowy PH: Incorporation in vitro of labeled amino acids into proteins of rabbit reticulocytes. *J Biol Chem* 196:669–694, 1952.

242 Nienhuis AW, Benz EJ Jr: Regulation of hemoglobin synthesis during the development of the red cell. *N Engl J Med* 297:1318–1328, 1371–1381, 1430–1436, 1977.

CHAPTER 12

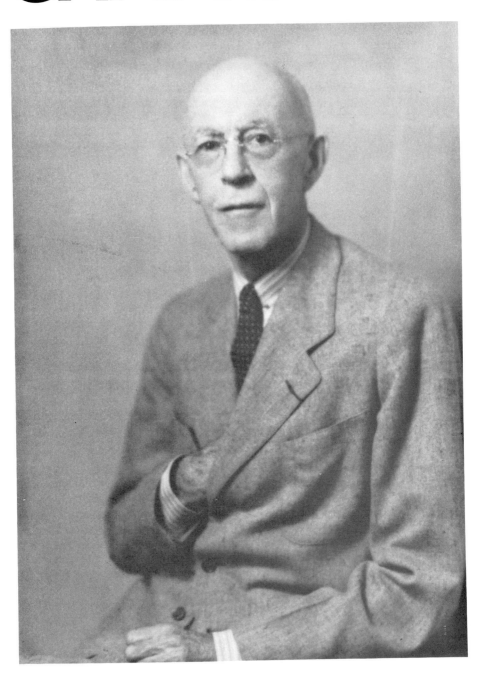

TOWARD AN UNDERSTANDING OF THE MOLECULAR BIOLOGY OF SOME COMMON INHERITED ANEMIAS: THE STORY OF THALASSEMIA

D. J. Weatherall

T he thalassemias are a group of anemias which result from inherited defects in the production of the respiratory protein hemoglobin. When the condition was first recognized in 1925, it was thought to be rare and restricted to certain Mediterranean races. Now it is known that the thalassemias occur throughout the world and that they are among the commonest inherited diseases of human beings. Furthermore, it has been realized recently that an understanding of the basic genetic defects which underlie these disorders promises to tell us a great deal about how mammalian genes work and about the genetic mechanisms that cause many human diseases. Indeed, the recent elucidation of the fundamental genetic defects in some forms of thalassemia has probably been the first real application of the "new" science of molecular biology to an understanding of human pathology.

The history of how we arrived at our present state of knowledge about thalassemia is extremely complex and is hidden in a massive literature, mainly

Chapter Opening Photo   A portrait of Thomas B. Cooley of Detroit. (*Reproduced by courtesy of Dr. Wolf Zuelzer.*)

from Europe, North America, and Southeast Asia. Because of the difficulties of language and the lack of scientific communication between Europe and North America during World War II, it is often impossible to assign correct priorities for key discoveries and to develop an accurate historical picture of the precise order in which they were made.

The development of knowledge about thalassemia seems to fall into four main phases. Between 1925 and 1940, the first clinical descriptions of the disease appeared. From 1940 to 1960, there was an amalgamation of information from Europe and the United States which gradually clarified the pattern of inheritance of the disease. In the next decade, it was realized that thalassemia is not a single condition but a heterogeneous group of disorders which result from different genetic defects of hemoglobin synthesis. Furthermore, it became apparent that these conditions have a widespread distribution and are not confined to Mediterranean populations. Finally, since 1960, steady progress has been made in clarifying the molecular basis for the different forms of thalassemia.

1925–1940

THE EARLY HISTORY OF THALASSEMIA

Thalassemia is such a common condition, particularly in the Mediterranean region and Southeast Asia, that it must have been seen frequently by physicians before the first clinical description was published in 1925. However, there is very little evidence that it was recognized as a specific entity before that time.

The Greek physician Caminopetros noted one possible reference to thalassemia in Hippocrates' *Coan Prognosis*. Dr. Robin Bannerman, who has contributed so much to our understanding of the history of thalassemia, quotes a recent English edition as follows: "When children of seven years of age show weakness, a bad colour, and rapid respiration on walking, together with a desire to eat earth, it denotes destruction of the blood and asthenia."[1] However, it seems quite possible that this was a description of iron-deficiency anemia in early childhood; a desire to eat dirt, a condition known as pica, occurs in iron-deficiency anemia and is not characteristic of children with thalassemia.

Early Italian writings on familial anemia with enlargement of the spleen may have included some cases of thalassemia. Bannerman has analyzed some of the reports in the Italian literature which Silvestroni and Bianco thought might be early descriptions of the disease.[1] He concludes that most of these dealt with conditions such as leishmaniasis, tuberculosis, or congenital syphilis, and in no case was there clear evidence that the authors had recognized a condition that would now be accepted as a form of thalassemia.

An interesting approach to the question of whether thalassemia occurred in historic or prehistoric times is the study of peculiar bone changes in skulls found in ancient burial places or belonging to mummies in a good state of preservation. There is a condition well known to anthropologists called *porotic hyperostosis* (Chapter 2), in which the changes in the skull are very similar to those demonstrable radiologically in the skulls of children with severe forms of thalassemia. Bone changes of this type have been found in skulls excavated in Sicily and Sardinia as well as in those of the ancient native populations of America, the Incas of Peru, Indians from Columbia, the Aztecs from Mexico, the Mayan Indians from the Yucatan, and from many other sites.[2] Indeed, several students of paleontology believe that the extinction of some of these ancient populations resulted from a blood disease, possibly a genetic hemolytic anemia similar to thalassemia. It should be remembered, however, that many of these skulls are from adults and that there probably are other hemolytic or nutritional anemias which can produce bone changes similar to porotic hyperostosis. The controversy over the pathological basis for these extraordinary skulls still rages and the relationship (if any) of porotic hyperostosis to thalassemia remains undefined. Perhaps it will be clarified in the future by analyzing blood samples from mummies using some of the newer techniques of scanning electron microscopy and by detailed analysis of the protein composition of mummified red cells. Certainly the finding of porotic hyperostosis cannot be regarded as unequivocal evidence for the presence of thalassemia.

By the beginning of this century, clinicians were becoming aware of a syndrome of anemia in infancy associated with enlargement of the spleen. One such disorder was the condition called "anaemia infantum pseudoleucaemica," which was described by von Jacsch, of Prague, in 1889.[3,4] Bannerman[1] gives a delightful pen sketch of von Jacsch, who was one of the earliest clinicians to recognize the importance of chemical and x-ray investigations in clinical medicine. His book *Klinische Diagnostik Innerer Krankheiten* was first published in Vienna in 1887, and the fifth edition was edited by Garrod, who later was the author of the famous *Inborn Errors of Metabolism* and who became Regius Professor of Medicine at Oxford. Von Jacsch described a young boy with anemia, a raised white cell count, enlargement of the spleen, and fever in whom a subsequent autopsy did not show changes of leukemia. He described additional cases later. However, it seems unlikely that he actually was seeing thalassemia in Prague at that time. Many other descriptions of von Jacsch's anemia appeared over the next 25 years, Whitcher's (1930)[5] and Capper's (1931),[6] for example; in reading these accounts, one is struck by the extraordinary diversity of the conditions described. There is no doubt that they included leukemia, nutritional deficiency, tuberculosis, congenital syphilis, and other infections. However, for 30 years or more after the turn of the century, it was common practice to describe any unusual anemia in infancy as "von Jacsch's anemia." It was not until 1925 that the condition which later became known as thalassemia was separated from this heterogeneous collection of anemias of infancy.

THE FIRST DESCRIPTION OF THALASSEMIA; THOMAS B. COOLEY OF DETROIT

There are two intriguing questions that must occur to any student of the history of thalassemia. First, why was the first clinical description of this disorder made in the United States, where the disease is rare, rather than in the Mediterranean, where it is common? Second, why was it first recognized by a rather obscure pediatrician, Thomas Cooley? The answer to the first question is probably quite simple—familiarity. Although hematology was very active in Italy at the beginning of the century, it may be that the frequent occurrence of thalassemia prevented it being noticed, whereas in the United States, where the condition was rare, it stood out as an interesting clinical oddity. Furthermore, the Italian hematologists at that time were particularly concerned with the study of morphology, and the subject was most actively pursued in such places as Pavia and Sienna, where there was relatively little thalassemia.[1] Whatever the reason, it was left to a pediatrician working in Detroit to provide the first clinical description.

Thomas Cooley, of Detroit (Chapter Opening Photo), is an enigmatic character; perhaps the best insight into his personality is found in an essay by Wolf Zuelzer.[7] The picture that emerges is of an austere and even arrogant man who was never truly appreciated in his time. Cooley was born in Ann Arbor, Michigan and graduated in medicine in 1895. After postgraduate work in Boston, he studied in Germany for a year and then returned to Boston to work on contagious diseases. Following this, after a short period in Ann Arbor, he moved to Detroit, where he built up a large private practice. However, he gradually withdrew from the latter to build up a full-time practice at the Childrens' Hospital at a time when most of his colleagues were more interested in their private work. He was appointed professor of pediatrics at Wayne University and director of the Childrens' Hospital in 1936. Zuelzer points out that Cooley's approach to the organization of clinical research was years ahead of his time. However, many of his ideas did not catch on during his years as professor of pediatrics. Possibly, this was because of his austere personality and difficulty in communicating with his colleagues, particularly during his later years. It is clear that he was a clinical investigator with a flair for accurate description of clinical syndromes, a brilliant teacher, and a man of broad cultural interests.

Cooley's first description of what became known as thalassemia appears on a single page of the *Transactions of the American Pediatric Society* in 1925 (Figure 12-1).[8] It is entitled "A series of cases of splenomegaly in children with

SECOND SESSION

A SERIES OF CASES OF SPLENOMEGALY IN CHILDREN, WITH ANEMIA AND PECULIAR BONE CHANGES. Presented by DR. THOMAS B. COOLEY and DR. PEARL LEE.

Five cases are reported, four from the Children's Hospital of Michigan and one from Dr. Abt's clinic.

All five presented the clinical syndrome ordinarily known as Von Jaksch's disease or pseudoleukemic anemia. There was anemia, splenomegaly, and some enlargement of the liver, discoloration of the skin, and in some of the sclerae, without bile in the urine. The blood showed normal or increased resistance to hypotonic solutions. There was moderate leukocytosis in all, not of the leukemic type, nucleated red cells, chiefly normoblasts, and in two, many reticulated cells. In all of these cases the symptoms were noted by the parents as early as the eighth month, when they were apparently well advanced   Rickets was not probable in any, and in only one was there definite ground for believing that syphilis might be a contributing factor.

In addition to the splenomegaly and the blood picture, in the four cases from the Children's Hospital attention was called to a peculiar mongoloid appearance, caused by enlargement of the cranial and facial bones, combined with the skin discoloration. In Dr. Abt's patient the cranial enlargement was also noted. Roentgen-ray examination of the skulls showed peculiar alterations of their structure, which the roentgenologist considered pathognomonic of this condition. The long bones also showed striking changes. These changes were identical in kind, varying only in degree in all four of the Detroit cases, while gross and microscopic examination in Dr. Abt's case showed a condition which would have given a similar picture.

Three of the patients died. One, who went through a course of antisyphilitic treatment because of a not thoroughly substantiated diagnosis of congenital syphilis, began to improve nearly a year after cessation of all treatment, and seems to be on the road to recovery. The fifth is living, after splenectomy, which is not believed to have improved his condition. He had, in addition to the ordinary symptoms, achlorhydria and some peculiarities in calcium and phosphorus metabolism, which could not be shown to be related to the anemia. He shows frequent hemoglobinuria and hemoglobin is constant in the blood serum. Since splenectomy he has had, for seven months, enormous numbers of nucleated red cells in his blood, reaching as high as 200,000. The only results in treatment have been with a mixture of spleen and red bone marrow, combined with administration of hydrochloric acid. One transfusion caused only slight, transient blood change, and urine examination showed that the transfused blood underwent rapid hemolysis. A more recent transfusion was followed by a better blood picture and less hemolysis.

Microscopic study of the tissues shows fibrous hyperplasia of the spleen, pigment deposit in the liver, and general leukoblastic hyperplasia of all of the bones, with erythroblastic aplasia. This general aplasia of the red cell-forming tissue seems probably to be the cause of the clinical manifestations, and from the early period at which they were noted, and apparently well advanced, it is suggested that the aplasia is congenital, and the disease to be considered a form of myelophthisic anemia. Case 3 may be considered to show that the body may compensate, through secondary hematopoietic areas, for the primary aplasia.

The desirability of roentgen-ray studies of the bones in other forms of anemia with splenomegaly is suggested.

Acknowledgments are made to Drs. P. F. Morse, E. R. Witwer and Lawrence Reynolds for pathologic and roentgenologic studies, and to Drs. A. Abt and O. T. Schlutz for the loan of their material. with Dr. Schlutz's complete analysis.

Figure 12-1 The first description of Cooley's anemia. (*From Trans Am Pediatr Soc* 37:29, 1925)

anemia and peculiar bone changes" and is written with a collaborator, Dr. Pearl Lee. In this short paper, there is an accurate description of the disease in four young children who had anemia, enlargement of the spleen and liver, discoloration of the skin and sclerae, and no bile in the urine. The red cells showed increased resistance to hypotonic solutions, and there was a moderate leukocytosis with nucleated red cells in the peripheral blood. In addition, the children had a peculiar mongoloid appearance caused by enlargement of the cranial and facial bones. In one case, the spleen had been removed without improvement. In this report, and in a more detailed account in a later paper,[9] Cooley gave a complete description of what would today be regarded as homozygous β-thalassemia. He thought that the disease was congenital but probably not hereditary. Cooley's great contribution was to describe a series of children with a specific clinical syndrome and to separate clearly the disorder from the heterogeneous group of childhood anemias that had hitherto gone under the general name of von Jacsch's anemia.

Over the ensuing 10 years, many reports of Cooley's anemia appeared in the medical literature, both in North America and Europe. Although some of these continued to use the term von Jacsch's anemia, it is clear that many of them were describing Cooley's anemia. Over the next few years, it became accepted that the disease occurs predominantly in Mediterranean populations. An extensive bibliography of the literature of this period is given in the review by Chini and Valeri.[2]

The term *thalassemia* was first used by Whipple and Bradford in 1932 in their classical paper on the pathology of the condition.[10] The word is taken from the Greek "Θαλαθθα," meaning "the sea." In a delightful essay on the life and work of George Whipple, Diggs describes his (Dr. Diggs') attempts to determine how the term thalassemia actually arose.[11] He writes:

> I have always blamed Bradford rather than Whipple for suggesting a seemingly erudite but less meaningful and less understood word. Bradford was from a small town in Missouri. He knew the batting averages of the St. Louis Cardinals, was quite familiar with the north end of south bound mules and the ways of quail and pheasant. He was a sluggish left handed first batsman on the Strong Memorial baseball team in Rochester while I covered the left field. In addition I knew that he did not know a word of Greek. When I wrote recently to ask him why in the name of heaven he changed the name of the disease to thalassemia, a term which did not identify the sea involved, he replied that a good baseball player does not argue with the umpire.

This reply leaves little doubt that the term thalassemia must be credited to George Whipple!

Further insight is provided by Dr. George W. Corner, who was at Rochester at the time when Whipple and Bradford were doing their early pathological work on Cooley's anemia. He has written:[12]

Because I was perhaps the most bookish of the young Rochester faculty, Dean Whipple made me his informal consultant on literary matters, several times asking my opinion on questions of nomenclature and etymology. Wishing to avoid the eponymic title 'Cooley's anemia,' he sought a name that would associate the disease with the Mediterranean area, all the cases known at the time having occurred in families originating there. He had . . . studied Greek at Phillips-Andover Academy, and he recalled the great story in the *Anabasis* of Xenophon's army coming over the mountain and gazing at last upon the sea, the Ten Thousand shouting as one man, 'Thalassa, thalassa!'

Whipple sent for me and asked whether I thought the name 'thalassic anemia' correct and appropriate. I had in fact never studied Greek, but of course I knew about the retreat of the Greek army from Persia and could at least tell the Dean that both words of his proposed name were from Greek roots and therefore properly associated. I gave no thought to the geographic aspects of the problem. Not until long afterward did I learn that the view hailed so joyfully by the homeward-bound Greeks was actually of the Black Sea. The weary men still had a voyage before them, and the Bosphorus to pass before reaching the Mediterranean Sea.

As a matter of fact, however, recent work suggests that it really does not matter whether thalassemia was named after the Mediterranean Sea or the Black Sea! The disease is extremely common in Turkey and in the southern U.S.S.R. Hence, the Black Sea is surrounded with a belt of thalassemia. Perhaps for this reason, it was even more appropriate to name the disease after the Black Sea, despite the fact that this was not actually in Dr. Whipple's mind.

By the late 1930s, the clinical picture of thalassemia had been completely defined. However, the idea that it was a genetically determined disorder was not formally proposed until the paper by the Greek clinician Caminopetros was published in 1936.[13] Interestingly, descriptions of the heterozygous state for thalassemia had appeared in the Italian literature as early as 1925, although it was 15 years before it was realized that the condition which was described by the early Italian writers was related to the disorder described at the same time in the U.S.A. by Cooley.

EARLY DESCRIPTIONS OF HETEROZYGOUS THALASSEMIA

In 1925, the Italian worker Rietti described a mild form of hemolytic jaundice in which the red cells showed increased osmotic resistance.[14] This was a very important observation because it clearly distinguished the disorder from the other common hemolytic anemia, hereditary spherocytosis. Indeed, the increased osmotic resistance of the thalassemic red cell has been an important diagnostic tool ever since Rietti's first description. Similar descriptions were published shortly afterward by other Italian workers, including Greppi and Micheli.[15,16] Short biographical sketches of these early Italian hematologists are given in Bannerman's monograph.[1] Interestingly, Micheli mentioned that he had noted abnormalities of the red cells of this type in the parents of a child with Cooley's anemia, but, as Bannerman points out, it is very unlikely that these early Italian authors understood the true relationship of what became known as malattia di Rietti-Greppi-Micheli to Cooley's anemia. In fact, Bannerman quotes Professor Baserga, of Ferrara, as saying that Rietti was unwilling to accept this idea even toward the end of his life. There seems little doubt, however, that these workers were describing various forms of heterozygous thalassemia. There is an extensive Italian literature on the Rietti-Greppi-Micheli syndrome, which was also called "Mediterranean hematologic disorder" by Chini and "microcytemia" by Silvestroni and Bianco. An excellent review and bibliography about the disorder was published by Chini and Valeri in 1949.[2]

It is interesting to reflect that it took 15 years from Rietti's first description of hemolytic jaundice with decreased red cell fragility for it to be realized that this was the heterozygous carrier state for the disease described by Thomas Cooley. Perhaps this is not too surprising, however. Much of the Italian literature was not easily accessible to the American workers and certainly in the period just before and during World War II, communication must have been difficult. Whatever the reason, it was not until 1940 that the true genetic basis of thalassemia was finally established.

1940–1949

It seems likely that the first definite evidence that Cooley's anemia is genetically determined was provided by Caminopetros in his important papers in 1936 and 1938[13,17] and by Angelini in Italy at about the same time.[18] Both these workers noticed that relatives of patients with Cooley's anemia have red cells with increased osmotic resistance.

A year or two later, and quite independently, several groups of American workers described heterozygous thalassemia in the U.S. for the first time. Max Wintrobe and his colleagues described typical blood changes in 40 members of three Italian families attending the Johns Hopkins Hospital, Baltimore, several of whom showed splenomegaly and mild icterus.[19] They realized that this was a mild form of thalassemia and, in a footnote to their famous paper, pointed out that they had seen this condition in both parents of a child with Cooley's anemia. Interestingly, the index case in Wintrobe's paper of 1941 is still alive, and a further clinical description of this patient, with comments by Dr. Wintrobe, appeared in a paper by Conley and Wintrobe in 1976.[20] Wintrobe attributes the discovery of this important family to the astute observations of his senior laboratory technician Regina Weistock (would that all of us were so honest!). Similar observations were made quite independently at about the same time in the U.S. by Dameshek[21] and by Strauss and his colleagues[22] and in Italy by Silvestroni and Bianco.[23]

More formal genetic studies followed, notably by Gatto,[24,25] Smith,[26] Silvestroni and Bianco,[23,27,28] and Valentine and Neel.[29,30] Valentine and Neel[30] named the mild form of Cooley's anemia "thalassemia minor," Gatto called it "thalassemia minima," and Silvestroni and Bianco used the term "microcytemia." Dameshek pointed out that the microcytic anemia in these cases is often accompanied by the presence of large, pale macrocytes and target cells and called the condition "leptocytosis" or "target cell anemia."

By 1949, it was clear that Cooley's anemia is the homozygous state for a partially dominant Mendelian gene and that the heterozygous state is identical to the condition described by Rietti and the early Italian workers, and later by Wintrobe, Dameshek, and others in the U.S. Excellent reviews drawing together all the early work in Europe and the U.S. were published in 1948 by Marmont and Bianchi,[31] in 1949 by Chini and Valeri,[2] and in 1952 by Bianco and her colleagues.[32] These established beyond any doubt that the Rietti-Greppi-Micheli syndrome is identical to the thalassemia minor of the American workers and to the microcytemia of Silvestroni and Bianco. These are particularly valuable historical papers, partly because they provide such an extensive bibliography of the earlier Italian literature but also because they indicate that many of the early Italian workers in the field were puzzled by the clinical variability of the disorder, particularly in its heterozygous state. Indeed, by 1949 it was already clear that thalassemia is not a single genetic disorder but a complex syndrome resulting from the interaction of more than one, and probably many more, genetic disease. Hence, workers in the field needed a new approach for the further analysis of the thalassemias. This came in 1949 with the discovery of simple techniques for studying human hemoglobin.

1949–1960

The period between the late 1940s and 1960 was one of rapid progress in all aspects of the human hemoglobin field. By 1960, it was possible for Ingram and Stretton to set out their famous theoretical model for the genetic basis of thalassemia. The background information which allowed them to develop their ideas was derived from many sources. These included the rapid accumulation of knowledge about the structure and genetic control of human hemoglobin and, in particular, knowledge from studies of the hemoglobin of patients with different types of thalassemia.

THE GENETIC CONTROL OF HUMAN HEMOGLOBIN

It had been known since 1866 that human hemoglobin is heterogeneous. Körber,[32a] in his doctoral dissertation, showed that the hemoglobin of human placental blood is more resistant to denaturation with alkali than that of adult blood. It was confirmed subsequently that the hemoglobin of fetal life is different in structure from that of adults, and it was established that many other species have both fetal and adult hemoglobins.

The discovery of sickle-cell anemia by Herrick in 1910 is described in detail in the preceding chapter. In 1949, Pauling and his associates in California, following a suggestion by William Castle, of Boston, studied the hemoglobin of patients with sickle-cell disease and showed that it has an electrophoretic mobility different from that of normal adult hemoglobin.[33] Furthermore, they showed that all the hemoglobin of individuals with sickle-cell disease is abnormal while that of symptomless carriers consists of both normal and abnormal types. Normal adult hemoglobin was called hemoglobin A and sickle-cell hemoglobin, after initially being called hemoglobin B, was called hemoglobin S. Elegant genetic studies of families with sickle-cell anemia by Neel,[34] Beet,[35] and the Lambotte-Legrands,[36] taken together with the findings of Pauling and his coworkers, suggested that the structure of human hemoglobin is controlled by a pair of genes and that the sickle-cell gene is a mutant allele of the hemoglobin A allele. Hemoglobin C (Chapter 11) was described by Itano and Neel in 1950[37] and shown to be an allele of hemoglobin S by Ranney in 1954.[38] The discovery of other hemoglobin variants followed, and these were shown to follow a simple Mendelian pattern of inheritance; several were shown to be alleles of hemoglobin S. However, in 1958 Smith and Torbert[39] described a large Baltimore family in which several members carried two abnormal hemoglobins, S and Hopkins 2, in addition to hemoglobin A. This important pedigree suggested that there must be nonallelism between the genes responsible for hemoglobin S and Hopkins 2 and, thus, that there must be two genetic loci involved in the control of adult hemoglobin.

In 1955, Kunkel and Wallenius demonstrated a minor hemoglobin fraction in normal adult red cells which they called hemoglobin A_2.[40] A variant of hemoglobin A_2 called hemoglobin B_2 (later renamed hemoglobin A_2') was described very shortly after this by Ceppellini.[41] These findings suggested that there must be a third locus involved in the control of the adult hemoglobins.

At the same time as these genetic studies were being carried out, the protein chemistry of human hemoglobin became an equally active field. In 1956, Ingram separated the peptides produced by tryptic hydrolysis of adult hemoglobin; this divides polypeptide chains only at the lysine and the arginine residues. Although arginine and lysine account for 60 amino-acid residues per mole of hemoglobin, Ingram only obtained 30 tryptic peptides, suggesting that hemoglobin consists of two identical half-molecules.[42] Shortly after this, groups led by Rhinesmith and Braunitzer confirmed that the globin fraction of hemoglobin A consists of two pairs of identical peptide chains, one with the terminal amino-acid structure valine-leucine, called the α chains, and the other with the terminal structure valine-histidine, called the β chains.[43,44] These findings agreed beautifully with Max Perutz's x-ray crystallographic analysis of horse hemoglobin, which he had shown to be an ellipsoid composed of two identical pairs, each half-molecule having two pairs of different peptide chains.[45] This work earned Perutz a Nobel Prize in 1962. At about the same time, Schroeder and Matsuda[46] found that fetal hemoglobin consists of two different pairs of peptide chains, one identical to those of the α chains of hemoglobin A; the others were found to be quite different from the β chains and, hence, were called γ chains. By the late 1950s, the complete amino-acid sequence of the α, β, and γ chains had been established. Furthermore, it was found that hemoglobin A_2 consists of α chains combined with a pair of globin chains which are similar to, but structurally distinct from, β chains. These were called δ chains.

By the early 1960s, a clear picture of the genetic control of the human hemoglobins had emerged. It appeared that there were at least four structural loci involved, i.e., α, β, γ, and δ. The α loci direct α-chain production, and in fetal life, α chains combine with γ chains to produce hemoglobin F ($\alpha_2\gamma_2$). In adult life, α chains combine with β chains and δ chains to produce hemoglobins A ($\alpha_2\beta_2$) and A_2 ($\alpha_2\delta_2$). The discovery by Weatherall and Baglioni[47] and Minnich and her coworkers[48] that patients who had inherited α-chain variants ($\alpha_2^x\beta_2$) had abnormal fetal hemoglobins ($\alpha_2^x\gamma_2$) at birth, and in later life had abnormal α-chain variants ($\alpha_2^x\beta_2$), indicated that a single α-chain locus controls α-chain synthesis both in fetal and adult life.

At the same time as the genetic control of hemoglobin was being worked out, there was a steady accumulation of information about changes in the hemoglobin pattern of patients with thalassemia.

HEMOGLOBIN PATTERN IN PATIENTS WITH THALASSEMIA

In 1946, the Italian worker Vecchio[49] noted that the hemoglobin of patients with Cooley's anemia was more resistant to alkali than normal adult hemoglobin. This suggested that these patients have more fetal hemoglobin than is usually present after the first year of life. Vecchio and others extended and confirmed these findings, and in 1952, Rich suggested that thalassemia results from a defect in hemoglobin A synthesis with persistent production of hemoglobin F.[50]

The next clue to the general nature of thalassemia came from the study of the hemoglobin patterns of patients with sickle-cell thalassemia. This condition was first described by Silvestroni and Bianco in 1944 and called "microdrepanocytic disease."[51] These Italian workers, who have made so many important contributions to the thalassemia field, collected additional cases between 1944 and 1955 and recorded their total experience in a valuable monograph in 1955.[52] The condition was first recognized in the United States by Powell and his colleagues.[53] The hemoglobin pattern of patients with this condition was first analyzed by Sturgeon, Itano, and Valentine[54] and by Singer and his colleagues.[55] They found that patients who received the thalassemia gene from one parent and the sickle-cell gene from the other had about 70 to 80 percent hemoglobin S and about 20 to 30 percent hemoglobin A, i.e., the reverse of what is found in the sickle-cell trait. This critically important observation suggested that the action of the thalassemia gene is to reduce the amount of hemoglobin A relative to hemoglobin S; i.e., there is "interaction" between the two genes.

However, it soon became evident that the interaction between hemoglobin variants and thalassemia does not always occur, and it was this observation that provided the first indication of the heterogeneity of thalassemia. In 1954, Zuelzer and Kaplan[56] described a patient with hemoglobin C-thalassemia in whom the relative amounts of hemoglobins A and C were similar to those found in the heterozygous state for hemoglobin C alone. In 1959, Zuelzer and his colleagues[57] reported a family in which there was a form of sickle-cell thalassemia that did not result in reversal of the hemoglobin A/S ratio. Furthermore, although in most families with sickle-cell thalassemia, the thalassemia gene appeared to behave as an allele of the sickle-cell gene, this was not the case in this family, where the two genes segregated independently. The recognition of this "noninteracting" form of thalassemia and its nonallelism with the sickle-cell gene indicated that there must be at least two genetic loci involved in the production of thalassemia (Figure 12-2).

Another key observation on the alteration of the hemoglobin patterns in patients with thalassemia was made in 1955, when Kunkel and Wallenius demonstrated an elevated level of hemoglobin A_2 in thalassemia heterozygotes.[40] This was confirmed by Gerald and Diamond in 1958[58] and subsequently by many other workers. However, in a later paper, Kunkel and his colleagues[59] noted that in 2 out of 34 parents of children with thalassemia major, there were normal levels of hemoglobin A_2. Again, this suggested the existence of more than one type of thalassemia.

Further evidence for the heterogeneity of thalassemia appeared during the mid-1950s. In 1955, Rigas and his colleagues observed a rapidly migrating hemoglobin variant in the blood of two members of a Chinese family, both of whom had the clinical picture of thalassemia.[60] At that time, new hemoglobins were being assigned letters of the alphabet; the next available one being H, this rapidly migrating variant was called hemoglobin H. A similar hemoglobin was noted, independently, in a Greek patient with thalassemia in the same year.[61] Further reports of the association of hemoglobin H with thalassemia came from Southeast Asia in 1957, and it was noted that the form of thalassemia in these families was not usually associated with an elevated level of hemoglobin A_2. Chemical analysis of hemoglobin H showed that it consists of a tetramer of four apparently normal β chains; i.e., it has the molecular formula β_4.[62] Thus, hemoglobin H was, up to that time, a unique variant in that it had no α chains. However, in 1957, Fessas and Papaspyrou described an abnormal hemoglobin

Figure 12-2 The concept of interacting and noninteracting thalassemia, which was so critical in the evolution of ideas about the action of the thalassemia genes in reducing the rate of globin chain synthesis. (*A*) The genotype and hemoglobins of an individual with the sickle-cell trait. Because hemoglobin S is produced less efficiently than hemoglobin A, carriers of the sickle-cell gene have less hemoglobin S than hemoglobin A. (*B*) Sickle-cell thalassemia. In this case, the individual has received both the sickle-cell gene and the β-thalassemia gene. The action of the latter is to reduce the amount of β-chain production, and, therefore, such compound heterozygotes have less hemoglobin A than hemoglobin S. (*C*) The compound heterozygous state for hemoglobin S and α-thalassemia. Here, α-chain synthesis is retarded, and the levels of hemoglobins A and S remain the same, but these red cells show the picture of thalassemia.

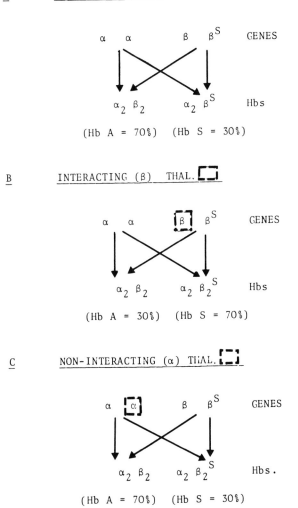

in the umbilical cord blood sample of an infant whose parents showed evidence of thalassemia.[63] In 1958, a similar variant was reported by Ager and Lehmann[64] in a 9-month-old infant with the blood picture of thalassemia who was a patient in St. Bartholomew's Hospital, London. Because there were no letters of the alphabet left for new hemoglobins, this was called hemoglobin Bart's, and it was recognized subsequently that hemoglobin Bart's and the variant described by Fessas and Papaspyrou are the same. Chemical studies showed that hemoglobin Bart's consists of four γ chains with the molecular formula γ_4.[65] Thus, hemoglobin Bart's appeared to be the fetal counterpart of hemoglobin H, i.e., a fetal hemoglobin without α chains.

Thus, it is clear that several key observations were made between 1950 and 1960. First, it was established that many thalassemia carriers, but not all, have elevated levels of hemoglobin A_2. The thalassemia gene associated with an increased level of hemoglobin A_2 "interacts" with the sickle-cell gene. However, there are forms of thalassemia with normal levels of hemoglobin A_2 which do not interact with the sickle-cell gene, nor do their genetic determinants behave as though they are alleles of the sickle-cell gene. Finally, hemoglobins H and Bart's seemed to be associated with a form of thalassemia with low levels of hemoglobin A_2, and both these variants were unusual in that they have no α chains and consist of tetramers of normal β or γ chains.

It now required someone to put all this together into a working hypothesis on the general nature of the defect in thalassemia which would account for the genetic heterogeneity of the disorder.

THE CONCEPT OF α- AND β-THALASSEMIA

Itano first pointed out that the level of hemoglobin S in the sickle-cell trait is less than that of hemoglobin A and that it falls into several modes, which appear to be inherited.[66] These observations led him to propose his *structure-rate hypothesis,* in which he suggested that the primary structure of a hemoglobin is responsible for its rate of synthesis. In his Harvey lecture delivered on April 29, 1954,[67] Linus Pauling developed the idea that thalassemia might result from the production of an abnormal hemoglobin with properties so similar to that of normal adult hemoglobin that the differences could have escaped detection. He suggested that because the thalassemia allele interferes with the production of normal hemoglobin, but does not interfere seriously with the manufacture of abnormal hemoglobins, as observed in patients with sickle-cell thalassemia, it must occupy the same locus on the chromosome as the alleles for other abnormal hemoglobins. He went on to suggest that the thalassemia gene might be responsible for the production of an abnormal hemoglobin of such a nature as to interfere with the inclusion of heme into the molecule. He further postulated that it should be possible to show a chemical difference between "thalassemia hemoglobin" and normal adult hemoglobin. Based on these ideas, Itano extended and refined his structure-rate hypothesis and its relationship to thalassemia, and in 1955, he wrote, "Thalassemia mutants at the hemoglobin locus are analogous to the mutants for abnormal hemoglobins, differing in their failure to alter the net charge of adult hemoglobin and in the greater inhibition they exert on the net rate of synthesis."[68]

In 1959, Ingram and Stretton[69] extended these ideas in their now classical paper on the genetic basis of thalassemia. They suggested that there are two major classes of thalassemia, the α-thalassemias and the β-thalassemias, in the same way that there are two major types of structural hemoglobin variants,

α-chain variants and β-chain variants. They examined published pedigrees and explained quite elegantly the interaction between β-thalassemia and β-chain hemoglobin variants and α-thalassemia and α-chain variants (Figure 12-2). Furthermore, they explained the production of hemoglobin H as the result of an inherited defect in α-chain synthesis, allowing excess β-chain production. Like Pauling and Itano, they believed that the reduced rate of α- or β-chain synthesis might be due to a "silent" electrophoretic mutation of the hemoglobin. They also proposed an alternative explanation, called the "tap hypothesis," in which they suggested that the defect might not be in the structural gene but in the DNA in the connecting unit preceding it. They felt that the genetic data available at that time were compatible with either hypothesis.

It is difficult to give clear-cut priorities for the beautiful work carried out in the 1950s, which allowed Ingram and Stretton to write their theoretical paper. In 1961, Itano and Pauling wrote a letter to *Nature,* in which they pointed out that the chemical studies on hemoglobin reported since 1957 had not substantially altered their inferences regarding the general nature of thalassemia.[70] This, they argued, was evidenced from the conclusions expressed by Ingram and his associates in their papers in the late 1950s, and they added that these papers were remarkable for the extent to which the custom of giving pertinent references to the ideas and findings of previous workers had been ignored! It seems to the present author, having reread the literature of the period, that the working out of the genetic basis for thalassemia depended on the work of many individuals. There is no doubt that Pauling and Itano had, more or less, got it right in the mid-1950s and that Ingram and his colleagues were able to put together a clearer and more complete picture at the end of the decade once it was established that the structure of hemoglobin is directed by the α- and β-globin genes. As mentioned in the acknowledgment section of Ingram and Stretton's paper,[69] several other workers must have played key roles in the evolution of these ideas, in particular Hermann Lehmann of Cambridge and Park Gerald of Boston.

Although subsequent work has shown that the "silent" amino-acid substitution hypothesis was incorrect, there is no doubt that the genetic model for thalassemia which was proposed in 1959 was correct, at least in outline. Indeed, much of it has been substantiated by subsequent studies of hemoglobin synthesis at the molecular level.

1960–1970

The stage was now set for rapid progress on several fronts. A good working model of the genetics of the disease was available, and relatively simple analytical techniques had been developed for analyzing the levels of hemoglobins A_2 and F and for detecting hemoglobins H and Bart's. Consequently, hematologists in hospital laboratories throughout the world could begin to apply these techniques to study thalassemic patients. It was soon realized that the thalassemias are diseases of worldwide distribution and remarkable genetic heterogeneity. Furthermore, a picture of the pathophysiology started to emerge.

THALASSEMIA IS NOT CONFINED TO THE MEDITERRANEAN REGION

Even as early as the 1930s, sporadic case reports started to appear which indicated that thalassemia-like disorders are not confined to individuals of Mediterranean background. Chernoff, in his excellent review of 1959, gave a very complete historical picture of the known distribution of thalassemia up to that time.[71] Even by then, it was clear that thalassemia occurs with a high frequency in Southeast Asia, the Indian subcontinent, and in parts of the Middle East. Information regarding the distribution of the thalassemia genes is still being obtained. Many groups of workers throughout the world have attempted to estimate the gene frequencies in their populations. An early start was made in Thailand through the help given to the Thai hematologists by the group at St. Louis led by the late Dr. Carl Moore. Dr. Moore's assistant Virginia Minnich made several visits to Thailand and in the 1950s, together with the Thai group and Amos Chernoff, published several classical papers dealing with the occurrence of hemoglobin H disease and hemoglobin E-thalassemia in Thailand.[72,73] The Thai group have subsequently carried out extensive population surveys, and an extraordinary picture has emerged regarding both the frequency and heterogeneity of thalassemia in Thailand. Indeed, the Thais have described over 50 different interactions of α- and β-thalassemia genes and hemoglobin E.[74] Other workers in Southeast Asia, notably Vella and Wong, in Singapore, and Lie-Injo Luan Eng, in Indonesia, have provided further evidence that both α- and β-thalassemia are relatively common disorders in the populations of the Malay peninsula and Indonesia. Chatterjee and his colleagues have shown that the β-thalassemia genes are common in many Indian populations,[75] and Aksoy has shown that the disease is common in Turkey. The thalassemia gene frequencies in these populations are summarized by Weatherall and Clegg.[76]

Meanwhile, work continued on the analysis of the frequency and heterogeneity of thalassemia in the Mediterranean region. Over many years, Silvestroni and Bianco have carried out large-scale population surveys in various parts of Italy,[77] and Fessas and his colleagues have both estimated the gene frequencies and defined the different forms of thalassemia in Greece.[78] β-Thalassemia was recognized in the American black population in the early 1950s, and it has become evident that both α- and β-thalassemia occur in individuals of African origin throughout the world.[76]

It is beyond the scope of this chapter to give detailed figures of the gene frequencies for the thalassemias, but taken as a whole, they probably represent the commonest group of single-gene disorders in the world population.[76] In parts of Italy and other Mediterranean countries, the carrier rate for β-thalassemia is as high as 15 to 20 percent. In Thailand, 20 percent of the population carry one form or another of α-thalassemia. The reasons for these remarkable gene frequencies have not yet been completely explained. Following the early interest in the protective effect of the sickle-cell trait against falciparum malaria, it was suggested that thalassemia carriers might also have enjoyed relative protection against the parasite.[76] This has been borne out by limited population studies, although the precise mechanism whereby the thalassemic red cell is protected against *Plasmodium falciparum* is not yet certain.

Hence, what had originally seemed to Cooley to be a relatively unusual disorder in individuals of Mediterranean background is now known to be an extremely common genetic disorder with a widespread distribution throughout many world populations. It causes a major public health problem, particularly in the underdeveloped countries. In Cyprus, for example, about one percent of all newborn infants are affected with a severe form of thalassemia. These infants will only survive if given regular blood transfusion. This puts a tremendous strain on blood transfusion services, and, in many cases, it is not possible to maintain these children with regular transfusion. This problem is equally severe in parts of India, Pakistan, and Southeast Asia. Indeed, once the anemias of infection and malnutrition are overcome in these countries, the thalassemia problem will become even more marked.

THE GENETIC HETEROGENEITY OF THE THALASSEMIAS

With the availability of relatively simple methods for hemoglobin analysis and with a good working model upon which to base the results of family studies, progress in the elucidation of the heterogeneity of the thalassemias was rapid in the period immediately after 1960.

It was soon realized that α-thalassemia is a heterogeneous disorder. In 1959, Lie-Injo Luan Eng made an extremely important observation.[79] She described a stillborn hydropic Indonesian infant whose red cells contained almost entirely hemoglobin Bart's; thus, the condition became known as the hemoglobin Bart's hydrops syndrome. Subsequently, it was realized that this was a very frequent cause of intrauterine death, not only in Indonesia but in Thailand and down the Malay peninsula. Early reports suggested that both the parents of such infants have a mild thalassemia-like disorder with normal levels of hemoglobin A_2 but do not have any hemoglobin H demonstrable in their red cells. Meanwhile, hemoglobin H disease, a moderately severe form of thalassemia in which hemoglobin H can be found in the red cells, was being found frequently in Oriental populations, and cases were being described in

Europe and the United States. The genetic basis of hemoglobin H disease was puzzling, however. Ingram and Stretton had suggested that it was the homozygous state for a form of α-thalassemia, but genetic analysis soon showed that this was incorrect.

The genetics of α-thalassemia was gradually clarified in the late 1960s, due not in the least to the extensive pedigree analyses carried out by the group in Thailand.[74] It became evident that there are two types of α-thalassemia genes, severe and mild, called α-thalassemia-1 and -2, respectively. The hemoglobin Bart's hydrops syndrome is the homozygous state for the α-thalassemia-1 gene and hemoglobin H disease results from the inheritance of both α-thalassemia-1 and α-thalassemia-2. In the newborn period, α-thalassemia-1 carriers have about 5 to 10 percent hemoglobin Bart's and α-thalassemia-2 carriers, approximately 2 to 3 percent of hemoglobin Bart's.

Although the genetics of α-thalassemia in Oriental populations had been clarified by 1970, it had also become apparent that the disease is not restricted to these peoples and that it occurs frequently in other populations, such as Arabs and African blacks.[76] Although the disease is well documented in these groups, the genetics have proved very difficult to work out and are still not understood.

Progress was equally rapid in recognizing the genetic heterogeneity of β-thalassemia. The first real indication of this came from studies of the hemoglobin pattern of patients with sickle-cell thalassemia. Usually there is a reduction in the amount of hemoglobin A as compared with hemoglobin S, but significant amounts of hemoglobin A are present. However, some patients with sickle-cell thalassemia were found to produce only hemoglobins S and A_2, with a small amount of hemoglobin F. This indicates that this form of β-thalassemia has completely suppressed β-chain synthesis. Similarly, it was found that some patients with homozygous β-thalassemia synthesize no hemoglobin A. This variety of β-thalassemia became known as β^0-thalassemia and the type in which some hemoglobin A (i.e., β chain) is produced as β^+-thalassemia.[76]

Further evidence of the heterogeneity of β-thalassemia was established when it was found that some patients with apparent β-thalassemia had normal levels of hemoglobin A_2 but unusually high levels of hemoglobin F. It was suggested that this condition resulted from a genetic defect in both β- and δ-chain synthesis, and the condition was called $\delta\beta$-thalassemia. Genetic analysis of families with β- and $\delta\beta$-thalassemia indicated that within each group, there might well be additional heterogeneity, but it was difficult to confirm this by simple pedigree analysis.[76]

Another important contribution to our understanding of the heterogeneity of β-thalassemia was made in 1958. Park Gerald and Louis Diamond noticed that one parent of a child with typical Cooley's anemia had thalassemia trait associated with a low level of hemoglobin A_2 and about 10 percent of a structural hemoglobin variant with electrophoretic properties similar to hemoglobin S.[58] They called the latter hemoglobin Lepore, Lepore being the family name of the propositus. In 1961, Baglioni analyzed the structure of hemoglobin Lepore and showed that it has normal α chains combined with non-α chains which consist of the amino terminal ends of the δ chains and the carboxyl terminal ends of the β chains.[80] Baglioni, using the model proposed by Oliver Smithies for the production of the α chain of haptoglobin, suggested that the $\delta\beta$ chain of hemoglobin Lepore had arisen by misalignment during meiosis of the homologous chromosomes carrying the δ and β genes followed by abnormal crossing over such that a $\delta\beta$-fusion gene was produced (Figure 12-3). A hemoglobin Lepore carrier would have one chromosome carrying β and δ loci, and the other of the homologous pair would have a single $\delta\beta$-fusion gene. Because hemoglobin Lepore is synthesized inefficiently, carriers have a blood picture identical to the β-thalassemia trait. This model predicted that persons homozygous for hemoglobin Lepore would make no hemoglobin A and A$_2$; this turned out to be the case.[81] Although hemoglobin Lepore thalassemia is rare, this was an important contribution because it was the first time that a form of thalassemia was explainable at the molecular level.

THE PATHOPHYSIOLOGY OF THALASSEMIA

In the early literature on thalassemia, the hemolytic basis for the anemia was stressed; indeed, Cooley first described the condition as a hemolytic anemia.[8] In their early paper on the pathophysiology of thalassemia,[10] Whipple and Bradford suggested that the disorder might result from a defect in the metabolism of pigment, although they did not expand on this idea. It was not until techniques for the study of red cell survival and turnover with radioactive isotopes became available that some insight into the pathophysiology of the disorder was obtained.

Sturgeon and Finch, in Seattle, were the first workers to carry out careful erythrokinetic studies on patients with thalassemia major.[82] Their studies showed that there was a marked degree of ineffective erythropoiesis in this condition, very similar to that found in pernicious anemia. This was confirmed by in vivo studies of hemoglobin turnover by Grinstein, Bannerman, and others.[83] In summarizing his total experience with erythrokinetic studies, Finch suggested that the degree of ineffective erythropoiesis in thalassemia is probably greater than in any other disorder.[84] These findings imply that there is extensive destruction of red cell precursors in the bone marrow as well as a shortened survival in the peripheral blood. In other words, the anemia of thalassemia is the result of defective production of red cells as well as shortened survival of those cells that are produced.

A clue to the basis for the ineffective production and premature destruction of the red cells in thalassemia came in 1963 from the elegant studies of

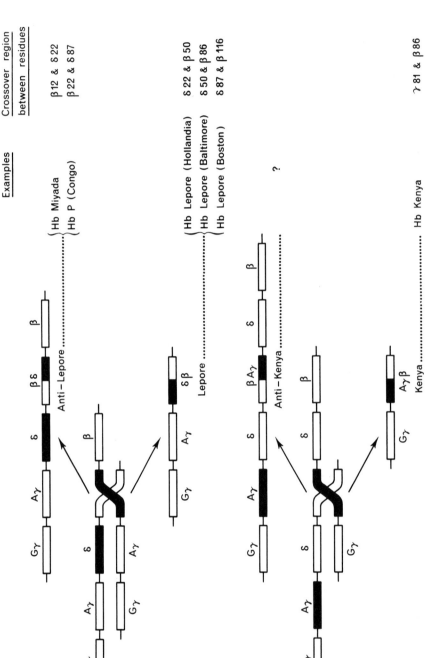

Crossover region between residues

β 12 & δ 22	} Hb Miyada
β 22 & δ 87	} Hb P (Congo)

Anti–Lepore

Lepore

δ 22 & β 50	} Hb Lepore (Hollandia)
δ 50 & β 86	} Hb Lepore (Baltimore)
δ 87 & β 116	} Hb Lepore (Boston)

?

Anti–Kenya

Hb Kenya

Kenya ...... γ 81 & β 86

Figure 12-3 The molecular mechanisms for the production of crossover variants, such as hemoglobin Lepore and hemoglobin Kenya. The concept of chromosomal misalignment with abnormal crossing over and the production of a δβ fusion gene as the basis for the production of hemoglobin Lepore was the first molecular mechanism to be worked out as a basis for a thalassemia disorder. Not only do studies of this type provide evidence about the molecular basis for different forms of thalassemia, but, until gene mapping techniques were developed, they provided the best indication that we had about the likely order of the hemoglobin genes on their respective chromosomes.

Phaedon Fessas, of Athens.[85] He showed that there are large, ragged inclusion bodies in the red cell precursors in the bone marrow of patients with β-thalassemia. These are also found in the peripheral blood, but only after splenectomy. Fessas suggested that these inclusions are precipitated α chains, which are produced because of the deficiency of β chains in thalassemic cells. He postulated that the inclusions might interfere with erythroid maturation and, so, cause ineffective erythropoiesis. Large single inclusion bodies are also observed in the red cells of patients with hemoglobin H disease after splenectomy. This suggests that hemoglobin H precipitates in older red cells and that the hemolysis of this disorder is due to the trapping in the spleen of cells containing large inclusion bodies. A similar mechanism presumably occurs in β-thalassemia, and, consequently, this is why inclusion bodies are only seen after splenectomy.

The idea of the thalassemias being primarily diseases of imbalanced globin chain production was extended in 1967 by Nathan and Gunn, who suggested that the abnormalities of red cell maturation and survival can be ascribed entirely to the effects of unbalanced globin chain production with precipitation of those chains that are produced in excess.[86] They argued that in β-thalassemia, those cells which continue to produce γ chains would be relatively protected from the deleterious effects of α-chain precipitation because in these cells some of the excess α chains could combine with γ to make hemoglobin F ($\alpha_2\gamma_2$). About this time, several workers showed that cells containing hemoglobin F survive relatively longer than cells containing hemoglobin A in the blood of patients with β-thalassemia. Nathan and Gunn further developed their model and suggested that, in addition to causing abnormalities of cellular maturation, the precipitating globin chains might interfere with red cell membrane function and that this might also contribute to the hemolysis observed in all the thalassemia syndromes.

All these ideas about the pathophysiology of thalassemia required experimental verification, and to achieve this, it was necessary to develop methods to study hemoglobin synthesis in thalassemic red cells.

Hemoglobin Synthesis in Thalassemia—1960–1970

It had been known for many years (since the pioneer experiments of London, Shemin, Borsook, and others) that it is possible to incorporate radioactive amino acids into hemoglobin in red cells incubated in vitro provided there are sufficient reticulocytes present in the blood sample. Several groups of workers in the late 1950s and early 1960s made use of these techniques to try to pinpoint the defect in hemoglobin synthesis in thalassemia. The earliest studies were carried out by Bannerman and Grinstein, working with Carl Moore, in St. Louis.[83] These workers showed that there is a defect in heme synthesis in thalassemic red cells, but it was difficult to equate this finding with the interaction observed between the thalassemia and sickle-cell genes, which was much more in keeping with the idea that thalassemia results from a primary defect in globin synthesis. For this reason, it seemed likely that the defect in heme production was secondary to one in globin synthesis.

The earliest attempts to study globin synthesis in thalassemic red cell precursors were made by Paul Marks and his colleagues at Columbia University.[87,88] In a series of elegant experiments, they were able to show that hemoglobin A synthesis is defective but that ribosomal function is normal in thalassemic cells. In 1964, Heywood and his colleagues demonstrated unequal labeling of the α and β chains of hemoglobin after incubation of thalassemic reticulocytes[89] with radioactive amino acids. Unfortunately, however, the rather crude methods which were available for separating α and β chains at that time made it impossible to assess the relative rates of production of these chains in normal or thalassemic red cells.

The technique that enabled further progress to be made in the field was developed by John Clegg, Michael Naughton, and the present author at Johns Hopkins University between 1964 and 1965.[90,91] These workers evolved a simple method for separating α, β, γ, and δ chains of hemoglobin which yielded almost 100 percent of the starting material. Therefore, if reticulocytes were first incubated with radioactive amino acids in vitro it became possible to measure the total amounts of α and β chains synthesized during the period of incubation. Over the next 2 or 3 years, this technique was applied by several groups to the study of different types of thalassemia, and it was possible to define many of these conditions in terms of defective α- or β-chain synthesis.[91] These in vitro studies demonstrated unequivocally that the α- and β-thalassemias are disorders that are characterized by imbalanced globin chain production. The final problem was to try to discover the cause for the defective rate of production of the α or β chains. It was at this stage of the story that thalassemia moved rather tentatively into the world of molecular biology.

The Molecular Biology of Thalassemia—1965–1978

The period between 1950 and 1970 saw the rapid growth of what became known as molecular biology. Crick[92] has pointed out that this is an unfortunate term because it has two meanings. In the broad sense, it encompasses an explanation for any biological phenomenon in terms of atoms and molecules. However, as it is currently used, it is mainly applied to work on the interactions of proteins and nucleic acids, especially to studies of gene structure, replication, and expression, including protein synthesis and structure. Crick also claims that he was forced to call himself a molecular biologist because it was more convenient to do so when asked what he did by inquiring clergymen, rather than to explain that he was a mixture of crystallographer, biophysicist, biochemist, and geneticist!

The nucleic acids were first discovered by Miescher, who in 1871 reported the isolation of an acid material he called "nuclein" from the nuclei of pus cells. However, for many years, their chemical structure was considered to be too simple to be the basic genetic material of cells. In 1950 Chargaff[93] described the chemical composition of DNA and showed that in addition to sugar and phosphate, DNA contains four bases, adenine (A), guanine (G), thymine (T), and cytosine (C), in amounts such that the ratios A/T and G/C are equal to one. Armed with this information, and the knowledge that DNA is a helical molecule, from the work of Wilkins and Franklin, it was possible for Watson and Crick to propose their now famous model for the molecular structure of DNA in 1953.[94] During subsequent years, the way in which DNA replicates itself and stores the information necessary to direct the primary structure of proteins, the mechanisms whereby this information is transferred to the cell cytoplasm, and the way in which proteins are synthesized by cells have been worked out, at least in general terms.

The way in which the flow of information from DNA to protein is organized has become known as the "central dogma" of molecular biology. This can be summarized as follows. DNA is not itself the direct template which orders the amino-acid sequence. The genetic information of DNA is transferred to messenger RNAs, large polymeric molecules with bases exactly complementary to the DNA upon which they are synthesized. These RNA molecules are the definitive templates for protein synthesis. This relationship is written

$$\text{DNA} \xrightarrow{\text{transcription}} \text{RNA} \xrightarrow{\text{translation}} \text{protein}$$

The amino acids are transported to the messenger RNA templates on specific adaptor molecules or transfer RNAs.

By the end of the 1960s, a general scheme of how protein synthesis is organized had been worked out[76] (Figure 12-4). The genetic information for the structure of a particular peptide chain, the α or β chains of hemoglobin, for example, is determined by the sequence of nucleotide bases in the DNA of the structural gene for that chain on a particular chromosome in the cell nucleus. Each amino acid is specified by a sequence of three bases, called a codon. This genetic information is relayed to the cell cytoplasm by the synthesis of a strand of RNA on the DNA template of the structural gene. Because of the rules of base pairing, the RNA strand, or messenger RNA, will be a "mirror image" of the DNA from which it is transcribed. The messenger RNA moves from the nucleus to the cytoplasm, where it binds to the ribosomes, on which peptide chains are synthesized. The initial step in peptide-chain synthesis is a complex reaction that brings together an initiation codon (AUG) at the 5' end of the messenger RNA, a specific initiation transfer RNA that "recognizes" the initiation codon, the ribosomal subunits, and several protein initiation factors.

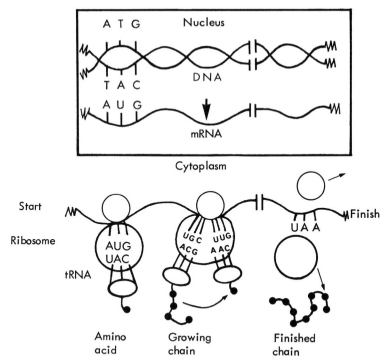

Figure 12-4 A diagrammatic representation of the main steps in protein synthesis. The genetic information for the structure of a protein is determined by the sequence of nucleotide bases in the DNA of the structural gene. In the diagram, each nucleotide base is designated by a letter (A, T, etc.). The nucleus is represented by the oblong box. (*From Weatherall DJ: The molecular basis for some genetic disorders of the red cell, in Weatherall, DJ (ed): Advanced Medicine. Kent, England, Pitman Medical, 1978, 385 pp, pp 327–339.*)

Once initiation has occurred, the process of translation follows. The ribosomes move along the messenger RNA from 5' to 3'. Each amino acid is carried to the template on a specific transfer RNA, which has a sequence of three bases, the anticodon, which can only bind to the appropriate codon of the messenger RNA. The nascent peptide chain, which is attached to the transfer RNA already in position, is successively transferred to each new incoming transfer RNA, and a peptide bond is formed with each new amino acid. In this way, a peptide chain gradually grows in length as the ribosome travels down the messenger RNA until a specific terminating codon (UAA or UAG) is reached, whereupon the process terminates, and the completed chain is released from the ribosomes to combine with other chains to form a protein.

This oversimplified story explains how genes control the structure of a protein. Obviously, there must be genetic mechanisms involved in the control of the rate of protein synthesis, the switching on and off of genes, and the many other complex metabolic activities that are operative in mammalian cells. However, nothing is known about these genetic control mechanisms in humans.

POTENTIAL MOLECULAR MECHANISMS
FOR THE THALASSEMIA SYNDROMES

Between 1960 and 1965, many theoretical models for the molecular basis for thalassemia were proposed. When hemoglobin A from patients with sickle-cell thalassemia was shown to have a normal structure, the "silent" amino-acid substitution theory was discarded. It was then suggested that at least some forms of thalassemia might be due to mutations at controller gene loci and, thus, would not involve structural genes. Borrowing freely from the elegant work of Jacob and Monod[95] on the control of gene expression in microorganisms, a series of models were proposed in which it was suggested that thalassemia might result from mutations at hypothetical "operator" or "regulator" loci, as defined in bacterial systems. Although it always seemed likely that the control of protein synthesis in human beings might be considerably more complex than in *Escherichia coli* these models stimulated much discussion, if little experimental work!

In 1963, Nance proposed quite a different mechanism for the basis of thalassemia based largely on Smithie's work on haptoglobin genetics and Baglioni's interpretation of how hemoglobin Lepore had arisen (Figure 12-3). Nance suggested[96] that there might have been a whole series of unequal but homologous crossovers at the globin complex, and, based on this mechanism, he was able to derive many of the thalassemia genotypes and phenotypes. Nance's paper is now largely forgotten, but recent work on the molecular basis for thalassemia indicates that he may have suggested the correct molecular mechanism for at least some forms of thalassemia.

In the early 1960s, it was easier to produce theories for the molecular basis for thalassemia than to design experiments to test the theories! The major problem was to decide at which level protein synthesis is abnormal. It was apparent that the abnormality could be anywhere between the structural gene and the globin chain. For example, it was possible that in those forms of thalassemia in which there is no globin chain synthesis, the globin genes might be deleted. On the other hand, the genes might be present, but there might be a defect in the mechanism of transcription or of processing of the messenger RNA. It was also possible that the lesion occurs at the cytoplasmic level in the mechanisms of chain initiation, translation, or termination. A defect of the latter type could arise from any one of several potential types of structural abnormality of the messenger RNA.

In the mid-1960s, the whole problem looked much too complicated, and it would have been a supreme optimist who would have predicted that within 10 years, many of these problems would be solved. The break came with the development of better techniques for studying hemoglobin synthesis in human red cell precursors.

GLOBIN CHAIN SYNTHESIS IN THALASSEMIA
IN INTACT CELLS AND CELL-FREE SYSTEMS

Once it became possible to study the synthesis of α and β chains of human hemoglobin in vitro in a quantitative way, it was possible to design experiments to look at the processes of globin chain initiation, elongation, and termination, both in normal and thalassemia reticulocytes. The earliest of these studies were based on techniques developed by Howard Dintzis[97] for studying the assembly of rabbit globin chains. Experiments of this type showed that the rates and patterns of assembly of thalassemic β chains were identical to those in normal individuals. This suggested that the β^+-thalassemias result from a reduced output of β-chain messenger RNA, but such messenger RNA that is made is functionally normal.[98] These and subsequent experiments seemed to rule out defects in the processes of chain initiation, translation, or termination as a cause for β^+-thalassemia. Such was the position in 1970.

The next major advance came when it became possible to isolate mammalian messenger RNA and to assess its activity in heterologous cell-free systems. This was first achieved by Schapira and his colleagues[99] using a rabbit reticulocyte system and by Lockard and Lingrel, who were able to stimulate mouse globin chain synthesis in a cell-free system derived from rabbit reticulocytes.[100] In 1971, Nienhuis and Anderson[101] and Benz and Forget[102] reported that they obtained human hemoglobin synthesis after adding either thalassemic or normal messenger RNA to a rabbit or to an Erlich's-ascites-tumor cell-free system, respectively. The same pattern of imbalanced globin chain that had been observed in the intact thalassemic cell was directed by thalassemic messenger RNA in the heterologous cell-free system. This provided further evidence that there is reduced β-chain messenger RNA activity in β-thalassemic cells. Similar methods were used to show that there is a deficiency of α-chain messenger RNA in the cells of patients with hemoglobin H disease.

All these experiments suggested that there is a deficiency of messenger RNA in the thalassemia syndromes. However, the techniques used could not distinguish between a reduced output of *normal* messenger RNA or the presence of normal amounts of an *abnormal* messenger RNA, which, for some reason, could not be utilized effectively for globin synthesis. The answer to this problem had to await the development of additional new technology, and this came in the early 1970s from the field of molecular hybridization.

MOLECULAR HYBRIDIZATION APPLIED TO THE THALASSEMIA PROBLEM

In 1964, Temin predicted that enzymes must exist for synthesizing DNA on RNA templates. Such an enzyme, reverse transcriptase, was isolated simultaneously in 1970 by Temin and Mizutani[103] and by Baltimore,[104] work which led to Baltimore and Temin receiving the Nobel Prize. This discovery has been of immense practical importance in the thalassemia field.

Once reverse transcriptase became available, it could be used to make DNA copies from specific messenger RNA templates. Thus, using relatively pure α- or β-chain messenger RNA, it was possible to copy complementary DNA (cDNA$_\alpha$ or cDNA$_\beta$) from these templates, and, if radioactive nucleotides were incorporated into the reaction, a radioactively labeled cDNA$_\alpha$ or cDNA$_\beta$ could be obtained. These techniques opened the way to two types of experiments (Figure 12-5). If DNA or double-stranded RNA is heated, the strands come apart and reanneal on cooling. If after denaturation, a radioactively labeled cDNA is added to the mixture of reannealing DNA or RNA, because of the rules of base pairing, it will only bind to the DNA or RNA if it finds identical base sequences. Thus, radioactive cDNA can be used as a sensitive "probe" to examine DNA or messenger RNA for the presence of complementary base sequences. Using the method of cDNA-RNA hybridization, several groups showed that there is a reduced amount of hybridizable β-chain messenger RNA in the cells of patients with homozygous and heterozygous β-thalassemia and that there is a reduced amount of hybridizable α-chain messenger RNA in the reticulocytes of patients with hemoglobin H disease.[105–107]

The next few years saw rapid progress in this field, particularly in the analysis of globin genes in different forms of thalassemia by cDNA-DNA hybridization. From these studies, the final answer to the molecular basis for at least some forms of thalassemia was obtained almost exactly 50 years after its first description by Cooley.

THE MOLECULAR BIOLOGY OF α-THALASSEMIA

The hemoglobin Bart's hydrops syndrome was the first form of thalassemia in which the molecular basis was completely worked out. Groups working independently in England and the United States designed the following experiment.[108,109] It was reasoned that if it were possible to obtain DNA from an infant with the hemoglobin Bart's hydrops syndrome and to make a relatively pure cDNA$_\alpha$ probe, i.e., cDNA copied from purified α-chain messenger RNA, by using the cDNA-DNA hybridization approach, it should be possible to ask whether DNA from the affected infant has any α-globin gene

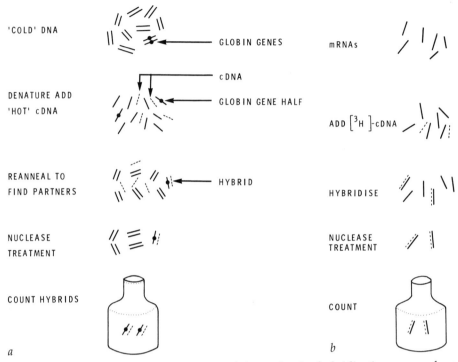

Figure 12-5 A simplified representation of the molecular hybridization approach as applied to the problem of thalassemia.

(a) An experiment using cDNA-DNA hybridization to determine whether there are any specific α- or β-chain globin genes in the total DNA of an individual with thalassemia. Radioactive cDNA is mixed with total DNA and allowed to hybridize under standard conditions. The presence or absence of hybridization indicates whether the globin genes are present or absent in the total DNA.

(b) An attempt to determine whether inactive globin messenger RNA is present in the cytoplasm of an individual with α- or β-thalassemia. Total RNA from peripheral blood cells is mixed with radioactive cDNA, and if inactive globin messenger RNA is present, this will hybridize; if no messenger RNA is present, no hybridization will occur.

sequences. Although this is asking whether the α-gene sequences are present in perhaps 10 million other sequences of similar size, this experiment is feasible because of the large amount of radioactivity that can be incorporated into the cDNA probes as shown in Figure 12-6. The results of this study showed that the α genes are largely deleted in DNA prepared from the liver of infants with hemoglobin Bart's hydrops syndrome (Figure 12-6). Because on genetic grounds it seems likely that normal individuals have two α-chain genes per haploid genome (that is, four genes in all),[110] these findings suggested that α-thalassemia-1 results from a deletion of both pairs of these genes. Therefore, homozygotes with the hemoglobin Bart's hydrops syndrome have no α-chain genes. Kan and his group went on to show that in hemoglobin H disease, there is a deletion of three out of the four α-globin genes.[111] This suggests that hemoglobin H results from the inheritance of α-thalassemia-1, in which both α genes are lost, and α-thalassemia-2, in which one of the linked pair of α genes is lost.

The final chapter in the story of the elucidation of the molecular basis of these common types of α-thalassemia came from a completely different approach. In 1970, Dr. Paul Milner, then working in Jamaica, studied a family in which three members had typical hemoglobin H disease. However, each of them had traces of an unusual hemoglobin variant in their red cells.[112] Genetic

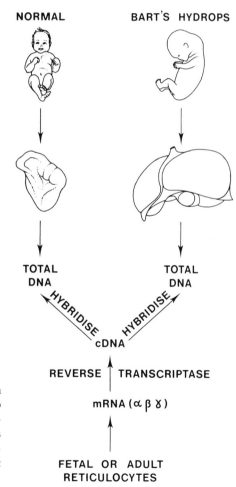

Figure 12-6 A schematic representation of the original experiment designed to answer whether the total DNA from infants with the hemoglobin Bart's hydrops syndrome contains any α-chain gene sequences. The details of this experiment are described in the text.

analysis of this family suggested that one parent of each of the affected siblings had typical α-thalassemia-1 while the other had a very mild thalassemia-like disorder together with an abnormal hemoglobin. This family came from a suburb of Kingston, Jamaica, called Constant Spring, and, hence, after its chemical characterization, the variant was named Constant Spring. Interestingly, trace amounts of an abnormal hemoglobin with properties similar to hemoglobin Constant Spring had been found quite independently in the blood of patients with hemoglobin H disease by Fessas' group in Athens, by Wasi and his colleagues in Thailand, and by Lie-Injo in Malaysia. Indeed, subsequent population studies indicated that about 2 percent of the population of Thailand carry hemoglobin Constant Spring.[113]

Hemoglobin Constant Spring turned out to be an unusual α-chain variant in that it has 31 additional amino acids at its C-terminal end. The α chain is normal up to position 141, where it usually ends, has glutamine at position 142, and a further 30 residues which do not resemble the sequence of any known protein. To explain this bizarre finding, it was suggested that it is caused by a mutation (i.e., a single base change) in the chain termination codon (UAA $\rightarrow$ CAA); thus, instead of reading "stop," glutamine (which is coded by CAA) is inserted, and then, a length of messenger RNA that is not normally utilized is translated until another "stop" codon appears. It was further postulated that the very low rate of synthesis of this variant (and hence the associated thalassemic blood picture) must be in some way connected with the "reading through" of this extra genetic material[114] (Figure 12-7). In the last few years, proof that this interpretation is correct has come from a variety of sources. Indeed, a whole family of these so-called α-termination mutant hemoglobins has been discovered, all associated with α-thalassemia.[114]

Thus, a relatively clear picture of the molecular basis of the α-thalassemia disorders, at least as they occur in Southeast Asia and parts of the Mediterranean, can now be put together. α-Thalassemia-1 is due to a loss of *both* α-chain genes, and the homozygous state produces the hemoglobin Bart's hydrops syndrome. The simultaneous inheritance of α-thalassemia-1 and α-thalassemia-2, or α-thalassemia-1 and hemoglobin Constant Spring, causes hemoglobin H disease. Hemoglobin Constant Spring, because of its slow rate of synthesis, produces an almost identical phenotype to α-thalassemia-2 (Figure 12-7).

While the molecular basis for the α-thalassemia disorders, as outlined in the previous sections, forms the basis for the varieties of the conditions seen in Southeast Asia and parts of the Mediterranean, this may not be the case in Africa and in the Middle East. The genetics of α-thalassemia in these populations is not yet worked out, and there is increasing evidence that there may be different underlying molecular mechanisms within these races. In particular, it is becoming clear that not all α-thalassemias are due to gene deletions.

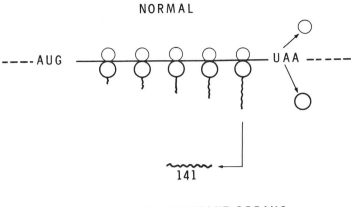

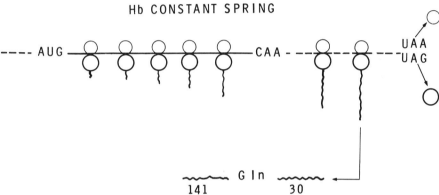

Figure 12-7 The molecular basis for the production of elongated α-chain variants, such as hemoglobin Constant Spring. A single base mutation in the chain termination codon allows extra messenger RNA to be translated with the production of an elongated α-chain variant. This is produced inefficiently and gives rise to the clinical phenotype of α-thalassemia.

THE MOLECULAR BIOLOGY OF β-THALASSEMIA

The molecular basis for the different forms of β-thalassemia has not proved so easy to sort out as that for α-thalassemia. The β-thalassemias are obviously an extremely heterogeneous group of conditions, and this is reflected at the molecular level just as it is by their remarkable clinical variability.

In β^+-thalassemia, there is a reduced amount of β-chain messenger RNA, but, as might be expected, the β chains are intact. So far, no further progress has been made in sorting out why the messenger RNA is produced at a reduced rate. Certainly such messenger RNA as is produced seems to function normally in all respects.

The molecular biology of β^0-thalassemia is extremely puzzling. Perhaps rather unexpectedly, it has been found that the β-globin genes are intact.[115] However, using the techniques of mRNA-cDNA hybridization, there is evidence for considerable molecular heterogeneity.[116–118] In some cases, no hybridizable β messenger RNA is present, while in others, β-globin messenger RNA is present but is not utilized for protein synthesis. This suggests that it is structurally abnormal. It should not be too long before enough of this material is available for chemical analysis so that the precise defect in its structure can be worked out.

$\delta\beta$-thalassemia has turned out to be more amenable to analysis by molecular hybridization. The homozygous state is rare, but DNA has been made from two affected individuals, and the β- and, probably, the δ-globin genes are deleted.[119]

THE ARRANGEMENT OF THE HUMAN HEMOGLOBIN GENES AND THEIR CONTROL AREAS

The production of hemoglobin Lepore by abnormal crossing over between the δ- and β-gene loci has already been described. This observation suggested that these loci must lie close together on the same chromosome (i.e., be closely linked). In 1972, a variant called hemoglobin Kenya was discovered.[120] This has a non-α chain which consists of the N-terminal residues of the γ chain and the C-terminal residues of the β chain. It is likely that this arose just like hemoglobin Lepore except that the abnormal crossing over was between the γ- and β-chain genes (Figure 12-3). This indicates that the γ chains must be linked to the δ and β chains in a tight cluster, i.e., γ-δ-β.

Another important milestone in the human hemoglobin story came in 1968 with the discovery by Schroeder and Huisman that normal human fetal hemoglobin is heterogeneous.[121] They showed that it is a mixture of molecules with the formula $\alpha_2\gamma_2^{136\text{-glycine}}$ and $\alpha_2\gamma_2^{136\text{-alanine}}$. The γ chains which contain glycine or alanine at position 136 are called $^G\gamma$ and $^A\gamma$, respectively. Genetic analysis of γ-chain variants has provided clear evidence that these $^G\gamma$ and $^A\gamma$ chains are the products of separate gene loci and, hence, that the human γ chains are controlled by two distinct structural loci.

When hemoglobin Kenya was discovered, it was found that heterozygous carriers had persistent hemoglobin F synthesis and that this was all of the $^G\gamma$ type. Thus, it was suggested that the human hemoglobin genes are linked in the order $^G\gamma$-$^A\gamma$-δ-β and that part of the $^A\gamma$, the whole of the δ, and part of the β chain are deleted during the crossing over "accident," which produces the $\gamma\beta$ fusion gene, which gives rise to hemoglobin Kenya (Figure 12-3). The fact that carriers of hemoglobin Kenya have persistent $^G\gamma$-chain production in adult life suggests that there is an area of the γ-δ-β gene cluster near the γ-chain locus which is involved in the suppression of γ-chain synthesis in adult life.

During the years when the thalassemias were being characterized, a related disorder, hereditary persistence of fetal hemoglobin (HPFH) was described. It was first observed in Africa by Edington and Lehmann in 1955[122] and studied extensively in the Baltimore black population by Conley and his group at the Johns Hopkins Hospital in the early 1960s.[123] Heterozygotes have about 25 percent fetal hemoglobin, while homozygotes have 100 percent fetal hemoglobin; there are no clinical abnormalities. These observations suggest that in HPFH, there is an absence of β- and δ-chain production and persistent γ-chain production, which totally compensates for the lack of β and δ chains. Like thalassemia, HPFH is a very heterogeneous condition, and the best characterized variety is found in Africans. In 1974, several groups independently showed that African HPFH is due to a deletion of the β and δ chains.[119,124,125] This finding, together with those in the carriers of hemoglobin Kenya, provides unequivocal evidence that there are areas in the γ-δ-β gene cluster that are involved in the suppression of fetal hemoglobin production in adult life. How these control areas operate and how they are related to neonatal switching from fetal to adult hemoglobin production remain the major unsolved problems in the human hemoglobin field.

The Present Position and Future Perspectives

It has taken just over 50 years to progress from Cooley's first description of thalassemia to our present state of knowledge. We now know that the thalassemia syndromes are among the commonest group of single-gene disorders in the world population and that they represent a very heterogeneous group of disorders of protein synthesis. Almost all the defects in the genetic machinery of a cell which have been described by microbial geneticists have now been found in humans as the basis for the different forms of thalassemia. These include single base substitutions both in the coding genes and in such critical control areas as the termination codons; deletions of genetic material, including whole genes or individual codons; abnormal crossing over, with the production of fusion genes; the production of structurally abnormal messenger RNA; the complete failure of transcription of structural genes; and a variety of defects in the control of the rate of messenger RNA synthesis which still remain to be fully defined. Indeed, even while this essay was being written some remarkable advances were being made in the elucidation of the basic molecular defects in thalassemia. By means of the very recently developed techniques of gene mapping, it has been possible to actually visualize the gene deletions which produce various forms of the disease. Even more remarkable is the news that it has been possible to isolate the human hemoglobin genes and insert them into the DNA of plasmids and hence to allow them to grow in clones of bacteria. Already, genes from thalassemic patients have been successfully grown in this way, and it is only a matter of time before they are fully sequenced. These developments will not only provide a ready source of DNA probes but should also allow structural studies to be carried out on the DNA of the α- and β-globin genes in both normal and thalassemic persons, including studies of some of the forms of β-thalassemia in which the genes seem to be intact. In addition, this technology should enable us to produce a map of the human hemoglobin genome. Clearly then, the thalassemias provide a model system for understanding the molecular genetics of any human disease that is caused by defective protein synthesis.

A question which may have occurred to the reader is whether all this rather esoteric science is of any value to patients suffering from thalassemia. Indeed, a similar question occurred to MacFarlane Burnet when he wrote *Genes, Dreams and Realities*.[126] In this book, he argued that molecular biology, while an amusing pastime for the intellectually gifted, is of no practical value whatever, and he extends his thesis with the theme that understanding cellular mechanisms is unlikely to produce anything of practical use in the fields of genetics or cancer. It is of interest to note that sickle-cell anemia gets a single mention as a "rare disease found only in Africa." Thalassemia is not mentioned at all!

While there is no doubt that the thalassemia field has not moved as rapidly at the practical level as at the fundamental level, perhaps some of the basic knowledge is not entirely wasted. By knowing the pathophysiology well, the clinician is able to organize his supportive management of the disease much more logically even though there is still no cure for any of the thalassemia disorders. The methods which were designed to study the rate of globin chain synthesis in vitro have been used recently to study intrauterine hemoglobin synthesis both in normal and thalassemic fetuses. As a direct extension of this work, a method for the prenatal diagnosis of thalassemia has been developed and is showing considerable promise.[127] If this becomes generally available, then much of the technology described in this chapter will come into its own, particularly in the area of genetic counseling and for the more accurate diagnosis of the complicated thalassemia syndromes. For this reason, and simply because most of the information about the molecular basis of these diseases has only been available for a few years, it seems much too early to predict how much of this work will be of practical value in the future.

The great unsolved problem in the field of hemoglobin is that of the control of the switch from fetal to adult hemoglobin. This is a challenging area because there is clear evidence that if it were possible either to prevent the switch or to reactivate fetal hemoglobin production, the β-chain hemoglobinopathies could be controlled. Perhaps the idea of making use of fetal genes to replace those that are structurally or functionally abnormal in adult life is the most exciting potential application of the molecular approach to human disease that we have.

Lessons from the Thalassemia Story for Medical Research in General

The thalassemia story has most of the ingredients present in any area of progress in medical research. It started with careful clinical descriptions and classifications, continued through an era of discovering the pathophysiology by the application of the standard methods of clinical research, and finally moved into the realm of molecular biology, where, because of the peculiarities of the red cell precursor, it has been possible for the first time to apply techniques from this relatively new discipline to human disease. The story has been interspersed with the usual blind alleys, personality clashes, strokes of good luck, and the general chaotic pattern of development which characterizes most medical research. There are, however, one or two particularly interesting points about the way the subject has developed.

Perhaps the major reason for the rapid progress in the thalassemia field in recent years has been the application of techniques from a wide range of often unrelated disciplines to the unraveling of the story of the disease. Certainly, none of the work that was done in the hemoglobin field between 1950 and 1960 was directly related to furthering our understanding of thalassemia. Moreover, the advances in molecular biology that have resulted in a better understanding of the molecular basis of thalassemia were all made by molecular biologists, most of whom had never heard of thalassemia! Probably nobody would have been more surprised than Temin or Baltimore if he had been told that their discovery of reverse transcriptase would help to sort out the genetic basis of some common inherited disorders of hemoglobin long before it provided any real insight into the cellular basis of cancer! Although those who administer research funds must be thoroughly confused by a story of this type, it is perhaps worth reminding them that the support of good basic research often has a fallout that is totally unpredictable. The thalassemia story is a perfect example of how good basic science in one field may have a profound effect on a totally unrelated field.

Another question raised by the thalassemia story is who should carry out the fundamental work on the cellular genetics of human disease. It is interesting to note that, until very recently, most of the progress in the thalassemia field has been made by medically orientated research groups with the occasional advice of basic scientists. In 1970, the Symposium on Molecular Hematology was held in Cambridge, and many of the problems of protein synthesis in thalassemia and related disorders were reviewed. In summing up, Sidney Brenner said that all these problems could be solved in a very short time with the techniques then available to molecular biologists. In fact, few molecular biologists have shown any interest whatever in the thalassemia field until the last year or so. This is because many of the problems that interest them can be worked out more easily in microbial systems, and they consider protein synthesis in human red cells to be a relatively "dirty" model system.

The lesson to be drawn from the thalassemia field is that it is essential to have medical scientists sufficiently well educated in the field of molecular biology so that they can at least initiate experiments and communicate well enough with molecular biologists to be able to ask the right questions relating to human disease. Clearly, the problem of bringing together the clinical and basic sciences is one which is not going to be solved easily; even in a relatively clear-cut field like that described in this essay, there have been (and still are) many difficulties in the organization of research in the "no man's land" between the patient and his DNA.

Acknowledgments

The author is indebted to Dr. Robin Bannerman for the excellent account of some aspects of the early history of thalassemia which appears in his monograph. It is also a pleasure to acknowledge the help of many authors who have provided reprints of their early work, in particular, Professor Ezio Silvestroni and Dr. Ida Bianco. An extensive bibliography of their early work in Italy can be found in Il Policlinico—Sezione Practica 75:1645–1669, 1969 (Edizioni Luigo Pozzi, Roma).

References

1 Bannerman RM: Thalassemia. A Survey of Some Aspects. New York and London, Grune and Stratton, 1961, 138 pp.
2 Chini V, Valeri CM: Mediterranean hemopathic syndromes. Blood, 4:989–1013, 1949.
3 Jacsch, R von: Über leukämie und leukocytose im kindesalter. Wien Klin Wochenschr 2:435–456, 1889.
4 Jacsch R von: Uber diagnose und therapie der erkrankungen des blutes. Prague Med Wochenschr 15:389, 403, 414, 1890.
5 Whitcher BR: Erythroblastemia of infants. Am J Med Sci 179:1–6, 1930.
6 Capper A: The nature of von Jaksch's anemia and the effect of splenectomy. Am J Med Sci 181:1–10, 1931.
7 Zuelzer WW: Thomas B. Cooley (1871–1945). J Pediatr 49:642–650, 1956.
8 Cooley TB, Lee P: A series of cases of splenomegaly in children with anemia and peculiar bone changes. Trans Am Pediatr Soc 37:29, 1925.
9 Cooley TB, Witwer ER, Lee P: Anemia in children with splenomegaly and peculiar changes in bones; report of cases. Am J Dis Child 34:347–363, 1927.
10 Whipple GH, Bradford WL: Mediterranean disease-thalassemia (erythroblastic anemia of Cooley); associated pigment abnormalities simulating hemochromatosis. J Pediatr 9:279–311, 1936.
11 Diggs LW: Dr. George Hoyt Whipple. Johns Hopkins Med J 139:196–200, 1976.
12 Corner GW: Personal communication.
13 Caminopetros J: Kliniki vol 12, no 5, 1936.
14 Rietti F: Ittero emolitico primitivo. Atti Accad Sci Med Nat Ferrara 2:14–19, 1925.

15 Greppi E: Ittero emolitico familiare con aumento della resistenza dei globuli. *Minerva Med* 8:1–11, 1928.

16 Micheli F, Penati F, Momigliano LG: Ulteriori richerche sulla anemia ipocromica splenomegalica con poichilocitosi. *Atti Soc Ital Ematol Haematologica* (*Pavia*) 16(suppl):10–13, 1935.

17 Caminopetros J: Recherches sur l'anemie érythroblastique infantile des peuples de la Mediteraneé orientale, étude anthroloogique, étiologique et pathogénique; la transmission héréditaire de la maladie. *Ann de Med* 43:104–125, 1938.

18 Angelini V: Primi risultati di richerche ematologiche nei familiari de ammalati di anemia di Cooley. *Minerva Med* 28:331–332, 1937.

19 Wintrobe MM, Mathews E, Pollack R, Dobyns BM: Familial hemopoietic disorder in Italian adolescents and adults resembling Mediterranean disease (thalassemia). *JAMA* 114:1530–1538, 1940.

20 Conley CL, Wintrobe MM: Thalassemia in the "D" family: case presentation: Mr. D. *Johns Hopkins Med J* 139:201–204, 1976.

21 Dameshek W: "Target cell" anaemia. An erythroblastic type of Cooley's erythroblastic anemia. *Am J Med Sci* 200:445–454, 1940.

22 Strauss MB, Daland GA, Fox HJ: Familial microcytic anemia. Observations on 6 cases of a blood disorder in an Italian family. *Am J Med Sci* 201:30–34, 1941.

23 Silvestroni E, Bianco I: Prime osservazioni di resistenze globulari aumentate in soggetti sani e rapporto fra questi soggetti e i malati di cosidetto ittero emolitico con resistenze globulari aumentate. *Boll Atti Accad Med* (*Roma*) 69:293–306, 1943–1944.

24 Gatto L: Thalassemia (microcarterocitosi). *Giorn di Med* 4:287–289, 1947.

25 Gatto L: Sulle ereditarieta della malattia di Cooley. *Minerva Med* 39:I 194–198, 1948.

26 Smith CH: Detection of mild types of Mediterranean (Cooley's) anemia. *Am J Dis Child* 75:505–527, 1948.

27 Silvestroni E: Microcitemia e malattie a substrato microcitemico, falcemia e malattie felcemiche. *50° Congresso Soc Med Int Roma* 3:108, 1949.

28 Silvestroni E, Bianco I: Ricerche sui familiari sani di malati di morbo di Cooley. *Ric Morfol* 22:217–221, 1946.

29 Valentine WN, Neel JV: A statistical study of the hematologic variables in subjects with thalassemia minor. *Am J Med Sci* 215:456–462, 1948.

30 Valentine WN, Neel JV: Hematologic and genetic study of transmission of thalassemia. *Arch Intern Med* 74:185–196, 1944.

31 Marmont A, Bianchi V: Mediterranean anaemia: clinical and haematological findings, and pathogenetic studies in milder forms of disease (with report of cases). *Acta Haematol* (*Basel*) 1:4–28, 1948.

32 Bianco I, Montalenti G, Silvestroni E, Siniscalso M: Further data on genetics of microcythaemia or thalassaemia minor and Cooley's disease or thalassaemia major. *Ann Eugenics* 16:299–314, 1952.

32a Körber E: Inaugural Dissertations, Dorpat 1866. Cited by Bischoff H: Untersuchungen über die Resistenz des Hämoglobins des menschenblutes mit besonderer berüchsichtigung des Sauglingalters, *Ztschr fd ges Exper Med* 48:472–489, 1926.

33 Pauling L, Itano HA, Singer SK, Wells IS: Sickle cell anemia; a molecular disease. *Science* 110:543–548, 1949.

34 Neel JV: Inheritance of sickle-cell anemia. *Science* 110:64–66, 1949.

35   Beet EA: Genetics of sickle-cell trait in Bantu tribe. *Ann Eugenics* 14:279–284, 1949.

36   Lambotte-Legrand J, Lambotte-Legrand C: L'anémie à hématies falciformes chez l'infant indigène du Bas-Congo. Étude génétique, clinique et hématologique basée sur 88 cas. *Mem Acad R Soc Colon Clin Sci Nat Med* 19:1–93, 1950.

37   Itano HA, Neel JV: A new inherited abnormality of human hemoglobin. *Proc Natl Acad Sci USA* 36:613–617, 1950.

38   Ranney HM: Observations on the inheritance of sickle-cell hemoglobin and hemoglobin C. *J Clin Invest* 33:1634–1641, 1954.

39   Smith EW, Torbert JV: Study of two abnormal hemoglobins with evidence for a new genetic locus for hemoglobin formation. *Bull Johns Hopkins Hosp* 102:38–45, 1958.

40   Kunkel HG, Wallenius G: New hemoglobin in normal adult blood. *Science* 122:288, 1955.

41   Ceppellini R: L'emoglobina normale lenta A_2. *Acta Genet Med Gemellol (Roma)* 8(suppl 2):47–68, 1959.

42   Ingram VM: A specific chemical difference between the globins of normal human and sickle-cell anaemia haemoglobin. *Nature* 178:792–794, 1956.

43   Rhinesmith HS, Schroeder WA, Pauling L: A quantitative study of hydrolysis of human dinitrophenyl (DNP) globin: the number and kind of polypeptide chains in normal adult human hemoglobin. *J Am Chem Soc* 79:4682–4686, 1957.

44   Braunitzer G, Hilschmann N, Rudloff V, Hilse K, Liebold B, Müller R: The haemoglobin particles. Chemical and genetic aspects of their structure. *Nature* 190:480–482, 1961.

45   Perutz MF, Rossmann MG, Cullis AF, Muirhead H, Will G, North ACT: Structure of haemoglobin. *Nature* 185:416–422, 1960.

46   Schroeder WA, Matsuda GJ: N-terminal residues of human fetal hemoglobin. *J Am Chem Soc* 80:1521, 1958.

47   Weatherall DJ, Baglioni C: A fetal hemoglobin variant of unusual genetic interest. *Blood* 20:675–685, 1962.

48   Minnich V, Cordonnier JK, Williams WJ, Moore CV: Alpha, beta and gamma hemoglobin polypeptide chains during the neonatal period with description of fetal form of hemoglobin $D_{\alpha St.Louis}$. *Blood* 19:137–167, 1962.

49   Vecchio F: Sulla resistenza della emoglobina alla denaturazione alcalina in alcune sindromi emopatiche. *Pediatria (Napoli)* 54:545–549, 1946.

50   Rich A: Studies on the hemoglobin of Cooley's anemia and Cooley's trait. *Proc Natl Acad Sci USA* 38:187–196, 1952.

51   Silvestroni E, Bianco I: Microdrepanocitoanemia in un sogetto di razza bianca. *Boll Atti Accad Med (Roma)* 70:347–362, 1944–1945.

52   Silvestroni E, Bianco I: *La malattia microdrepanocitica.* Il Pensiero Scientifico. Editore, Roma. 1955, 138 pp.

53   Powell WN, Rodarte JG, Neel JV: The occurrence in a family of Sicilian ancestry of the traits for both sickling and thalassemia. *Blood* 5:887–897, 1950.

54   Sturgeon P, Itano HA, Valentine WN: Chronic hemolytic anemia associated with thalassemia and sickling trait. *Blood* 7:350–357, 1952.

55   Singer K, Singer L, Goldberg SR: Studies on abnormal hemoglobins. XI. Sickle cell-thalassemia disease in the Negro. The significance of the S+A+F and S+A patterns obtained by hemoglobin analysis. *Blood* 10:405–415, 1955.

56 Zuelzer WW, Kaplan E: Thalassemia hemoglobin C-disease; a new syndrome presumably due to the combination of the genes for thalassemia and hemoglobin C. *Blood* 9:1047–1054, 1954.

57 Cohen F, Zuelzer WW, Neel JV, Robinson AR: Multiple inherited erythrocyte abnormalities in an American negro family: hereditary spherocytosis, sickling and thalassemia. *Blood* 14:816–827, 1959.

58 Gerald PS, Diamond LK: The diagnosis of thalassemia trait by starch block electrophoresis of the hemoglobin. *Blood* 13:61–69, 1958.

59 Kunkel HG, Ceppellini R, Müller-Eberhard U, Wolf J: Observations on the minor basic hemoglobin component in blood of normal individuals and patients with thalassemia. *J Clin Invest* 36:1615–1625, 1957.

60 Rigas DA, Koler RD, Osgood EE: New hemoglobin possessing a higher electrophoretic mobility than normal adult hemoglobin. *Science* 121:372, 1955.

61 Gouttas A, Fessas P, Tsevrenis H, Xefteri E: Description d'une nouvelle variete d'anaemie hemolytique congenitale. (Etude hematologique, electrophoretique et genetique.) *Sang* 26:911–919, 1955.

62 Jones RT, Schroeder WA: Chemical characterization and subunit hybridization of human hemoglobin H and associated compounds. *Biochemistry* 2:1357–1367, 1963.

63 Fessas P, Papaspyrou A: A new fast hemoglobin associated with thalassemia. *Science* 126:1119, 1957.

64 Ager JAM, Lehmann H: Observations on some "fast" hemoglobins: K, J, N and "Bart's". *Br Med J* i:929–931, 1958.

65 Hunt JA, Lehmann H: Abnormal human haemoglobins. Haemoglobin "Bart's": a foetal haemoglobin without α-chains. *Nature* 184:872–873, 1959.

66 Itano HA: Qualitative and quantitative control of adult hemoglobin synthesis: a multiple allele hypothesis. *Am J Hum Genet* 5:34–45, 1953.

67 Pauling L: Abnormality of hemoglobin molecules in hereditary hemolytic anemias, in *The Harvey Lectures 1954–55*. New York, Academic Press, 1954, pp 216–241.

68 Itano HA: The human hemoglobins: their properties and genetic control. *Adv Protein Chem* 12:216–268, 1957.

69 Ingram VM, Stretton AOW: Genetic basis of the thalassaemia diseases. *Nature* 184:1903–1909, 1959.

70 Itano HA, Pauling L: Thalassaemia and the abnormal human haemoglobins. *Nature* 191:398–399, 1961.

71 Chernoff AI: The distribution of the thalassemia gene: a historical review. *Blood* 14:899–912, 1959.

72 Chernoff AI, Minnich V, Na-Nakorn S, Tuchinda S, Kashemsant C, Chernoff RR: Studies on hemoglobin E. I. The clinical, hematologic and genetic characteristics of the hemoglobin E syndromes. *J Lab Clin Med* 47:455–489, 1956.

73 Minnich V, Na-Nakorn S, Tuchinda S, Pravitt W, Moore CV: Inclusion body anemia in Thailand (hemoglobin H-thalassemia disease), in *Proc. 6th Cong. Int. Soc. Hemat, Boston.* New York, Grune and Stratton, 1958, p 743.

74 Wasi P, Na-Nakorn S, Pootrakul S, Sookanek M, Disthasongchan P, Pornpatkul M, Panich V: Alpha- and beta-thalassemia in Thailand. *Ann NY Acad Sci* 165:60–82, 1969.

75 Chatterjee JB: Haemoglobinopathy in India, in Jonxis JHP, Delafresnaye JF (eds):

   Abnormal Haemoglobins. Oxford, Blackwell Scientific, 1959, 427 pp, pp 322–339.

76 Weatherall DJ, Clegg JB: *The Thalassaemia Syndromes,* 2d ed. Oxford, Blackwell Scientific, 1972, 374 pp.

77 Silvestroni E, Bianco I: The distribution of the microcythaemias (or thalassaemias) in Italy. Some aspects of the haematological and haemoglobinic picture in these haemopathies, in Jonxis JHP, Delefresnaye JF (eds): *Abnormal Haemoglobins.* Oxford, Blackwell Scientific, 1959, 427 pp, pp 242–259.

78 Fessas P: Thalassaemia and the alterations of the haemoglobin pattern, in Jonxis JHP, Delefresnaye JF (eds): *Abnormal Haemoglobins.* Oxford, Blackwell Scientific, 1959, 427 pp, pp 134–155.

79 Lie-Injo LE, Jo Bwan Hie: Hydrops foetalis with a fast-moving haemoglobin. *Br Med J* ii:1649–1650, 1960.

80 Baglioni C: The fusion of two peptide chains in hemoglobin Lepore and its interpretation as a genetic deletion. *Proc Natl Acad Sci USA* 48:1880–1886, 1962.

81 Neeb H, Beiboer JL, Jonxis JHP, Sijpesteijn JAK, Müller CJ: Homozygous Lepore haemoglobin disease appearing as thalassaemia major in two Papuan siblings. *Trop Geogr Med* 13:207–215, 1961.

82 Sturgeon P, Finch CA: Erythrokinetics in Cooley's anemia. *Blood* 12:64–73, 1957.

83 Bannerman RM, Grinstein M, Moore CV: Haemoglobin synthesis in thalassaemia: in vitro studies. *Br J Haematol* 5:102–120, 1959.

84 Finch CA, Deubelbeiss K, Cook JD, Eschbach JW, Harker LA, Funk DD, Marsaglia G, Hillman RS, Slichter S, Adamson JW, Ganzoni A, Giblett ER: Ferrokinetics in man. *Medicine (Baltimore)* 49:17–53, 1970.

85 Fessas P: Inclusions of hemoglobin in erythroblasts and erythrocytes of thalassemia. *Blood* 21:21–32, 1963.

86 Nathan DG, Gunn RB: Thalassemia: the consequences of unbalanced hemoglobin synthesis. *Am J Med* 41:815–830, 1966.

87 Marks PA, Burka ER: Hemoglobin synthesis in human reticulocytes: a defect in globin formation in thalassemia major. *Ann NY Acad Sci* 119:513–522, 1964.

88 Marks PA, Burka ER, Rifkind RA: Control of protein synthesis in reticulocytes and the formation of hemoglobin A and F in thalassemia syndromes and other hemolytic anemias. *Medicine (Baltimore)* 43:769–778, 1964.

89 Heywood JD, Karon M, Weissman S: Amino acids: incorporation into alpha- and beta-chain of hemoglobin by normal and thalassemic reticulocytes. *Science* 146:530–531, 1964.

90 Clegg JB, Naughton MA, Weatherall DJ: Abnormal human hemoglobins. Separation and characterisation of the α- and β-chains by chromatography, and the determination of two new variants, *J Mol Biol* 19:91–108, 1966.

91 Weatherall DJ, Clegg JB, Naughton MA: Globin synthesis in thalassaemia: an in vitro study. *Nature* 208:1061–1065, 1965.

92 Crick FHC: Recent research in molecular biology: Introduction. *Br Med Bull* 21:183–186, 1965.

93 Chargaff E: Chemical specificity of nucleic acids and the mechanism of their enzymatic degradation. *Experientia* 6:201–209, 1950.

94 Watson JD, Crick FHC: Molecular structure of nucleic acids. A structure for desoxyribose nucleic acid. *Nature* 171:737–738, 1953.

95   Jacob F, Monod J: Genetic regulatory mechanisms in the synthesis of proteins. *J Mol Biol* 3:318–356, 1961.

96   Nance WE: Genetic control of hemoglobin synthesis. *Science* 141:123–130, 1963.

97   Dintzis HM: Assembly of the peptide chains of hemoglobin. *Proc Natl Acad Sci USA* 47:247–261, 1961.

98   Clegg JB, Weatherall DJ, Na-Nakorn S, Wasi P: Haemoglobin synthesis in β-thalassaemia. *Nature* 220:664–668, 1968.

99   Schapira G, Dreyfus JC, Maleknia N: The ambiguities in rabbit haemoglobin: evidence for a messenger RNA translated specifically into haemoglobin. *Biochem Biophys Res Comm* 32:558–561, 1968.

100   Lingrel JB, Lockard RE, Jones RF, Burr HE, Holder JW: Biologically active messenger RNA for haemoglobin. *Ser haematol* 4:37–69, 1971.

101   Nienhuis AW, Anderson WF: Isolation and translation of hemoglobin messenger RNA from thalassemia, sickle cell anemia, and normal human reticulocytes. *J Clin Invest* 50:2458–2460, 1971.

102   Benz EJ, Forget BG: Defect in messenger RNA for human hemoglobin synthesis in beta thalassemia. *J Clin Invest* 50:2755–2760, 1971.

103   Temin HM, Mizutani S: RNA-dependent DNA polymerase in virions of Rous sarcoma virus. *Nature* 226:1211–1213, 1970.

104   Baltimore D: RNA-dependent DNA polymerase in virions of RNA tumour viruses. *Nature* 226:1209–1211, 1970.

105   Kacian DL, Gambino R, Dow LW, Grossbard E, Natta C, Ramirez F, Spiegelman S, Marks, PA, Bank A: Decreased globin messenger RNA in thalassemia detected by molecular hybridization. *Proc Natl Acad Sci USA* 70:1886–1890, 1973.

106   Houseman D, Forget BG, Skoultchi A, Benz EJ: Quantitative deficiency of chain specific messenger ribonucleic acids in the thalassemia syndromes. *Proc Natl Acad Sci USA* 70:1809–1813, 1973.

107   Forget BG, Baltimore D, Benz EJ, Housman D, Lebowitz P, Marotta CA, McCaffrey RP, Skoultchi A, Swerdlow PS, Verma IM, Weissman SM: Globin messenger RNA in the thalassemia syndromes. *Ann NY Acad Sci* 232:76–87, 1974.

108   Ottolenghi S, Lanyon WG, Paul J, Williamson R, Weatherall DJ, Clegg JB, Pritchard J, Pootrakul S, Wong Hock Boon: The severe form of α thalassaemia is caused by a haemoglobin gene deletion. *Nature* 251:389–392, 1974.

109   Taylor JM, Dozy A, Kan YW, Varmus HE, Lie-Injo LE, Ganeson J, Todd D: Genetic lesion in homozygous α thalassaemia (hydrops fetalis). *Nature* 251:392–393, 1974.

110   Lehmann H, Carrell RW: Difference between α- and β-chain mutants of human haemoglobin and between α- and β-thalassaemia. Possible duplication of the α-chain gene. *Br Med J* 4:748–750, 1968.

111   Kan YW, Dozy AM, Varmus HE, Taylor JM, Holland JP, Lie-Injo LE, Ganeson J, Todd D: Deletion of α-globin genes in haemoglobin-H disease demonstrates multiple α-globin structural loci. *Nature* 255:255–256, 1975.

112   Clegg JB, Weatherall DJ, Milner PF: Haemoglobin Constant Spring—a chain termination mutant? *Nature* 234:337–340, 1971.

113   Fessas P, Lie-Injo LE, Na-Nakorn S, Todd D, Clegg JB, Weatherall DJ: Identification of slow-moving haemoglobins in haemoglobin H disease from different racial groups. *Lancet* i:1308–1310, 1972.

114   Weatherall DJ, Clegg JB: The α chain termination mutants and their relationship to the α thalassaemias. *Phil Trans Roy Soc* 271:411–455, 1975.
115   Tolstoshev P, Mitchell J, Lanyon G, Williamson R, Ottolenghi S, Comi P, Giglioni B, Masera G, Modell B, Weatherall DJ, Clegg JB: Presence of gene for β globin in homozygous β^0 thalassaemia. *Nature* 260:95–98, 1976.
116   Kan YW, Holland JP, Dozy AM, Varmus HE: Demonstration of non-functional β-globin mRNA in homozygous β^0-thalassemia. *Proc Nat Acad Sci USA* 72:5140–5144, 1975.
117   Ramirez F, O'Donnell JV, Marks PA, Bank A, Musumeci S, Schiliro G, Pizzarelli G, Russo G, Lippio B, Gambino R: Abnormal or absent β mRNA β^0 in Ferrara and gene deletion in $\delta\beta$ thalassaemia. *Nature* 263:471–475, 1976.
118   Temple GF, Chang JC, Kan YW: Authentic β-globin mRNA sequences in homozygous β^0-thalassemia. *Proc Nat Acad Sci USA* 74:3047–3051, 1977.
119   Ottolenghi S, Comi P, Giglioni B, Tolstoshev P, Lanyon WG, Mitchell GJ, Williamson R, Russo G, Musumeci S, Schiliro G, Tsistrakis GA, Charache S, Wood WG, Clegg JB, Weatherall DJ: $\delta\beta$-thalassemia is due to a gene deletion. *Cell* 9:71–80, 1976.
120   Huisman THJ, Wrightstone RN, Wilson JB, Schroeder WA, Kendall AG: Hemoglobin Kenya, the product of a fusion of γ and β polypeptide chains. *Arch Biochem Biophys* 153:850–853, 1972.
121   Schroeder WA, Huisman THJ, Shelton R, Shelton JB, Kleihauer EF, Dozy AM, Robberson B: Evidence for multiple structural genes for the γ-chain of human fetal hemoglobin. *Proc Nat Acad Sci USA* 60:537–544, 1968.
122   Edington GM, Lehmann H: Expression of the sickle-cell gene in Africa. *Br Med J* 1:1308–1311 and 2:1328, 1955.
123   Conley CL, Weatherall DJ, Richardson SN, Shepard MK, Charache S: Hereditary persistence of fetal hemoglobin: a study of 79 affected persons in 15 Negro families in Baltimore. *Blood* 21:261–281, 1963.
124   Forget BG, Hillman DG, Lazarus H, Barell EF, Benz EJ, Caskey CT, Huisman THJ, Schroeder WA, Housman D: Absence of messenger RNA and gene DNA for β-globin chains in hereditary persistence of fetal hemoglobin. *Cell* 7:323–329, 1976.
125   Kan YW, Holland JP, Dozy AM, Charache S, Kazazian HH: Deletion of the β-globin structure gene in hereditary persistence of foetal haemoglobin. *Nature* 258:162–163, 1975.
126   Burnet M: *Genes, Dreams and Realities*. Aylesbury, Medical and Technical Publishing, 1971, 136 pp.
127   Kan YW: Prenatal diagnosis of hemoglobin disorders, in Brown EB (ed): *Progress in Hematology*, vol X. New York, Grune and Stratton, 1977, 421 pp, pp 91–104.

CHAPTER 13

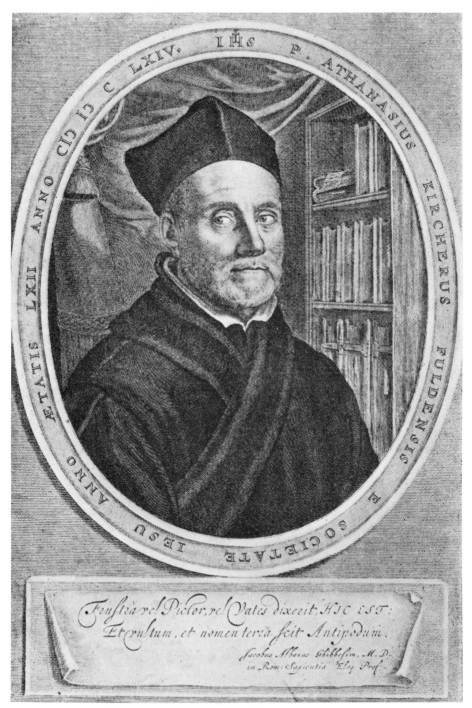

Frustra vel Pictor, vel Vates dixerit, HIC EST:
Et vultum, et nomen tercia fecit Antipodum.

Jacobus Albanus Ghibbesius. M.D.
in Rom: Sapientia Eloq Prof.

DEFENSES OF THE BODY:
THE INITIATORS OF DEFENSE,
THE READY RESERVES, AND
THE SCAVENGERS

Charles G. Craddock

O ur understanding of the sophisticated, multicellular systems involved in the defenses of the body has evolved from the microscopic recognition of the white blood corpuscles (leukocytes) in the eighteenth century (Senac and Hewson) and the demonstration in 1886 by Ilya (or Elie) Metchnikov (or Metchnikoff) of phagocytosis, the means whereby cells absorb and destroy waste or harmful material as a fundamental mechanism of defense. Metchnikov's investigations represent the watershed in this aspect of hematology. Prior to the advent of cellular staining for morphological study of leukocytes, there was confusion as to the source, behavior, and function of these cells; leukocytes were considered as a group. Ehrlich's contributions (see Chapter 1) provided the techniques for delineating the major leukocytic varieties. Recognition of the fundamental role of lymphocytes and lymphatic tissue in immunological defense is a relatively recent development and is the subject of another chapter. This chapter deals with the historical steps in the recognition of leukocytes as essential elements in the

Chapter Opening Photo   Athanasius Kircher (1602–1680). (*Courtesy of National Library of Medicine, Bethesda, Md.*)

417

defensive roles of microbial ingestion (phagocytosis), digestion (microbicidal action), and initiation of the immune response.

Metchnikov's brilliant observations were made in the same time period that Koch and Pasteur were describing the microbial causation of infectious diseases. The manifestations of microbial disease and of other disorders marked by inflammation naturally depend upon the body's interaction with the cause, such as the response to invading microbes by the defense systems of the body; the latter evoke the fever, swelling, and pain associated with inflammation. Therefore, the historical developments concerning cellular defense are interwoven with the history of microbial and other processes associated with inflammation. Whether the inflammatory process and its manifestations are always favorable to the body's integrity, whether the destructive consequences of inflammation work at times to the body's disadvantage, and whether the inflammatory process should be suppressed in the treatment of disease are questions which have spanned the history of medicine even to the present day.

Early Concepts of Illness

Prior to the time of Hippocrates, disease was accepted as a divine infliction, the physician a mere delegate of the gods. The patient could recover only through faith and participation in mystic rites presided over by temple priests. Ultimately illness came to be regarded as being due to an imbalance of the four humors, as was discussed in Chapter 1. Treatment consisted of attempts to correct this imbalance. For example, for symptoms of excessive phlegm (cold), a hot remedy (e.g., spiritous liquor) was called for. Fever was associated with a surplus of blood, and a cold remedy was indicated, e.g., cucumber seeds (hence, "cool as a cucumber"). Alterations in the blood were considered to be central to the development of illness. Although he accepted the doctrine of the four humors, Hippocrates also promulgated the revolutionary view that disease is a natural process and looked upon the patient as an individual whose "constitution" would react to disease in its own way. This concept, however, was not a popular one.

Until the nineteenth century, the practice of medicine as it related to inflammatory states was based on attempts to modify the patient's imbalance of humors. The lesions occurring in such diseases as cholera, smallpox, and pneumonia were conceived as sites for the discharge of the ill humors in the form of diarrhea, skin vesicles, or bloody phlegm, respectively. Incredibly complex rituals were devised to alter body heat or bowel and urinary function, or the festering of skin lesions. Following the example of Galen, the mixing of botanicals and the writing of elaborate prescriptions reached almost undecipherable heights. These concoctions came to be termed "galenicals." In addition, in almost all conditions associated with fever, bloodletting was employed as a means of venting the foul humor. According to the Salerno school of medicine, "Bleeding soothes rage, bringing joy to the sad, and saves all lovesick swains from going mad."[1]

A few physicians questioned the rationality of these practices. Paracelsus (Aureolus Phillipus Theophrastus Bombastus von Hohenheim, 1493–1541) spent most of his adult life thundering against the destructive practices of his colleagues. Jean Baptiste van Helmont (1577–1644) cried, "A bloody moloch sits president in the chairs of medicine." Nevertheless, venesection continued to be a major clinical practice into the middle of the nineteenth century (affecting the terminal illness of George Washington and many others). Thomas Sydenham (1624–1689), the "English Hippocrates" of the seventeenth century, also argued against the falseness of established practice "entangled in the obscurity of notions taken up by booke men and fitted to hypotheses where with they had prepossessed themselves in their closets" because he, unlike most, made detailed observations of patients sick with various diseases and observed the deterioration caused by the regimens of the day. He recognized the "purulence" of the clotted blood in such diseases as pneumonia and pleurisy and used descriptive language to imply the movement of pus ("peccant matter") from the blood to the "membrans" of the lung and pleura in the pathogenesis of such disorders long before pus was recognized microscopically as being derived from the blood. Although Sydenham resorted to phlebotomy in certain conditions, he used it sparingly and not at all in "nonpurulent" conditions, such as smallpox, saying of the existing regimens:

> I doubt not but that by such means as these, greater slaughters are committed and more havock made of mankind every yeare than hath been made in any age by the sword of the fiercest and most bloudy tyrant that the world ever produced, and which makes it yet more sad, this distraction lights not upon any so much as the youth and flourishing part of mankinde amongst whom likewise the richest, as being the best able to be at the charges of dyeing according to the art, suffer most under this calamitty.[2]

The sophistry and rigidity of medical practice, including bloodletting in its various forms, did not begin to yield to knowledge for more than a century to come. In 1836, Pierre Charles Alexandre Louis (1787–1872), the remarkable French clinician and pioneer in the statistical compilation of biomedical findings, was able to compile sufficient data to prove that venesection was not only useless but harmful in the medical management of such disorders as lobar pneumonia.[3] Louis, a physician of international scope and experience, methodically correlated symptoms and physical findings as well as therapeutic maneuvers with disease progression and autopsy findings. He studied disease firsthand, having practiced for some years in Russia, traveled to Malta with the British (to study yellow fever), and visited the United States on several occasions. He helped to delineate the clinical spectrum of tuberculosis, typhoid fever, and yellow fever. His approach to the tabulation and formulation of findings into constellations of disease had particular influence on the development of clinical disciplines by his many students and admirers in North America, as was noted by Sir William Osler in 1897.[4]

The centuries before Metchnikov yielded few discoveries to illuminate the nature of inflammation. One near breakthrough occurred in 1657 when Athanasius Kircher (1602–1680) (Chapter Opening Photo) put a few drops of blood from a plague victim (Rome epidemic of 1656–1657) under his 32X microscope. This Jesuit priest, mathematician, physicist, politician, and Egyptologist was astonished to observe "innumerable swarms of worms." From that observation he concluded that animate corpuscles cause and carry contagion. Although he was probably seeing leukocytes rather than bacteria, he proposed that these "worms" were causative of the disease. He described the "living parasite" as a "thin, elusive vermicle, invisible to the naked eye." However, the time was not propitious for exploration of this startling concept of disease. The idea of microbial contagion, as well as leukocytic defense, lay dormant for two centuries.[1]

Hewson's Observations

The one scientist in the pre-Metchnikov era who stands out in bold relief is William Hewson (1739–1774), some of whose fundamental contributions to blood clotting and red blood cell morphology are discussed in Chapter 1. Hewson was especially interested in the lymphatic system. His treatise on that subject,[5] dedicated to Benjamin Franklin, described physiological experiments involving microscopy, both in vitro and in vivo (e.g., in the webbing of the frog's foot), in a wide variety of animals (fishes, birds, amphibia, and mammals, including humans). Employing dye injection and dissection, he studied the lymphatic vessels of many species and, specifically in humans, the regional lymphatics in most body areas. He proved that lymphatic vessels are not simply extensions of arteries, a contention held by many at that time, and studied the anatomy and absorptive function of the veins and lymphatics of intestinal mucosa. He observed that lymph nodes (whose basic architecture and dual circulation, vascular and lymphatic, he described) were stopping stations along lymphatic vessels and concluded that the body cavities, peritoneal, pleural, and pericardial, are drained by the lymphatic system. The entire lymphatic system, not just the lacteals of the small intestine, he regarded as forming a system of "absorbents" to drain the body cavities as well as the intestines and the subcutaneous regions. He also recognized the significance of the lymphatic "absorbents" as a route of entry for noxious agents into the blood, as in boils, syphilis, and cancer. Thus, he pointed out that "the axillary glands are likewise frequently observed to swell in consequence of cancers in the breast, and it is found to be of no use to extirpate the breast itself, unless the infected glands can likewise be removed; for otherwise the cancerous humor left in the glands may renew the disease."[5]

Hewson noticed that the cellular content of the lymph (chyle) was nucleated (he used the term "central particles") and believed that these structures were formed in lymph nodes and were transported to the blood through the thoracic duct, mainly by passive compression of the lymphatics by muscular contraction, gravity, arterial pulsation, respiration, and cardiac action. He also showed that the thymus discharges huge numbers of cells into the thoracic duct and into the blood. Recognizing the normal involution of the thymus with age, he called attention to the accelerated reduction in thymus weight and cellularity with acute and chronic disease. Raising interesting questions as to why the thymus normally should be larger and most active early in life, he suggested that the gland is mainly required at that stage of life and that its function, once dispersed by cellular export, later is carried on elsewhere. He was convinced that the thymus serves a vital function, as reported by Gulliver:[6] "Nay, some have been led into very unphilosophical conjectures, viz., that perhaps it [thymus] was useless, or that if it did perform any office, it was so obscure as to escape investigation. But the ingenious author [Hewson] entertained too exalted an idea of Nature to suppose that any part of the animal frame was useless." Hewson observed white cells in the blood and believed they all entered the blood from the lymph. With the equipment available to him he could not know that several varieties of white cells existed. Unfortunately, he also came to the mistaken conclusion that the nucleated cells of the lymph which enter the blood are transformed into red blood cells in the spleen. Indeed, he presented detailed arguments to support this transformation as the raison d'être of the spleen. Although he recognized that removal of the spleen did not shorten life in experimental animals, he explained this on the assumption that some other tissue supplants the spleen's role in this "vital process." Perhaps this mistaken concept, not illogical at the time, accounts for the long neglect of Hewson's other observations.

The Meaning of Pus

Whether the inflammatory reaction in tissues in response to known trauma or unknown factors is harmful or helpful was the subject of protracted debate. The cellular constituents of pus, early recognized as colorless and nucleated, were considered to arise spontaneously within the matrix of "coagulable lymph" or "blastema." J. E. de Senac in his *Traité de la structure du coeur* (1749)[7] mentioned the "globules blanc du pus" as belonging to the chyle (à la Hewson). Their possible origin from similar cells in the blood was not considered. Later this concept of the plasmatic extravascular source of pus was modified to include the fibrous connective tissue (intracellular "ground substance" or Grundsubstanz of Virchow and others).

The defensive nature of inflammation with respect to known observable events, such as the expulsion of a foreign body like a thorn, was recognized. As summarized by C. J. B. Williams in 1844:[8] "There is in organized beings a certain conservative power which opposes the operation of noxious agents and labours to expel them when they are introduced." This "power" was the "archaeus" of van Helmont (1577–1644), the "anima" of Stahl (1660–1734), the "vis medicatrix naturae" of Cullen (1712–1790). Indeed, the thorn in the flesh became widely used as a metaphor to highlight the defensive nature of inflammation in the containment of contagious diseases, in which invisible noxious agents were likened to thorns. Nevertheless, acceptance of the inflammatory process as salutary in terms of wound and fracture repair and foreign body rejection was more than offset by the tissue destruction, pain, sickness, and even death which were seen also to be related to inflammation. Consequently, modification of the manifestations of inflammation comprised the basis for most medical interventions in the ancient era and extended through most of the nineteenth century.

Understanding of the true nature of inflammation and of the relation of the constituents of the blood to pus was hampered by the incomplete anatomical definition of the microcirculation. Capillaries interconnecting the arterial and venous blood circuits were not observed by William Harvey (1578–1657) in his famous treatise *De Motu Cordis*. Early observers of the microcirculation in such tissues as the web of a frog's foot were uncertain about the completeness of the wall surrounding the capillaries. For example, George Ernst Stahl (1660–1734), in his *Theoria Medica Vera*,[9] rejected the idea of complete capillary vessels connecting arteries and veins and envisioned the blood as flowing along tiny open-faced channels in the interface of blood with solid tissue (rather like rain water flowing in rivulets on the earth). Accordingly, he envisioned the development of inflammation as being promoted by an obstruction to blood flow in the venous circuit, a sort of damming of the flow, thereby promoting a discharge of "blastema" or "coagulable lymph." The investigations of Wilson Philip in 1799 and of John Thomson and Charles Hastings in the opening decades of the nineteenth century, as well as other studies in Germany and France, demonstrated the closed microcirculation of fish, amphibia, and mammals. C. F. Koch, in reviewing the subject of the mechanisms of inflammation in 1832,[10] precluded the origin of extravascular (pus) cells from the circulation because of the now convincing demonstration of capillary integrity. Thus, the hemic origin of pus was temporarily laid to rest in spite of the similarity of the "coulourless cells" in the blood and in pus.

In the mid-nineteenth century, confusion and contradictory opinion were rife as to the origin, nature, and value of the inflammatory response. The renowned founder of cellular pathology Rudolf Virchow (1821–1902) for a long time adhered to the view that pus cells arise from precursor cells located in the mesenchyme of various connective tissues and not from the white blood corpuscles, even in the face of mounting evidence to the contrary.[11] On the other hand, William Addison (1802–1881) (Figure 13-1), a medical practitioner in Malvern and a man of prominence, being physician to the Duchess of Kent, in 1843[12–14] insisted that the colorless corpuscles of the blood are identical with those of pus and that the former move from the circulation into tissues to form pus. His evidence was twofold. First, thin blood smears made from "blood just drawn from an inflamed surface, such as a pimple or the base of a boil" showed more abundant colorless corpuscles containing granules than did blood from a noninflamed site. He used dilute acetic acid to rid the preparations of red corpuscles so as to better compare the cells of the blood and of pus. He concluded that "pus corpuscles of all kinds are altered colourless corpuscles." Secondly, by examining the microvascular response in the web of the frog's foot to the external irritant of a crystal of salt, he noted that white cells accumulated within the initially accelerated, and later slowed, circulation. He described the engorgement of vessels by these cells and the appearance of

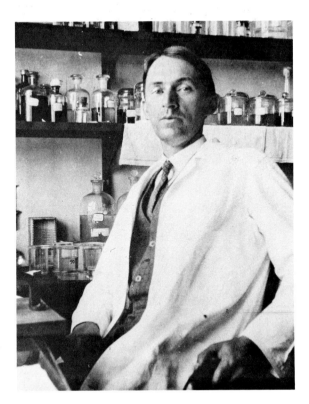

Figure 13-1 William Addison (1802–1881). (*Courtesy of National Library of Medicine, Bethesda, Md.*)

similar cells outside the vessels. However, he did not actually observe cells moving across the endothelial walls; indeed, he assumed the vessel walls to be incomplete and, like Stahl, regarded the ''spill-over'' of leukocytes into tissue as being secondary to venous congestion.

Addison's view of the hemic origin of pus cells was, in many respects, confirmatory of an earlier view propounded by René Dutrochet (1776–1847),[15] but Dutrochet later retracted his claim that these ''vagabond'' cells could migrate across vascular channels, having become convinced of the completeness of vascular enclosures.

Addison's contention of the hemic sources of pus cells, although initially received with enthusiasm, fell into disrepute after the demonstration that capillaries are completely enclosed structures. Unlike his namesake Thomas Addison, William Addison became the subject of controversy, and his concept of leukocyte diapedesis was rejected, primarily because of Virchow's conviction that inflammatory ''pus'' cells arose from extravascular sources. Ignored were the observations of another English scholar, Augustus Volney Waller (1816–1870) (Figure 13-2), who had patiently watched leukocyte diapedesis

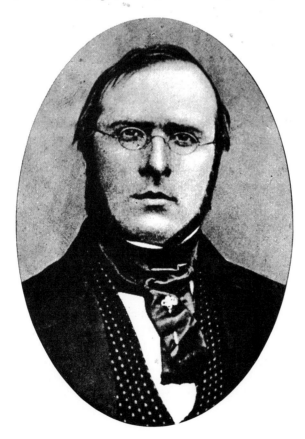

Figure 13-2 Augustus Volney Waller (1816–1870). (*Courtesy of National Library of Medicine, Bethesda, Md.*)

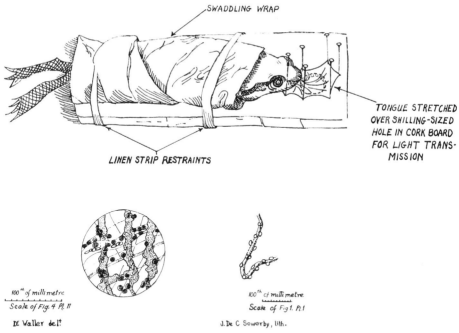

Figure 13-3 Three of August Waller's drawings of 1846, showing his hyperextended frog tongue model for microscopy of the microcirculation. In the microscope field to the left, he has omitted the cell structure of the tongue to emphasize the vasculature, showing "vessels of the inferior surface after the escape of (nucleated) corpuscles but not discs" (erythrocytes). The vessels "appear deformed and indented at the points of escape, near which the corpuscles are generally found." The remainder of this figure was covered with membranous muscular striae, which, to avoid complication, are not represented. To the right, he shows a small vessel beaded with corpuscles in various stages of "extravasation." He denotes this "extrafibrination of a vessel." (*Reproduced from Waller AV: Phil Mag 29 [series 3]:271–287, 297–405, 1846.*)

over a span of 4 hours (1846).[16,17] Waller recognized the significance of William Addison's concepts of leukocyte diapedesis. He studied the microvasculature of the hyperextended frog's tongue, fixed in position for prolonged microscopy (Figure 13-3), and submitted explicit drawings of leukocytes halfway through small pores between adjacent endothelial cells, there "by means of their own propulsive efforts." He stated that his observations had shown "the admirable manner in which nature has solved the apparent paradox of eliminating from a fluid circulating in closed tubes, certain particles floating in it, without causing any rupture or perforation in the tubes, or allowing the escape of the red particles, which are frequently the smaller of the two, or that of the fluid part of the blood itself." He later transferred his investigative talents to neurology, being remembered for his description of neuronal axon ("Wallerian") degeneration.

A major milestone in the conceptualization of the inflammatory process as a manifestation of body defense was Julius Cohnheim's description in 1867 of white cell migration through vascular walls. The observation filled a crucial "missing link" in the chain of events explaining the hemic origin of inflammation. Cohnheim was an assistant to Virchow at the latter's Institute of Pathology in Berlin. His work was an extension of that of another of Virchow's assistants, Friedrich Daniel von Recklinghausen (1833–1910) (Figure 13-4). Von Recklinghausen devised a method for the microscopic study of a bit of living tissue under conditions that maintained the humidity and temperature necessary for microscopic examination of such tissue over a period of many hours.[18] He was fully cognizant of the observations of earlier workers (Wharton Jones in 1844,[19] Davaine in 1850,[20] von Kolliker in 1852,[21] and Lieberkühn in 1854[22]) who had called attention to the similarity of amoebae and algae to white cells in terms of their contractile and "distinct protean movements, like those of the colourless corpuscle." With his improved technique, von Recklinghausen was able to establish to his own satisfaction, if not that of Virchow, the complete identity of the "wandering" (as he called them) white cells in the blood and the white cells in pus. He studied the normally avascular cornea of

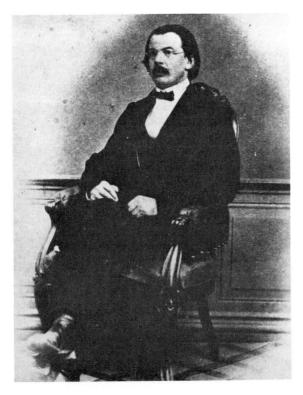

Figure 13-4 Friedrich Daniel von Recklinghausen (1833–1910). (*Courtesy of National Library of Medicine, Bethesda, Md.*)

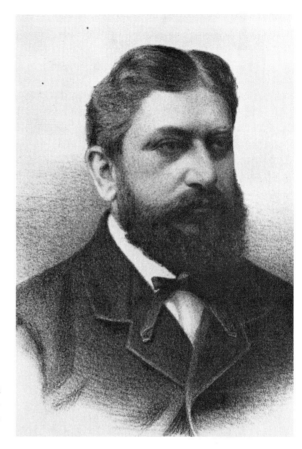

Figure 13-5 Julius Cohnheim (1839–1884). (*Courtesy of National Library of Medicine, Bethesda, Md.*)

rabbits and fragments of cornea implanted into the subcutaneous lymph sac of frogs and stained the leukocytes with carmine and vermilion. He showed that the leukocytes of the frog picked up the dye which had been deposited in the area and then moved into the implanted corneal tissue as it decayed. He did not trace stained cells as they passed from the circulation into the cornea; apparently he was more interested in where these amoeboid cells went than in their origin.

Cohnheim (Figure 13-5) used the model of the inflamed cornea and the exposed mesentery of the frog as well as various dyes and vital staining techniques. Four years after von Recklinghausen's report, Cohnheim's observations in frogs led him to conclude[23] that "some pus corpuscles in the inflamed cornea were formerly colourless blood corpuscles; they forced their way into the cornea from blood vessels." He described cells that had been vitally stained while in the circulating blood migrating through vascular walls into the exudate caused by exposure of the frog mesentery to air. He documented the protrusion of a white cell through a capillary wall, the cell's extension into the extravascular area while still fixed to the capillary wall by a long projection, and, finally, the free form of the diapedesed leukocyte. Cohnheim graciously acknowledged Addison's precedence in the discovery of diapedesis, recognition that was actually undeserved because Addison had not observed the phenomenon but had concluded its validity on circumstantial evidence. Waller's observations were overlooked.[24]

By 1873 Cohnheim[25] had decided that the basic cause of the margination of white blood cells along the walls of the blood vessels and their outward movement were due to a "molecular lesion" of the vascular wall; the exudation of white cells was a "secondary phenomenon." He was aware of the concepts concerning the microbial causation of inflammatory disease (commenting that in the "bacteria-happy" ["bacterienfroh"] year of 1873, there existed investigators who assigned to bacteria the role of agents of inflammation), but he regarded the hypothesis as "hardly probable." He conceived of the exudation of leukocytes as beneficial in the sense of fibrous union or encapsulation but did not suggest its uniformly defensive nature in response to microbial invasion, capitulating to the existing precepts, particularly those of Virchow. He seemed to miss the crucial significance of leukocyte exudation as a defense against microbial invasion. Others, however, postulated that white cell exudation, as shown by Cohnheim, was a fundamental defensive posture mobilized by the body. For example, a pathologist in Philadelphia, Joseph G. Richardson, wrote in 1869[26] that he had confirmed Cohnheim's "equation of white cells in blood, pus, mucus and salivary secretions." He further stated that if the recently proposed hypothesis of bacterial causation of infectious disease was correct, "the white corpuscles . . . collect during their amoeba-form movements those germs of bacteria which my own experiments . . . indicate always exist in the blood to a greater or lesser amount." Although one may question the credibility of the last part of this statement, one can only admire the nearness of Richardson's bold shot to the target. He considered that the movement of bacteria-laden phagocytes into saliva, the intestinal lumina, and so on underlay the "beneficial and rational" practices of the day, such as induced irritation, application of mercurials to surfaces, or the use of the seton,* tartar emetic, and purging.

Metchnikov and Phagocytosis

The crucial observations which provided convincing evidence of the pitting of white cells against invading microorganisms as the raison d'être of inflammation were made by a man who was entirely outside the ranks of the medical

---

*The seton was a strip of linen or similar material passed through the skin to provoke pus and allow escape thereof.

profession. Ilya Metchnikov (1845–1916) (Figure 13-6), while a professor of zoology at the University of Odessa, investigated the digestive process in lower animals. In 1878, he published his first paper dealing with the behavior of wandering amoeboid cells in the tissues of the marine sponge.[27] He was building upon the observations of Lieberkühn, who showed that these amoeboid cells ejected the undigestible residues of food particles (1857).[28] Metchnikov's interest in these and other cells with similar digestive activities came to dominate his life. He designated these specialized cells as "phagocytes" (Greek: phagein, to eat). In 1882, following the assassination of Czar Alexander II and the consequent political unrest involving campus life, Metchnikov resigned his post at Odessa and traveled to Sicily with his wife and children. At Messina, he pursued his studies on marine organisms. The crucial observation leading to his conclusions regarding the role of phagocytosis in body defense has been described graphically by him.[29] He was alone, his family enjoying the performance of a visiting circus. He turned to his microscopy of the wandering amoeboid cells of the transparent larval starfish. The thought arose, borne from many previous studies, that perhaps these cells served to defend the starfish's interior from harmful intruders, utilizing their inherent migratory ability to approach an intruder in this small creature without a

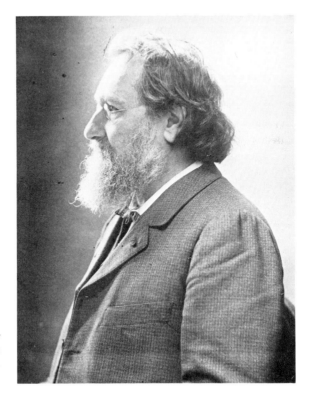

Figure 13-6 Ilya Metchnikov (1845–1916). (*Courtesy of Los Angeles County Medical Society.*)

vascular system. "From the small garden of our house, a small garden in which we had set up a Christmas tree on a little tangerine tree a few days before, I took several thorns from a rose in order to introduce them beneath the skin of these superb larval starfish, as transparent as water." After a sleepless night of anticipation, he arose early and observed that which he had already predicted; the thorn was surrounded by mobile phagocytic mesenchymal cells. This experiment, he said, "served as the foundation of the theory of phago-cytosis to the development of which I devoted the following twenty-five years of my life." It is noteworthy that such a brilliant illumination of this basic defense mechanism should have come about from the straightforward obser-vation of the effect of a rose thorn. One can only conjecture that he had in mind the analogy of microbial invasion of tissues with the metaphorical thorn of earlier times.

Virchow visited Messina in the spring of 1883. Metchnikov explained his concepts of inflammatory defense and showed the great pathologist prepara-tions of starfish larvae, elaborating that in these avascular creatures, the white corpuscles would chase and destroy microorganisms by virtue of their capacity for amoeboid movement, independently of a vascular system for transport. Virchow, with his customary mixture of critical skepticism and recognition of an important concept, reminded Metchnikov that, insofar as mammalian leukocytes were concerned, the prevailing opinion among pathologists was that microorganisms exploited leukocytes as sites favorable for their prolifera-tion, transport, and dissemination to tissues. Robert Koch, for example, had pointed out in 1878[30] that the relationship of certain microorganisms to white blood cells was puzzling at best: "They penetrate them and multiply in their interior," an aspect far removed from the concept of a protective role for blood leukocytes. Nevertheless, Virchow published Metchnikov's papers in his own journal and favorably assessed the Russian's contentions as to the importance of phagocytosis in body defense.[31]

Metchnikov previously had traced the phagocytic activities of cells in plasmodia, water fleas (*Daphnia*), and larval starfish. Although he had not pursued any medical studies until shortly before leaving for Messina, he had become acquainted with Cohnheim's *Lectures on General Pathology*. He was impressed with Cohnheim's description of the passage of white corpuscles through vessel walls, but he found Cohnheim's theory of a "molecular lesion" of the capillary wall as an explanation of diapedesis in response to infection "extremely vague and nebulous [in] character." Other than this, he knew relatively little of the discordant views of physicians and pathologists as to the value or destructiveness of the inflammatory process. His naivete in this respect probably made easier his forceful presentation of phagocytosis as a basic mechanism of defense. This led him in 1882 to state:[32] "Diapedesis and accumulation of white corpuscles in inflammatory diseases must be regarded as modes of defense of the organism against microorganisms, the leukocytes in this struggle devouring and destroying the parasites." He marshaled his extensive evidence for the independent amoeboid activity of phagocytes in creatures lacking a vascular system and coupled this with the recorded data dealing with human disease in, for example, E. Ziegler's treatise on pathological anatomy[33] so as to provide "a great number of observations fitted to facilitate the acceptation of the new hypothesis on inflammation and healing."

Metchnikov was not alone in the discernment of the white corpuscles in the blood of human beings as fulfilling a defensive role; Richardson, of Philadelphia, has been mentioned. Another American, the bacteriologist George Sternberg, according to Brieger,[34] wrote in 1883: "It has occurred to me that possibly the white corpuscles may have the office of picking up and digesting bacterial organisms when by any means they find their way into the blood." Further, the "propensity exhibited by the leukocytes for picking up inorganic granules is well known, and that they may be able not only to pick up but to assimilate, and so dispose of, the bacteria which come in their way does not seem to be very improbable in view of the fact that amoebae, which resemble them so closely, feed upon bacteria and similar organisms." Sternberg claimed that he had expressed these ideas verbally at a meeting of the American Association for the Advancement of Science in August 1881.

Whether or not such claims to precedence for conceptualizing the role of white cells in body defense are justified, Metchnikov, no doubt, deserved recognition and acclaim for his studies. With Paul Ehrlich, he was awarded the Nobel Prize in Medicine and Physiology in 1908. With single-minded dedication and vigor, Metchnikov promoted and propounded a biological doctrine of cellular defense which has persisted to the present time.

Delineation of the Different Types of White Blood Cells

In Chapter 1, the many contributions of Paul Ehrlich are described. As mentioned there, his staining techniques completely changed the course of hematology. It is worth remembering that until his time, with the exception of the use of certain vital staining techniques, such as those described in the work of von Recklinghausen and Cohnheim, students of the blood worked with unstained fresh material, preferably in the living animal. The techniques introduced by Ehrlich, which necessitated fixation and, consequently, death of the cells, captured the attention and energy of hematologists and hematopathologists to such an extent that for almost 50 years thereafter, the study of living cells was greatly overshadowed. It seems likely, in retrospect, that the fundamentally important observations of Metchnikov might have been delayed if the information concerning the amoeboid behavior of leukocytes in vivo had not been acquired by observers of living cells.

On the basis of the presence or absence of granulation and amoeboid movement, Thomas Wharton Jones had described more than one variety of blood leukocyte by 1850.[19,35,36] Max Schultze elaborated on Jones' findings and described four types of white cells in human blood, providing surprisingly accurate descriptions of small lymphocytes, large lymphocytes, polymorphonuclear granulocytes, and basophils (or eosinophils).[37] Moreover, these early students of the microcirculation had a reasonably clear view of blood flow (rheology). The axial flow of red cells and the margination of white cells were observed in the microcirculation of the web of the frog's foot by Thomas Wharton Jones in 1842.[35] He described how the "colourless" corpuscles may be seen accumulating at "the inner surfaces of small vessels, along which they move very slowly in comparison with the red corpuscles, which occupy the axis of the current." The white cells "roll along like round pebbles at the bottom of a stream. . . . When the current of blood is slow, a number of corpuscles are observed to be stationary, giving the vessel an appearance as if it were lined with an epithelium of globular corpuscles, a few of which are every now and then becoming detached from the rest and roll along." It would be a century later before Sabin, Vejlens, Beeson, Wood, and J. S. Lawrence would reexamine the microscopy of the microcirculation and amplify the singular behavior of circulating granulocytes, monocytes, and other leukocytes.

Ehrlich's aim in the application of stains to blood cells was to utilize the known chemical structure of the dye so that it would interact with the cellular constituents, thereby heightening the anatomical characteristics of the cell. (His "Farbenanalyse" was philosophically different from modern histochemistry, which defines the chemistry of the cellular constituents.) Aniline dyes were classified as basophilic or acidophilic; acid radicals, such as fuchsin, safranin, and Bismarck brown, combined with the hydroxyl ions in the cells. Basic dyes, such as eosin, benzaline, and nigrosin, combined with hydrogen ions. He found that neutral dyes (e.g., picric acid-rosaniline) had an affinity for the granules in the majority of blood leukocytes. In a definitive paper in 1880,[38] he introduced the terms acidophil, neutrophil, and basophil. (The term eosinophil subsequently replaced acidophil.) On the basis of these cytoplasmic staining qualities and the configuration of the nucleus, he divided the cells of the blood into categories of lymphocytes, large mononuclears (large lymphocytes), large mononuclears with an indented nucleus (later called monocytes), and polymorphous nucleated cells with neutrophilic (the majority), acidophilic (eosinophilic), or basophilic granules.

Ehrlich termed the varieties of leukocytic granules "specific," meaning that these cell constituents are manufactured within cells of a defined lineage and are the functional units of the particular cell. He emphasized that the different varieties of cell types in the blood are identifiable by the staining qualities of these granules, and he developed a "triacid solution" after "a trial of many hundreds of combinations" to permit easy applicability to the study of blood. Although he knew that accurate chemical identification of the compounds contained in these granules "would lie in the distant future," he recognized the process of degranulation in abscesses and stated, "the granules of the wandering cells are destined to be surrendered to the environment. This elimination of the granules is probably one of the most important functions of the polynuclear leukocytes." As described in Chapter 1, the development of methods to determine leukocyte numbers, combined with differential staining, led to the study of alterations in the white blood cells in disease. Ehrlich was impressed with the significance of granulocytic leukocytosis in the many types of infection as representing "an active chemiotactic reaction of the polynuclear elements." Specific conditions could elicit specific leukocytotic responses. For example, he summarized his own and others' observations of conditions associated with eosinophilia, such as bronchial asthma, pemphigus, acute and chronic dermatitides, helminthiasis, and malignant tumors. He believed the marrow to be the site of origin of all varieties of granulated leukocytes, which respond to "special chemiotactic stimuli" associated with certain disorders. In disorders associated with eosinophilia, "the specific substances [in these disorders] are absorbed, reach the blood and impart to it the chemiotactic property. The direct cause, then, of most forms of eosinophilia thus seems to lie in the products of tissue breakdown."

Lymphocytes, which arose entirely within the lymph nodes and spleen, according to Ehrlich's view, do not have the amoeboid, migratory capacity of granulocytes. Like students of the blood for many years to come, Ehrlich assigned no function to lymphocytes, believing that lymphocytosis is a "mechanical process," unrelated to infection in the same sense as polynuclear leukocytosis. One gains the impression, reading Ehrlich's comments about lymphocytes, that the lack of specific stainable features to characterize these cells led him, as it would many others, to feel a certain sense of frustration concerning the function of lymphocytes. He took issue with the opinions of many of his contemporaries and predecessors, who described lymphocytes as precursors of other cell types. He contended that various cell lineages are distinct. The enigma of the lymphocytes, cells without any apparent function, would continue to confound hematologists for many years. The theme would recur many times, however, that these morphologically undistinguished cells, ubiquitously present in most tissues, serve as precursors of other cell types.

Ehrlich described the leukocytosis of infectious disease as entirely consistent with the views of Metchnikov. However, he had reservations about accepting the view that phagocytosis is the keystone of body defense. He had in mind the mounting evidence that antibodies are elaborated by tissues to neutralize the toxic products of microorganisms, an area of work which would occupy most of his attention, energy, and productivity for years to come. In his paper "Histology of the Blood," he states:[39]

> Limitations to this engaging theory of Metchnikov have come to light. . . . Denys, Buchner, Martin, Hahn, Goldschneider, Jacob, Lowy and Richter, and many others have demonstrated that the most important weapon of the leukocytes is not the mechanical one of their pseudopodia, but that of their chemical products ("alexins", Buchner, *or antibodies*). By the aid of bactericidal or antitoxic substances which they secrete, they neutralize the toxins produced by the bacteria, and thus render the foe harmless by destroying his weapon of offense, even if they do not exterminate him.

Thus, Ehrlich attributed to phagocytic cells and, later, to *all* body cells the capability of responding to certain microbial toxins through membrane receptors which elicit the generation of neutralizing secretions (i.e., antibodies) specific for the particular toxin. Of course, we know now that antibody production and secretion is a property restricted to the body's lymphoreticular system. One can only imagine the surprise and delight that Ehrlich would experience if he were alive today to witness the emergence of the many varieties of lymphocytes as the providers of the immunological specificity which he recognized as being so critical to body defense.

Clinical Recognition of the Effects of Severe Neutropenia— the Dreaded Affliction Agranulocytosis

The imperative role which leukocytes play in the defense of the body against bacterial infection was demonstrated dramatically by studies of severe neutropenia (reduction in the number of neutrophilic granular leukocytes) in a syndrome that became known as agranulocytosis. Between the two world wars and extending through World War II, the major advance of nonsurgical medicine was in the area of the body's defense mechanisms against microbes; the discovery of penicillin by Fleming in 1928 and of the sulfonamides by Domagk in 1935 were major achievements in this field. Fleming's discovery was developed and applied clinically by Florey and his colleagues in 1940. These and subsequent advances in antibiotic technology and treatment provided a chemical means for suppressing the virulence of infectious diseases caused by bacteria and fungi. Simultaneously with these events, the imperative need for the cellular defense systems to maintain the body's integrity was emphasized forcefully by the consequences of a severe reduction in the number of circulating neutrophilic granulocytes.

Agranulocytosis, as a clinical entity of unknown etiology, was first described by Philip King Brown, of San Francisco, in 1902,[40] but general interest in this disorder was not aroused until the report of six cases by Werner Schultz in 1922.[41] The clinical picture was dramatic; the victim, often a woman 30 to 50 years of age, would develop a severe sore throat accompanied by great prostration and high fever. Death often followed in 2 or 3 days. This was associated with an absence of granular leukocytes. The syndrome was being reported particularly in Germany, Scandinavia, and the United States. The number of cases increased rapidly, particularly between the years 1929 and 1934. During the mid-1930s, the association of agranulocytosis with the taking of the analgesic drug aminopyrine began to be suspected.[42] This drug had been patented in Germany in 1907 as Pyramidon and was used as such or in combination with barbiturates in such products as Allonal and Peralga. Kracke in 1931[43] reported at a meeting the production of a syndrome resembling agranulocytosis in rabbits by giving drugs containing a modified benzene ring. The idea that the mysterious clinical syndrome might be due to the use of coal tar–derived drugs, such as Pyramidon, was supported by the studies of Plum in Denmark.[42,44] He compared the increasing use of these drugs from the time of their introduction with the growing incidence of cases of agranulocytosis until 1934 and contrasted this with the decreasing number of cases as sales of the drug decreased when suspicion began to be aroused and became publicized. The most frequently encountered victims of agranulocytosis, it was observed, were persons who had occasion to use pain-relieving drugs such as aminopyrine and those who had access to it and could afford it.

Conclusive evidence that aminopyrine could cause agranulocytosis was provided in 1934 by Madison and Squier, who showed that one could produce transient neutropenia by readministering small doses of the drug to subjects who had recovered from aminopyrine-induced agranulocytosis.[45] Thus, it was shown that in persons sensitive to such an agent, when the first line of defense against bacterial infection—the granulocytes—disappeared, a fulminating infection could develop from which the victim would not recover unless these cells became available again. Meanwhile, reports of agranulocytosis associated with a variety of other medications accumulated.

Today, depression of the available numbers of polymorphonuclear neutrophilic leukocytes (granulocytes) is recognized as a life-threatening condition even though ever more effective antibiotics are becoming available. Serious neutropenia can occur in association with various chronic disease states and, as a result of environmental exposure to hematotoxins, or as the effect of agents which suppress bone marrow blood cell production or delivery. Hematotoxins include certain viruses, chemicals in industrial environments, ionizing radiation, drugs which injure marrow tissue in rare individuals sensitive to the drugs, and chemicals which directly damage rapidly renewing tissues in all persons exposed to them. Many chemicals used to treat cancer in its various forms are in the last category. Elucidation of the mechanisms whereby neutropenia occurs (injury to marrow cells that produce neutrophils or accelerated removal of neutrophils by immunologic or splenic effects in the periphery) has developed into one of the more demanding arenas of hematology.

Normal Neutrophil Production, Maturation, Circulation, and Fate (Neutrophil Granulocyte Kinetics)

For many years after the development of methods for counting and staining leukocytes, hematologic information about the varieties of leukocytes was mainly descriptive. The study of leukocytes in terms of their kinetics, their biochemical behavior, and the mechanisms that cause alterations in cell numbers and function languished behind the progressive and logical delineation of the mechanisms involved in the development of anemia. With the development of various techniques, some simple (e.g., cell separation technology), some extremely complex and emanating from such fields as radioisotopic technology, biochemistry, bacteriology, pharmacology, and electron microscopy, further advances in these directions were made.

From observations about the rates of development of neutropenia in animals after marrow injury (e.g., from ionizing radiation or toxic chemicals, such as nitrogen mustard),[46] it became clear that normal neutrophils have a brief life span in the blood. However, fluctuations in the numbers of circulating granulocytes occur with such suddenness and after such a variety of stimuli that little insight could be obtained concerning the nature of leukopenia or leukocytosis in terms equivalent to the understanding of anemia as due to the diminished production or increased loss or destruction of red cells. In the 1950s, studies of neutrophil kinetics began with the quantification of cells in the blood entering and leaving organs such as the lung and spleen[47] and the response of the blood granulocyte level to the mechanical removal of cells (i.e., leukopheresis or leukapheresis from the Greek *apheresis* meaning to withdraw or remove).[48] These observations were soon coupled with the use of radioactive isotopes, particularly ^{32}P-orthophosphate incorporated into the nuclear deoxyribose nucleic acid (DNA) of precursor cells as they doubled their genetic complement preparatory to cell division. Because the total amount of DNA contained in nucleated cells, such as leukocytes, is a fixed entity for the life span of the particular cell, isotopic incorporation into the DNA structure affords a reliable means of tagging cells as they are produced in the marrow or elsewhere. This technique of ^{32}P labeling of DNA had been applied in bacterial systems and shown to be a reliable method for counting bacterial replication in culture. In 1954, the Norwegian Ottesen described the appearance and disappearance of ^{32}P-DNA–labeled neutrophils in the blood of two hematologically normal human subjects who had received the isotope.[49] Using innovative techniques for separating neutrophils from other blood cells and quantifying the specific activity of the ^{32}P-labeled DNA, he showed that neutrophils appeared in the blood after a delay of 5 to 6 days, circulated very briefly, and entered the tissues by diapedesis.

These observations led Craddock and his associates to use ^{32}P labeling of the DNA of replicating marrow cells in the study of normal and irradiated dogs subjected to leukopheresis,[50] endotoxin administration (which causes neutropenia followed by neutrophilic leukocytosis), or sterile exudates induced to attract huge numbers of neutrophils.[51] Their investigations showed that reserves of maturing, nondividing neutrophils in the normal marrow are the principal source of neutrophils for release into the blood and for transport to body areas requiring neutrophils to mount an inflammatory response.

Radioactive phosphorus was being used as a therapeutic agent in the management of certain hematologic disorders, and these workers, as well as Osgood and others,[52] applied these techniques to human beings. In 1959, Athens, Cartwright, Wintrobe, and their associates applied another isotope technique to the study of neutrophil kinetics in human subjects.[53] ^{32}P-labeled diisopropyl fluorophosphate (^{32}P-DFP), an inhibitor of cellular cholinesterase, had been developed in the toxicological study of insecticides and was known to form an irreversible bond with maturing neutrophils beyond the myelocyte stage of maturation. Lymphocytes are not labeled by the compound. ^{32}P-DFP was used by these investigators to label neutrophils in vitro, the labeled cells being then transfused back into the donor; or the tracer compound was injected into the subject, and in samples of neutrophils after they had been separated from other blood elements, the quantity of ^{32}P was determined at intervals. In addition to clarifying many features of neutrophil kinetics, these studies defined the very brief sojourn of normal polymorphonuclear neutrophils in the circulating blood (random disappearance with half-life of 6 to 7 hours). They also permitted determination of those neutrophils which were free-flowing in the blood and those which Wharton Jones, in 1842, had observed as being transiently adherent to vascular endothelium (the marginated or marginal pool). Application of these principles to the study of various pathological states followed.

The determination of blood and marrow compartments (total quantities) of neutrophils and their precursors in normal humans was accomplished by Donohue, Gabrio, and Finch using radioactive iron to determine the marrow erythropoietic mass as a standard against which the quantity of granulocyte-producing cells could be estimated.[54] The movement of cells into cutaneous sites of induced inflammation was coupled with isotopic labeling to assess the migratory capacity of neutrophils responding to chemotactic (attracting) stimuli. The application of this technology to abnormal states followed apace.

Another radioisotopic technique, tritium (^{3}H) labeling of compounds metabolized by living cells, provided high-resolution radioautographic preparations suitable for light and electron microscopy. The radioactivity, localized in the labeled cell, could be visualized and counted in fixed, stained blood films and tissue sections overlaid with photographic film or emulsion to detect the isotopic emissions. The development of techniques to determine tritium by liquid scintillation spectrophotometry rapidly expanded and simplified the applicability of DNA labeling as a means of assessing the proliferative behavior of tissues. It was found that replicating mammalian cells incorporate tritiated (or carbon 14–labeled) thymidine into the thymidylic acid moiety of DNA. Also, it was found that cells incubated in the presence of ^{3}H-thymidine incorporate the isotope rapidly into newly produced DNA. ^{3}H-thymidine injected into animals was incorporated into the DNA of dividing cells. By timed observations of the behavior of precursor (dividing) cells, Lajtha[55] and others examined the phases in the regenerative cycle (i.e., the G_0 or G_1 postmitotic "gap" phase, the DNA synthesis or S phase, the premitotic "gap" or G_2 phase, and the mitotic or m phase). Labeled cells or their labeled progeny could, thereby, be traced through developmental sequences in the marrow and into blood and tissues. The technique, as applied in planned procedures to experimental animals and to patients with nonhematological as well as hematological disorders, such as leukemia, permitted accurate in vivo assessment of neutrophil production from stem-cell precursors, serial proliferative and maturational sequences, and other kinetic data.[56] The contributions of Cronkite and his associates were particularly lucid in this respect.

One important consequence of such studies of granulopoiesis was the demonstration of impaired or delayed rates of replication by leukemic ("blast") cells as compared with normal granulocytic precursor cells. When combined with other assessments of cellular proliferation, such as mitotic index, in in vivo and in vitro studies of leukemic cells, it was found, surprisingly, that, as suggested in 1953 by Astaldi and Mauri,[57] most acute leukemic blast cells replicate themselves more slowly than their normal counterparts rather than at an accelerated rate, as had been assumed. Leukemic blast cells display a marked proliferative advantage and accumulate in the body because of the high fraction of blast cells which are capable of cell division, though delayed, and because of the failure of these cells to mature and carry out the "death-related" functions of normal neutrophils, which are associated with brief survival (rapid turnover).[58] The concept of myeloblastic leukemia being a condition of imposed maturational block or failure rather than simply overproduction of tumor cells was both revolutionary and important in the conceptualization of the disease. Mauer and his associates subsequently showed that leukemic blasts in various locations differed in their replicative activity and rates.[59] The concept of acute leukemic tissue as being in a resting state (i.e., "out of cell cycle"), the G_0 or prolonged G_1 state (to a variable degree), modifiable by treatment has been found to have considerable relevance in the treatment of acute leukemia.

Humoral Control of Granulopoiesis

Attempts to elucidate humoral mechanisms of granulopoietic control were pursued with increasing intensity once the enormity of ongoing neutrophil production became measurable. Early efforts to demonstrate "leukopoietin(s)" (i.e., stimulators of granulopoiesis) had been frustrated by rapid fluctuations in blood neutrophil concentration in response to many and varied stimuli. It was shown that any manipulation that produced neutropenia, whether by removal of neutrophils, by causing increased margination, by accelerated clumping, or by adherence and extravascular migration of these cells, would be followed by accelerated release of cells from marrow reserves and blood leukocytosis. In spite of several experimental systems which suggested the liberation of "releasing factors(s)" or leukopoietin(s) in response to neutropenia, reproducible techniques for their demonstration were not available until in vitro methods of assessing granulopoiesis were developed.

The independent demonstration in two separate laboratories[60,61] that normal murine and human marrow tissue can be induced to form colonies of newly formed granulocytes and monocytes when cultured in semisolid media under controlled environmental conditions was a technological milestone. In Donald Metcalf's laboratory in Melbourne, this breakthrough occurred against the background of many attempts by Metcalf and Bradley to culture normal and leukemic mouse thymus tissue. Layers of normal and leukemic thymus cells and other tissues, including bone marrow, were studied in attempts to promote lymphopoiesis. Bone marrow as an underlayer was found to promote growth. On microscopic examination, the colonies contained the ringed nuclei characteristic of mature mouse granulocytes in the marrow layer. The system was reversed with marrow in the overlayer, and it was found that a variety of tissues and tissue extracts in the underlayer would promote the growth of granulocytic and macrophage cells in the overlayer. "By chance," said Metcalf,

> at a meeting in Philadelphia in October 1965, Leo Sachs and I were discussing work in our laboratories and it became clear that Dov Pluznik and he had been working on granulocyte-monocyte (GM) colony formation by spleen cells in simultaneous studies in Israel. As described by Leo Sachs, their colonies were composed of mast cells whereas I knew that ours were composed of granulocytes and macrophages. However, we too had encountered difficulty in assuring ourselves that the macrophages were not mast cells, since virtually all macrophages grown in agar contained phagocytosed metachromatic agar particles.[61]

A complex stimulatory activity (colony-stimulating activity, CSA) was shown by these and other workers to promote the formation of colonies of monocytes and granulocytes that emanate from precursor cells (colony-forming units in culture, CFU-C). CSA appears to be heterogeneous in molecular structure, and it is probable that different factors are derived from various tissue sources.[62] The content and high rate of secretion of CSA by macrophages[63,64] pointed to close interrelationships between phagocytic cells derived from granulocytic and monocytic tissue. Although direct proof is lacking that CSA is a physiological stimulator of granulopoiesis, the findings of many investigators point to crucial interactions between cells of different lineages in eliciting increased granulopoiesis by tissues throughout the body as the local inflammatory reaction is generated. For example, bacterial products, particularly endotoxin, elicit both CSA production and granulopoiesis. These observations hark back to Cohnheim and others in their consideration of bacteria and bacterial products as direct controllers of neutrophil behavior. Perhaps equally important as mechanisms for control of cell production are the inhibitors or modulators of granulopoiesis, also amenable to study in culture systems.

Metabolic Reactions Associated with Granulocytic Function

In the appropriate development of an inflammatory response to defend the body against invading microbes, to remove damaged tissue, and to promote tissue repair, granulocytes must be available in sufficient numbers and must be responsive to the signals generated to attract them to the site of infection or injury. The directional amoeboid movement of granulocytes in response to such signals is chemotaxis. Clarification of the nature of chemotactic signals comprises a critical area in understanding the inflammatory response and relates granulocytic cells to soluble plasmatic components. Chambers consisting of two compartments separated by a micropore filter were devised by Boyden for this type of study.[65] Normal neutrophils, monocytes, or eosinophils placed on one side of the filter membrane will respond to chemotactic signals on the other by migrating into and through the filter. By such techniques, components of complement and certain factors involved in blood coagulation were shown to play a role in chemotaxis.[66] As presently conceived, complement consists of a group of soluble protein constituents, largely produced by macrophage tissue throughout the body, which circulate in the plasma and lymph as latent enzymes. These latent enzymes, if activated through a complex sequence of proteolytic cleavage (peptide-splitting) steps, provide a number of active enzymes (esterases) capable of damaging the structural phospholipids in cell membranes. Neutrophilic and eosinophilic granulocytes (as well as certain B lymphocytes [see Chapter 14] and monocytes) have receptor molecules on their surfaces that combine with constituents of complement activation in a way that promotes chemotaxis. Phenomena now recognized as promoting complement enzyme activation include the formation of complexes between the microbial antigen (Ag) and the lymphocyte-plasma cell–produced antibody (Ab), bacterial products, such as endotoxin, and foreign surfaces (which may activate the clotting enzyme sequence as well). Complement activation, therefore, generates components that can directly damage cell membranes (microbial and somatic) as well as eliciting the build-up of granulocytes and the other cells that participate in inflammation.

After moving to and localizing in areas of infection or inflammation, granulocytes ingest and kill bacteria by mechanisms to be mentioned shortly. These complex functions require energy. As is so often the case, it was a deficiency state that first emphasized the importance of cell function. Dr. Moises Chediak, of Havana, Cuba, beginning in 1940 at medical and other scientific meetings, called attention to anomalous leukocytic granulations which characterize the disorder now associated with his name (Chediak-Higashi-Steinbrinck syndrome). The patient studied by him, an 11-month old infant (who died of a blood dyscrasia 2 years later), had three other siblings with the disorder (in a family of 15 children). Chediak showed the blood smears to many prominent American and European hematologists, none of whom recognized the condition. In 1952, Chediak published his observations and proposed that the syndrome represented a disease entity;[67] an autosomal recessive genetic disorder with anomalous leukocytic granulation, oculocutaneous albinism, and a propensity to serious, often fatal infection or lymphoma-like disease. In Germany, W. Steinbrinck independently reported a similar condition in 1948,[68] and in 1954, Higashi[69] described a third family in which three of seven siblings had the fatal affliction. The case reported in 1957 by Donohue and Bain[70] was the first on the North American continent.

As noted earlier, Ehrlich had recognized that "elimination of the granules is probably one of the most important functions of the polynuclear leukocytes." Metchnikov proposed in 1887 that leukocytes may be involved in the liberation of substances which damage adjacent tissues.[71] In retrospect, the proclivity of children with the Chediak-Higashi-Steinbrinck syndrome to serious infection should have been recognized as a defect in "degranulation," a process that is essential for the antimicrobial activity of these phagocytic cells.

In 1955, de Duve and his associates in Belgium described a distinct class of granules in rat liver tissue, granules containing acid phosphatase, enzymes (nucleases) that degrade ribonucleic acid and deoxyribonucleic acid, cathepsin, and beta glucuronidase.[72] They proposed the term "lysosomes" for these granules, thus calling attention to "their richness in hydrolytic enzymes." They likened these granules to the digestive vacuoles in amoebae. In 1960, Cohn and Hirsch isolated and characterized the hydrolytic enzymes in the so-called specific cytoplasmic granules of rabbit polymorphonuclear leukocytes.[73] They described how the plasma membrane surrounding the engulfed particle fuses with the lysosomal membrane[74] to form a phagosome or digestive vacuole like a tiny stomach. In 1965, Hirshhorn and Weissmann described similar lysosomal granules and events in human neutrophilic leukocytes,[75] thus completing the anatomical description of the process whereby these cells engulf and digest viable bacteria. Later, Bainton and her associates defined the time of appearance and the partial chemical content of the azurophil and the cell-specific granules that appear as granulocytes develop from precursor cells in normal human bone marrow.[76]

Studies of the biochemistry of living blood leukocytes had actually begun with the demonstration in 1911 that these cells consume oxygen.[77] The breakdown of sugar (glycolysis) by leukocytes was observed to occur under both aerobic (in the presence of oxygen) and anaerobic conditions. The demonstration of continued glycolysis under aerobic conditions was the first established exception to Warburg's postulate that this was a characteristic of tumor tissue.[78] It was not, however, until the early 1950s that a systematic analysis of the activity of the enzymes of glycolysis in normal and leukemic leukocytes was begun by Valentine, Beck, and their associates.[79-82] Study of their nucleic acid, protein, and lipid metabolism followed. Although therapeutically exploitable differences between leukemic and normal cells or their precursors at similar stages of cell development were not found, differences in the formation of certain cytoplasmic enzymes, notably alkaline phosphatase, were discovered; these differences would become important diagnostic features in certain leukemic states.[82]

The metabolic behavior of normal blood granulocytes during phagocytosis was described by Sbarra and Karnovsky in 1959.[83] They found that a striking elevation in glycolysis via the hexose monophosphate shunt pathway as well as an increased breakdown of glycogen to glucose (glycogenolysis) occurs during the process. Subsequently, it was shown that a defect in this metabolic activity prevents phagocytic cells from killing certain ingested bacteria in the condition known as chronic granulomatous disease. Characterized by recurring infection and inherited in one form of the disease as a sex-linked recessive trait affecting the male offspring of carrier mothers, this disorder was described as an entity by Berendes, Bridges, and Good[84] and by Landing and Shirkey[85] in 1957.

Since then, many additional disorders related to some defect in the complex cellular machinery of granulocytes that is required for body defense have been described. Some of these involve deficiencies of a specific enzyme that is required for bacterial killing while others involve defects in the chemical events that provide energy for the cell to function.

Tissue Destruction by Granulocytes

That the inflammatory response with the formation of pus is double-edged, often causing damage to body tissues, continues to be an important consideration in the management of disease, as it was in the sixteenth century. In the tissue destruction produced experimentally in the 1950s in the form of the "Arthus" and "Shwartzman" reactions to injected bacterial products,[86,87] the participation of neutrophils was demonstrated. In 1964, Thomas provided the first direct evidence that lysosomes per se are capable of initiating the hemorrhagic necrosis characterizing these reactions.[88] By 1965, Dixon, Cochrane, and their associates had demonstrated the role of polymorphonuclear leukocytes and complement in the nephrotoxic nephritis induced by immune sera in rabbits[89] as well as in experimental serum sickness.[90] These experimental observations afforded animal models that could be used to clarify the destructive effects of leukocytes on body tissues in certain diseases of human beings (some nephritides, necrotizing arteritis, gout, rheumatoid arthritis). It was even shown that an inborn deficiency of an enzyme inhibitor, α-antitrypsin, that neutralizes the tissue-destructive effects of trypsin released from phagocytes may be associated with a form of lung tissue destruction and emphysema.[91] Investigations of alterations in the granulocytic component of inflammation by time-honored agents such as cinchona, aspirin, and colchicine have opened new avenues for the pharmacologic manipulation of inflammation for the benefit of patients.

Fever is the foremost manifestation of bacterial infection. Body temperature is regulated by a small cluster of thermosensitive neurons located in a region near the floor of the brain's third ventricle. In 1948, Beeson described a pyrogenic material released from rabbit leukocytes.[92] Subsequently, Atkins and Wood showed that this pyrogen, called endogenous or leukocytic pyrogen, is the same as the material released into blood plasma following injection of typhoid vaccine.[93,94] Later, pyrogenic material of somewhat different physicochemical characteristics was shown to be contained in monocytes and macrophages.[95] This substance alters body temperature through an effect on the thermoregulatory center of the central nervous system.

Various leukocytic constituents causing still other manifestations of inflammation, such as changes in blood flow, stasis, cell breakdown, blood clotting, and so forth, had already been studied extensively by Menkin in the 1930s.[94] He demonstrated that substances generated at sites of pus formation evoke marked changes in the vascular system, but he did not relate these products to granulocyte-contained factors. Specific vasoactive chemicals, particularly histamine, contained in basophils and tissue mast cells, were shown by others[96] to be pathogenetic in certain body reactions (e.g., allergic reactions). A series of substances from neutrophils may interact with plasma factors to generate potent kinins, and some of these, when activated in sufficient amounts, can lead to anaphylactic shock, widespread clot formation, tissue necrosis, and even death. These events have been ably described by Weissmann.[97]

Thus, the inflammatory response, designed for the body's defense, can be extremely harmful; granulocytes and derivatives of monocytes are crucial to most of these events. Study of the events occurring in the inflammatory response and the search for methods to control or direct these events for the benefit of sick people constitute a major portion of current biomedical research. The ability to alter the inflammatory process by chemical means has finally progressed to intelligent intervention, replacing the empiricism of the past (e.g., bloodletting).

The Macrophages Are More Than Scavengers:
The Monocyte-Macrophage (Reticuloendothelial) System

The terms *reticuloendothelium* and *reticuloendothelial system* (RES) evolved from Metchnikov's concepts early in the twentieth century but were used first by Aschoff in 1924[98] to designate the varieties of macrophagic cells that have the properties of removing and storing certain particulate materials and dyes from the blood and lymph. These cells are distributed throughout most of the body, and their structure varies according to their activity. They are involved in a great variety of the body's diseases as well as in the reaction to injury.

Reticulo (or reticular) refers to the tendency of large phagocytic cells in various organs to form a lattice or reticulum by cytoplasmic extensions; *endothelial* refers to the cells' proximity to vascular endotheliocytes, from which they sometimes seem to arise. Trapping and removing unwanted particulate material in the blood and lymph were considered to be the function of the RES and formed the unifying property linking the widely dispersed components. Phagocytosis of large particles is characteristic (hence, the name macrophages, as contrasted to the microphagic polymorphonuclear granulocytes). The engulfed particles may be microbes or foreign materials; the remnants of somatic cells being removed after a normal life span or cells broken down in an accelerated fashion, as in disease; or the products of lipid metabolism. The extent of macrophagocytosis can vary from that normally seen, for example, in the germinal centers of gut-associated lymphatic nodules to the markedly increased macrophagocytosis that is seen in disease, as in disseminated tuberculosis. Depending upon the nature of the material engulfed by macrophages, it may be visible within them for prolonged periods of time, thus constituting a major difference from the transient sojourn of material engulfed by polymorphonuclear leukocytes. The component of the RES showing increased macrophagocytosis varies depending upon the nature and location of the disease process. An array of descriptive terms has evolved to designate macrophages, depending on their structure and function, the nature of the engulfed material, the location, the affected organ, and its relationship to other structures, particularly the vascular and lymphatic endothelium. When the macrophages contained somatic tissue remnants they were called *histiocytes*; histiocytes might be either fixed within the particular organ (sessile) or mobile (as in the splenic red pulp). Other terms imbued the cells with some function, usually hypothetical, other than the removal of microbial or cellular structures or products. For example, Ranvier coined the term "clasmatocyte"[99] to convey the idea that the large amoeboid cells of the mesentery give off small pieces of cytoplasm, which serve as food for other connective tissue cells. In an article published in 1958, discussing the "tower of Babel" which had developed in the terminology of the RES, Gall listed over 30 terms[100] for macrophage constituents of the system.

Equally confusing were the opinions about the origin of RES macrophages. These were fairly and lengthily presented by Richard Jaffe in Downey's *Handbook of Hematology* in 1938.[101] As an example, the pulmonary alveolar macrophage was believed by some (Maximow[102] and Lang[103]) to arise locally from extravascular mesenchymal tissue; others believed these macrophages evolved from blood monocytes,[104] and still others contended that alveolar macrophages arose from the endothelium of blood capillaries.[105] Blood monocytes, according to about half of the authors cited by Jaffe, were considered to be circulating products of similar cells in the RES throughout the body. The other half believed that blood monocytes were derived from such precursors as "the common vascular endothelium," the lymphocyte, "undifferentiated mesenchymatous cells," hemocytoblasts, or myeloblasts. Maximow contended[106] that the "non-phagocytic reticular cell" (in the adventitia of small arteries) was endowed with "complete mesenchymal cytopoietic potencies." This cell was probably the same as the reticular cell (the fixed stem cell or "clasmatocyte") of Cunningham, Sabin, and Doan (1925);[107] it probably was the cell postulated as "the ruhende Reticuloendothelien" by Masugi (1927),[108] and the "mesenchyme cell" by Seemann (1931).[109] Calling it a polyblast, Maximow believed that it evolved from lymphocytes, arising from a "perivascular germinal layer of undifferentiated mesenchymatous cells." Thus, in the view of many prestigious authorities, the RES reproduced not only itself and varieties of macrophages and circulating monocytes but also formed the ultimate pluripotential stem cell which is the source of all hemic cellular elements. The ongoing debate over terminology and the origin and function of the cells that comprise the RES consumed much time and journal space, but it contributed little substantive knowledge, as these two paragraphs indicate.

It will be recalled that Virchow long contended (from 1859) that the cells forming pus in tissues originated from "mesenchymal tissues" at extravascular sites. The hematogenous origin of blood granulocytes finally altered his view insofar as these most common constituents of pus were concerned. However, macrophages were observed to undergo mitosis in local tissues. Moreover, in certain disease states, extravascular proliferation of macrophages was noted to occur to such an extent that tumorous destruction of organs resulted. A disease marked by great enlargement of the spleen and liver and involving other tissues that exemplifies such destruction was originally described by Gaucher as a primitive epithelioma in 1882.[110] It was later recognized that the expanding tumorous masses of lipid-laden macrophages characterizing this disease were not malignant. Only recently has it been shown that the basic defect in this disorder (Gaucher's disease) is a hereditary cerebrosidase deficiency, the accumulation and tumorous hyperplasia of macrophages being a compensatory response, sequestering undegraded lipid in phagocytic tissue. Such disorders, so mysterious when not understood, provided evidence to support Virchow's concept of the production of the macrophage constituents of pus in extravascular and extramedulllary sites.

With the development of improved techniques to identify, quantify, and trace migratory cells (as described for granulocytes), much of the confusion and controversy concerning the RES is being clarified. Whereas derivatives of monocytes in peripheral locations do indeed have the proliferative capacity to provide more macrophages, the marrow (in the adult mammal) is the sole provider of pluripotential stem cells (although some cells with this capability leave the marrow, circulate, and enter various other organs). Isotopic kinetic studies, combined with marker chromosome analysis in irradiated animals, have established that the bone marrow is the source of circulating monocytes.[111,112] According to assessments of marrow cell production (i.e., colony formation) in vitro,[63] monocytes are produced in the marrow from precursors which also produce granulocytes. Consequently, the macrophages and the microphages are close relatives in terms of origin as well as function. Monocytes, however, are exported from the marrow as immature cells with a retained proliferative capability, unlike their polymorphonuclear granulocytic "cousins." The commonality of the precursor cell with immature granulocyte precursors and the lack of monocyte storage and maturation in the marrow account for the paucity of identifiable monocytes and their precursors in normal marrow, in contrast to neutrophilic granulocytes and their precursors. Whereas granulocytes complete their morphologic and functional maturation in the marrow, monocytes complete their maturation to macrophages after leaving the marrow and the blood. Maturation to macrophages, the monocyte-macrophage transition, first clearly described in the blood of lower vertebrates by Lewis and Lewis in 1926,[113] is accompanied by the full development of amoeboid motility, phagocytic capacity, and cytoplasmic and lysosomal equipment.[114] Mobile macrophages develop special esterases and other enzymes which can attack the lipid-rich capsules of bacteria such as the tubercle bacillus, a property early recognized as special to macrophages. They also generate special membrane receptor immunoglobulin and complement receptor sites, which are believed to impart to these cells their ability to phagocytize antibody-coated (opsonized) particles (e.g., microbes or somatic cells), a property imperative to body defense.[115]

The similarities in the behavior and function of monocytes and polymorphonuclear neutrophilic granulocytes ceases when these cells migrate into extravascular sites. The neutrophil, being an end stage cell, expires soon after leaving the blood. Some monocytes, on the other hand, can divide to provide more monocytes. Furthermore, compelling evidence was presented in 1968 supporting the view that some fixed tissue macrophages are replaced (perhaps in some instances after very long intervals) by marrow-produced, bloodborne mononuclear cells.[116] Because the renewal rates of normal tissue macrophages (e.g., Kupffer cells) may be very slow, the required rate of replacement may be quite slow. In other locations, e.g., in granulomas sequestering tubercle bacilli or fungi, the renewal of macrophages may be more rapid.

Some of the maturational events occurring in the monocyte-to-macrophage transition can be assessed in cultures of monocytes as they develop into mature macrophages. In fact, a major portion of the rapidly expanding body of knowledge over the past two decades has been derived from in vitro investigations concerned with interactions of macrophages and the immune (lymphatic) system in body defense and recognition of "self," i.e., the body's own cells (see Chapter 14 and below).

The macrophage system, with its highly developed equipment for macrophagocytosis and killing of viable foreign cells as well as clearing of damaged or defective "self" cells, has a great potential for tissue destruction. If misdirected or misguided by a defective or disordered immune system, it is not difficult to envision how the macrophage system could mount autoimmune aggressive destruction of somatic (self) tissues.

Antigen-specific antibody molecules, produced by a lymphocytic clone generated in response to the specific foreign antigen coat of the foreign cell (opsonin effect), direct the macrophage to the antigenic site and facilitate phagocytosis and killing or sequestration of the unwanted cell(s). Another example of how the immunological apparatus (lymphatic tissue) interacts with the macrophage system to provide the latter with selectivity involves a number of secretions produced by antigen-sensitized thymus-derived (T) lymphocytes known as lymphokines (as described by Dr. Ford in Chapter 14). The influence of one of these secretions, known as migration-inhibition factor (MIF), is particularly illustrative. Rich and Lewis, in 1932, demonstrated in animals inoculated with tuberculosis that the protein antigen tuberculin inhibited the migration of macrophage cells taken from animals showing immunity (delayed hypersensitivity or "cellular" immunity not involving circulating antibody).[117] In 1964, David, Al-Askari, and Lawrence[118] developed an in vitro method of assessing this activity by the inhibition of cells migrating into capillary tubes, the macrophages being obtained from the peritoneal cavity of guinea pigs inoculated with tuberculosis. Subsequently various in vitro modifications have made possible the study of this interaction between lymphocytes and phagocytic cells in humans using a wide variety of sensitizing antigens. Assay of MIF has emerged as the most sensitive and reliable means of assessing cellular immune capability (or delayed hypersensitivity), both terms signifying T-cell-directed immune specificity.

Interaction of macrophages with products or components of the lymphatic system such as antibodies and MIF serves to remove foreign or unwanted material or metabolic products. Macrophages also are essential for the *initiation* of immunological defenses, involving, for example, complex antigens on viable pathogenic microorganisms. Interplay between T lymphocytes (thymus-derived "helper" cells) and macrophages is necessary to "process" antigen in such a way as to elicit the development of lymphocytic clones to express immunity.

Also of great interest to students of the body's defense mechanisms are findings that suggest a major role of the macrophage system in the humoral control of granulopoiesis (as described earlier in this chapter). The putative leukopoietin CSA is produced in large amounts by monocytes and macrophages, and the secretion of this material by macrophages is augmented by bacterial endotoxin. These findings, as well as the results of in vivo studies of the endotoxin effect, imply that CSA, perhaps generated in the RES incident to infection or trauma, may signal the marrow to provide more granulocytes or monocytes. Normally reactive macrophages may well be central to effective function of both the lymphatic tissue and the granulocytes.

Thus, the macrophage, as proposed by Metchnikov in his studies of larval starfish reacting to an impinging rose thorn, probably represents the central cellular unit in the body's defense. This type of cell is common to all multicellular creatures, even to those without a vascular system. The sophisticated features of specialized varieties of microphages and the elaborate immunologic apparatus of mammals were added later in the course of evolution. In effect, if macrophages are not present to engulf and digest the invading microbe or foreign tissue and to process the cellular antigens somehow, immunocytes will not be induced to elaborate the specific antibody or to manifest cellular immunity. Moreover, in the absence of functional macrophages, microbes, even if coated with antibody, may not be killed. Macrophages produce and secrete plasma-soluble substances which are critical to lymphocyte induction (e.g., "processed antigen") and function (e.g., complement components). They also secrete substances which are critical to granulopoiesis (e.g., CSA) and granulocyte function (e.g., complement components).

Thus, the monocyte-macrophage system today is believed to be central to body integrity, being necessary for the initiation of defense and for the mobilization of ready reserves, as well as serving as mere scavengers. Moreover, its interaction with other cellular components appears necessary to provide the diversity of defensive mechanisms required in complex organisms. Finally, the refinement provided by immunologic specificity is crucial in determining whether the inflammatory response is beneficial in terms of ridding the body of unwanted material or harmful in terms of damaging the tissues of the host.

References

1   Bettmann OL: *A Pictorial History of Medicine*. Springfield, Charles C Thomas, 1956, 336 pp.
2   Dewhurst K: *Dr. Thomas Sydenham (1624–1689). His Life and Original Writings*. London, The Wellcome Historical Medical Library, 1966, 191 pp.
3   Louis PCA: *Researches on the Effect of Bloodletting in Some Inflammatory Diseases, and*

on the Influence of Tartarized Antimony and Vesication in Pneumonitis, Putnam CG (trans). Boston, Hilliard and Grey, 1836, 171 pp.

4   Osler W: Influence of Louis on American medicine. *Bull Johns Hopkins Hosp* 8:161–167, 1897.

5   Hewson W: *Experimental Inquiries, Part II, A Description of the Lymphatic System in the Human Subject and Other Animals.* London, J Johnson, 1774, 239 pp, p 152. (In Latin, appears in English in ref. 6.)

6   Gulliver G (ed): *The Works of William Hewson, F.R.S.* London, Sydenham Society, 1846, 360 pp.

7   de Senac J: In Traité de la structure du coeur, Ed. Baron A. Portal (1742–1832), 2:91, 661–664, 1749.

8   Williams, CJB: *Principles of Medicine.* Philadelphia, E Barrington and JD Haswell, 1844, 395 pp, pp 212–215.

9   Stahl GE: in Chaulant L (ed): *Theoria Medica Vera.* Leipzig, 3 vol, 12° Lipsiae, Sumpt L Vossii, 1831–1833, vol 1, pp 252–264.

10 Koch CF: Ueber die Entzuendung nach mikrospopischen Versuchen. *Arch Anat Physiol* 6:121–260, 1832.

11 Virchow R: Ueber die Reform der pathologischen und therapeutichem Anschanungen durch die mikrosckopschen Untersuchungen. *Arch Pathol Anat Physiol Wissensch Med* I:205–235, 1847.

12 Addison W: Colourless globules in the buffy coat of the blood. *Lond Med Gaz* 27:479–481, 1840–1841.

13 Addison W: On the colourless corpuscles and on the molecules and cytoblasts in the blood. *Lond Med Gaz* ii:144–148, 1841–1842.

14 Addison W: Experimental and practical researches on the structure and function of blood corpuscles; on inflammation and on the origin and nature of tubercles in the lungs. *Trans Prov Med Surg Assoc* 11:236–306, 1843.

15 Dutrochet R: Recherches anatomiques et physiologiques sur la structure intime des animaux et vegetaux, et su leur motilité. Paris, JB Ballière, 1824, 233 pp, pp 164–169, 172, 214–216.

16 Waller AV: Microscopic examination of some of the principal tissues of the animal frame, as observed in the tongue of the living frog, toad, etc. *Phil Mag* 29 (3d series):271–287, 1846.

17 Waller AV: Microscopic observations on the perforation of the capillaries by corpuscles of the blood, and on the origin of mucus and pus-globules. *Phil Mag* 29(3d series):397–405, 1846.

18 Recklinghausen FD von: Über Eiter-und Bindegewebeskoerperchen. *Arch Pathol Anat Physiol Klin Med* 28:157–197, 1863.

19 Jones TW: Report on the changes in the blood in inflammation and on the nature of the healing process. *Br For Med Rev* 18:225–280, 1844.

20 Davaine, CJ: Recherches sur les globules blancs du sang. *Seanc Mem Soc Biol (Paris)* ii:103–105, 1850.

21 Kolliker RA von: *Manual of Human Histology,* Busk G, Huxley T (trans and eds). London, The Sydenham Society, 1852, vol 1, p 46.

22 Lieberkühn, JN: Über die Psorospermien. *Arch Anat Physiol Wissensch Med* 21:1–24, 1854.

23 Cohnheim JF: Über entzuendung und Eiterung. *Arch Pathol Anat Physiol Klin Med* 40:179–264, 1867.

24   Rather LJ: *Addison and the White Corpuscles: An Aspect of Nineteenth-Century Biology.* Berkeley, University of California Press, 1972, 287 pp.

25   Cohnheim J: *Neue Untersuchungen uber die Entzuendung.* Berlin, Hirschwald, 1873, 85 pp.

26   Richardson JG: On the identity of the white corpuscles of the blood with salivary, pus and mucus corpuscles. *Pa Hosp Rep* 2:249–254, 1869.

27   Metchnikov I: Spongiologische Studien. *Z Wissensch Zool* 27:115–126, 1878. Cited in Starling FA, Starling EH (trans): *Lectures of the Comparative Pathology of Inflammation.* New York, Dover, 1968, 244 pp.

28   Lieberkühn N: Beitrage zur Anatomie der Spongien. *Arch Anat Physiol Wissensch Med* 24:376–403, 1857.

29   Metchnikov I: Uber die Beziehung der Phagocyten zu Milzbrandbacillen. *Arch Pathol Anat* 97:502, 1884.

30   Koch R: *Untersuchungen uber die Aetiology der Wundinfectionskrankheiten.* Leipzig, F Barth, 1878, 80 pp.

31   Virchow R: Der Kampf der Zellen und der Bakterien. *Arch Pathol Anat Physiol Klin Med* 101:1–13, 1885.

32   Metchnikov, I: Immunity in infective diseases, in Starling FA, Starling EH (trans): *Comparative Pathology of Inflammation.* New York, Dover, 1968, 244 pp.

33   Ziegler E: *Lehrbuch der Allgemeinen und Speciellen Pathologischen Anatomie und Pathogenese,* 2d ed, Jena, G. Fisher. 1882, 382 pp.

34   Brieger GH: Introduction, in Metchnikov I: Immunity in infective diseases, Binnie FG (trans). *J Hist Med* 24:368, 1969.

35   Jones TW: The blood-corpuscle considered in its different phases of development in the animal series. *Philos Trans R Soc Lond,* vol 133, pt I, pp 63–87, 1842.

36   Jones TW: Observations on some points in the anatomy, physiology and pathology of the blood. *Br For Med Rev* 14:585–600, 1842.

37   Schultze M: Ein heizharer Objekttisch und seine Verwendung bei untersuchungen des Blutes. *Arch Mikr Anat* I:1–42, 1865.

38   Ehrlich P: Methodologische Beitrage zur Physiologie und Pathologie der verschisdenen Formen der Leukocyten. *Z Klin Med* I:553–558, 1880.

39   Ehrlich P: *Gesammelte Arbeiten zur Immunitäts Forschung.* Berlin, A. Hirschwald, 1904, 776 pp, p 342.

40   Brown PK: A fatal case of acute primary infectious pharyngitis with extreme leukopenia. *Am Med* 3:649–652, 1902.

41   Schultz W: Ueber eigenartige Halserkrankungen. *Dtsch Med Wochenschr* 48:1495–1498, 1922.

42   Plum P: Agranulocytosis due to aminopyrine; experimental and clinical study of 7 new cases. *Lancet* 1:15–18, 1935.

43   Kracke RR: Experimental production of agranulocytosis. *Am J Clin Pathol* 2:11–15, 1932.

44   Plum P: *Clinical and Experimental Investigations in Agranulocytosis.* London, H.K. Lewis, 1937, 410 pp.

45   Madison FW, Squier TL: Etiology of primary granulocytopenia (agranulocytic angina). *JAMA* 102:755–758, 1934.

46   Lawrence JS, Dowdy AH, Valentine WN: Effects of radiation on hemopoiesis. *Radiology* 51:400–418, 1948.

47 Ambrus CM, Ambrus JL, Johnson GC, Pockman EW, Chernick WS, Back N, Harrison JWE: The role of the lungs in regulation of the white blood cell level. *Am J Physiol* 178:33–38, 1954.

48 Craddock CG, Adams WS, Perry S, Skoog WA, Lawrence JS: Studies of leukopoiesis. The technique of leukopheresis and the response in normal and irradiated dogs. *J Lab Clin Med* 45:881–886, 1955.

49 Ottesen J: On the age of human white cells in peripheral blood. *Acta Physiol Scand* 32:75–78, 1954.

50 Craddock CG, Perry S, Lawrence JS: The dynamics of leukopoiesis and leukocytosis as studied by leukopheresis and isotopic techniques. *J Clin Invest* 35:285–288, 1956.

51 Craddock CG, Perry S, Lawrence JS: Control of the steady state proliferation of leukocytes, in Stohlman F (ed): *The Kinetics of Cellular Proliferation.* New York, Grune and Stratton, 1963, 456 pp, pp 242–263.

52 Osgood EE, Li JG, Tivey H, Duerst ML, Seaman AJ: Growth of human leukemic leukocytes in vitro and in vivo as measured by uptake of P^{32} deoxyribose nucleic acid. *Science* 114:95–98, 1951.

53 Athens JW, Mauer AM, Ashenbrucker H, Cartwright GE, Wintrobe MM: Leukokinetic studies. I. A method for labeling leukocytes with di-isopropyl fluorophosphate (DFP^{32}). *Blood* 14:303–307, 1959.

54 Donohue DM, Gabrio BW, Finch CA: Quantitative measurements of hemopoietic cells of the marrow. *J Clin Invest* 37:1564–1567, 1958.

55 Lajtha LG: On DNA labeling in the study of the dynamics of bone marrow cell populations, in Stohlman F (ed): *Kinetics of Cellular Proliferation.* New York, Grune and Stratton, 1959, 456 pp, pp 173–187.

56 Cronkite EP, Fliedner TM: Granulopoiesis. *N Engl J Med* 270:1347–1351, 1964.

57 Astaldi G, Mauri C: Recherches sur l'activite proliferative de l'hemocytoblaste de la leucemie aigue. *Rev Belge Pathol* 23:69–71, 1953.

58 Craddock CG, Nakai GS: Leukemic cell proliferation as determined by in vitro deoxyribonucleic acid synthesis. *J Clin Invest* 41:360–364, 1962.

59 Mauer AM, Fischer V: Comparison of the proliferation capacity of acute leukemia cells in bone marrow and blood. *Nature* 193:1085–1088, 1962.

60 Pluznik DH, Sachs J: The cloning of normal mast cells in tissue culture. *J Cell Comp Physiol* 66:319–321, 1965.

61 Metcalf D: Personal communication to C.G. Craddock, February 21, 1978.

62 Bradley TR, Metcalf D: The growth of mouse bone marrow cells in vitro. *Aust J Exp Biol Sci* 44:287–289, 1966.

63 Chervenick PA, LoBuglio AF: Human blood monocytes: stimulators of granulocyte and mononuclear colony formation in vitro. *Science* 178:164–166, 1972.

64 Golde DW, Cline MJ: Identification of the colony-stimulating cell in human peripheral blood. *J Clin Invest* 51:2981–2984, 1972.

65 Boyden S: The chemotactic effect of mixtures of antibody and antigen on polymorphonuclear leukocytes. *J Exp Med* 115:453–457, 1962.

66 Ward PA, Cochrane CG, Muller-Eberhard HG: The role of serum complement in chemotaxis of leukocytes in vitro. *J Exp Med* 122:327–331, 1965.

67 Chediak M: Nouvelle anomalie leucocytaire de caractere constitutionnel familial. *Rev Hematol* 7:362–366, 1952.

68 Steinbrinck W: Uber eine neue Granulations-anomalie der Leukocyten. *Dtsch Arch Klin Med* 193:577–579, 1948.

69 Higashi O: Congenital gigantism of peroxidase granules. First case ever reported of qualitative abnormality of peroxidase. *Tohoku J Exp Med* 59:315–318, 1954.

70 Donohue WL, Bain HW: Chediak-Higashi syndrome. A lethal familial disease with anomolous inclusions in the leukocytes and constitutional stigmata: report of a case with necropsy. *Pediatrics* 20:416–420, 1957.

71 Metchnikov I: Sur la lutte des cellules de l'organisme contre l'invasion des microbes. *Ann Inst Pasteur* I:321–328, 1887.

72 de Duve C, Pressman BC, Gianetto R, Wattiaux R, Appelmans R: Tissue fractionation studies. 6. Intracellular distribution patterns of enzymes in rat liver tissue. *Biochem J* 50:604–608, 1955.

73 Cohn ZA, Hirsch JG: The isolation and properties of the specific cytoplasmic granules of rabbit polymorphonuclear leukocytes. *J Exp Med* 112:983–986, 1960.

74 Cohn ZA, Hirsch JG: The influence of phagocytosis on the intracellular distribution of granule-associated components of polymorphonuclear leukocytes. *J Exp Med* 112:1015–1020, 1960.

75 Hirschhorn R, Weissmann G: Isolation and properties of human leukocyte lysosomes in vitro. *Proc Soc Exp Biol Med* 119:36–38, 1965.

76 Bainton DF, Ullyot JL, Farquhar MG: The development of neutrophilic polymorphonuclear leukocytes in human bone marrow: origin and content of azurophil and specific granules. *J Exp Med* 134:907–912, 1971.

77 Graefe E: Die Steigerung des Stoffwechsels bei chronischer leukämie und ihre Ursachen (Augleich ein Beitrag zur Biologie der weissen Blutzellen). *Dtsch Arch Klin Med* 102:406–409, 1911.

78 Warburg O: *Uber den Stoffwechsels der Tumoren.* Berlin, Springer Verlag, 1926, 263 pp.

79 Valentine WN, Beck WS: Biochemical studies on leukocytes. I. Phosphatase activity in health, leukocytosis, myelocytic leukemia. *J Lab Clin Med* 38:39–42, 1951.

80 Beck WS: A kinetic analysis of the glycolytic rate and certain glycolytic enzymes in normal and leukemic leukocytes. *J Biol Chem* 216:333–338, 1955.

81 Beck WS: A kinetic analysis of the glycolytic rate and certain glycolytic enzymes in normal and leukemic leukocytes. *J Biol Chem* 216:333–340, 1955.

82 Valentine WN, Follette JH, Solomon DH, Reynolds J: The relationship of leukocyte alkaline phosphatase to "stress," to ACTH and to adrenal 17-OH-corticosteroids. *J Lab Clin Med* 49:723–728, 1957.

83 Sbarra AJ, Karnovsky ML: The biochemical basis of phagocytosis. I. Metabolic changes during the ingestion of particles by polymorphonuclear leukocytes. *J Biol Chem* 234:1355–1357, 1959.

84 Berendes H, Bridges RA, Good RA: A fatal granulomatosis of childhood: the clinical study of a new syndrome. *Minn Med* 40:309–312, 1957.

85 Landing BA, Shirkey HS: A syndrome of recurrent infection and infiltration of viscera by pigmented lipid histiocytes. *Pediatrics* 20:431–433, 1957.

86 Stetson CA: Studies on the mechanism of the Shwartzman phenomenon: certain factors involved in the production of the local hemorrhagic necrosis. *J Exp Med* 93:489–494, 1951.

87 Stetson CA, Good RA: Studies on the mechanism of the Shwartzman phenome-

non: evidence for the participation of polymorphonuclear leukocytes in the phenomenon. *J Exp Med* 93:49–52, 1951.

88   Thomas L: Possible role of leukocyte granules in the Shwartzman and Arthus reactions. *Proc Soc Exp Biol Med* 1115:235–237, 1964.

89   Cochrane CG, Unanue ER, Dixon FJ: A role for polymorphonuclear leukocytes and complement in nephrotoxic nephritis. *J Exp Med* 122:99–105, 1965.

90   Kniker WT, Cochrane CG: Pathogenic factors in vascular lesions of experimental serum sickness. *J Exp Med* 122:83–87, 1965.

91   Eriksson S: Pulmonary emphysema and alpha$_1$-antitrypsin deficiency. *Acta Med Scand* 175:197–199, 1964.

92   Beeson PB: Temperature-elevating effect of a substance obtained from polymorphonuclear leukocytes. *J Clin Invest* 27:524–527, 1948.

93   Bennett IL Jr, Beeson PB: Studies on the pathogenesis of fever. II. Characterization of fever-producing substances from polymorphonuclear leukocytes and from the fluid of sterile exudates. *J Exp Med* 98:493–497, 1953.

94   Menkin V: Studies on inflammation; isolation of a factor concerned with increased capillary permeability to injury. *J Exp Med* 67:129–135, 1938.

95   Valentine WN, Pearce ML, Lawrence JS: Studies on the histamine content of blood with special reference to leukemia, leukemoid reactions and leukocytosis. *Blood* 5:623–627, 1950.

96   Valentine WN, Pearce ML, Lawrence JS: Studies on the histamine content of blood with special reference to leukemia, leukemoid reactions and leukocytosis. *Blood* 5:623–628, 1950.

97   Weissmann G (ed): *Mediators of Inflammation.* New York, Plenum, 1974, 205 pp.

98   Aschoff L. Das reticulo-endotheliale System. *Ergeb Inn Med Kinderheilk* 26:1–8, 1924.

99   Ranvier L: Des clasmatocytes. *C/R Acad Sci (Paris)* 110:165–170, 1890.

100 Gall EA: The cytochemical identification and interrelation of mesenchymal cells of lymphoid tissue. *Ann NY Acad Sci* 73:120–123, 1958.

101 Downey H (ed): *Handbook of Hematology.* New York, Hoeber, 1938, vol II, 887 pp, pp 973–1271.

102 Maximow AA: Bindegewebe und blutbildende Gewebe, in Mollendorff V (ed): *Handbuck der Mikroskopischen Anatomie des Menschen.* Berlin, Springer, 1927, vol 2, pt 1, p 23.

103 Lang FJ: Über die Alveolar-phagozyten der Lunge. *Arch Zellforsch* 2:93–98, 1930.

104 Foot NC: On the origin of the pulmonary "dust cells." *Am J Pathol* 3:413–417, 1927.

105 Permar HH: The mononuclear phagocytes in experimental pneumonia. *J Med Res* 44:27–29, 1923.

106 Maximow A: Morphology of the mesenchymal reactions. *Arch Pathol* 4:557–562, 1927.

107 Cunningham RS, Sabin FR, Doan CA: The development of leucocytes, lymphocytes and monocytes from a specific stem cell in adult tissues. Contrib. to Emryol. No. 84. Carnegie Inst., Carnegie Inst., Washington, Publ. 361–365, 1925.

108 Masugi M: Über die Beziehungen zwischen Monozyten und Histiozytem. *Beitr Pathol Anat* 76:396–399, 1927.

109 Seemann G: *Histologie der Lungenalveole.* Jena, Fischer, 1931, 88 pp.

110 Gaucher E: De l'épithéliome primitif de la rate, hypertrophie idiopathique de la rate sans leucemie. Thèse de Paris, 1882, 31 pp.

111 Volkman A, Gowans JL: The origin of macrophages from bone marrow in the rat. *Br J Exp Pathol* 46:62–66, 1965.

112 Virolainen M: Hematopoietic origin or macrophages as studied by chromosome markers in mice. *J Exp Med* 127:943–948, 1968.

113 Lewis MR, Lewis WH: Transformation of mononuclear blood cells into macrophages, epitheloid cells, and giant cells in hanging drop blood cultures from lower vertebrates. Carnegie Inst., Washington. Publ. 96, Contrib. to Embryol. 18:95–98, 1926.

114 Cohn ZA, Benson B: The differentiation of mononuclear phagocytes: morphology, cytochemistry and biochemistry. *J Exp Med* 121:153–160, 1965.

115 Huber H, Polley MJ, Linscott WD, Fudenberg HH, Muller-Eberhard HJ: Human monocytes: distinct receptor sites for the third component of complement and for immunoglobulin G. *Science* 162:1281–1284, 1968.

116 Boak JL, Christie GH, Ford WL, Howard JG: Pathways in the development of liver macrophages; alternative precursors contained in populations of lymphocytes and bone marrow cells. *Proc R Soc Lond (Biol)* 169:307–310, 1968.

117 Rich AR, Lewis MR: The nature of allergy in tuberculosis as revealed by tissue culture studies. *Bull Johns Hopkins Hosp* 60:115–121, 1932.

118 David JR, Al-Askari S, Lawrence HS: Delayed hypersensitivity in vitro. I. The specificity of inhibition of cell migration by antigens. *J Immunol* 93:264–268, 1964.

CHAPTER 14

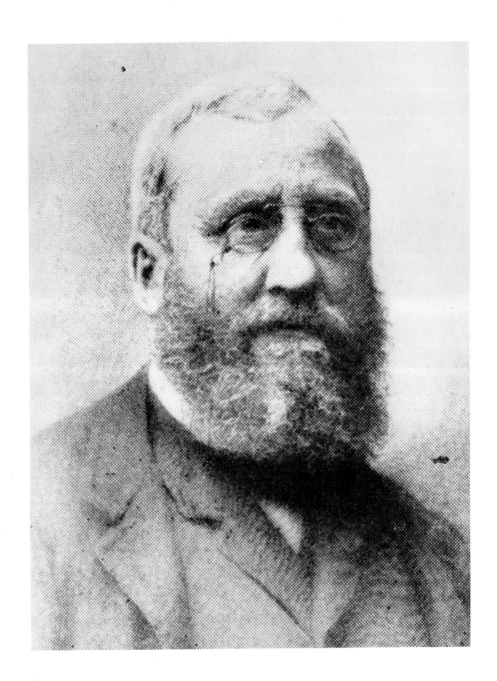

THE LYMPHOCYTE—ITS TRANSFORMATION FROM A FRUSTRATING ENIGMA TO A MODEL OF CELLULAR FUNCTION

William L. Ford

The lymphocyte is the second most abundant type of white cell in human blood (after the neutrophil); yet in appearance it seems to be nothing more than a round nucleus surrounded by a thin rim of featureless cytoplasm. Throughout two centuries of frustration over the obscurity of its function, the plainness of its appearance seemed appropriate to the apparent insignificance of its performance. Only very recently has it been learned how misleading is its stark simplicity and how this contrasts with its extraordinarily intricate role in the formation of antibodies and in the expression of other immune responses.

The lymphocyte is found not only in the blood but is also by far the preponderant cell in the lymph nodes, the white pulp of the spleen, the thymus, the tonsils, and the appendix. Many lymphocytes are present in the bone marrow, and smaller numbers are found in almost all other organs, such as the skin, gut, and liver. The lymphocyte obtained its name because it is

Chapter Opening Photo   Antoine Ranvier (1835–1922).

457

almost the only cell type present in lymph, the watery fluid that flows in the system of vessels known as the lymphatic system. The early story of this ubiquitous cell is intertwined with the discovery of the lymphatic system. However, its recent history falls within the mainstream of immunology.

It is only in the last 20 years that it has become apparent that the lymphocyte *is* the immune system. In 1956, William Boyd[1] included only one reference to the lymphocyte in his comprehensive textbook *Fundamentals of Immunology*. His intent was merely to dismiss the candidacy of the lymphocyte as an antibody-producing cell in favor of the plasma cell. In the 1950s, the evidence linking lymphocytes with immune responses was unsatisfactory, and it was still sensible to regard the function of the cell as enigmatic. It was mainly in the decade from 1958 to 1968 that decisive advances were made, so that now there is probably a deeper knowledge of the lymphocyte than about any other cell type in the body apart from possibly the much simpler red cell. The lymphocyte has become a paradigm of many fundamental cellular processes, such as the organization of the cell membrane and the mechanism by which specific protein is assembled according to genetic instructions and then is packaged and secreted across the cell membrane.

Although the era of the lymphocyte thus appears to have been launched explosively around 1960, the seeds of the unprecedented advances in lymphocytology were planted in the 1930s and 1940s, when several approaches were initiated that were to lead to hard evidence implicating lymphocytes in immune reactions. A crucial development was Medawar's work in the 1940s,[2,3] which associated the study of transplant rejection and immunology. Until then, immunology had consisted largely of the study of antibodies and macrophages. Equally important was the fusion of a classical series of essentially physiological studies on the life history of the lymphocyte with the mainstream of immunology. For this, Gowans' work between 1957 and 1962 was largely responsible[4-7] (Figure 14-1).

In Chapter 13, the history of the defenses of the body as reflected in the role of lymphocytes as well as monocytes, macrophages, and all three types of granulocyte was described. These cells play their individual defensive roles against a multitude of infections and other harmful agents. In its most general sense, immunology includes the study of all these defenses, but after the discovery of antibodies in 1890, immunologists focused most of their attention on the *specific* immune response, the reaction to a microbial infection. Thus, for example, when infected with tetanus, the body will adapt itself to resist the organism. The response usually contributes to recovery from the infection and will persist so that the body is less susceptible to that infection for a prolonged period. However, such acquired resistance does not extend to another organism, e.g., diphtheria. By contrast, the *nonspecific* defenses, for which granulocytes and monocytes are responsible, are present before an infection starts.

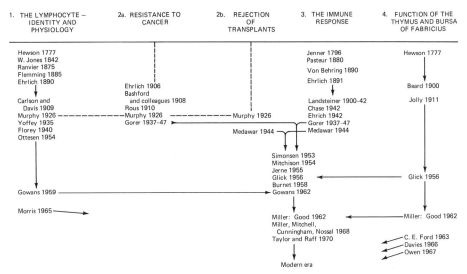

Figure 14-1 Some of the contributors to current knowledge of the lymphocyte are grouped according to streams of research that extend over long periods. The horizontal lines indicate names of individuals whose contributions have led to the convergence of streams.

These cells may become somewhat more effective in the course of an infection, but this increased efficiency applies to all microorganisms and is not tailor-made for each individual invader.

As described in earlier chapters, Paul Ehrlich is a crucial figure in the early phases of our story; first, because he introduced and developed selective staining methods for lymphocytes (1879–1890[8,9]) and later, from 1890 until about 1903, because of his studies of antibody formation.[10,11]

The Lymphocyte up to Paul Ehrlich

THE LYMPH AND ITS CELLS

Before Ehrlich entered the scene, it was appreciated that there is a system of lymphatic vessels distinct from arteries and veins. This conducts a one-way stream of a watery fluid named lymph (Latin, *lympha*—"clear spring water") into the venous side of the blood circulation. Lymph contains a variable number of cells, but only a few of these are recognizably red cells; most are "lymph corpuscles." Some but not all of the white cells in the blood are identical in appearance with these lymph corpuscles or lymphocytes. The small round cells that predominate in the thymus, lymph nodes, and white pulp of the spleen also are classified as lymphocytes, and all of these organs produce lymphocytes and contribute them to the blood, sometimes via the lymphatics.

The lymphatic system was discovered in the seventeenth century, when curiosity about body structure and formation was revived. This was soon aided by the first primitive microscopes. By 1722, Leeuwenhoek (Chapter 1) had seen rounded corpuscles in lymph, as did several other observers later in the 1700s.[12] The lymphatics of the intestine (lacteals) had attracted attention because after a meal fat is partly absorbed by this route, causing these vessels to appear milky.[13] In 1622, Gasparo Aselli in Pavia near Milan traced these lymph vessels to the lymph nodes in the mesentery. Jean Pecquet in 1651 found that, like veins, fine lymphatics combine to form larger trunks, and eventually these form a larger vessel, the thoracic duct, which collects lymph from a large area of the body and discharges it into the subclavian vein.[13]

The huge contribution of William Hewson to knowledge of the lymphatic system and of white blood cells has been acknowledged in Chapters 1 and 13. An imaginative investigator, he carried out numerous experiments on many different species. Some quotations from Gulliver's edition of Hewson's work[14] will show that his insights underlay all the early discoveries regarding the lymphocyte, although some of these were not fully accepted until the twentieth century.

In 1773 he stated,

> By the lymphatic system and its appendages we mean the lymphatic vessels, the lymphatic glands (nodes), the thymus and the spleen. At the first view it may seem extraordinary that nature should have given so many and so complicated organs to form only part of the blood, when she effects other secretions by organs apparently more simple; but our surprise must cease when we reflect, that upon a due formation of these particles, not only the various functions of the body but the very existence of the animal, in a great measure, depends.

This clearly expresses the notion of a unified lymphoid system. However, Hewson thought that all white cells were derived from lymphoid tissue, and indeed in describing lymph corpuscles as "central particles" he implied that they were transformed into red cells in the spleen. This he seems to have inferred because red cells have a pale central area, which under a primitive microscope resembles a white cell. Since he would not have been able to see any structure within a lymphocyte, he assumed these featureless spheres to be naked nuclei.

Hewson's ideas on the role of the thymus and the fate of the lymphocyte ("central particle") in the blood are partially conveyed in the following passages.

The thymus gland then, we consider as being an appendage to the lymphatic glands, for the more perfectly and expeditiously forming the central particles of the blood in the foetus, and in the early part of life.

We have proved that vast numbers of central particles made by the thymus and lymphatic glands, are poured into the blood vessels through the thoracic duct and if we examine the blood attentively we see them floating in it. Nature surely would not make so infinitely many particles to answer no purpose! What then becomes of these particles after they are mixed with the circulating blood; are they immediately destroyed? No. They are, we believe, carried with the blood to the spleen, not that the spleen has any elective attraction over them; but that being equally and uniformly diffused through the general mass of blood, a due proportion of them is received by the spleen with its arterial blood, and that when arrived there, the spleen has the power of separating them from other parts of the blood. . . .

Hewson was right in regarding the thymus as a major primary source of lymphocytes. Many of these cells do enter the blood and are rapidly redistributed to other lymphoid organs, the spleen taking about 50 to 60 percent. Hewson misinterpreted the relationship between red and white cells because microscopes were so imperfect in the eighteenth century and staining methods were yet to be invented.

The first half of the nineteenth century was a fallow period for advances in understanding lymphocyte function. As microscopes improved it was seen that the white cells in the blood were not uniform. Wharton Jones[15] made the important observation that some white cells were granular while others were not, adding that the granular type predominated in the blood but most of the cells in lymph were nongranular. The credit he deserves for this astute description is sullied by his unfortunate guess that the different forms of leukocyte are merely different ages or phases of the same cell type—an idea which continued to be misleading until well into the twentieth century.

THE HISTOLOGICAL OBSERVATIONS OF RANVIER AND FLEMMING

In the last quarter of the nineteenth century, in addition to Ehrlich, major contributions to knowledge of the lymphocyte were made by Louis Antoine Ranvier (1835–1922) (Chapter Opening Photo), of Paris, and Walther Flemming (1843–1905) (Figure 14-2), of Prague and later, Kiel. In 1875, Ranvier published his 1100 page *Traité Technique d'Histologie.*[16] This authoritative work included not only detailed descriptions of the structure of lymph nodes and lymphatic vessels but also reported extensive experiments on lymphocytes and farsighted discussions as to their function.

The serious study of lymphocytes in vitro was initiated by Ranvier. He described in accurate detail the way in which lymphocytes move fitfully and

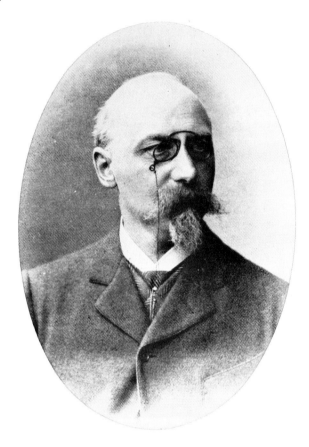

Figure 14-2 Walther Flemming (1843–1905).

sluggishly across a glass slide, and he compared the deformations of the cells as they moved with the motility of amoebae. More importantly he undertook a comprehensive series of experiments to define the conditions under which lymphocytes move in vitro. He found that mammalian lymphocytes are motile when the medium is heated to 30 to 37°C but do not move at 20°C, and above 40°C they round up and die. The oxygen requirement for movement was emphasized as well as the importance of the humidity of the gaseous phase (no doubt affecting the osmolarity of the medium). Also, lymphocytes do not move in suspension but require a solid surface to crawl over.

Ranvier obtained lymphocytes from dogs or rabbits by thoracic duct cannulation with a glass tube. He also did some experiments with pericardial fluid from rabbits and, in the case of frogs, took lymph from the dorsal lymph sac. His technical ingenuity is exemplified by a method which he used to harvest lymph cells from the frog that consisted of implantation of the pith of an elder twig; the interstices became infiltrated with cells of which a high yield could thus be obtained. However, it is unfortunate that Ranvier sometimes used fluid from a *serous* cavity like the pericardium because it is known to contain a high proportion of macrophages as well as lymphocytes.

Although as Ranvier acknowledged, lymphocyte movement was first observed by Wharton Jones in 1842,[15] and Ranvier's observations were soon confirmed by Renaut,[17] Ehrlich[18] failed to observe this phenomenon, and he, and later Maximov,[19] denied that lymphocytes had this ability. This controversy dominated the study of lymphocytes for about 40 years and probably diverted attention from other more important properties of the cell. Between 1875 and 1920, many papers were published supporting one side or the other. Following the work of W.H. Lewis and L.T. Webster,[20] the view prevailed that under defined conditions of temperature and composition of culture medium, lymphocytes would consistently move in vitro (reviewed by Harris[21]). Possibly the obsession with lymphocyte motility in vitro arose because of the general impact made by Metchnikov's observations on large phagocytic cells (Chapter 13). Macrophages and granulocytes both move more quickly than lymphocytes, and their movement is subject to attraction by products of bacteria, degenerating blood cells, and other chemotactic material. Lymphocytes are not phagocytic and show a rather different pattern of movement.

Ranvier[16] asserted that lymphocytes play a considerable role in the body, as suggested by their two essential characteristics—migration and diapedesis. The migration of lymphocytes throughout the entire body and their ability to cross the walls of blood vessels into tissues (diapedesis), especially at sites of inflammation, led Ranvier to the belief that lymphocytes contribute to healing and repair. He suggested that to fulfill this role, lymphocytes were consumed in many tissues and, thus, a constant production of new cells either in the lymph nodes or connective tissues was necessary to maintain the level in the lymph and the blood.

Ranvier believed that local oxygen tension was the factor that determined the migration of lymphocytes within lymph nodes and their discharge into the lymph, as well as influencing the site of their diapedesis from the blood. It will be impossible to judge this proposal finally until we have some clue as to the mechanisms determining the unique migratory pattern of lymphocytes. Ranvier was outstanding for seizing on the really important histological observations when speculating about function.

Flemming was another anatomist who made good use of the improved microscopes and the newly devised methods for staining tissues. His name is usually associated with the discovery of secondary follicles in the spleen, lymph nodes, and tonsils. These consist of a pale central area of large cells surrounded by a rim of small dark lymphocytes. Flemming called the pale areas germinal centers because of the abundance of dividing cells in these situations. He also noted "tingible bodies"; these are now known to be macrophages stuffed with the debris of dead cells.

In 1885, Flemming[22] published his ideas about the fact that lymph leaving a lymph node in the efferent vessel was always found to be much richer in cells than lymph arriving at the node in afferent lymphatic vessels. Apparently a large number of cells are added to lymph while it passes through a lymph node within a closed labyrinthine system.[16] He proposed a new way of looking at this fact; namely, that only two processes could account for the huge discrepancy between the cell influx and efflux. Either cell division in the node makes a major contribution to the high output of cells in the efferent lymph or alternatively lymphocytes enter from the blood by continuously or intermittently crossing the walls of blood vessels within the nodes so that a continuous circulation of these cells from blood into lymph and back again to the blood could occur. He emphasized that no evidence existed at that time to favor one possibility or the other. Considering his extensive work on cell division in germinal centers as well as in other areas of lymph nodes his open mindness on this point excites as much wonder as the rigorous logic of his compartmental analysis of the lymph node. Precisely the same balance sheet with the same items of credits and debits to the lymphocyte population of a lymph node was applied by Hall and Morris in 1965.[23] The conceptual basis of their experiment on the popliteal lymph node of the sheep was that of Flemming but they had available tritiated thymidine which enabled them to show that only about 4 percent of the cells in efferent lymph are formed by division within the resting node. Consequently, immigration of cells from the blood within the node *must* be the major source of the cells in the efferent lymph.

THE SIGNIFICANCE OF EHRLICH'S WORK

The profound influence of Ehrlich's staining methods on the concept of the lymphocyte, especially from the viewpoint of the hematologist has already been stressed here and in Chapters 1 and 13. His work on the subject from 1879 until 1891 established the lymphocytes as a class of leukocyte accounting for 22 to 25 percent of cells in normal blood.[8,9] Following this work, they were called lymphocytes rather than lymph corpuscles or lymphatic elements. Ehrlich drew a distinction between lymphocytes and other leukocytes by emphasizing their different origins. He proposed that lymphocytes originate in the lymph nodes and spleen while other classes of leukocyte are produced in the bone marrow. He insisted that the lymphocyte represented a separate cell lineage rather than being a precursor of other cell types, as asserted by Wharton Jones.[15] As evidence he cited patients with a selective deficiency of lymphocytes in the blood as a consequence of widespread malignant involvement of lymph nodes. One patient with lymphosarcoma had only 0.6 percent of lymphocytes among his white cells but normal levels of other leukocytes.[9] This did not suggest that lymphocytes and other leukocytes readily transformed into each other. Eventually in the twentieth century this sort of evidence was obtained from animal models in more clear-cut form, and it was proved decisively that the lymphocyte is an independent cell line.

Ehrlich turned his attention to the formation of antibodies shortly after they were discovered by von Behring and Kitasato in 1890.[24] Although this chapter is not intended to be a history of immunology, it is appropriate to set in context some of Ehrlich's practical and theoretical contributions to the subject.

At the end of the 1700s, Jenner[25] had proved the effectiveness of smallpox vaccination, and in the 1880s, Pasteur[26] developed vaccines by attenuating microorganisms. The contribution of von Behring and Kitasato was to show that the acquired resistance to diphtheria or tetanus organisms resided in the blood serum. For this key advance, von Behring was awarded the first Nobel Prize for Physiology and Medicine in 1900. In 1891, Ehrlich[11] published elegant experiments on immunity to two plant toxins—ricin and abrin. He found that by injecting small, sublethal doses, the dose could be gradually increased until the animal would survive injections of several hundred times the previously lethal dose. Later, Ehrlich demonstrated that immunity could be transferred to suckling offspring in the milk—an important mechanism for protecting the young at a susceptible stage.

In his publications from 1896, Ehrlich developed a theory of antibody production, which was given in detail in his Croonian Lecture of 1900.[10] The theory had many facets and included three concepts which are particularly important:

1 The cellular machinery for making a given antibody is present before the cell first experiences the particular antigen.
2 Cells are able to react with antigen because they display on their surface an accurate sample of the antibody they are capable of manufacturing. Antibody formation is stimulated when antigen selects the appropriate receptor (his famous "side chain theory").
3 One cell may express many or all antibody specificities.

The first two ideas are now well established as cornerstones of the selective theory of immunity. The third idea turned out to be wrong because what is selected by antigen is a cell rather than a subcellular unit. As proposed in the 1950s and proved in the 1960s, the cell selected is none other than the lymphocyte. As it turned out, the nineteenth century research ultimately of the greatest significance for the lymphocyte was the work on antibody formation, but, paradoxically, it seems that Ehrlich himself never associated lymphocytes with immune responses.

Ehrlich's conception of immunity was built upon the neutralization of toxins by antibody, and he apparently assumed that this should be a general property of all cells. He failed to appreciate the significance of the work of

Pfeiffer and Marx[27] and of Deutch[28] at the very end of the century indicating that the capacity to form antibodies is a property of specialized tissues such as the spleen.

The side chain theory gradually fell out of favor throughout the first few decades of this century. Initially this was partly because to overcome particular objections, Ehrlich put forward ad hoc elaborations divorced from experimental evidence. Later, Landsteiner's work[29] on the chemical modification of protein antigens led to some understanding of the chemical basis of antigenicity. He showed that not only toxins were antigens and that the number of possible different antigens to which the body can respond might be in the order of hundreds of thousands or millions; it seemed unlikely that during its development the body would produce the machinery necessary for the manufacture of each and every one of this multitude of antigens. Landsteiner showed that antibodies may even be produced against antigens which include chemical groupings apparently not found in nature. It had been thought such a faculty would not have any selective advantage and, therefore, would be unlikely to have evolved. Even more inconceivable was the notion that each cell could express about a million different receptors on its surface.

Gradually, Ehrlich's model was discarded in favor of a radically different one which proposed that the antigen itself was part of the machinery for making antibody protein. The simplest form of this idea was that antigen acted as a template on which the amino-acid sequence of an antibody molecule was built up. When the antibody molecule was finished, it was somehow dissociated from the antigen and secreted from the cell so that the process could begin again. This "instructive theory" implied that the cell making antibody contained sufficient antigen over the long period that antibody synthesis continued. The rational consequence of this was to examine the cells in which antigens localized. This approach was adopted by many workers in the early 1900s. They used colored dyes linked to proteins to trace their fate after injection.[30] It was found that most of an antigenic protein was taken up by macrophages in the liver, spleen, bone marrow, and, after subcutaneous injection, in lymph nodes. These macrophages were a major component of the "reticuloendothelial" system, as had been defined by Aschoff.[31] Throughout the first half of the present century it was thought reasonable to assume that antibodies were made within the macrophages of the reticuloendothelial system. The events within the cell which were thought to lead to antibody secretion were described by Sabin.[32] Thus, until the last few decades, the lymphocyte was largely ignored in the context of antibody responses because labeled antigens did not localize within these cells. Later it became apparent that the small lymphocyte was not a major antibody producer either. These two facts provide the clue to the long delay in identifying the lymphocyte as a key cell in immune responses. In recent years, the instructive mechanism of antibody formation has been discarded, but in the process some of Ehrlich's ideas have been vindicated.

OTHER NOTIONS OF THE FUNCTION OF THE LYMPHOCYTE

Until the lymphocyte was shown to be responsible for immune responses, there were two main strands of speculation regarding its function—the lymphocyte as a precursor cell and the lymphocyte as a supplier of nutrients (the "trephocyte" theory). In the 1800s, the lymphocyte was thought to be an early phase in the development of erythrocytes or of other leukocytes. Perhaps most persistent has been the idea that the lymphocyte is a precursor of macrophages.[18] The explanation for the abundance of evidence that has been put forward in favor of these essentially misleading ideas may be the resemblance between the appearance of the lymphocyte and some of the precursor cells. For example, in the bone marrow there is a substantial number of "transitional cells," which Yoffey and his colleagues showed to be precursors of the red cell series.[33] However, the similarity of these transitional cells to lymphocytes may be coincidental. The immediate precursors of macrophages are monocytes, but in the blood these cells have a variable appearance. Some of them are round cells almost as small as lymphocytes, thus accounting for many investigations which have shown that when lymphocyte-like cells are isolated from the blood and maintained in culture, unmistakable macrophages appear within a few days.

The idea that lymphocytes are simply packages of protein and nucleic acids designed for the distribution of metabolites to all tissues was elaborated by Ranvier,[16] who regarded lymphocytes as carrying around the body a reserve of essential metabolites which were available to any tissue with an exceptional requirement. This idea was bolstered by the short time lymphocytes spent in the bloodstream and the misconception that they have an exceptionally short life span. The theory was extended in several directions, including the idea that the lymphocyte has a function in controlling the size and growth of organs.[34] No rigorous evidence has ever been provided in favor of this role, but neither is any single observation decisively against it. The formal burial of the theory has yet to be arranged.

Four Convergent Pathways Leading to the Immunological Role of the Lymphocyte

The rapid progress in elucidating the function of the lymphocyte from 1960 onward resulted from the convergence of several lines of research, some of which were directed towards other objectives (Figure 14-1). These can be discussed in turn.

WHY TRANSPLANTS OF BOTH TUMORS AND NORMAL TISSUES GENERALLY FAIL TO THRIVE IN THEIR NEW HOST

One of the most significant convergences involved the study of cancer by transplanting tumors and the study of the mechanism by which normal tissues are rejected after they are grafted to new hosts. It was not until the 1940s that it was fully established that the rejection of grafts of cancer tissue between animals of the same species or different species was governed by the same set of rules that apply to normal tissues such as skin and that both general examples of rejection had the features of a specific immune response akin to antibody formation, although neither depended on the appearance of antibodies in the serum.

In the nineteenth century, Hanau observed that malignant tumors could sometimes be transmitted from one animal to another by transferring living cells from the tumor.[35] In the early twentieth century transplantation became a popular method of studying cancer. C.O. Jensen[36] and Paul Ehrlich[37] found that experimental cancers arising in mice usually failed to grow in another mouse. Also, the growth and survival of the tumor were curtailed sooner if the mouse had been inoculated with the same tumor at an earlier stage. Ehrlich supposed that transplanted cancer cells regressed because of "athrepsia" or starvation. He speculated that the tumor failed to obtain nutrients from the host because it lacked the appropriate "side-chains"; the increased resistance to a second inoculation of cancer cells was attributed to depletion of nutrients by the first tumor. However, Bashford and his colleagues at the Cancer Research Fund Laboratories in London pointed out that the general resistance of animals to a transplanted tumor had much in common with an immune response.[38-40] They recorded the invasion of tumors by lymphocytes, plasma cells, and fibroblasts and concluded that the rapid accumulation of lymphocytes in transplanted tumors must follow their massive emigration from the blood vessels within the tumor.[39] A further important discovery was that when a recipient had been grafted with normal tissue, its resistance to a tumor graft was sometimes increased as effectively as if it had received an inoculation of cancer cells.[40] As later became clear, this was because tumors generally bear the same antigens as do normal tissues, and, therefore, grafts provoke the same type of acquired resistance whether they are cancerous or not.

The culmination of this line of work, at least from the point of view of the lymphocyte, came in the beautifully designed and lucidly described experiments of James B. Murphy published in collected form in 1926.[41] Working at the Rockefeller Institute in New York with only an occasional colleague, Murphy applied a wide range of ingenious methods mainly to the mechanism of resistance, or immunity, to transplants of tumors. He also experimented on grafts of normal tissue and resistance to tuberculosis. He was ahead of his time in associating these phenomena, which we now know to be examples of "cell mediated immunity." His evidence that the lymphocyte was not just involved but played a decisive role in these processes was as follows:

1 Exposure of rats and mice to x-rays kills lymphocytes throughout the body and dramatically lowers resistance to cancer grafts.

2 Tumors can usually be grafted into embryos successfully. The lack of resistance of embryos can be overcome if along with the tumor a graft of spleen or bone marrow from an adult is included, but grafts of kidney or liver are ineffective. Thus, adult organs containing lymphocytes confer resistance to the cancer.

3 When tumors are grafted into resistant mice, not only are they invaded by lymphocytes but this is accompanied by a large increase in the numbers of lymphocytes in the blood and is associated with the proliferation of lymphocytes in the spleen and lymph nodes.

4 Lymphoid tissues could be stimulated, and at the same time the resistance of rats and mice to tumor grafts was increased in three ways: (a) a small dose of soft x-rays, which did not penetrate far beyond the skin, (b) exposure of rats or mice to "dry heat"—an ambient temperature of about 60°C, and (c) injection of olive oil. Later workers, however, have found these particular results difficult or impossible to repeat.

Murphy's studies of experimental tuberculosis in mice also yielded a battery of convincing though circumstantial evidence of the defensive role of the lymphocyte.[41] He acknowledged previous work that correctly indicated that antibody formation is not an important factor in resistance to tuberculosis and concluded that antibodies are likewise unimportant in destroying tumor grafts.

Looking back on Murphy's enormous contribution after half a century, the intriguing question is why it was not followed by a rapid expansion of lymphocyte studies in the 1920s. Although widely known and highly regarded, Murphy's work was not followed up as it deserved to be. One reason for this is that in their attempts to analyze the mechanism of resistance, Murphy and his contemporaries transferred fragments of complex organs rather than dissociated cells teased out of lymphoid organs. As will be recounted later, it was the transfer between animals of dissociated lymphoid cells that established the concept of cell mediated immunity in the 1940s and 1950s. In the 1920s, the necessary equipment—needles, syringes, and salt solutions—were readily available, but experimentalists had an *idée fixe* that even gentle disruption of a tissue into single cells would not allow the cells to function after transfer. Another reason is that Murphy did not go quite far enough in clarifying his concepts. He discussed resistance to tumor grafts and to tuberculosis in terms of "immunity" and gave reasons for believing that antibody production was not involved. However, the notion that immunity could be defined by criteria other than the detection of serum antibody was not developed further until Medawar's publications in the 1940s.

Murphy and Hektoen[42] deserve particular credit for their exploitation of x-rays to investigate immunity, although Heineke[43] had already shown much earlier that lymphocytic tissue is exquisitely sensitive to radiation. However, x-rays damage many other tissues, including most precursor cells in the bone marrow, and so it was not certain that x-rays inhibit the capacity to make antibody *because* they destroy lymphocytes until, much later, Gowans corrected the deficiency of x-rayed rats by replenishing lymphocytes alone.[44]

Following Murphy's contribution, Snell[45] and Gorer[46] performed classical experiments on the rules governing the acceptance or rejection of tumor transplants.[47] They developed and exploited inbred strains of mice, which were becoming available in larger numbers following the initiative of Little[48] and found that tumors could readily be transferred from one member of an inbred strain to another; such individuals were genetically uniform, like identical twins. The resistance to tumors was analyzed by transferring tumors between strains and to and from hybrids. Inherited factors were found to be all important, particularly certain attributes of the tumor determined by a complicated system of linked genes named the H-2-locus. In 1933, J.B.S. Haldane[49] proposed that these attributes were in fact antigens, that is, they act by stimulating the immune system as do the blood-group antigens on red cells. The implication of these discoveries for the lymphocyte eventually turned out to be of the utmost significance and justifies this digression into what was regarded as primarily cancer resarch.

The second confluence of independent lines of research was the integration of immunology and transplantation research, which is largely due to the work of Peter B. Medawar (1915–   ). As a young zoologist in Oxford during World War II, he pursued a number of approaches to the treatment of burns. While a visiting worker in Tom Gibson's Burns Unit in Glasgow, he studied the mechanism by which skin grafts transferred from one individual to another were eventually rejected, because the possibility of delaying or preventing this rejection was of obvious practical importance. The problem was that although an area of skin can be successfully transplanted from one part of an individual to a distant site on the same individual, a graft of skin to another individual inevitably contracted and died after a latent interval of around 2 weeks, even though it had healed in and gained a new blood supply perfectly well.[2]

The history of tissue transplantation extends far back into the nineteenth century,[47] but until Medawar's research, the notion that graft rejection might be an example of an immune response was only one of several ideas under consideration. Medawar studied the survival of skin grafts between outbred rabbits of differing genetic makeup.[3] He found that first grafts were always rejected after 14 to 16 days. A second graft from the same donor was rejected after only 7 to 8 days, but if the graft came from a different donor it was rejected with the slower "first-set" tempo. Medawar had thus shown a form of memory which was specific for the foreign tissue with which the animal had come in contact. This form of specific memory had been long established as a hallmark of the antibody response. Thus, Medawar drew a crucial distinction between the *innate* capacity of animals to reject grafts sooner or later and the *acquired* capacity for accelerated rejection, which follows either a preliminary graft or the injection of living cells of the same constitution.[3,50]

After the war, Medawar became professor of zoology at Birmingham and later moved to University College, London. Then, along with Billingham and

Brent, he undertook an illuminating series of studies of immunity to tissue grafts. They developed a concept of the accelerated rejection of a second graft as a reflection of a state of "homograft sensitivity," analogous to delayed-type hypersensitivity to the tubercle bacillus, that is, the inflammatory response found at 24 hours after injection of tuberculin into the skin of a subject who has encountered the bacillus. In 1954, they reported the transfer of homograft sensitivity (accelerated "second-set" rejection) from one animal to another by transferring living cells. They found that a cell suspension produced from the lymph node reacting to a skin graft was the most effective source of cells, and they called this *adoptive* immunization to distinguish it from *passive* immunization following transfer of antibody.[51] The point of the term adoptive is that living lymphocytes generally have to be adopted by their host for successful transfer of their immune function.

In fact, the first experiment to show the adoptive transfer of transplantation immunity by lymphoid cells had been done a few months earlier in Oxford by N.A. Mitchison[52] using a transplantable tumor. Nicolas Avrion Mitchison (1928–) had been a pupil of Medawar and is the nephew of J.B.S. Haldane. Throughout the past 25 years, Mitchison and his pupils have continued to make key contributions in immunology, as will become clear. The substantial British contribution to this field is very largely due to the interwoven careers of four Oxford scientists—Florey, Medawar, Gowans, and Mitchison.

DEVELOPMENTS IN IMMUNOLOGY OF RELEVANCE
TO THE LYMPHOCYTE

The discovery of the adoptive transfer of accelerated graft rejection by Mitchison and Medawar was the second piece of evidence that graft rejection is an immune process. To understand its crucial importance, it is necessary to go back in time and outline developments in the mainstream of immunology.

The model of antibody formation proposed by Ehrlich[10] in 1900 flared like a comet and then died gradually over the first decade of the century. The notion that antigen triggered antibody responses by selecting preformed receptors became unattractive because the work of Karl Landsteiner[29] on haptens (chemical groups which can alter an antigenic protein so that a different antibody is produced against it) suggested that the number of possible antibodies must be in the order of millions rather than a few hundred or thousand. It seemed incredible that the machinery for the synthesis of all these different proteins could be developed in each organism before they had ever encountered the antigens. The prevailing view for half a century was that the notion of developing a capacity to produce antibodies which might never be needed was too extravagant to contemplate.

Karl Landsteiner (1868–1943) was an Austrian who moved from Europe to the Rockefeller Institute in New York in 1923. As recounted in Chapter 20, he was awarded the Nobel Prize in 1930 for his early work on human blood-group antigens on red cells.[53] However, his work on the chemical modification of protein antigens would surely also have deserved the award, and, like other prize winners in immunology, he did not rest on his laurels. In 1933, he started a systematic study of contact sensitivity to picryl chloride and other simple chemicals painted on the skin.[54] This apparently had an immune component because a greatly increased inflammatory reaction was elicited by a given compound when it was applied some time after a previous exposure to the same compound. Landsteiner was puzzled that despite these features of an immune response, contact sensitivity differed from antibody formation in that the latter cannot be provoked by small molecules unless they have been linked to proteins as haptens; there is a minimum size for an antigen that corresponds roughly to the size of small protein molecules.

Merrill W. Chase (1905–   ) joined Landsteiner's team in 1936. Their systematic attempts to transfer contact sensitivity from one guinea pig to another using serum proved difficult, although occasionally they had some apparent success, which in retrospect is difficult to explain. In 1942, they reported in only two pages an experiment which had been performed in 1940.[55] They had found that by harvesting the inflammatory exudate, consisting of living cells and fluid, from the peritoneal cavity of a sensitized guinea pig and injecting it into a second guinea pig which had never had contact with the antigen until challenged, they also transferred the contact sensitivity. The novel finding was that only the cells in the exudate and not the fluid component were effective in the transfer. When the cells were killed by gentle heat, the recipient did not become sensitive to the chemical.

Landsteiner died in 1943, 10 years after starting work on contact sensitivity. It is uncertain to what extent he realized the far-reaching importance of the finding that a class of immune responses can be transferred by cells but not by serum, as contrasted to antibody responses, for which serum transfer had been shown in the 1890s to be effective. Landsteiner had assumed that contact sensitivity must be due to some unusual class of antibody response.[54] This turned out to be wrong, but the principle of the transfer experiment he and Chase pioneered was to lead by the 1950s to the established concept of two fundamentally different mechanisms for implementing immune responses, one of which is antibody formation and the other, later called cell mediated immunity. Fortunately, Chase took seriously the advice he had received from Michaelis, "You do not need to understand *first*. Just keep working, working hard and the prepared mind will see."[54]

The idea that some immune responses might be implemented by effector *cells* rather than by antibody had been heralded by Murphy's studies on the role of lymphocytes in resistance to tuberculosis and skin grafting.[41] By the 1950s, contact sensitivity, delayed type sensitivity to tuberculosis, and rejection of skin grafts from another individual had been grouped together under the umbrella of cell mediated immunity.[56] It was later established that all these responses are implemented by a population of effector lymphocytes ultimately derived from the thymus and newly generated in response to the sensitizing antigenic stimulus. Several events in the 1940s underlie this conceptual development, which is one of the most important in cellular immunology.

The fact that animals which have been infected with tuberculosis develop altered reactivity to tuberculoprotein had been known since Robert Koch's experiments[57] in the nineteenth century. A small dose of tuberculoprotein injected into the skin elicits an inflammatory reaction in a sensitized subject which differs in two ways from allergic reactions mediated by antibody; first, it does not reach a maximum intensity until 24 to 48 hours after the antigenic challenge, and second, at the height of the reaction the cells in the area are mostly lymphocytes and macrophages. It had also been known for many years that delayed-type hypersensitivity to tuberculoprotein was in most circumstances associated with resistance to infection. The proof that this resistance is achieved by cell mediated immunity is that it can be conferred on a naive recipient by the transfer of immune lymphocytes.[58] Chase made a start on the long road to proving this by showing in 1945 that resistance to tuberculosis could be transferred by peritoneal exudate cells (including lymphocytes) but not by serum.[59]

Mounting Suspicion of the Role of the Lymphocyte in Antibody Formation
At about the same time as Landsteiner and Chase's work was published, a different line of research was concerned with the organs and cells responsible for antibody synthesis. We have already noted evidence from 1898 that the capacity to form antibodies is limited to certain cells and tissues.[27,28] The next significant experiment on the subject was performed by McMaster and Hudack in 1935.[60] By introducing the principle of comparing lymph nodes on one side of the body with lymph nodes on the other, they showed that most of the antibody formed in response to injection of antigen into the ear skin was produced in the lymph node draining the site of injection. After injection, antigenic particles were borne to the lymph node in fine lymphatic vessels and were then filtered out within the node and taken up by macrophages. However, the cell population of both the lymph nodes and the spleen (long regarded as the "the lymph node of the blood" [Chapter 5]) includes lymphocytes and plasma cells as well as macrophages and other cell types. The common-sense assumption—that the cell type which took in the bulk of the antigen would be the same cell that made antibody—inculpated the macrophage as the producer of antibody. However, several clues emerged around 1940 which suggested that lymphocytes and plasma cells were also intimately involved.

In 1939, Rich, Lewis, and Wintrobe studied the cells in the spleen responding to an intravenous injection of foreign protein.[61] There was a marked increase in the number of large lymphocytes, which could be identified and clearly distinguished from macrophages by studying their mode of locomotion in vitro. They realistically observed, "Since the function of the lymphoid cells is so dark a mystery, most of those who regard the acute splenic tumor cells as lymphoblasts refrain from speculation regarding the function which these cells serve." They went on to point out, "There are, indeed, a number of facts which render the possibility that the lymphocyte may play a role in antibody formation worthy at least of consideration and study," and they concluded that one function of the lymphocyte is concerned with the body's reaction to foreign protein.

W.E. Ehrich had been impressed for some years by the observation that small doses of antigen, sufficient to elicit a respectable antibody response, did not provoke any perceptible change in macrophages.[62] Along with T.N. Harris, he made a comprehensive study of the response of the rabbit popliteal lymph node to particulate antigens.[63] They stressed the proliferation of lymphocytes within the stimulated lymph node, which started throughout all the compartments of the node but later was concentrated in the germinal centers described by Flemming in 1885.[22] A substantial increase in the numbers of lymphocytes released into the efferent lymphatic coincided with the rise of antibody concentration in the lymph. As Ehrich and Harris concluded, "The fact that the tissue response accompanying the formation of antibodies was chiefly a lymphocytic one points to the lymphocyte as a factor in the formation of antibodies." They did not commit themselves to the view that lymphocytes secreted most of the antibody but suggested that lymphocytes play an active role following the processing of antigen by phagocytes.[63]

Ehrich and Harris went on to publish in 1946 an experiment in which they extracted the antibody from the cells in efferent lymph of the popliteal node 6 days after stimulation with antigen.[64] They found that the concentration of antibody in the cells was six times higher than was present in the fluid component of lymph, indicating that the cells in efferent lymph included active antibody producers. Since almost all of these cells were lymphocytes, the candidacy of the lymphocyte as the producer of antibodies was promoted, particularly since very few of the other leading candidate—the macrophage—were present.

A Digression to the Plasma Cell   Because of the world war, Ehrich and Harris were unaware of the line of research in Scandinavia which was soon to attribute to the plasma cell the responsibility for the bulk of antibody secretion. This began with Bing and Plum's clinical observations in 1937 that myeloma—a tumor of the plasma cell line—was generally associated with excess production of antibody globulin.[65] They also observed that in chronic lymphocytic leukemia, a large excess of lymphocytes might be present in the blood and tissues without any increase in antibody globulin in the serum. This lead was followed up experimentally by Bjørneboe and Gormsen,[66] who repeatedly immunized rabbits with multiple antigens and noted a marked increase in the number of plasma cells in the lymphoid tissues and bone marrow. Astrid Fagraeus, at first in cooperation with Bing[67] during the war, devised a number of approaches, which built up a convincing body of circumstantial evidence that the plasma cell was the main producer of antibody.[68] One approach was to culture small fragments of splenic red pulp at the peak of an antibody response, when the main cell type in the red pulp was the plasma cell. The quantity of antibody produced per milligram of tissue was found to be correlated with its concentration of plasma cells. This work became widely accepted as indicating that antibody is produced not by macrophages or lymphocytes but by plasma cells.

Seven years later, the perfection of a new approach not only provided definitive proof of antibody secretion by the plasma cell but, perhaps equally important, enabled this to be visualized directly. This was the application of fluorescent protein tracing to the study of antibody formation by Albert Coons, Leduc, and Connolly[69] at Harvard. Coons had previously studied the fate of injected antigen by conjugating a fluorescent dye to antibody. The technique was extended so that sections of lymphoid tissue could be treated in vitro with soluble antigen which bound only to antibody-containing cells. The tissue sections were then treated with fluorescent antibody, which was bound in turn to the free antigenic sites on the antigen molecules. Thus, with appropriate controls, cells containing *specific* antibody could be identified. This work consolidated Fagraeus' view[68] that a great deal of antibody was secreted by large, immature plasma cells, still capable of cell division, rather than by the mature end cell, with a highly condensed nucleus.

When W.E. Ehrich, T.N. Harris, and their colleagues in Philadelphia became aware of the Scandinavian work, they studied the sequential changes in lymph nodes after antigenic stimulation by measuring the content of RNA and DNA using the methods pioneered by Brachet and Caspersson.[70,71] Small lymphocytes possess rather little RNA, but plasma cells have a great deal. They found that antibody synthesis correlated in time with the RNA content of lymph nodes and also with plasma cell accumulation. In 1949, they retracted their suggestion that lymphocytes secreted antibodies and stated explicitly their agreement with Fagraeus. Cellular immunology had reached its first milestone with the identification of the plasma cell as the antibody-forming cell, but that milestone now seems like a pebble on the shore. There was no worthwhile evidence as to the origin of plasma cells, and Fagraeus' idea that they were derived from a "primitive reticulum cell"[68] was hardly verifiable because of the ill-defined nature of that cell. Furthermore, antigen had never been observed to enter plasma cells. What was the connection between the antigen-engulfing macrophage and the plasma cell, and what role if any did the lymphocyte play?

These questions were tackled by T.N. Harris and his wife Susanna in a long series of experiments on the formation of antibody to *Shigella* bacilli in rabbits.[72,73] They exploited the principle of cell transfer from a donor to a recipient, which has already been referred to in the account of the role of the lymphocyte in cell mediated immunity. After injecting a donor rabbit with the antigen, they removed the local lymph node, made a cell suspension, and injected the lymph node cells into a recipient. Later, they discovered that the lymph node cells could be exposed to the antigen in vitro before injection into an x-irradiated recipient, then washed almost free of antigen, and still produce an effective antibody response.[72] The conclusion to which these experiments appeared to lead was that the antigen, either directly or after macrophage processing, induced lymphocytes to differentiate into plasma cells in the passive recipient. Unfortunately, the Harris's were never able to establish their point conclusively because of the presence of small numbers of macrophages and perhaps "reticulum cells" in their lymph node suspensions. Nevertheless, their work was influential in pointing the way to the lymphocyte as the antigen-sensitive cell.

Again, the Lymphocyte in Graft Rejection   Meanwhile, in the 1950s, the study of graft rejection as an immune reaction was making steady progress. In 1955, Algire, Weaver, and Prehn[74] reported an ingenious experiment in which small grafts were placed in plastic diffusion chambers to allow the access of serum antibody while preventing access by cells. When such diffusion chambers were placed in a suitable site within recipients of a different strain, grafts that would normally be promptly rejected survived and prospered. Clearly, antibody was not sufficient to reject grafts; the direct access of host cells to the graft was necessary. In the same year, Mitchison[75] described an attempt to trace immune lymph node cells in a graft on the assumption that they have to enter the grafted tissue in order to cause rejection. He labeled the cells in vitro with acriflavine to make them fluorescent. Disappointingly he could not find any of the cells in the graft after intravenous injection. This was the first of a long series of similarly conceived experiments which in the end showed that only small numbers of the immune lymphocytes migrate from the blood into a graft or, indeed, into other sites of cell mediated immunity.[76]

From the time of Medawar and Mitchison's work in the 1950s to the present, the immunology of tissue transplantation has influenced cellular immunology in general to an extent which can scarcely be exaggerated. Another major example of this was the idea and the proof of immunological tolerance, for which Burnet and Medawar shared the Nobel Prize of 1960. Ehrlich[11] had given thought to "horror autotoxicus"—the problem of why the body did not produce antibodies against its own molecules, which would be antigenic if injected into another animal—but the first substantial observation was the famous report of R.D. Owen[77] in 1945 that nonidentical cattle twins which shared the same blood circulation before birth continued in adult life to foster blood cells from their twin partners even though they were genetically different and would normally be promptly rejected by an immune reaction. On the basis of this observation, Burnet and Fenner[78] predicted that nonresponsiveness to one's own body constituents depended on their presence at a critical stage of embryonic development.

The chance of solving a practical problem again aroused the interest of Peter Medawar.[79] He was told that cattle breeders needed a method for distinguishing identical from nonidentical twins soon after birth. Being then unaware of Owen's work, Medawar pointed out that a sure and simple solution would be to exchange skin grafts between pairs of calves; the grafts would be rejected in the case of nonidentical (dizygotic) twins. Contrary to his assumption, the skin grafts nearly always survived indefinitely whether the twins were identical or not.[79] Ultimately it was realized that nonidentical twins may be made tolerant of antigens common to skin and other tissues by exposure to bloodborne cells before birth.

Medawar conceived that the next step was to try to produce this tolerance (or selective unresponsiveness) experimentally. In 1956, Billingham, Brent, and Medawar[80] injected lung and kidney cells from mice of one strain into newborn mice of another strain. As predicted, this enabled the mice to accept grafts from that strain throughout their life; they had been deceived into regarding these antigens as "self." Although this work was cited in Medawar's Nobel award, it may be that his earlier experiments on the immune nature of graft rejection[3] and on adoptive transfer of immunity[51] were of even greater significance. Credit for the discovery of tolerance may be shared by several additional researchers, especially Owen[77] and Hasek.[81] Owen supervised Sherman Ripley, who had succeeded by 1952 in producing tolerance artificially in a small number of rats. After finishing his Ph.D. work, Ripley returned to South Africa from California; unfortunately, the publication of their findings was delayed and finally abandoned. In Prague, Hasek[81] independently demonstrated immunological tolerance in chickens by fusing embryos in parabiosis for several days to allow a mutual exchange of bloodborne cells.

These experiments all followed the principle of presenting a set of antigens belonging to another individual at the critical time in development; the other side of the coin was to remove an organ normally present at this crucial phase of development and put it back later. If Burnet and Fenner were right, the animal should not in these circumstances recognize the organ as "self" and should reject it. This challenging experiment was not in fact done until 1962, when Triplett[82] did it in the tree frog. It is one of the few pieces of evidence to support the view that natural tolerance of self components and artificially induced tolerance are basically similar processes. Yet it is an experiment which stands on its own, for neither in Triplett's work nor in that of others did it lead to a new line of experimentation.

The notion of immunological tolerance was soon extended beyond transplantation immunology to embrace several examples of depressed antibody formation which had been long regarded as enigmatic.[83] It quickly became apparent that tolerance to many antigens could be produced by administering the material in the appropriate dose, route, and at the appropriate time in the animal's development.

Burnet's Theory of Immunity Implicates the Lymphocyte   The key concepts of cell mediated immunity and immunological tolerance had been inferred from astute observations and critical experiments. By contrast, the clonal selection theory of "acquired immunity" presented by McFarlane Burnet[84] in 1958 was not inspired by any single finding but depended on fitting a number of already established facts into a conceptual framework that was partly old and partly new. Burnet's blend of ideas revolutionized the course of immunology as radically as physics had been changed by Einstein. Almost all original research in immunology over the last decade has been conceived within Burnet's framework although probably none of the present applications of the subject need take his ideas into account, just as the majority of engineers need not be concerned with relativity.

Sir Frank McFarlane Burnet (1899–   ) (Figure 14-3) is an Australian who had already achieved distinction in virology and bacteriology when in 1944 he became head of the Walter and Eliza Hall Institute in Melbourne. He had been intrigued by antibody formation and published several provocative monographs on the subject from 1941. His experience in the processes of genetic mutation and natural selection among populations of microorganisms attracted him to certain aspects of Ehrlich's side chain theory of 1900 and also to a revival of selective theories in 1955.[85]

This is to the credit of Niels K. Jerne, who had proposed that very small amounts of all possible antibodies were produced at a steady rate *before* the body experienced any antigen. The only role of antigen was to select the appropriate antibody and carry it to a specialized system of antibody-producing cells. Entry of the antibody into this particular type of cell led to the production of more of that antibody.[85] The originality of Jerne's model was that it stressed the need to generate an enormous diversity of antibodies early in development. Its weakness was the lack of any conceivable mechanism by which the entry of antibody into a cell could initiate the production of multiple copies of that particular antibody.

The most significant new idea in Burnet's comprehensive theory was the proposal that the structure selected was a cell or more explicitly one clone of identical cells out of a large number of different clones. The cellular response to selection by antigen involved cell multiplication, thereby increasing the pro-

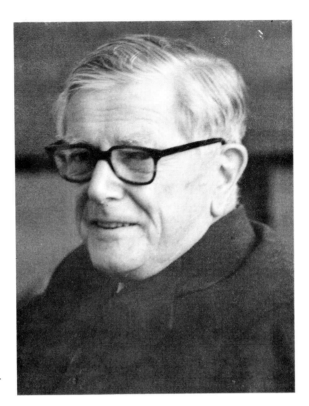

Figure 14-3 Sir Frank McFarlane Burnet (1899–   ).

portion of cells specific for that antigen within the whole population of
antigen-reactive cells. Burnet made two courageous assumptions—first, that
each cell could respond to only one antigen, so that its daughters would
produce only one antibody, and second, that there arose in the course of
development many thousands or millions of potentially reactive clones.[84] This
diversity of cells was accounted for by postulating *somatic mutation* of the
genes responsible for antibody production during the multiplication of the
precursor cells throughout early development. However, it is now clear that
somatic mutation alone cannot wholly account for the diversity of lymphocytes.

In 1958, Burnet was reasonably rather hesitant in specifying the cell type
selected by antigen. He proposed that the lymphocyte was the most likely
candidate, citing work on cell migration by J.L. Gowans[4] in favor of this view.
However, it was not until the early 1960s that lymphocytes were shown to be
antigen-reactive cells and not until even later was it proved repeatedly that
each antigen does indeed select a particular clone of lymphocytes. In 1958, the
major influence that gave credibility to Burnet's revolutionary theory was no

doubt the advances in the molecular biology of DNA, RNA, and protein synthesis that led to Crick's dogma[86]—genetic information flows from DNA to RNA to protein. The information required for synthesis of a specific protein has never been found to come directly from either DNA or another protein; it invariably comes via RNA. Is it conceivable that antibody formation is an exception in that the information is partly or wholly obtained from a protein antigen? In the 1950s, biologists rightly suspected that the answer would be negative. Soon, antibody synthesis was drawn into the mainstream of molecular biology, and recently much attention has been devoted to the genetic control of antibody synthesis on the assumption that it will reveal information relevant to protein synthesis in general.

THE LIFE HISTORY AND FATE OF THE LYMPHOCYTE

In 1909, Davis and Carlson of the University of Chicago published a thorough study of the number and types of leukocytes in the blood and major lymph trunks of the dog.[87] Like their predecessors in lymphatic cannulation since Ranvier,[16] they were impressed by the large numbers of lymphocytes conveyed to the blood by the major lymphatic trunks. By measuring (1) the number of lymphocytes entering the blood per hour and (2) the number of lymphocytes in the blood, they calculated that the lymphocytes in the blood must be replaced "at least once and possibly three or four times" every 24 hours. In view of the fact that the level in the blood remains approximately constant, they suggested four possibilities for the fate of this army of lymphocytes:

> (1) They may be rapidly destroyed. (2) They may develop into . . . 'more advanced' forms. (3) Lymphocytes may be 'reserve cells' . . . used in repair processes. (4) They may circulate from lymph to blood, and from blood, through capillary endothelium, into the tissue lymph, and thence back into the lymph of the larger lymphatic trunks.

The enigma of the fast turnover of lymphocytes in the bloodstream provoked a great deal of experimentation,[12] but virtually nothing was added to Carlson and Davis' masterly analysis of the problem for almost 50 years. Bunting and Huston elaborated the first possibility by proposing that lymphocytes migrated like lemmings into the gut, where they were digested.[88] This was based on the presence of lymphocytes between the epithelial cells of the small intestine; the lymphocytes were supposed to be en route from the blood to the cavity of the intestine. Despite the apparent wastefulness of producing large numbers of lymphocytes to be dumped into the gut a few hours after reaching the bloodstream, this idea remained in favor for many decades.

The notion that lymphocytes might recirculate from blood to lymph via tissue spaces and afferent lymphatics was revived by Sjövall in 1936[89] but was dismissed by Yoffey and Drinker[90] on the grounds that only 1 in 30 of the lymphocytes leaving a node in efferent lymph could be accounted for by cells arriving at a lymph node in the afferent lymph. They overlooked Flemming's suggestion[22] that lymphocytes might leave blood vessels within a lymph node to account for the much greater numbers in lymph leaving the node.

The enigma of the fast replacement of lymphocytes in the blood was one of the many research interests of Howard Walter Florey (1898–1968),[91] who as well as sharing the Nobel Prize for the discovery of penicillin made outstanding contributions to the study of peptic ulceration and, later, arterial disease. Florey paid a brief visit to A.J. Carlson's laboratory in 1925, following which he studied many aspects of lymph and lymphborne cells at the London Hospital and later at Sheffield, where he was the first experimentalist to be Professor of Pathology. After experiencing some difficulty in trying to wrest that department from the dominating influence of morbid anatomy, he moved to Oxford to head the Sir William Dunn School of Pathology, where he inspired a succession of younger collaborators to work on lymphocytes. A particularly active period was around 1940, when Florey and his colleagues published one paper (their first) on penicillin and three papers on lymphocytes obtained from the thoracic duct of cats or rabbits. The results section of one paper begins with a distinct Oxford flavor: "During the course of some hot summer days of 1939 lymphocytes were recognized in our rabbits' ear chambers. . . ."[92] In the circumstances of that summer at the start of World War II and when substantial progress on penicillin was being achieved in Oxford, it is remarkable that Florey could devote any time to observing or writing about lymphocytes. The pressure on the Oxford group to drop everything except penicillin must have been intense, but Florey had a long-standing love affair with the lymphocyte, which was poignant in that his personal contribution was minor in comparison with the achievements of those who came under his influence.

The Oxford workers followed many approaches to the study of the lymphocyte, including observations made on living lymphocytes under the most favorable conditions of culture they could devise. It was found that lymphocytes tended to degenerate and die after about 24 hours outside the body—an observation which seemed to be consistent with their supposedly short life span in the body. Jean Medawar (who had married Peter Medawar in 1937) did not observe any transformation of lymphocytes into other cell types[93] and criticized Bloom's claim[94] to have observed the transformation of lymphocytes into phagocytes. She attributed Bloom's observations to the presence of a substantial proportion of phagocytic cell precursors in his starting population because of the traumatic method he used to collect lymph. Although her arguments were persuasive, the question of whether lymphocytes are precursors of macrophages remained a bone of contention until the 1960s, when it was clearly established that lymphocytes and monocytes/macrophages are distinct cell lines with only a remote ancestral relationship.[95]

After World War II, Jesse Bollman and his colleagues at the Mayo Clinic introduced a number of techniques that facilitated the study of lymphocyte physiology.[96,97] The plastic tubing now available was much more suitable for the cannulation of lymphatic vessels than the glass or rubber tubing previously used. Bollman cannulated the main lymphatic vessel of the rat in the upper abdomen by exploiting the broad "thoracic duct" before it pierces the diaphragm to enter the chest. This abdominal operation proved to be an easier routine procedure than cannulation of the thoracic duct in the neck before it enters the great veins. Bollman also designed a restraining cage in which rats could be maintained with an indwelling cannula for several days. The findings of the Mayo Clinic group[97] on the cell output in lymphatics from the liver and intestine as well as the thoracic duct proved to be useful, but they were not revolutionary. However, the technical advances were such that since then the rat has been the main species for the study of lymphocyte physiology, although more advances in the immunological role of lymphocytes have been made in the mouse.

Another technical development which burgeoned after 1945 was the availability and application of radioactively labeled compounds for biological research. As has been described in the preceding chapters, the age and life span of cells can be measured by using radioactive precursors of DNA since it is, in general, synthesized at only one point in the generation cycle of the cell. In 1954, Ottesen used radioactive phosphorus to estimate the life span of lymphocytes in human blood.[98] By injecting ^{32}P and measuring the persistence of the compound in the DNA of blood lymphocytes, he calculated that the majority of lymphocytes had an average life span of 100 to 200 days. Since the prevailing opinion was that the life span of lymphocytes is measurable in hours or a few days at most, this seemed an astonishing conclusion. We now know that many small lymphocytes in the blood have a life span of several years.

The notion that lymphocytes are produced in large numbers, only to be destroyed within a few hours after entering the blood, was decisively overturned by James Learmonth Gowans (1924–   ) (Figure 14-4) in the Dunn School of Pathology at Oxford. Having been infected with Florey's enthusiasm for the lymphocyte, Gowans adopted Bollman's method of cannulating the thoracic duct of the rat below the diaphragm.[4] An apparently trivial but in fact important modification was to bend the cannula through 180° so that it emerged from the rat through the back rather than the belly, where it was vulnerable to the animal's teeth. Gowans concentrated on the consistent fall in the thoracic duct output between 1 and 5 days after cannulation. By the end of this period, the output of cells is only 15 to 20 percent of the initial output. Gowans found that the decrease in output could be effectively prevented by collecting the cells in the lymph and reinjecting them into the blood.[4] He initially favored the conventional explanation for the decreased

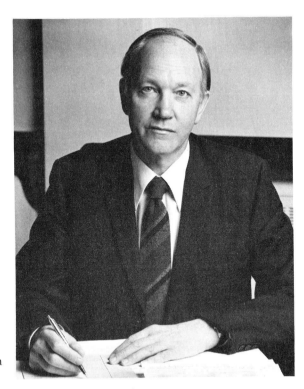

Figure 14-4 James Learmonth Gowans (1924–   ).

output, which was that cell production in the lymph nodes fell during drainage of the thoracic duct due to lack of essential nutrients, which had been depleted when cells were lost from the animal. However, Gowans found that when lymphocytes were killed before reinfusion, the drop in lymphocyte output was just as spectacular as if the cells have been flushed down the sink. Since the reinfusion of dead cells should have prevented the depletion of nutrients, an alternative explanation was required. The proposition that lymphocytes leaving the blood continuously recirculate through the tissues into lymph would account for all the results since loss of cells from a thoracic duct cannula could then be regarded as slow drainage of a large pool of recirculating lymphocytes. Gowans proved this explanation to be correct by radioactively labeling lymphocytes and reinjecting them into the bloodstream.[5] After a few hours, large numbers of the injected lymphocytes appeared in the thoracic duct of the recipient, indicating that these cells could travel from blood to tissue to lymph. Normally they would have returned to the blood to complete their circuit.

The studies of Ottesen and of Gowans in the 1950s gave us a radically new conception of the lymphocyte. The small lymphocyte is now established as a predominantly long-lived cell which follows a remarkable migration pathway involving its continuous redistribution between the spleen, lymph nodes, and other organs via the blood and lymph.

Confirmation that most small lymphocytes in human blood were long-lived cells came from an unexpected source. Karen Buckton and other cytogeneticists in Edinburgh were concerned that following treatment with moderate doses of x-rays, patients had an increased tendency to develop leukemia. They were interested in the relationship between leukemia and the high frequency of chromosomal abnormalities found in the white blood cells of the irradiated patients. From a study of unstable chromosome aberrations, they concluded that the average small lymphocyte must have a "lifetime" of several years between cell divisions.[99] Finally, the application of improved methods of estimating the life span of cells with radioactive isotopes firmly established that most lymphocytes in blood, spleen, and lymph nodes had a life span of weeks or months although some cells are "short-lived."[100] By contrast, in the bone marrow and thymus, most lymphocytes became labeled after 3 to 5 days of tritiated thymidine infusion, thus showing that these cells have recently been produced from precursors and are "turning over" rapidly.[101] The majority of small lymphocytes outside the bone marrow and thymus are nondividing cells and have come to be regarded as dormant cells waiting to be activated.

The most telling confirmation of Gowans' conclusions on recirculation was achieved in Australia by another pupil of Florey—Bede Morris—who with Joe Hall studied the cell kinetics of a single popliteal lymph node in the sheep.[23] In that species, both the efferent and afferent lymphatics of a single node can be cannulated so that the arrival and departure of cells can be studied at the same time. By infusing a radioactive precursor of DNA, they were also able to estimate the rate at which new lymphocytes were produced by cell division within the lymph node. The cells arriving in afferent lymph and the new production of cells within the node could only account for a small minority of the cells leaving the node. By the same reasoning as that applied by Flemming in 1885,[22] they concluded that at least 85 percent of the small lymphocytes in efferent lymph must have entered the node from the blood perfusing its vessels.[23] In support of this, Hall and Morris found that killing almost all the lymphocytes in a lymph node by x-irradiation confined to the node is followed within 24 hours by replenishment of the cells in the node and the restoration of the traffic in efferent lymph.[102] That these lymphocytes must have recently come from the blood was beyond doubt.

The route by which lymphocytes migrate into lymph nodes was defined by Gowans and Julie Knight.[103] They labeled lymphocytes in vitro with a radioactive compound and then reinjected them into the bloodstream. Removing lymph nodes and other tissues from the injected animals, they cut sections for microscopy, and by coating the sections with a photographic emulsion they were able to pinpoint the precise location of the migrating lymphocytes. At only 10 minutes after injection, most of the lymphocytes were in or around the walls of peculiar blood vessels in a particular compartment of the lymph node—the deep zone of the cortex—which Delphine Parrott and her colleagues were soon to describe as a thymus dependent area because it became depleted of lymphocytes when the thymus was removed from mice at birth.[104] Lymphocytes leave the blood flowing within lymph nodes by migrating across the walls of small venules lined by plump endothelial cells that contrast with the flat lining cells of small veins elsewhere.[103] The presence of lymphocytes in the walls of these specialized blood vessels had been remarked on by Zimmermann in 1923, who suggested that their function was to conduct a stream of lymphocytes in the opposite direction—from lymph node into blood.[105] This idea was developed into the notion of two alternative routes of entry into the blood of lymphocytes produced in the lymph node: (1) "direct entry"—across the walls of small blood vessels and (2) "indirect entry"—via efferent lymphatics.[12] It was not until radioactive labels became available—both to measure lymphocyte life span and to trace their migration pattern—that it became clear that lymphocytes were leaving rather than entering the blood across these small veins. The lesson to be learned is that study of static sections with the microscope cannot give reliable information regarding the direction of cell migration.

THE MYSTERIES OF THE THYMUS AND THE BURSA OF FABRICIUS

Once more we must go far back in time to trace a line of work which became integrated with cellular immunology and lymphocyte studies in the 1960s. The thymus was regarded by Hewson as the main source of "lymph corpuscles."[14] This notion was amplified by Beard, of Edinburgh, who, without false modesty, claimed in 1900 to have discovered the true function of the thymus.[106] He proposed that it was the source of all white cells and assumed that the distinction between different types of leukocyte was trivial because they were merely stages of the same cell line. To his credit, he took into account the fact that the thymus is not essential to life because it can be removed from adults, children, or experimental animals without obvious harm. Also, the thymus had long been known to reach its maximum size relative to body weight around birth and to regress after puberty. Beard suggested that the thymus seeds cells to the blood and other organs early in life. He described the dispensability of the thymus in adulthood thus, "The thymus . . . no more ceases to exist than would the Anglo-Saxon race disappear, were the British Isles to sink beneath the waves."[106]

For almost a century, progress in understanding the thymus was hampered by a remarkable misconception. In children dying suddenly from injury, the thymus appeared to be abnormally large, and it was assumed that a large thymus (status thymolymphaticus) increased susceptibility to injury. Gradually it was realized that what had been thought to be a large thymus was often normal and what had been thought at postmortem to be a normal thymus was in fact shrunken as a result of the stress of chronic illness before death. The confusion was cleared away by some very simple experiments. Andreasen showed that starvation of rats causes the thymus to shrink drastically,[107] and Thomas F. Dougherty and Abraham White, of Yale, noted that large doses of adrenal cortical hormones cause the death of most of the lymphocytes in the thymus within a few hours.[108]

The logical test of Beard's ideas was to remove the thymus from an animal as early in life as possible before the seeding of precursor cells had occurred. However, this was not achieved until 1961, when it was found that removal of the thymus from mice or rabbits immediately after birth leads to a deficiency in their capacity to mount immune responses.[109,110] Of the many examples of a discovery being made simultaneously by two or more groups working independently, few could have been more remarkable than the train of events surrounding the discovery of the function of the thymus. Within a few months of each other, Jacques Miller, of the Chester Beatty Institute in London, and Archer and Pierce, working in Robert Good's laboratory in Minneapolis, published preliminary papers on the effect of thymectomy performed on newborn mice and rabbits, respectively. During the following year, each group published definitive papers on the immunological deficit in such animals,[111,112] and Byrom Waksman and his colleagues at Yale reported similar findings in rats.[113] The last group found clear evidence that delayed hypersensitivity and graft rejection were particularly impaired; antibody responses were rather variably affected.

Different paths had led Jacques Miller and the Minneapolis group to remove the thymus from rodents at birth. From 1958, Miller had become interested in the leukemia induced by injection of the Gross virus into newborn mice. He found that removal of the thymus after weaning prevented the development of the leukemia. Was this because the virus could only multiply in the thymus? The virus had to be given on the day of birth, and so to answer this question the thymus had to be removed at birth. He found that this led to a fatal wasting disease when the mice were 4 to 8 weeks of age whether the virus had been injected or not. When the mice were protected from infection, significantly fewer died. Miller found that the neonatally thymectomized mice gave poor immune responses; particularly, the rejection of grafts was dramatically delayed. Moreover, their spleens lacked the normal amount of lymphoid tissue.[110,112]

Robert Good and his team of clinical and experimental workers had been studying inherited disorders of the immune system throughout the 1950s. Varco and Good had in 1955 described an association between tumors of the thymus and defective antibody formation in children.[114] They had been impressed by the discovery of Bruce Glick, published in 1957, that removal of the bursa of Fabricius from chickens within 2 weeks of hatching leads to an inability to produce antibodies in later life.[115] The bursa of Fabricius is a lymphoid organ which develops as an outgrowth from the posterior wall of the bird's cloaca (rectum). Its similarity to the thymus is that both are lymphoid organs with structural elements derived from gut epithelium, as had been pointed out by Jolly in 1914.[116] By 1960, removal of the thymus from newborn animals had become a logical next step in the substantial program of Good's team. However, Archer and Pierce's preliminary paper[109] was less decisive than was Miller's first paper,[110] largely because the consequences of removing the thymus from the newborn rabbit are less clear cut; the rabbit is slightly more mature at birth than is the mouse.[111]

The discovery of the immune function of the thymus in early life was the most important ever made in understanding that organ. Jacques Miller, working alone, though in contact with Medawar and Gowans, had made the discovery almost as a digression from his objectives in leukemia research. Bob Good and his team had built up a momentum toward the thymus which, with hindsight, was bound to carry them to success. The two discoverers would have been less than human if they had been completely unconcerned with priority and credit. The important thing is that each has continued to make outstanding contributions to cellular immunology.

The relationship of the bursa of Fabricius to antibody formation had been discovered accidentally by Glick and his colleagues.[115] The bursa reaches its maximum size relative to body weight before hatching and regresses even faster and more completely than does the thymus. This suggested that the bursa is only required at a certain stage of development and so it was logical to test the effect of removal of the bursa as early as possible. Glick removed the bursa by surgery from a group of chickens within 2 weeks of hatching and was disappointed to find that they survived to adulthood with no obvious abnormalities. However, because of a shortage of birds for teaching, they were used in a class exercise to demonstrate antibody formation to *Salmonella*. The chickens failed to produce antibody. By 1960, it was firmly established that the presence of the bursa in early life is necessary for the development of antibody responsiveness.[117]

In the years following 1961, the roles of the thymus and bursa became dominant themes for experimentation. The work of most far-reaching significance was published by Burnet and his colleagues Warner and Szenberg in 1962.[118] They studied chickens that had been injected with testosterone in embryonic life. This either prevented the development of both the bursa and thymus or it impaired the bursa alone. In retrospect, their most significant finding was that graft rejection occurred with the usual tempo in birds without a bursa but was deficient in birds lacking a thymus as well. On the basis of these findings, they proposed that the bursa of Fabricius and the thymus each gives rise to a major population of lymphocytes; the cells derived from the bursa are precursors of antibody-forming cells, while the thymus gives rise to the cells responsible for graft rejection. This finding was the morning star of the lymphocyte reformation—the identification in the late 1960s of two major populations, the thymus-derived (T) and thymus-independent (B) lymphocytes.

The Emergence of the Lymphocyte as the Immunologically Competent Cell

By 1961, several convergent lines of research had established that the lymphocyte is deeply involved in both antibody production and in cell mediated immunity; that most lymphocytes are long-lived nomadic cells; and that at least some lymphocytes are dependent on the activity of the thymus in early life. Although the role of lymphocytes in antibody formation was still obscure, the evidence that they were crucially important had become inescapable. It had been known since early in the century that the small lymphocyte was exceptionally vulnerable to x-irradiation and that whole-body x-irradiation of animals depressed their ability to form antibodies to an antigenic stimulus given a day or two later.[41,42]

Radiation with x-rays is as precise as a blunderbuss in that it damages all cells more or less, but in 1963, Gowans and McGregor in Oxford showed that a more selective method of depleting the body's population of lymphocytes also reduced its capacity to form antibodies.[119] They exploited Gowans' modified technique of thoracic duct cannulation of rats by maintaining the cannulated rats for 5 days. The cells in the lymph were lost from the rat and because most of these were recirculating lymphocytes, the spleen, lymph nodes, and blood all became depleted of lymphocytes. When stimulated with an antigen, these rats failed to produce a normal antibody response, but when lymphocytes were given back to them, full antibody responses were restored. Gowans also found that x-irradiated rats could produce a nearly normal antibody response provided that after the x-rays, they were replenished with lymphocytes.[44] This underlined the need for lymphocytes in the formation of antibody but did not deny the possibility that macrophages might also have an essential role because macrophages are resistant to much higher doses of x-rays than can be given to a whole animal if it is to survive.

In 1961, Marvin Fishman[120] proposed on the basis of his experiments on antibody formation in vitro particular roles for the lymphocyte and the macrophage which were radically different from Burnet's notions. Even with hindsight, it is difficult to decide whether Fishman's work should be regarded as a digression or as an obligatory phase in the development of cellular immunology. Fishman achieved the technical tour de force of producing an antibody response in tissue culture from start to finish. Antigenic virus particles were fed to a culture of peritoneal exudate cells, in which macrophages predominate. These cells were then killed, and RNA was extracted and fed to a culture of lymph node cells. After a few days of culture, a significant but small amount of antibody was detectable in the fluid of the cell culture. The antibody formed was specific for the virus, and the inductive material produced in the first culture was destroyed by an enzyme specific for RNA. Fishman suggested that following the engulfment of an antigen, macrophages produce and secrete a specific sequence of RNA. This is transferred to lymphocytes where it acts as a messenger RNA, conveying the information necessary for the manufacture of antibody. The key notion was that the important step ultimately leading to the production of a specific antibody takes place in the macrophage; the lymphocyte/plasma cell was only a factory operating on a blueprint supplied from another cell.[120]

These experiments were taken very seriously, and attempts to repeat them using other antigens were set up in many laboratories throughout the world. However, there were several difficulties in interpreting Fishman's results. First, both the initial culture of peritoneal exudate cells and the second culture of lymph node cells included several cell types. Second, the titers of antibody produced were low compared to the response to these antigens by an intact animal. The most important difficulty did not emerge for a few years. It was clearly shown by Ita Askonas and Joan Rhodes that Fishman's method of extracting RNA with phenol produced material that included at least part of the protein antigen.[121] The complexing of RNA to an antigen somehow augmented the antibody response it provoked after injection, but the sequence of nucleotides in the RNA is now thought to be immaterial. However, by this time, attempts to induce antibody synthesis in vitro with purified RNA had been abandoned, and most immunologists no longer interpret Fishman's results as evidence for the transfer of information that passes in the form of nucleic acid molecules between the different cells involved in antibody formation.

The gradual eclipse of the notion of macrophage RNA instructing antibody formation in the lymphocyte came about because of accumulating evidence that an interaction between the lymphocyte and some antigens at least was sufficient to initiate an immune response. To give an account of this evidence we must digress from antibody formation and return again to transplantation immunity.

In 1953, Morten Simonsen had suggested on the basis of 5 years of transplantation experiments in dogs that the large lymphocytes in the recently transplanted spleen or kidney might be lymphoid cells of the transplanted organ reacting against antigens of the host.[122] He tested this notion experimentally by injecting adult spleen cells from chickens or mice into embryos or newborns. In each case, the hosts became ill and died after a latent period of a few days.[123] This is an example of *graft-versus-host reaction,* in which the usual roles of graft and host are reversed. Instead of the host rejecting the graft, it was found that under certain circumstances grafts will react against and may reject their hosts. Murphy[124] had observed such a reaction in 1916 but had unfortunately failed to grasp its significance.

Graft-versus-host reactions were cleverly exploited to solve many problems, including the identification of the cells that initiate this immune reaction.[125] Billingham and Brent[126] found that injection of cells from one strain of mouse into newborns of another strain was frequently followed by a fatal wasting, which they called runt disease. They showed that this was an example of a graft-versus-host reaction and that it could be produced by lymphoid cells, such as cells from lymph nodes or blood leukocytes. This narrowed down the search for the "immunologically competent cell," as it was to be entitled by Medawar.[127] In 1962, Gowans showed that small lymphocytes *alone* could initiate a full-blown graft-versus-host reaction in a susceptible recipient. Moreover, some of the small lymphocytes transformed within 24 hours into much larger dividing cells.[6] This was rigorously proved by the use of chromosome markers.[128] After many decades of wild speculation, this was the first unequivocal proof that the common lymphocyte, a cell that had for so long been regarded as doomed and expendable, could transform into at least one other cell type.

Many agents are now known to induce this process of "lymphoblastic transformation" from a small lymphocyte to a large basophilic cell which proceeds to divide repeatedly.[129] Three years before Gowans' demonstration in intact animals, Hungerford and Nowell in Philadelphia had used phytohemagglutinin (PHA) to clump and remove red cells from blood samples in order to separate leukocytes for chromosome studies.[130] They obtained a higher yield of dividing leukocytes than had previously been found with other methods of separating leukocytes. It soon became clear that PHA stimulates certain cells to go into division. This was a bonus for the chromosome studies but proved to be an even greater boon to immunologists because in 1965 it was shown by direct cinematographic observation that PHA stimulates the small lymphocyte to enlarge and then to undergo successive divisions.[131] About the same time, Dutton and Pearce[132] found that DNA synthesis by spleen cells from immunized rabbits could be stimulated by adding protein antigens to a tissue culture of the cells. Only an antigen to which the rabbits had been immunized was effective. They assumed rightly that antigens stimulated "memory" lymphocytes in the immune population to divide so that the system could be regarded as initiating a secondary antibody response in vitro.

A more decisive experiment in clarifying the function of the lymphocyte was the finding by Jim Gowans and Jonathan Uhr[133] that the capacity to mount a secondary antibody response could be conferred on a naive rat by giving it a pure population of small lymphocytes from an immunized rat; in other words immunological memory was carried by small lymphocytes. These and many other experiments in the 1960s firmly established the lymphocyte as the antigen-sensitive cell,[134] but no one had yet succeeded in attaching a suitable label to lymphocytes to prove their conversion to plasma cells, and Burnet's suggestion that each lymphocyte only responds to one antigen or a restricted range of antigens still was unsupported.

Another unsolved problem was the enigmatic relationship between lymphocytes and macrophages. This had been highlighted by studies of the fate of radioiodinated antigens within lymphoid tissue. Almost all the material was taken up by macrophages and by peculiar dendritic cells in the germinal centers.[135,136] Later, Ita Askonas[137] and her colleagues at Mill Hill in London showed clearly what had long been suspected—that the cells making antibody are different from those ingesting antigens, and, in general, the two cells occupy different areas of the spleen and lymph nodes.

The Diversity of Lymphocytes

In the mid-1960s, many immunologists would have anticipated the role of the thymus to be the production of lymphocytes, which after seeding to the spleen and lymph nodes could differentiate into antibody-producing plasma cells.[137] Two facts gave credence to this view. First, the capacity to form antibodies could be fully restored to lymphocyte-deficient animals by replenishing them with thoracic duct lymphocytes. The obvious and, as it happened, correct interpretation was that the precursors of antibody-forming cells are included in the thoracic duct lymphocyte population.[7,44,119] The second fact was that most thoracic duct lymphocytes were produced in the thymus. This was first indicated by the deficit of these cells following removal of the thymus[139] and later was supported by labeling cells in situ within the thymus. By this technique, Weissman[140] showed that lymphocytes produced in the thymus do contribute to the recirculating pool of lymphocytes and seed to the spleen and lymph nodes, particularly to those areas which had been described as thymus dependent by Delphine Parrott, Maria de Sousa, and June East[104] in the previous year (1966). In the meantime, the ultimate origin of lymphocytes in the thymus had been settled after a long series of painstaking experiments mainly by exploiting the chromosome markers pioneered by C.E. Ford and Micklem.[141] These culminated in Moore and Owen's convincing evidence that the precursors of thymus lymphocytes originate in the bone marrow and enter the embryonic thymus from the blood.[142] The role of the thymic epithelial cell is somehow to control the differentiation of lymphocytes within the organ.

This view of thymus function in antibody formation now appears to have been unsatisfactory, especially with the benefit of hindsight. The evidence for two major subpopulations of lymphocytes in birds was not taken seriously enough until Henry Claman and his colleagues[143] reported an experiment in 1966, which might have been done many years previously. The results were not in themselves very revealing, but their experiment has barely been surpassed in the field of immunology in terms of the amount of subsequent work it stimulated. Claman's group studied the ability of different cell populations to restore the capacity of irradiated mice to form antibodies. They found, as expected, that spleen cells are efficient in restoration of this capability (like thoracic duct lymphocytes), but thymus cells and bone marrow cells each are very weak despite a high or moderate content of lymphocytes. However, a mixture of thymus cells and marrow cells produced a far larger response than the sum of the two populations. The finding of synergy between bone marrow cells and thymus cells indicated that at least two cell types are involved but gave no clue as to what role each plays. At that stage it was not even certain that both cells were lymphocytes, but within a few years these results were accepted as the first evidence of functional cooperation between thymus derived (T) lymphocytes and "bursa-equivalent" derived or thymus independent B lymphocytes.[144] (It is a misconception that the B stands for bone marrow; precursors of both B and T cells reside in the bone marrow.)

In some ways, Claman's finding was fortuitous because thymus cells include only a minority of mature T lymphocytes ready to help in antibody formation. Also, the bone marrow includes some T lymphocytes as well as B lymphocytes at several stages of maturation. Fortunately, in the mouse strain studied there were insufficient T cells in the marrow compared to the number of B cells to give an optimal response. Probably some T- and B-cell precursors had an opportunity to differentiate to mature antigen-sensitive cells in the recipient before the antigenic stimulus was given. In any event, the experiment did work consistently and provided a model to study the nature of cell cooperation in antibody responses.

A particularly useful event at this stage was the discovery of a system of antigens present in brain, thymus cells, and thymus derived cells in the spleen and lymph nodes of mice—the theta antigen or Thy-1, as it was renamed. This antigenic system had been discovered by Reif and Allen[145] in 1964, but it was not until 1969 that Martin Raff[146] and Michael Schlesinger[147] independently found evidence that Thy-1 could be used to distinguish thymus derived from other lymphocytes in peripheral sites, such as the spleen, lymph nodes, and blood. They also exploited anti-theta serum to selectively eliminate T cells from cell mixtures.

An experienced team at the Hall Institute in Melbourne, including Jacques Miller and Graham Mitchell, set out to define the roles of the two cells required for antibody formation.[148,149] They exploited two ways of marking the thymus derived and the bone marrow cells—by using transplantation antigens and chromosome markers. They decisively established that the antibody-forming cells are derived exclusively from the bone marrow cells. In addition, the relationship between lymphocytes and plasma cells had at last been clarified; some lymphocytes (B cells) responded to antigens by dividing and differentiating to plasma cells. Whatever role T cells were playing, it was not to act as precursors of plasma cells. However, it was soon established that both T and B cells could carry immunological memory and that both lymphocyte sets could be rendered tolerant under different circumstances.[150] It emerged that the "help" provided by T cells in the induction of B cells has all the characteristics of specific immunity.

The dichotomy between T and B lymphocytes aroused the enthusiasm of a wide spectrum of clinicians and biologists. Indeed, initial overenthusiasm led to almost every characteristic of the lymphocyte being contrasted between T and B cells.[151] Thus, it was proposed that T cells are long-lived and B cells short-lived; T cells recirculate, but B cells do not. Now we know that lymphocytes do vary in their life span and their ability to recirculate from blood to lymph, but these properties cut across the B–T division. The overenthusiasm was moderated by Bede Morris's suggestion that B and T were most appropriate as the first and last letters of "BullshiT."

There is another sense in which lymphocytes are diverse. At least for B lymphocytes, there now is good evidence that a given lymphocyte will respond to only one antigen. This implies the existence of as many different sets of B lymphocytes as antigens—on the order of a million. This discovery is as important as the B–T dichotomy, although it is more difficult to comprehend and to accept. To appreciate the development of this idea, we must return to Burnet, who had proposed that the structure selected by antigen was a cell and that the lymphocyte was the most likely candidate.[84] This selective theory gradually gained credibility, at first because of evidence against the alternative instructive theory. For example, it was shown that an antibody could be partly unfolded and on refolding would resume its previous configuration and ability to bind antigen; like other proteins, the shape and biological activity of an antibody depends on its sequence of amino acids.[152] This is clearly contrary to the idea that antigen is incorporated into a template on which the folding of a standard antibody sequence occurs.

The first positive evidence in favor of cell selection was the observation that when lymphocytes initiated a graft-versus-host reaction, only a minority of lymphocytes responded to a complement of transplantation antigens.[6] In the early 1960s, it was realized that a crucial test of the selective theory was to show that the set of lymphocytes responding to one antigen was distinct from the set of lymphocytes responding to another antigen. In 1962, Gowans suggested that I should test whether the 95 percent of donor lymphocytes that apparently did *not* respond in a graft-versus-host situation were capable of responding to another set of transplantation antigens, but Atkins and I did not succeed in this experiment until 1971.[153]

Of the many approaches tried, the one which first succeeded depended on advances in technique rather than in principle. In 1961, Stavitsky,[154] reviewing the many attempts to achieve antibody production entirely in vitro, pointed out that it was arguable whether or not a primary antibody response had ever been carried through from start to finish. Dutton and Mishell[155] found a culture medium in which an antibody response to sheep erythrocytes could be initiated and maintained for several days, in fact until the appearance of cells producing hemolytic antibody, as detected by the plaque-forming cell assay introduced by Jerne and Nordin in 1963.[156] Radioactive (^{3}H) thymidine was added to the cultures at a crucial stage in order to kill selectively the cells synthesizing DNA. The method was selective because only the cells proliferating in response to the antigen took tritiated thymidine into their nuclei. A high concentration of tritiated thymidine was used so that sufficient radiation built up in the cell nucleus to kill the radiosensitive lymphocytes. It was found that after several days of culture with the "hot pulse" of tritiated thymidine, the remaining population of lymphocytes had been rendered unresponsive to the antigen added to the culture but were fully responsive to another antigen. The experiment had exploited the requirement for lymphocyte proliferation after antigen stimulation and the radiosensitivity of dividing cells to show that there exist at least two lymphocyte subsets corresponding to the two antigens used in the experiment.[155]

After the application of much ingenuity, several other ways were found to "negatively select" lymphocyte populations so that they would become depleted in cells responsive to a particular antigen. Not only did these developments support this pillar of Burnet's theory; they also added important new information on the nature of lymphocyte diversity. In 1969, Wigzell[157] achieved practical realization of an idea which had been discussed for several years. By sticking a protein antigen to glass beads packed in a vertical column, he was able to select lymphocytes by passing them down the column so that they made extensive contact with a large antigen-coated surface. The passed cells were found to be depleted of cells responsive to the antigen on the column. This showed that lymphocytes have some structure *on their surface* that can recognize antigen, and, in consequence, the cell may be retarded or immobilized. This is the antigen-binding receptor envisaged by Ehrlich in 1900 as a "side chain."[10]

A third way of achieving negative selection harked back to the observation made by Wesslén in 1952 that after immunizing rabbits some antibody-forming cells appear in the thoracic duct lymph. Moreover, he noted that some lymphocytes from the thoracic duct could bind to their surface the antigen which had been injected.[158] In 1967, Naor and Sulitzeanu[159] noted that when even nonimmune spleen cells were incubated with radioactively labeled antigen, a small minority of cells bound antigen to their surface. Gordon Ada and his colleagues[160] at the Hall Institute in Melbourne showed that these cells were lymphocytes, and by using as antigen a radioactive protein heavily labeled with ^{125}I, they were able to deliver enough radiation to the lymphocyte to kill it after 24 hours in culture. This antigen-induced suicide technique selectively destroyed the clone of lymphocytes responsive to the antigen involved. The method uniquely permitted the enumeration and characterization of the antigen-binding lymphocytes and confirmed the existence of surface receptors for antigen.

From the first time that immunological competence had been attributed to the lymphocyte in the early 1960s, the burning question was how the lymphocyte recognizes antigen. With the demonstration of antigen-binding receptors, this question became more insistent. The most economical possibility was that each lymphocyte expresses on its surface an accurate sample of the antibody its daughters will secrete after antigenic stimulation. In other words, the receptor on the lymphocyte surface is antibody of which the specificity and other characteristics are identical with the antibody secreted by the plasma cells derived from it. Any other possibility involved two series of recognition molecules.

Sell and Gell,[161] in Birmingham, had shown in 1965 that antibodies directed against immunoglobulin can induce blast transformation of some lymphocytes. This implied that immunoglobulin was present at the cell surface. However, direct visualization of this was not achieved until 1969. Roger Taylor and Martin Raff, working in Avrion Mitchison's laboratory at Mill Hill, each became interested in antibodies on the surface of lymphocytes from a different viewpoint. They cooperated and used labeled anti-immunoglobulin to detect antibody on 20 to 50 percent of mouse lymphocytes, depending on their source. The material was not evenly distributed around the surface but was gathered into a cap at one pole of the cell.[162] The finding of immunoglobulin on the surface of some lymphocytes has turned out to be one of the most important discoveries of the last decade, and in retrospect it is extraordinary that it was not made earlier since labeled anti-antibodies had been available for more than 10 years. Raff later showed that almost all lymphocytes express either the theta antigen or surface immunoglobulin, but none express both.[163] Thus, surface immunoglobulin is a characteristic of thymus-independent B cells and has come to be accepted as the most important defining criterion.

Later, in 1969, Ben Pernis and his colleagues[164] confirmed the presence of surface immunoglobulin on a class of lymphocyte, but they did not observe caps—the fluorescent material was in patches all over the cell. The discrepancy was quickly resolved when Raff visited Pernis' laboratory in Genoa. They found that the difference in temperature at which the test was performed accounted for the observed difference in distribution of immunoglobulin. In metabolically inactive lymphocytes, anti-immunoglobulin identifies antibody receptors evenly distributed over the whole surface of the cell, and it is presumed that this is their natural state. However, at room temperature, anti-immunoglobulin induces the redistribution of antibody receptors first into patches and then into a single polar cap. This is an active process requiring the participation of microfilaments within the cell. Study of this process of capping has yielded clues to the organization of proteins in the cell membrane and the role of the cytoskeleton, including microfilaments and microtubules. This is an outstanding example of how in the past few years, the lymphocyte has fulfilled the role of a model cell; other cells that are less suitable for direct study are presumed to behave similarly.[165]

The evidence that the clonal selection theory of Burnet is correct, at least as applied to B lymphocytes, became entirely adequate in the early 1970s with, for example, the finding by Raff, Feldmann, and de Petris[166] that certain antigens can induce capping of the receptors of the corresponding clone of B lymphocytes. All the immunoglobulin of the cell is swept up into the cap, thus showing that the B lymphocyte expresses immunoglobulin of only one specificity. By a number of approaches, Klinman[167] has shown that only one in a million or fewer B lymphocytes are responsive to each antigen.

By contrast, the mechanism by which T lymphocytes recognize and respond to antigens has remained obscure. It has been established for a decade that T cells are necessary for cooperation with B cells in the majority of antibody responses and that cell mediated immune responses are initiated and finally executed by T cells without a requirement for B-cell activity. In both contexts, the role of T cells appears to be just as specific as the role of B cells in antibody formation.[168] An obvious possibility is that T cells recognize antigens by the same means as do B cells, that is, by antibody molecules on their membrane. Despite a great deal of effort in trying to prove this, the evidence still is unsatisfactory. The term "elusive T-cell receptor" was coined in 1972 by Simonsen,[169] and elusive it has remained. However, there have been a number of surprising twists to the story.

Much progress in understanding how T cells recognize antigens has been achieved by studying immune responses to transplantation antigens. In the early 1960s two methods were introduced which enabled certain aspects of the immune response of lymphocytes to transplantation antigens to be studied in vitro. Mixed lymphocyte culture allowed the proliferative response of mutually stimulating populations of lymphocytes to be readily measured.[170] The technique has been refined and applied to solve many basic immunological questions as well as aiding typing for kidney transplantation. A later stage of the immune response can be investigated by measuring the cytolytic activity of immune lymphocytes. This refers to the destructive effect observed in culture when lymphocytes from an immunized animal ("attacker cells") are brought into contact with the type of antigenic cells against which they have been immunized ("target cells"). A successful example of this principle was reported by Govaerts,[171] who in 1960 cultured dog kidney cells in vitro. Thoracic duct lymphocytes from another dog which had been immunized against these kidney cell antigens were added to the culture. As he had anticipated, Govaerts noted that the immune lymphocytes killed the kidney cells after 24 to 48 hours in culture. This can be regarded as a system for studying the implementation of graft rejection in vitro, and these findings were soon confirmed and extended to other target cells.[172] The most informative series of experiments were performed by Brunner, Cerottini, and their colleagues in Lausanne following their discovery that a certain tumor cell in DBA/2 mice (the mastocytoma P815) was particularly useful because extensive target cell disintegration was measurable after only 4 to 6 hours culture in the presence of immune lymphoid cells from mice immunized against DBA/2 antigens.[173]

Brunner and Cerottini proved that the killer cell was in fact a T lymphocyte. This cell had to make contact with the target cell but apparently did not act by releasing a toxic chemical mediator because "innocent bystanders" (unrelated cells added in to the culture of attackers and targets) were unaffected.[174] Killing by T cells did not require the action of complement, which is needed when lysis of a target cell is produced by antibody. In fact, when the target cells are coated with antibody directed against antigens on its surface, they are protected from the lethal effect of killer T cells.

The simple idea that grafts are rejected because they are infiltrated by cytolytic lymphocytes which kill the graft cells by direct contact in the same way as target cells may be killed in vitro has not been accepted as the only mechanism involved. A great deal of work has been concentrated on "lymphokines"—biologically active substances liberated when sensitized T cells encounter their specific antigen.[175] The best defined of these substances is *migration inhibition factor* (MIF), which retards the spontaneous migration of macrophages.[176] In a graft undergoing rejection, macrophages have the role of scavenging the debris released from the damaged cells. It, thus, makes biological sense to keep them around the area where the action is going on. However, the biological significance of the many other activities attributed to lymphokines remains uncertain.

The way in which T cells recognize antigen was naturally pursued by the same means as had been successfully applied to B lymphocytes. The killer T lymphocytes produced as a result of immunization could be depleted or enriched by allowing them to adhere to immobilized cells expressing the antigens recognized by the T cells.[177] By contrast, the helper T lymphocytes cooperating with B lymphocytes in antibody formation could *not* be enriched or depleted in this way or on Wigzell columns. As usual, negative findings of this kind make little impact, although they may be of great significance.

During the years around 1970, evidence accumulated that the recognition of antigens by T lymphocytes might be radically different from the recognition mechanism of B lymphocytes. A number of competent investigators failed to find any detectable antibody on the surface of T lymphocytes although a red herring was thrown across this trail by the capacity of some T cells to absorb small amounts of antibody made by other cells.[178] In the 1960s, Simonsen[179] had repeatedly made the point that the recognition of major transplantation antigens by T lymphocytes was anomalous in several ways. This included the high proportion of T cells in nonimmune animals precommitted to respond to each of these major antigens. Simonsen estimated this to be *at least* 1 to 2 percent compared to the proportion of about one in a million which the clonal selection theory would predict.[179]

A second discovery linking T cells to the major transplantation antigens or major histocompatibility complex (MHC) was equally unexpected and mysterious. McDevitt,[180] Benacerraf,[181] and others showed that in mice and guinea pigs, the antibody response to several different antigens is inherited, so that a given strain may be a high or low responder. The ability to give a high response resided in the T cells rather than the B cells, and the genes controlling these responses were almost always within the MHC.[181] A third way in which the T-cell receptor is linked to the MHC is equally intriguing. The generalization is emerging that for T cells to interact with other cells (e.g., B cells, macrophages, target cells), recognition by the T cells of part of the MHC of the other cell is necessary. For example, Katz and Benacerraf showed that T and B cells must share the same MHC for cooperation in antibody responses.[182] Zinkernagel, Doherty,[183] and others found that for T cells to be able to kill target cells expressing a viral or chemical antigen, identity at the MHC was again necessary. Jacques Miller and Vadas showed that for delayed hypersensitivity, MHC compatibility between T cells and macrophages is essential.[184] This finding also showed that the role of macrophages is to present the antigen in a particular way to T lymphocytes and is not easily reconcilable either with the possibility that informational RNA is transmitted between macrophages and lymphocytes or with the other extreme that the role of macrophages is simply to break down large antigens into smaller molecules to be spewed out in the vicinity of the lymphocyte. These three phenomena linking the T-cell receptor to the MHC clearly have to be taken into account when considering the means by which T cells recognize antigen. The empirical discovery that several important human diseases are strongly associated with certain genes in the HLA locus (the human MHC)[185] has added a heavy impetus to work in this field.

The intriguing finding that it is during its period of differentiation in the thymus that the T lymphocyte learns which MHC antigens to regard as "self"[186] is bound to stimulate another period of intense effort to understand what the thymus does at a more basic level than is appreciated at present.

The likelihood that there are several subsets of T cells has become established after many years of work by Harvey Cantor and Ted Boyse,[187] who sought laboriously for discriminating characteristics. Helper T cells and cytolytic or killer T cells certainly belong to different sets, and it is possible that suppressor T cells and those T cells that implement delayed hypersensitivity also belong to distinct sets. There has been a surge of work concerning the role of suppressor T cells as one mechanism of immunological tolerance or unresponsiveness ever since Richard Gershon[188] in 1972 produced concrete evidence for the existence of suppressor cells that can prevent or turn off specific immune responses. This came a long time after Michael Woodruff's suggestion[189] in 1959 that tolerance as recognized in a whole animal might be the consequence of the production of "tolerant cells."[47]

Conclusion

Until around 1960, the lymphocyte was regarded as "a poor sort of cell, characterized by mostly negative attributes." Our tardiness in appreciating the complex physiology of lymphocytes was partly because their rather uniform appearance does not reveal their astonishing diversity. Once the first substantial discoveries had been achieved, progress accelerated rapidly. This was partly due to the exploitation of new techniques but at least as important were ingeniously designed experiments and the blending of previously unrelated lines of research, particularly transplantation studies and immunology.

Over the last few years, the lymphocyte has emerged as a model cell in the sense that knowledge of some of its functions is so advanced that cell biologists will be occupied in asking whether other cells operate in a similar way. As well as the examples already given, the way in which the local environment of the thymus or bursa influences development, the generation of the enormous diversity of antibody specificities, and the way in which helper and suppressor T cells orchestrate the functions of several other cell types all seem to have wide implications in biology and medicine.

References

1 Boyd WC: *Fundamentals of Immunology,* 3d ed. New York, Interscience, 1956, 776 pp.
2 Gibson T, Medawar PB: The fate of skin homografts in man. *J Anat (Lond)* 77:299–310, 1943.
3 Medawar PB: The behaviour and fate of skin autografts and skin homografts in rabbits. *J Anat* 78:176–199, 1944.
4 Gowans JL: The effect of the continuous re-infusion of lymph and lymphocytes on the output of lymphocytes from the thoracic duct of unanaesthetized rats. *Br J Exp Pathol* 38:67–81, 1957.
5 Gowans JL: The recirculation of lymphocytes from blood to lymph in the rat. *J Physiol* 146:54–69, 1959.
6 Gowans JL: The fate of parental strain lymphocytes in F_1 hybrid rats. *Ann NY Acad Sci* 99:432–455, 1962.
7 Gowans JL, Gesner BM, McGregor DD: The immunological activity of lymphocytes, in *Biological Activity of the Leucocyte.* London, Churchill, Ciba Foundation Study Group no. 10, 1961, 120 pp, p 32.
8 Ehrlich P: *Farbenanalytishe Untersuchungen zur Histologie und Klinik des Blutes.* Berlin, Hirschwald, 1891, 137 pp.
9 Himmelweit F (ed): *The Collected Papers of Paul Ehrlich.* London, Pergamon Press, 1956, vol I, 653 pp.

10   Ehrlich P: On immunity with special reference to cell life. *Proc R Soc Lond (Biol)* 66:424–448, 1900.

11   Himmelweit F (ed): *The Collected Papers of Paul Ehrlich*. London, Pergamon Press, 1957, vol II, 562 pp.

12   Delamere G: *General Anatomy of the Lymphatic System*. Leaf CH (trans). London, Westminister Press, 1903, p 33.

13   Yoffey JM, Courtice FC: *Lymphocytes, Lymph and the Lymphomyeloid Complex*. London, Academic Press, 1970, 942 pp.

14   Gulliver G: *The Works of William Hewson F.R.S.* London, Printed for the Sydenham Society, 1846, 360 pp, pp 275, 280, 282.

15   Jones TW: The blood corpuscle considered in its different phases of development in the animal series. *Philos Trans R Soc Lond Part I*: 63–87, 1842.

16   Ranvier LA: *Traité Technique d'Histologie*. Paris, Librairie F. Savy, 1875, 1110 pp.

17   Renaut J: Recherches sur les éléments cellulaires du sang. *Arch Physiol Norm Pathol* 8:649–671, 1881.

18   Ehrlich P, Lazarus A: Anaemia. Histology of the blood normal and pathologic, in Ehrlich P, Noorden K von, Lazarus A, Pinkus F (eds): *Diseases of the Blood*. Philadelphia and London, Saunders, 1905, 216 pp.

19   Maximow AA: The lymphocytes and plasma cells, in Cowdry EV II (ed): *Special Cytology*. New York, Hoeber, 1932, vol 2, pp 603–650.

20   Lewis WH, Webster LT: Migration of lymphocytes in plasma cultures of human lymph nodes. *J Exp Med* 33:261–269, 1921.

21   Harris H: Role of chemotaxis in inflammation. *Physiol Rev* 34:529–562, 1954.

22   Flemming W: *Studien über Regeneration der Gewebe*. I. *Die Zellvermehrung in den Lymphdrusen und Verwandten Organen, und ihr Einfluss auf Deren Bau*. Bonn, Max Cohen und Sohn, 1885, 66 pp, pp 4–23.

23   Hall JG, Morris B: The origin of the cells in the efferent lymph from a single lymph node. *J Exp Med* 121:901–910, 1965.

24   Behring EA von, Kitasato S: Uber das Zustandekommen der Diphtherie-Immunität und der Tetanus Immunität bei Thieren. *Dtsch Med Wochenschr* 16:1113–1114, 1890.

25   Jenner E: *The Origin of the Vaccine Inoculation*. London, Printed by D.N. Sherry, Berwick Street, Soho, 1801, 8 pp.

26   Pasteur L: Méthode pour prévenir la rage après morsue. *C R Acad Sci (Paris)* 103:777–785, 1886.

27   Pfeiffer R, Marx KFH: Die Bildungstätte der Choleraschutzstoffs. *Z Hyg Infektkrankh* 37:272–297, 1898.

28   Deutch L: Contribution a l'étude de l'origin des anticorps typhiques. *Ann Inst Pasteur* 13:689–691, 1899.

29   Landsteiner K: *The Specificity of Serological Reactions*. Cambridge, Harvard University Press, 1945, 310 pp.

30   Gay FP, Clark AR: The reticulo-endothelial system in relation to antibody formation. *JAMA* 83:1296–1297, 1924.

31   Aschoff L: Das reticulo-endotheliale System. *Ergeb Inn Med* 26:1–118, 1924.

32   Sabin FR: Cellular reactions to a dye-protein with a concept of the mechanism of antibody formation. *J Exp Med* 70:67–82, 1939.

33   Yoffey JM: *Bone Marrow Reactions*. Baltimore, Williams and Wilkins, 1966, 152 pp.

34 Burwell RG: The role of lymphoid tissue in morphostasis. *Lancet* ii:69–74, 1963.

35 Hanau A: Erfolgreiche experimentelle Übertragung von Karzinom. *Fortschr Med* 9:321–339, 1889.

36 Jensen CO: Experimentelle Untersuchungen über Krebs bei Mausen. *Zentralbl Bakteriol* 34:28–122, 1903.

37 Ehrlich P: Experimentelle Carcinomstudien an Mausen. *Arb Inst Exp Ther Frankfurt* 1:77–81, 1906.

38 Bashford EF, Murray JA, Haaland M: *Resistance and Susceptibility to Inoculated Cancer.* London, Third Scientific Report of the Cancer Research Fund, 1908, 509 pp, p 359.

39 Da Fano C: *A Cytological Analysis of the Reaction in Animals Resistant to Implanted Carcinomata.* London, Fifth Scientific Report of the Cancer Research Fund, 1912, 94 pp, pp 57–58.

40 Higuchi S: *On the Immunizing Power of the Placenta, Blood, Embryonic Skin, Mammary Gland and Spleen of Different Species against Carcinoma of the Mouse.* London, Fifth Scientific Report of the Cancer Research Fund, London, 1912, 94 pp, pp 79–94.

41 Murphy JB: The lymphocyte in resistance to tissue grafting, malignant disease and tuberculous infection. *Monogr Rockefeller Inst Med Res* 21:1–168, 1926.

42 Hektoen L, Corper HJ: Effect of injection of active deposit of radium emanation on rabbits with special reference to the leucocytes and antibody formation. *J Infect Dis* 31:305–312, 1922.

43 Heineke H: Experimentelle Untersuchungen über die Einwirkung der Roentgenstrahlen auf innere Organe. *Mitt Grenzgeb Med Chir* 14:21–94, 1905.

44 Gowans JL, McGregor DD: The origin of antibody-forming cells, in *Immunopathology.* Basel, Schwabe, IIId Internation Symposium, La Jolla, 1963, 389 pp, pp 89–98.

45 Snell GD: Methods for the study of histocompatibility genes. *J Genet* 49:87–108, 1948.

46 Gorer PA: The genetic and antigenic basis of tumour transplantation. *J Pathol Bacteriol* 44:691–697, 1937.

47 Woodruff MFA: *The Transplantation of Tissues and Organs.* Springfield, Ill., Charles C Thomas, 1960, 777 pp.

48 Little CC: The genetics of tissue transplantation in mammals. *J Cancer Res* 8:75–95, 1924.

49 Haldane JBS: The genetics of cancer. *Nature* 132:265–266, 1933.

50 Medawar PB: The immunology of transplantation. *Harvey Lect* 52:144–176, 1956–1957.

51 Billingham RE, Brent L, Medawar PB: Quantitative studies on tissue transplantation immunity. II. The origin, strength and duration of actively and adoptively acquired immunity. *Proc R Soc Lond (Biol)* 143:58–80, 1954.

52 Mitchison NA: Studies on the immunological response to foreign tumor transplants in the mouse. I. The role of lymph node cells in conferring immunity by adoptive transfer. *J Exp Med* 102:157–177, 1955.

53 Landsteiner K: Zur Kenntnis der antifermentatiuen, lytischen und agglutinierenden Wirkungen des Blutserums und der lymphe. *Zentralbl Bacteriol* 27:357–362, 1900.

54   Chase MW: Hypersensitivity to simple chemicals. *Harvey Lect* 61:169–203, 1965–1966.
55   Landsteiner K, Chase MW: Experiments on transfer of cutaneous sensitivity to simple compounds. *Proc Soc Exp Biol Med* 49:688–690, 1942.
56   Lawrence HS: Similarities between homograft rejection and tuberculin-type allergy: a review of recent experimental findings. *Ann NY Acad Sci* 64:826–835, 1957.
57   Koch R: Weitere Mittheilungen uber ein Heilmittel gegen Tuberkulose. *Dtsch Med Wochenschr* 17:101–102, 1891.
58   Lefford MJ, McGregor DD, Mackaness GB: Properties of lymphocytes which confer adoptive immunity to tuberculosis in rats. *Immunology* 25:703–715, 1973.
59   Chase MW: The cellular transfer of delayed hypersensitivity to tuberculin. *Proc Soc Exp Biol Med* 59:134–135, 1945.
60   McMaster PD, Hudack SS: The formation of agglutinins within lymph nodes. *J Exp Med* 61:783–805, 1935.
61   Rich AR, Lewis MR, Wintrobe MM: The activity of the lymphocyte in the body's reaction to foreign protein, as established by the identification of the acute splenic tumor cell. *Bull Johns Hopkins Hosp* 65:311–327, 1939.
62   Ehrich WE: Studies of the lymphatic tissue. III. Experimental studies of the relation of the lymphatic tissue to the number of lymphocytes in the blood in subcutaneous infection with staphylococci. *J Exp Med* 49:347–360, 1929.
63   Ehrich WE, Harris TN: The formation of antibodies in the popliteal lymph node in rabbits. *J Exp Med* 76:335–348, 1942.
64   Harris TN, Grimm E, Mertens E, Ehrich WE: The role of the lymphocyte in antibody formation. *J Exp Med* 81:73–83, 1945.
65   Bing J, Plum P: Serum proteins in leucopenia. *Acta Med Scand* 92:415–428, 1937.
66   Bjørneboe M, Gormsen H: Experimental studies on the role of plasma cells as antibody producers. *Acta Pathol Microbiol Scand* 20:649–692, 1943.
67   Bing J, Fagraeus A, Thorell B: Studies on nucleic acid metabolism in plasma cells. *Acta Physiol Scand* 10:282–294, 1945.
68   Fagraeus A: Antibody production in relation to the development of plasma-cells. *Acta Med Scand (Suppl)* 204:1–122, 1948.
69   Coons AH, Leduc EH, Connolly JM: Studies on antibody production. I. A method for the histochemical demonstration of specific antibody and its application to a study of the hyperimmune rabbit. *J Exp Med* 102:49–72, 1955.
70   Ehrich WE, Drabkin DL, Forman C: Nucleic acids and the production of antibody by plasma cells. *J Exp Med* 90:157–168, 1949.
71   Harris TN, Harris S: Histochemical changes in lymphocytes during the production of antibodies in lymph nodes of rabbits. *J Exp Med* 90:169–180, 1949.
72   Harris S, Harris TN: Studies on the transfer of lymph node cells. X. Estimation of the amounts of shigella-trypsin antigen associated with the lymph node cells during in vitro incubation. *J Immunol* 80:316–323, 1958.
73   Harris TN, Harris S: Lymph node cell transfer in relation to antibody production, in *Cellular Aspects of Immunology*. London, Churchill, Ciba Foundation Symposium, 1960, 495 pp, p 172.
74   Algire GH, Weaver JM, Prehn RT: Growth of cells in vivo in diffusion chambers. I. Survival of homografts in immunized mice. *J Natl Cancer Inst* 15:493–507, 1954.

75 Mitchison NA, Dube OL: Studies on the immunological response to foreign tumor transplants in the mouse. *J Exp Med* 102:179–197, 1955.

76 Werdelin O: The origin, nature and specificity of mononuclear cells in experimental autoimmune inflammations. *Acta Pathol Microbiol Scand (A) (Suppl)* 232, 1972, 91 pp.

77 Owen RD: Immunogenetic consequences of vascular anastamoses between bovine twins. *Science* 102:400–401, 1945.

78 Burnet FM, Fenner FJ: *The Production of Antibodies*, 2d ed. Melbourne, MacMillan, 1949, 142 pp.

79 Medawar PB: Immunological tolerance, in *Nobel Lectures. Physiology of Medicine. 1942–62*. Amsterdam, Elsevier, 1964, pp 704–713.

80 Billingham RW, Brent L, Medawar PB: "Actively acquired tolerance" of foreign cells. *Nature* 172:603–606, 1953.

81 Hasek M, Hraba T: Immunological effects of experimental embryonal parabiosis. *Nature* 175:764–765, 1955.

82 Triplett EL: On the mechanism of immunologic self recognition. *J Immunol* 89:505–510, 1962.

83 Mitchison NA: Immunological tolerance and immunological paralysis. *Br Med Bull* 17:102–106, 1961.

84 Burnet FM: *The Clonal Selection Theory of Acquired Immunity*. Nashville, Vanderbilt University Press, 1959, 208 pp.

85 Jerne NK: The natural selection theory of antibody formation. *Proc Natl Acad Sci USA* 41:849–857, 1955.

86 Crick FHC: in *The Biological Replication of Macromolecules*. Symp Soc Exp Biol (Gt. Brit.), number 12, New York, Academic Press, 1958, 255 pp, p 138.

87 Davis BF, Carlson AJ: Contributions to the physiology of lymph. IX. Notes on the leucocytes in the neck lymph, thoracic lymph and blood of normal dogs. *Am J Physiol* 25:173–185, 1909.

88 Bunting CH, Huston J: Fate of the lymphocyte. *J Exp Med* 33:593–600, 1921.

89 Sjövall H: Experimentelle Untersuchungen uber das Blut und die blutbildenden Organe—besonders das lymphatische Gewebe—des Kaninchens bei wiederholten Aderlässen. Lund, Håken Ohlssons Buchdruckerei, 1936, 308 pp.

90 Yoffey JM, Drinker CK: The cell content of peripheral lymph and its bearing on the problem of the circulation of the lymphocyte. *Anat Rec* 73:417–427, 1939.

91 Abraham EP: Howard Walter Florey. *Biographical Memoirs of Fellows of the Royal Society* 17:255–302, 1971.

92 Ebert RH, Sanders AG, Florey HW: Observations on lymphocytes in chambers in the rabbit's ear. *Br J Exp Pathol* 21:212–218, 1940.

93 Medawar J: Observations on lymphocytes in tissue culture. *Br J Exp Pathol* 21:205–211, 1940.

94 Bloom W: Transformation of lymphocytes into granulocytes in vitro. *Anat Rec* 69:99–116, 1937.

95 Volkman A, Gowans JL: The production of macrophages in the rat. *Br J Exp Pathol* 46:50–61, 1965.

96 Bollman JL, Cain JC, Grindlay JH: Techniques for the collection of lymph from the liver, small intestine, or thoracic duct of the rat. *J Lab Clin Med* 33:1349–1352, 1948.

97 Mann JD, Higgins GM: Lymphocytes in thoracic duct, intestinal and hepatic lymph. *Blood* 5:177–190, 1950.

98 Ottesen J: On the age of human white cells in peripheral blood. *Acta Physiol Scand* 32:75–93, 1954.

99 Buckton KE, Court-Brown WM, Smith PG: Lymphocyte survival in men treated with X-rays for ankylosing spondylitis. *Nature* 214:470–473, 1967.

100 Little JR, Brecher G, Bradley TR, Rose S: Determination of lymphocyte turnover by continuous infusion of ³H-thymidine. *Blood* 19:236–242, 1962.

101 Everett NB, Tyler RW: Lymphopoiesis in the thymus and other tissues: functional implications. *Int Rev Cytol* 22:205–237, 1967.

102 Hall JG, Morris B: Effect of X-irradiation of the popliteal lymph-node on its output of lymphocytes and immunological responsiveness. *Lancet* i:1077–1080, 1964.

103 Gowans JL, Knight EJ: The route of recirculation of lymphocytes in the rat. *Proc R Soc Lond (Biol)* 159:257–282, 1964.

104 Parrott DMV, de Sousa MAB, East J: Thymus dependent areas in the lymphoid organs of neonatally thymectomised mice. *J Exp Med* 123:191–204, 1966.

105 Zimmermann F: Der feinere Bau der Blutcapillaren. *Z Anat Entwickl* 68:29–109, 1923.

106 Beard J: The source of leucocytes and the true function of the thymus. *Anat Anz* 18:550–560, 1900.

107 Andreasen E: Studies on the thymolymphatic system. *Acta Pathol Microbiol Scand (Suppl)* 49, 1943, 171 pp.

108 Dougherty TF, White A: Functional alterations in lymphoid tissue induced by adrenal cortical secretion. *Am J Anat* 77:81–116, 1945.

109 Archer OK, Pierce JC: Role of the thymus in development of the immune response. *Fed Proc* 20:26, 1961.

110 Miller JFAP: Immunological function of the thymus. *Lancet* ii:748–749, 1961.

111 Good RA, Dalmasso AP, Martinez C, Archer OK, Pierce JC, Papermaster BW: The role of the thymus in development of immunologic capacity in rabbits and mice. *J Exp Med* 116:773–796, 1962.

112 Miller JFAP: Effect of neonatal thymectomy on the immunological responsiveness of the mouse. *Proc R Soc Lond (Biol)* 156:410–428, 1962.

113 Arnason BG, Jankovic BD, Waksman BH, Wennersten C: Role of the thymus in immune reactions in rats. II. Suppressive effect of thymectomy at birth on reactions of delayed (cellular) hypersensitivity and the circulating small lymphocyte. *J Exp Med* 116:177–186, 1962.

114 Good RA, Varco RL: A clinical and experimental study of agammaglobulinemia. *Journal-Lancet* 75:245–271, 1955.

115 Glick B, Chang TS, Jaap RG: The bursa of Fabricius and antibody production in the domestic fowl. *Poult Sci* 35:224–225, 1956.

116 Jolly J: Sur les mouvements amiboides des petites cellules de la bourse de Fabricius et du thymus. *C R Soc Biol (Paris)* 77:148–150, 1914.

117 Mueller AP, Wolfe HR, Meyer RK: Precipitin production in chickens. XXI. Antibody production in bursectomized chickens and in chickens injected with 19 nortestosterone on the fifth day of incubation. *J Immunol* 85:172–179, 1960.

118 Warner NL, Szenberg A, Burnet FM: The immunological role of different lymphoid organs in the chicken. 1. Dissociation of immunological responsiveness. *Aust J Exp Biol Med Sci* 40:373–387, 1962.

119 McGregor DD, Gowans JL: The antibody response of rats depleted of lymphocytes by chronic drainage from the thoracic duct. *J Exp Med* 117:303–320, 1963.

120 Fishman M, Adler FL: The role of macrophage-RNA in the immune response. *Cold Spring Harbor Symp Quant Biol* 32:343–348, 1967.

121 Askonas BA, Rhodes JM: Immunogenicity of antigen containing ribonucleic acid preparations from macrophages. *Nature* 205:470–474, 1965.

122 Simonsen M: Biological incompatibility in kidney transplantation in dogs. *Acta Pathol Microbiol Scand* 32:1–84, 1953.

123 Simonsen M: The impact on the developing embryo and newborn animal of adult homologous cells. *Acta Pathol Microbiol Scand* 40:480–500, 1957.

124 Murphy JB: The effect of adult chicken organ grafts on the chick embryo. *J Exp Med* 24:1–6, 1916.

125 Simonsen M: Graft-versus-host reactions: their natural history and applicability as tools of research. *Prog Allergy* 6:349–469, 1962.

126 Billingham RW, Brent L: Quantitative studies on tissue transplantation immunity. IV. Induction of tolerance in newborn mice and studies on the phenomena of runt disease. *Philos Trans R Soc Lond (Biol)* 242:439–477, 1959.

127 Medawar PB: Introduction, in Wolstenholme GEW, Knight EJ (eds): *The Immunologically Competent Cell*. London, Churchill, Ciba Foundation Study Group no. 16, 1963, 110 pp, pp 1–3.

128 Gowans JL, McGregor DD, Cowen DM, Ford CE: Initiation of immune responses by small lymphocytes. *Nature* 196:651–655, 1962.

129 Ling NR, Kay JE: *Lymphocyte Stimulation*, 2d ed. Amsterdam, North Holland, 1975, 398 pp.

130 Hungerford DA, Donnelly AJ, Nowell PC, Beck S: The chromosome constitution of a human phenotypic intersex. *Am J Hum Genet* 11:215–236, 1959.

131 Marshall WH, Roberts KB: Continuous cinematography of human lymphocytes cultured with phytohaemagglutin including observations on cell division and interphase. *Q J Exp Physiol* 50:361–374, 1965.

132 Dutton RW, Pearce JD: Antigen-dependent stimulation of synthesis of DNA in spleen cells from immunized rabbits. *Nature* 194:93–94, 1962.

133 Gowans JL, Uhr JW: The carriage of immunological memory by small lymphocytes in the rat. *J Exp Med* 124:1017–1030, 1966.

134 Gowans JL, McGregor DD: The immunological activities of lymphocytes. *Prog Allergy* 9:1–78, 1965.

135 Nossal GJV, Austin CM, Pye J, Mitchell J: Antigens in immunity. XII. Antigen trapping in the spleen. *Int Arch Allergy Appl Immunol* 29:368–383, 1966.

136 Humphrey JH: The fate of antigen and its relationship to the immune response. *Antibiot Chemother* 15:7–23, 1969.

137 McDevitt HO, Askonas BA, Humphrey JH, Schlecter I, Sela M: The localization of antigen in relation to specific antibody-producing cells. *Immunology* 11:337–351, 1966.

138 Fichtelius KE: On the destination of thymus lymphocytes, in Wolstenholme GEW, O'Connor M (eds): *Ciba Foundation Symposium on Haemopoiesis*. London, Churchill, 1960, 490 pp, pp 204–236.

139 Schooley JC, Kelly LS: Influence of the thymus on thoracic duct lymphocyte output, in Good RA, Gabrielsen AE (eds): *The Thymus in Immunobiology*. New York, Hoeber-Harper, 1964, 778 pp, p 236.

140 Weissman IL: Thymus cell migration. *J Exp Med* 126:291–304, 1967.
141 Ford CE: Traffic of lymphoid cells in the body, in Wolstenholme GEW, Porter R (eds): *The Thymus. Experimental and Clinical Studies.* London, Churchill, Ciba Foundation Symposium, 1966, 538 pp, p 131.
142 Moore MAS, Owen JJT: Experimental studies on the development of the thymus. *J Exp Med* 126:715–726, 1967.
143 Claman HN, Chaperon EA, Triplett RF: Immunocompetence of transferred thymus-marrow cell combinations. *J Immunol* 97:828–832, 1966.
144 Roitt IM, Greaves MF, Torrigiani G, Brostoff J, Playfair JHL: The cellular basis of immunological responses. *Lancet* 2:367–371, 1969.
145 Reif AE, Allen JMV: The AKR thymic antigen and its distribution in leukemias and nervous tissue. *J Exp Med* 120:413–447, 1964.
146 Raff MC: Theta isoantigen as a marker of thymus-derived lymphocytes in mice. *Nature* 224:378–379, 1969.
147 Schlesinger M: Anti-theta antibodies for detecting thymus-dependent lymphocytes in the immune response of mice to serum red blood cells (SRBC). *Nature* 226:1254–1256, 1970.
148 Nossal GJV, Cunningham A, Mitchell GF, Miller JFAP: Cell to cell interaction in the immune response. III. Chromosomal marker analysis of single antibody-forming cells in reconstituted, irradiated or thymectomized mice. *J Exp Med* 128:839–853, 1968.
149 Miller JFAP, Mitchell GF: The thymus and antigen-reactive cells. *Transplant Rev* 1:3–42, 1969.
150 Miller JFAP, Sprent J: Cell-to-cell interaction in the immune response. VI. Contribution of thymus-derived cells and antibody-forming cell precursors to immunological memory. *J Exp Med* 134:66–82, 1971.
151 Davies AJS: The thymus and the cellular basis of immunity. *Transplant Rev* 1:43–91, 1969.
152 Buckley CE, Whitney PL, Tanford C: The unfolding and renaturation of a specific univalent antibody fragment. *Proc Natl Acad Sci USA* 50:827–834, 1963.
153 Ford WL, Atkins RC: Specific unresponsiveness of recirculating lymphocytes after exposure to histocompatibility antigen in F_1 hybrid rats. *Nature New Biol* 234:178–180, 1971.
154 Stavitsky AB: In vitro studies of the antibody response. *Adv Immunol* 1:211–261, 1961.
155 Dutton RW, Mishell RI: Cell populations and cell proliferation in the *in vitro* response of normal mouse spleen to heterologous erythrocytes. Analysis by the hot pulse technique. *J Exp Med* 126:443–454, 1967.
156 Jerne NK, Nordin AA: Plaque formation in agar by single antibody-producing cells. *Science* 140:405, 1963.
157 Wigzell H, Andersson B: Cell separation on antigen-coated columns. Elimination of high-rate antibody-forming cells and immunological memory cells. *J Exp Med* 129:23–36, 1969.
158 Wesslén T: Studies on the role of lymphocytes in antibody production (unpublished). 1952, Personal communication.
159 Naor D, Sulitzeanu D: Binding of radioiodinated bovine serum albumin to mouse spleen cells. *Nature* 214:687–688, 1967.

160 Ada GL, Byrt P, Mandel T, Warner N: A specific reaction between antigen labelled with radioactive iodine and lymphocyte-like cells from normal, tolerant and immunized mice or rats, in Sterzl J, Riha I (eds): *Developmental Aspects of Antibody Formation and Structure.* New York, Academic Press, 1970, p 503.

161 Sell S, Gell PGH: Studies on rabbit lymphocytes in vitro. 1. Stimulation of blast transformation with an antiallotype serum. *J Exp Med* 122:423–440, 1965.

162 Raff MC, Sternberg M, Taylor RB: Immunoglobulin determinants on the surface of mouse lymphoid cells. *Nature* 225:553–554, 1970.

163 Raff MC: Two distinct populations of peripheral lymphocytes in mice distinguishable by immunofluorescence. *Immunology* 19:637–650, 1970.

164 Pernis B, Forni L, Amante L: Immunoglobulin spots on the surface of rabbit lymphocytes. *J Exp Med* 132:1001–1018, 1970.

165 Lerner RA, Dixon FJ: The human lymphocyte as an experimental animal. *Sci Am* 228:82–91, 1973.

166 Raff MC, Feldmann M, de Petris S: Monospecificity of bone-marrow-derived lymphocytes. *J Exp Med* 137:1024–1030, 1973.

167 Klinman NR, Press JL: The B cell specificity repertoire: its relationship to definable subpopulations. *Transplant Rev* 24:41–83, 1975.

168 Greaves MF, Owen JJT, Raff MC: in *T and B lymphocytes, Origins, Properties and Roles in Immune Responses.* Amsterdam, Excerpta Medica, 1974, 316 pp.

169 Crone M, Koch C, Simonsen M: The elusive T cell receptor. *Transplant Rev* 10:36–56, 1972.

170 Bain B, Lowenstein L: Genetic studies on the mixed leucocyte reaction. *Science* 145:1315–1316, 1964.

171 Govaerts A: Cellular antibodies in kidney homotransplantation. *J Immunol* 85:516–522, 1960.

172 Rosenau W, Moon HD: Lysis of homologous cells by sensitized lymphocytes in tissue culture. *J Natl Cancer Inst* 27:471–483, 1961.

173 Brunner KT, Mauel J, Rudolf H, Chapius B: Studies of allograft immunity in mice. I. Induction, development and *in vitro* assay of cellular immunity. *Immunology* 18:501–515, 1970.

174 Cerottini JC, Brunner K: Cell-mediated cytotoxicity, allograft rejection and tumor immunity. *Adv Immunol* 18:67–132, 1974.

175 Dumonde DC, Wolstencroft RA, Panayi GS, Matthew M, Morley J, Howson WT: Lymphokines, non-antibody mediators of cellular immunity generated by lymphocyte activation. *Nature* 224:38–42, 1969.

176 David JR: Delayed hypersensitivity in vitro. Its mediation by cell free substances formed by lymphoid cell-antigen interaction. *Proc Natl Acad Sci USA* 56:72–77, 1966.

177 Golstein P, Svedmyr EAJ, Wigzell H: Cells mediating specific in vitro cytotoxicity. I. Detection of receptor-bearing lymphocytes. *J Exp Med* 134:1385–1402, 1971.

178 Hunt SV, Williams AF: The origin of cell surface immunoglobulin of marrow-derived and thymus-derived lymphocytes of the rat. *J Exp Med* 139:479–496, 1974.

179 Nisbet NW, Simonsen M, Zaleski M: The frequency of antigen-sensitive cells in tissue transplantation. *J Exp Med* 129:459–467, 1969.

180 McDevitt HO, Chinitz A: Genetic control of the antibody response: relationship between immune response and histocompatibility (H-2) type. *Science* 163:1207–1208, 1969.

181 Benacerraf B: The genetic control of specific immune responses. *Harvey Lect* 67:109–141, 1973.

182 Katz DH, Hamaoka T, Benacerraf B: Cell interactions between histoincompatible T and B lymphocytes. II. Failure of physiological cooperative interactions between T and B lymphocytes from allogeneic donor strains in humoral response to hapten-protein conjugates. *J Exp Med* 137:1405–1418, 1973.

183 Zinkernagel RM, Doherty PC: H-2 compatibility requirement for T cell mediated lysis of target cells infected with lymphocytic choriomeningitis virus. Different cytotoxic T cell specificities are associated with structures coded for in H-2K or H-2D. *J Exp Med* 141:1427–1436, 1975.

184 Miller JFAP, Vadas MA: Antigen activation of T lymphocytes: influence of major histocompatibility complex. *Cold Spring Harbor Symp Quant Biol* 41:579–588, 1977.

185 Dick HM: HLA and disease. Introductory review. *Br Med Bull* 34:271–274, 1978.

186 Zinkernagel RM, Callahan GN, Klein J, Dennert G: Cytotoxic T cells learn specificity for self H-2 during differentiation in the thymus. *Nature* 271:251–253, 1978.

187 Cantor H, Boyse E: Regulation of the immune response by T-cell subclasses. *Contemp Top Immunobiol* 7:47–67, 1977.

188 Gershon RK, Cohen P, Hencin R, Liebhaber SA: Suppressor T cells. *J Immunol* 108:586–590, 1972.

189 Woodruff MFA: Comment in discussion, in Albert F, Lejeune-Ledant G (eds): *Biological Problems of Grafting*. Liège, University of Liège Press, 1959, 453 pp, p 258.

CHAPTER 15

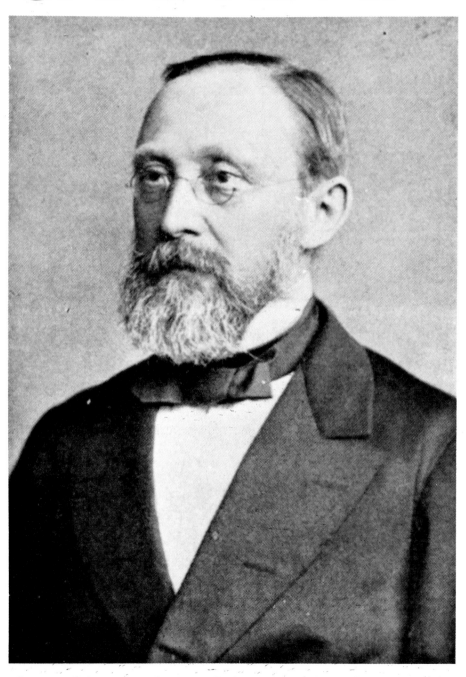

THE DREAD LEUKEMIAS AND THE LYMPHOMAS: THEIR NATURE AND THEIR PROSPECTS

Frederick W. Gunz

The word *leukemia* was coined in 1847[1] by Rudolf Virchow, the father of cellular pathology, some 2 years after he described the disease and the year before he lost his first university appointment in Berlin, a victim of his uncompromisingly radical political attitudes.[2] Leukemia was then a clinical and pathologic curiosity, to be catalogued and fought over by the experts and, for the patients, a condition that carried no hope of recovery. In the decades that followed, Virchow, having been restored to office, continued his long ascent to the very pinnacle of German medical science while maintaining his enlightened views on social and political problems.

Leukemia was discussed, subclassified, investigated from many angles, and eventually treated, with variable degrees of success. However, for many years, the condition received little public attention. The dread, the widespread fear of what was pictured as a sinister and ill-understood disease came much later largely as a consequence of its dramatization by the popular news and

Chapter Opening Photo   Paul G. Werlhofv (1699–1767): morbus maculosis Werlhofi. *Major RH: The History of Medicine, Springfield, Ill, Charles C Thomas, 1954, 2 vols, 1155 pp, p 807.*)

511

entertainment media, ironically at the very time when substantial progress was at last being made in understanding the nature of leukemia and the treatment of some of its forms.[3]

Beginnings

It is generally held that leukemia was discovered almost simultaneously by Virchow in Berlin[4] and by Bennett in Edinburgh.[5] Chronologically, Bennett's publication in October 1845 preceded Virchow's by some 6 weeks. Certainly, others had previously seen similar cases. In the flourishing French medical literature of the early nineteenth century, there are scattered reports of patients with large spleens and peculiar blood, some of whom probably had leukemia. Donné, in his *Cours de microscopie,* described the characteristic blood changes,[6] and in the same issue of the journal as Bennett's article, Craigie,[7] a Scot, gave an account of an undoubtedly genuine case which he had observed several years previously. However, it was Virchow and Bennett who recognized the significance of their first observations and immediately set to work defining this new and remarkable disease and its place in the spectrum of pathology.

Bennett

John Hughes Bennett (1812–1875) was 33 in the momentous year 1845. A native Englishman, he graduated from the Edinburgh medical school. His career as a student had been brilliant, and after qualifying, he went to Paris, where he came under the influence of the great microscopist Donné. Two years in France and another two in Germany saw him ready to return to his adopted home in Scotland, where he rapidly became known as an outstanding teacher. Indeed, he is credited with having given the first courses in practical physiology and pathology in Britain. In these he was undoubtedly helped by the use of the newly designed compound microscope (Chapter 1), with which he must have become thoroughly familiar during his years with Donné.

By 1845 he was already a Fellow of the Royal Society of Edinburgh, and three years later he gained the Chair at the Institutes of Medicine. However, the greater honor of the Chair of Physic at Edinburgh University eluded him, probably because of his temperament, which brought him into conflict with the medical establishment.[8] He was a man of brilliance but short temper, certain of his own virtues, pugnacious, and unable to suffer fools. In his obituary,[9] the eulogist states that "his tendency to indulge freely in critical and sarcastic remarks upon the works of others did not make him a general favorite with some of his professional brethren." Even without these defects, a thrusting young Englishman with a strong continental background might have found it difficult to reach the top in the solidly traditionalist climate which was then still prevalent in Edinburgh.

Virchow

Virchow (Chapter Opening Photo) was Bennett's junior by 9 years. In 1845, he was only 24 and just 2 years out of the Berlin army medical school. Even then, he had already shown signs of unusual ability. A pupil of Johannes Müller—who had just announced the discovery of the animal cell—Virchow became assistant to Professor Froriep, who had been in Paris at about the same time as Bennett. The first research project which Froriep gave to his assistant was the study of inflammation of the veins. This had two important outcomes: "It threw a clear light upon the previously obscure problems of thrombosis and embolism; and it led to the formulation of a new morbid concept, that of leukemia."[2]

Both Bennett and Virchow made their original observations at the autopsy table. Each man's patient had been sick for $1\frac{1}{2}$ or 2 years. In each case, symptoms had consisted of gradually increasing weakness, swelling of the abdomen, and a variety of troubles, including severe nosebleeds, shortly before death. Each examiner found two remarkable features: a great enlargement of the spleen and a most peculiar appearance of the blood, with changes in its color and consistency. To Bennett it seemed that the blood had pus mixed with it, and when he examined it microscopically, there were in fact huge numbers of the same corpuscles which he and many others were used to seeing in pus (Figure 15-1). Although he could find no source of inflammation that might have given rise to the pus, he nevertheless concluded that his patient had died from "the presence of purulent matter in the blood," and this diagnosis was duly incorporated in the title of his famous case report.

Virchow saw the same striking changes, but he interpreted them differently. He remembered that the normal blood contains colorless corpuscles quite similar to those in pus and in his patient's blood. The only difference was that the normal ratio of "pigmented" (i.e., red) and colorless (white) corpuscles seemed reversed in this instance. Virchow, too, could find no inflammation that might have led to the formation of pus, but, in contrast to Bennett, he was disinclined to call the condition "pyemia," i.e., blood containing pus. Instead, he contented himself with the descriptive name "white blood," which made no judgment on causation. White blood, translated into Greek, became *leukemia* 2 years later.

Controversy

The stage was now set for what was to turn into an unedifying quarrel between two leading investigators. It was conducted in the medical journals and concerned both the priority of their observations and the matter of their interpretation. Even the name of the condition, Virchow's "Leukämie" versus Bennett's rival "leucocythaemia"[10] was acrimoniously debated, and for years

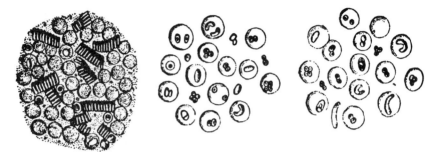

Figure 15-1 Microscopic appearance of blood in a case of leukemia reported by Bennett in 1852. (*Reproduced by permission from Rosenthal N: The lymphomas and leukemias. Bull NY Acad Med 30:583–600, 1954.*)

both designations continued to be used. Although century-old priorities are now unimportant, the controversy concerning the pathology of leukemia remains fascinating from the historic viewpoint and has occasional repercussions even today.

No one doubted that the main trouble in leukemia lay in the astonishing masses of colorless corpuscles in the blood. But what were they doing there in the first place, and whence had they come? "Wherever the colorless blood corpuscles may come from, that is whence those that are so immensely prevalent in leukemia must also be derived," said Virchow in 1856.[11] There seemed to be three possibilities: the corpuscles might arise in the blood, or get there from the lymph, or be torn from the walls of the blood vessels. Virchow was sure the second alternative was correct; the cells no doubt came normally from the lymph, but he also guessed there might be other sources, perhaps the spleen. Although initially he had tended to believe the corpuscles might be derived from the blood plasma, he was by now convinced that the cells could only come from other cells and not from fluids.

Early in his work and in line with most other physicians of his day, Virchow still accepted Hewson's eighteenth century views on the interrelationships of the various types of blood cells, according to which the red corpuscles were formed in the blood from colorless ones (Chapter 1)—perhaps, as Bennett thought, the red cells were their liberated nuclei. This theory accounted rather neatly for the fact that in leukemia there appeared to be too few red cells as well as too many white ones. This was understandable if the normal white-to-red transformation was slowed down in leukemia. Later,[11,12] Virchow came to doubt that the white corpuscles in the blood could ever be transformed into red ones. Instead, he thought they were "end products" that had no specific functions and met an early death in the circulation. The production of red from white cells, Virchow now believed, took place in the lymph nodes and probably the spleen. When we remember that neither Virchow nor Bennett nor any of their contemporaries could stain blood or count its constituents, we should not be surprised by their occasional exotic ideas about the blood cells. The marvel was how often their guesses were close to the truth!

Regardless of the precise origin of the colorless corpuscles, the question remained—and would remain for many years—in leukemia, what causes them to become almost as numerous as the red cells? Although Virchow had stumbled on leukemia in the course of his study of phlebitis, an inflammatory condition of the veins, he soon became convinced that inflammation was not the cause of leukemia. The colorless globules might resemble those in pus, but they had a different significance, and by 1856, Virchow thought the real trouble lay in the organs that he believed produce these cells, mainly the lymph nodes, the liver, and the spleen, which were of course much enlarged in many cases of leukemia. Many physicians besides Bennett and Virchow had by now described patients with the new disease, and some of them had studied the blood during life and found the same changes that had originally been seen postmortem. This discovery led even Bennett to accept the improbability of pus being mixed with blood in patients who might go on living for months. If, therefore, leukemia was not simply an inflammation of the blood but arose from abnormalities in the blood-forming organs, what then was the nature of these abnormalities?

Here there were great difficulties. Both the spleen and the lymph nodes were still "mystery organs," which were found enlarged in a variety of common diseases. It seemed probable that in leukemia the enlargement of the spleen had an origin different from that usually seen in malaria (known then as "intermittent fever"), and it was noted that there were differences in the pathology of leukemic and tuberculous ("scrofulous") lymph nodes. These, however, were negative statements, and positive conclusions were much more difficult to reach. Virchow decided eventually to call leukemia a disease *sui generis*,[12] but try as he would, he could discover no basic mechanism by which it was produced. Somehow there was an overgrowth (*hyperplasia*) of the tissues in the lymph nodes, spleen, and liver without evidence of a cause. Infection could not be entirely ruled out, but it seemed an unlikely explanation. This lack of certainty became the refrain of much of the published work of the ensuing period until eventually the balance of opinion swung from simple hyperplasia to *neoplasia* (new growth) as the probable mechanism.

Types of Leukemia

At this point we will anticipate the fact that in modern times it has become impossible to speak of leukemia as a single disease. Rather, we now recognize a number of different types, which differ from each other in many respects, such as their manifestations, response to treatment, and, probably, causation.[3] Some of these differences were observed soon after Virchow's and Bennett's original discoveries, others are only gradually emerging today.

The early authors spoke of *leukemia* and reported the presence of colorless or "white" corpuscles, which some equated with pus cells, as has been seen, while others called them lymph corpuscles or globules, for they were supposed to be derived from the lymph nodes and thence to enter the blood. Donné[13] believed the white corpuscles were actually formed from small chylous, i.e., fatty, particles and became transformed into red corpuscles in the spleen. Soon, however, Virchow decided that not all "lymph corpuscles" were the same—most were granular and had irregular trefoillike or even divided nuclei, but there were also some agranular ones with smooth round nuclei. The latter were increased in certain cases of leukemia in which the lymph nodes were particularly large. Therefore, Virchow proposed to subdivide leukemia into two forms, one characterized chiefly by great swelling of the spleen ("splenic" or "lienal" leukemia) and the other by enlargement of the lymph nodes ("lymphatic" leukemia), each with its own predominant variety of corpuscles. This basic distinction has held since Virchow's time, with one important qualification; in 1870, Neumann,[14] in Königsberg, first suggested that the colorless corpuscles are normally made in the bone marrow (Chapter 3), and that in so-called splenic leukemia, the marrow rather than the spleen is the major source of the excess corpuscles or, at least, is an equally important one. Later, many authors began to write of "splenomedullary leukemias," a term that eventually became simplified to "myeloid," that is, marrow-derived.

A further subdivision of the leukemias into acute and chronic forms was based on clinical grounds. In 1889, Ebstein[15] first used the term "acute" leukemia, but earlier authors, as far back as Virchow, had certainly seen patients with the acute forms and had described their characteristic symptoms. However, in 1879 the best-known account of leukemia in the English language[16] still treated "splenic leucocythaemia" as a chronic disease. The importance of Ebstein's new classification was soon realized, for the immediate outlook was particularly grim for patients who had the symptoms of the acute form of leukemia; they were found to be unresponsive to all forms of treatment that were tried, while those with chronic leukemia could often be temporarily relieved. Indeed, a diagnosis of acute leukemia began to carry with it the implication of death, usually within weeks if not days, and this somber picture remained substantially unaltered for nearly 60 years after Ebstein's original publication.

The problem of classifying leukemia became vastly simplified when Ehrlich introduced his new methods of staining blood cells (Chapter 1).[17] What had until then only been dimly realized became suddenly clear; the white blood cells were not identical but consisted of a great variety of forms, some probably precursors of others. The two basic types, granulocytes and lymphocytes, as Virchow had suspected, were, indeed, clearly distinguishable. Ehrlich was able to confirm the fact that granulocytes were the predominant type in both the splenic and myeloid forms of leukemia, which were therefore identical. At the turn of the century, Naegeli, the great Swiss hematologist, described a new cell, the myeloblast, which was shown to be the ancestor of all granular cells and was soon found to be grossly increased in number in many acute leukemias. From then on, the presence of primitive myeloblasts (and, later, lymphoblasts) came to be regarded as a hallmark of acute leukemia, which, thus, could be diagnosed by microscopy as well as on clinical grounds.

Myeloid and *lymphatic, acute* and *chronic,* are terms still in use for the classification of the leukemias. However, in 1865, another name, *pseudoleukemia,* was introduced by Julius Cohnheim.[18] This term created massive confusion among clinicians and among those who were trying to compile statistical information on leukemia. Cohnheim, then aged 26 and later a famous pathologist in the Virchow tradition, described a single case of what at first he thought was leukemia, with enlargement of the spleen and early death of the patient; indeed, the published protocol leaves little doubt that this was a genuine example of acute leukemia. However, because Cohnheim, working well before the introduction of staining methods, could not find the great increase in white blood corpuscles which then characterized leukemia, he decided to name the condition pseudoleukemia. Unfortunately, this term also suited a large variety of other conditions, many of which were not leukemia and some not even remotely related to it. In effect, pseudoleukemia soon came to be used as a label for any condition in which either the spleen or the lymph nodes were enlarged but the white corpuscles were not grossly increased in number and in which no other positive diagnosis could be made. This catchall term included many cases of tuberculosis, syphilis and other infectious diseases, some cancers, and a mixture of more or less vague conditions, as well, of course, as some genuine leukemias; but the group in which the greatest confusion arose was that of the lymphomas, especially Hodgkin's disease.

The Lymphomas

Lymphoma is a collective term which, over the years, has come and gone in the medical literature according to the fashion of the day and the nation. It was mentioned by Virchow and was certainly in use in the 1880s.[19] Since then, it has done battle with a large number of alternative designations. Today it seems to be the preferred name for a group of diseases which cause enlargement of the lymph nodes and are regarded as more or less distant relatives of the leukemias. They too are tumorous or neoplastic in nature, and the adjective *malignant* is therefore often added to the noun *lymphoma*.

Hodgkin's Disease

The first cases of what were later to be included among the lymphomas were published well before the first leukemias. In 1832, Thomas Hodgkin of Guy's Hospital, in London, gave an account[20] of seven patients who had come to the hospital shortly before death, all with great enlargement of lymph nodes and, usually, the spleen. At first it was believed that tuberculosis had caused these changes, but Hodgkin thought that there was an essential difference, even though in his day he could not study the microscopic picture. By nature generous and optimistic, perhaps because of his Quaker background, Hodgkin wondered if something could not have been done for these poor patients:

> Were patients thus affected to come under my care in an earlier and less hopeless period of their malady, I think I should be inclined to endeavour as far as possible to increase the general vigour of the system, to enjoin, as far as consistent with this object, the utmost protection from the inclemencies and vicissitudes of the weather, to employ iodine externally, and to push the internal use of caustic potash as far as circumstances might render allowable.

This note of compassion comes refreshingly from a field where the patient's interests were not often mentioned and where, somewhat later, therapeutic nihilism became the fashion.

Hodgkin's observations could not have attracted much attention, for the condition was, in effect, rediscovered in 1856 by the redoubtable Samuel Wilks, also of Guy's Hospital. At the end of his report[21] on "cases of a peculiar enlargement of the lymphatic glands frequently associated with disease of the spleen," Wilks noted that he had only just become aware of Hodgkin's previous work; in fact, three of Wilks' six cases (taken from the Guy's museum) had already been described by Hodgkin. The embarrassment felt by this English gentleman may be imagined, and in a second publication,[22] he hastened to bestow the credit which he realized should be Hodgkin's. The additional cases that Wilks now described in much greater detail than previously were given the eponym Hodgkin's disease and were clearly separated from cancer, tuberculosis, and "lardaceous" (amyloid) disease. But what the true nature of Hodgkin's 30-year-old disease might be, Wilks could not say, even though, in contrast to Hodgkin, he had some inkling of its microscopic features.

Wilks' account of Hodgkin's disease and Cohnheim's of pseudoleukemia were published during the same year. Both described patients with a fatal disease in which enlargement of the spleen was a prominent feature and in which some resemblance to leukemia existed but without there being an increase in the number of colorless corpuscles in the blood. Careless readers of the two papers overlooked the fact that there were many dissimilar features, notably the gross enlargement of the lymph nodes in Hodgkin's disease, which was certainly not mentioned in Cohnheim's case. Hodgkin's disease was almost immediately equated with pseudoleukemia, with consequent confusion that took many years to sort out. As late as 1931, in his famous textbook of hematology,[23] Naegeli grappled unsuccessfully with the convolutions of pseudoleukemia, and from 1929 to 1938, the official International List of Causes of Death included Hodgkin's disease among the pseudoleukemias.

Today pseudoleukemia is scarcely remembered while Hodgkin's disease has been defined with precision by multitudes of pathologists and discussed from every conceivable point of view.[24–26] It has been clearly separated from infectious causes of enlargement of the lymph nodes, such as tuberculosis and syphilis, which were common in the nineteenth and early twentieth centuries, but are much less so now in most Western countries, as well as from other conditions, notably the so-called lymphosarcomas, which have become well defined and which today are often grouped together as "non-Hodgkin's lymphomas."

Lymphosarcoma

It was Virchow once again who first wrote of lymphosarcoma.[27] In his textbook on tumors, he considered it a malignant neoplasm affecting the lymphatic tissue. Thirty years later, Kundrat[28] revived the term and defined it more sharply as a primary affection of the lymph nodes which sooner or later spreads to neighboring structures in the manner of malignant diseases and also progresses to other groups of lymph nodes. Kundrat thought he could distinguish this condition from leukemia, but later observers were not so sure.

It gradually appeared that there were a large variety of conditions with rather similar clinical features and that some—if not all—had a propensity to become transformed into leukemia, particularly into the chronic lymphatic type.[29,30] Where these conditions differed chiefly from each other and from Hodgkin's disease was in their microscopic appearances and, especially, in the nature of their predominant cells, whereas the clinical courses were much more alike. Not surprisingly, therefore, it was left to the pathologists to define the various entities and produce classifications; not unexpectedly, a large number of often conflicting classifications were suggested. Indeed, although more recently some consensus has been achieved, we still do not possess a classification of the lymphomas that is universally accepted. However, the remaining arguments are concerned with relatively technical minutiae, and the general outlines of the picture are distinct enough. These are briefly summarized in the section which follows.

Description of the Leukemias and Lymphomas

The basic subdivision of the diseases with which we are concerned is into two main groups, the leukemias and the lymphomas. The leukemias, as early as they can first be identified in any one patient, are found to be generalized throughout the body; they affect, primarily, the blood-forming organs, such as the bone marrow, liver, spleen, and lymph nodes, nearly always with consequent changes in the blood itself. The most obvious of the changes in the blood in leukemia are an increase in the number of white cells and the presence of immature or abnormal white cells as well as anemia. The lymphomas, by contrast, are usually localized, at least in their earlier stages, and show themselves as swellings, primarily of the lymph nodes and, less prominently, the spleen, liver, and, sometimes, other organs, without specific changes in the blood. In their later stages, some of the lymphomas have a tendency to invade the bone marrow and blood and, thus, they may become indistinguishable from leukemia.

Leukemias are subclassified either according to their predominant cells (myeloid or granulocytic, lymphatic, and so on) or according to their clinical course (acute or chronic). Thus, we speak, for example, of acute lymphatic or of chronic myeloid leukemia. The lymphomas are subdivided on the one hand into Hodgkin's disease and on the other a large group of so-called non-Hodgkin's lymphomas, which take their names from their predominant cell types and microscopic (histologic) structure. Hodgkin's disease has little tendency to spread to the blood, but many of the non-Hodgkin's lymphomas may turn into leukemias at some point in their course.

Who Gets Leukemia?

John Menteith was a slater aged 28, of dark complexion, previously healthy, and temperate; but, upon his admission to the Edinburgh Royal Infirmary on February 27, 1845, he was sick, listless, and had a huge tumor in the abdomen and several smaller tumors in the neck, groins, and under the arms. Marie Straide was a cook aged 50 when she was admitted to the Charité Hospital in Berlin on March 1 of the same year. She had lost much weight and had a hacking cough, painful abdomen, and other distressing symptoms. These were the first known patients with leukemia. They perished in misery and were quickly forgotten, except as "cases" of what might be a rare, new, and pathologically interesting complaint. True enough, 2 years later, Virchow wrote, "The physicians are the natural attorneys of the poor, and social problems should be solved by them,"[31] but by that time, the problems of poor Menteith and Straide had already been solved.

By 1977, leukemia had become one of the great examples of the sad ending; on television and in motion pictures, the young and attractive die from it whenever an author's plot requires an early demise. Leukemia in a public figure becomes instant news. Autobiographies of leukemia patients are published. As a result, it is widely thought that leukemia is far more common than it was formerly and that from it die chiefly the young, including many children. These are the beliefs that have made leukemia a "dread disease." They are also beliefs that are either partially or altogether false.

For many years after it was first described, leukemia remained an oddity, so much so that every case that was diagnosed was duly published in the medical literature. Statistics on its prevalence in the population were unavailable until well into the twentieth century, and then, the official classification, under the term pseudoleukemia, included Hodgkin's disease with leukemia. Various authors published series of cases; that is, collective accounts of what they or their colleagues had observed in practice, but these could give no more than a partial impression of the problem of leukemia, for there was no telling whether these cases were representative of cases in the wider community. Indeed, acceptable statistics could only be compiled after leukemia was officially recognized as a distinctive cause of death, and then, only for those deaths that were medically certified and recorded. Moreover, because the disease can only be diagnosed with certainty by laboratory tests, the statistics depend heavily on the quality of laboratory services; in other words, there is bound to be more leukemia diagnosed in places where there are better laboratories, or in places where more people can afford to have laboratory tests. If only for this reason, we would expect to find more leukemia today than 50 years ago, and more in the developed countries compared with the developing world, but we should interpret such differences largely as statistical artifacts. Naturally, this does not exclude the possibility that, in addition, there are also "real" differences, and this will be discussed later.

If we take the mortality from leukemia in the United States as an example, the *rate* of deaths per 100,000 or 1 million of the population per year, we find that it quadrupled between 1920 and 1950, but since the late 1950s, there has been little further increase. A similar pattern can be found in many other Western countries, and the question is: what does this mean? We have already seen that at least part of the increase can be attributed to better diagnosis, but we still do not know how large a part. The problem is crucial, for if there has been a *real* increase in leukemia, this must have resulted from an increase in whatever causes the disease; equally, the reasons for the recent slowing down must be explained. Only much more detailed and broadly based epidemiologic studies are likely to provide the answers to this all-important question, but it is quite clear that if there has been a real increase, it is nothing like as great as that suggested by the crude mortality records.

In the meantime, what is the risk of getting leukemia? This may depend to some extent on one's country of residence, unless, indeed, we accept the view that the published differences are due only to differences in the thoroughness of case finding. The risk certainly depends on one's age. About 20 percent of all leukemias occur in children, with the greatest mortality between the ages of 2 and 5. In older children and young adults, the mortality is relatively low, but it rises steadily from the fourth decade and peaks in old age. Contrary to popular belief, therefore, old people have the highest risk of dying from leukemia, which is, thus, by no means a disease only of the bright and beautiful. In one respect, however, the purveyors of medical folklore are correct; children and young people who develop leukemia are likely to have the acute rather than the chronic forms. In fact, in childhood, chronic leukemia is very rare, while in adults, all forms occur, still with more acute than chronic cases.

The statistics indicate that in Western countries, some six to eight persons per 100,000 population die each year from leukemia. We do not know with any certainty how many people *develop* leukemia because such statistics (termed *incidence*) are not usually recorded, whereas those for mortality are. In 1968, it was estimated that 19,000 Americans developed leukemia.[32] From such figures, one can calculate that the average individual at birth has a 1 in 200 chance of developing leukemia some time during a lifetime. This risk decreases as the individual becomes older.

Compared to leukemia, the lymphomas are collectively a little more common, though not much more so. They too occur at all ages, but Hodgkin's disease is unique in having two peaks at which it is most frequent—one in adolescence, the other in middle age. Many have speculated about the reasons, but as yet without success.

The Nature of Leukemia

Earlier in this chapter, the controversy between Bennett and Virchow concerning the cause of the peculiar "white blood" of their patients was mentioned. Was it pus—a sign of inflammation—or something else? Bennett must have regretted his rash commitment to the theory of pyemia, which he could soon see was untenable. But if not pus, then what gave rise to the enormous numbers of white corpuscles, and what caused the accompanying anemia? Bennett lived another 30 years, Virchow nearly 60, but neither could add much to Virchow's tentative view in 1856 that leukemia was a disease *sui generis*,[12] that is, of unknown origin or, in more modern parlance, *idiopathic*.

Today, human leukemia remains an idiopathic disease, but the term may now be qualified: although we cannot say exactly what causes the disease, or any of its types, we do know a good many factors that could and some that definitely do contribute to its causation in human beings.

Far more is known about the origin of leukemia in animals; an enormous amount of work has been done, mainly on specially bred strains developed in the laboratory, but lately also on free-living species, many of which do develop leukemia. These include rodents; domestic animals, such as cats, dogs, and cattle; birds, especially chickens and turkeys; and monkeys, apes, and some other primates. The outcome of all these studies is the unchallenged finding that leukemia never arises from a single cause. Rather, the disease comes about when several factors act together or, more commonly, in sequence; among these factors are genetic constitution, the animal's innate resistance, the activity of viruses, and the influence of a large variety of physical and chemical agents that are collectively known as *trigger factors*. Unquestionably, the development of leukemia in animals is always a very complex business; it is not likely to be any simpler in humans.

In his monograph *Leukemia and Allied Disorders*, published in 1938, Forkner[33] gave an excellent account of the various views held during the latter nineteenth and the earlier part of the present century regarding the etiology, transmission, and experimental production of leukemia. Basically, there were three alternatives; leukemia might result from an infectious cause; it might be a so-called metabolic disorder caused by either excessive or, more likely, deficient production of some essential substances in the body; or it could be akin to a malignant tumor or neoplasm. The same possibilities could be considered for the lymphomas.

Infection, although rejected in the form conceived by Bennett, continued to be canvassed as a possible cause of leukemia and lymphoma. Indeed, there was no question that many patients with leukemia developed infections, and a wide variety of microorganisms were isolated from them. However, it gradually became clear that these infections were the consequence rather than the cause of the disease; leukemia often predisposes those suffering from it to attacks by microorganisms because their natural defenses are lowered. Tuberculosis came under suspicion as late as 1936,[34] having previously been a strong candidate as the cause of Hodgkin's disease,[24] and, for about 50 years, there was a school that invoked malaria (which still occurred in many parts of Europe) as a predisposing cause of leukemia.[16] None of these theories was borne out, and, gradually, the advocates of infection fell back on the activity of "unidentified organisms" as a cause of leukemia. It was only a small step to substitute viruses for "unidentified organisms," and those who espoused this possibility could point to interesting supporting evidence from the experimental field. This will be further discussed below.

The theory that leukemia might occur because of the lack of some normal substance (or, possibly, an excess of such a substance) has been voiced from time to time. It received a powerful impetus when it was found in the 1920s that pernicious anemia, until then, a disease nearly as fatal as leukemia, could be controlled by the addition of a "liver factor" to the diet (Chapter 10). There were, indeed, certain similarities in the two diseases, for in both the blood cell precursors showed defective and atypical maturation. Could it not be, therefore, that in leukemia too, some maturation factor was missing, and was it possible that this disease also might be brought under control if only the factor were identified and administered? Cases were on record in which the transfusion of blood or merely of plasma had apparently caused startling, although transient, improvement in the symptoms of leukemia, and in the early 1950s, some authorities, like Sir Lionel Whitby,[35] in England, argued strongly for more research on the possibility of substitution therapy. Nothing came of these attempts, which were probably premature, because there was, then, next to nothing known about the factors that regulate the growth and maturation of blood cells. Such knowledge is only now beginning to emerge, and, perhaps as a result, there may one day be a renewed interest in experiments on substitution therapy for leukemia.

Tumors and Malignancies

A well-known medical dictionary[36] defines *tumor* as an abnormal mass resulting from the excessive multiplication of cells, and *malignant* as (1) endangering health or life or (2) pertaining to or denoting the progressive growth of certain tumors which, if not checked by treatment, spread to distant sites, terminating in death.

Many observers throughout the years, as they reviewed the features of leukemia, were struck by their similarity to the malignant tumors, but among those discussing the similarity, there has been a curious reluctance to designate leukemia as a malignancy. A number of reasons can be given for this reluctance. One is that some leukemias behave quite unlike malignant tumors in that their course is slow, long, and relatively benign. Yet in the end, a sudden change to a much more aggressive behavior often occurs in such cases. Much has been made, especially by pathologists,[24,37,38] of the fact that destruction of local tissues—one of the characteristics of malignant tumors—is usually absent in leukemia and even in most lymphomas. However, these objections have not always held up. Lymphomas often exhibit features that closely mimic those of cancers of the same organs. Even leukemias can cause marked local destruction before they become generalized. Such tumors (chloromas) were reported as early as 1811,[39] first by ophthalmologists because they tended to occur in or near the orbit. Later it became apparent that chloromas were early manifestations of leukemia.

Myeloma (also known as multiple myeloma) is clearly a malignant tumor of the bone marrow cells; it was first described[40] shortly before Bennett's and Virchow's accounts of leukemia. Myeloma has a tendency to destroy the bones it infiltrates. Like many of the lymphomas (from which, however, it differs in other respects), myeloma not infrequently invades the blood and can cause leukemia (plasma-cell leukemia). Lastly, leukemia in animals almost invariably resembles malignant tumors in its pathology and clinical characteristics. For all these and other reasons, most specialists have come to regard leukemia as either an actual or potential malignant tumor; that is, leukemia is a distinctive form of cancer.

Causes: Research on Animals

By itself, the addition of this designation does not add much to what has always been known, namely that leukemia is a particularly unfortunate disease to have and usually a fatal one. Of much greater importance would be a knowledge of the factors that cause normal marrow cells to become transformed into "cancerous" ones, for that, basically, is how leukemia is thought to arise. It is in this field of investigation that great strides have been made by experimental methods, especially in mice. Such animal work has one great advantage over the study of human disease; there are strains of mice which have been produced by inbreeding over many generations and which are, thus, genetically almost pure; that is, every individual is like every other, as though they were an endless family of identical twins. In some strains leukemia occurs in almost every individual, in others it is quite rare. This difference is largely accounted for by differences in the animal's *predisposition* toward the spontaneous development of the disease. But in strains with a low incidence of spontaneous leukemia, the rate can be greatly increased if the animals are exposed either to ionizing radiations or to certain chemicals. We therefore know that in these mice at least two factors are necessary before disease occurs: genetic predisposition, which is quite variable, and exposure to trigger factors, to which different strains are more or less susceptible.

Viruses are a third group of factors involved in the cause of leukemia in many animal species. The first clear indication of this came as early as 1908, when Vilhelm Ellermann and Oluf Bang,[41] two assistants in the bacteriological laboratory of the Royal Veterinary School in Copenhagen, found that they could transmit leukemia among chickens, which were "cheap and easily got" and quite suitable as experimental animals. They began by injecting cells from birds with leukemia into healthy ones, some of which thereupon developed the disease as the leukemic cells multiplied. However, much more exciting was the same authors' observation that in order to transmit leukemia it was not necessary to inject cells; some of the healthy birds developed the disease when they were injected with filtered cell-free extracts from a leukemic chicken. The cause of the disease, they concluded, must be a virus, that is, an organism small enough to pass through filters that prevent the passage of bacteria and other common originators of infections.

Ellermann and Bang's findings have been confirmed many times since, and several viruses have been identified in fowl leukemia. In mammals, however, similar experiments, although attempted many times, were unsuccessful until 1951, when Ludwik Gross (Figure 15-2), in New York, showed for the first time that leukemia could be transmitted by means of cell-free extracts provided the recipient animals were newborn rather than adult mice.[42] Gross, born and educated in Poland, was originally trained as a clinician, and his early studies were made in his spare time while he was on duty as a medical officer in various U.S. Army hospitals. For several years, his published findings were regarded with suspicion and even disbelief by experts in the field. Eventually, they were not only confirmed but it was recognized that Gross' work formed a landmark in cancer research. It opened an era of extremely active new virologic research, in the course of which viruses were identified in the leukemia of mice, rats, guinea pigs, cats, dogs, cattle, and,

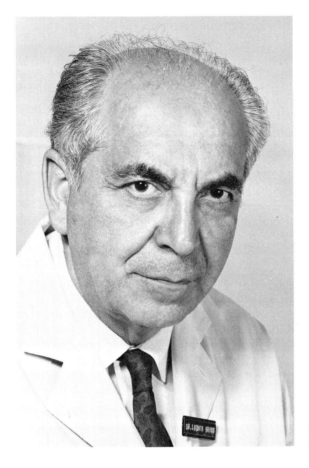

Figure 15-2   Dr. Ludwik Gross (1904–).

lately, primates. Most of these viruses are related to each other, and most are not infectious in the usual sense; that is, they do not spread from individual to individual in the manner of diseases such as poliomyelitis or influenza (*horizontal transmission*), but are transmitted from generation to generation through the germ cells (*vertical transmission,* a term coined by Gross). Exceptions to this rule are some fowl leukemias and leukemia of the domestic cat, which can spread horizontally, and is, thus, truly infectious, although it cannot ordinarily be passed to other species. In particular, it seems certain that humans do not catch leukemia from infected cats.[43]

The precise way in which viruses cause leukemia in animals is far from clear except for the fact that they do so in concert with many other factors, among them the subject's genetic susceptibility and the activity of triggers, such as radiation or chemicals.[44]

Causes of Leukemia in Human Beings

Compared with laboratory mice, humans have always been poor subjects for studying the cause of leukemia. Genetically, they are far from pure, and they cannot be experimented upon. Therefore, such knowledge as we have has come from more or less fortuitous observations together with a modicum of epidemiology. Even so, there is now a fairly impressive body of evidence which suggests that mice and humans may not be too far apart in the origins of their leukemias.

By far the best-known and most thoroughly established etiologic factors in human leukemia are *ionizing radiations:* x-rays, gamma rays, atomic radiation, and others. The event that brought this home to people everywhere was the dropping of the atom bomb on Hiroshima and Nagasaki, with its sequel in the form of a rise in the incidence of leukemia (Figure 15-3). This began about 3 years after the bombing, reached a peak in 6 years, and then slowly declined. Much the greatest incidence of leukemia was found among those closest to the explosion, whereas at a distance of 2000 m or more the risk was no greater than among the unirradiated people.[45] From this it could be concluded that ionizing radiations, including gamma rays and neutrons, could cause leukemia and that their effect depended on the size of the dose. Evidently it also depended on at least one additional factor, namely personal susceptibility, for only a small proportion of all those irradiated developed the disease. Altogether some 250 cases of leukemia occurred between 1946 and 1965 in the 183,000 people exposed to radiation in Hiroshima and Nagasaki.

Although this was the most spectacular demonstration, the relationship between radiation and leukemia had been strongly suspected long before the atomic bombings. As early as 1911, Jagić,[46] one of the luminaries of the Vienna School of Medicine, had reported cases of leukemia among radiologists, and there have been many similar case histories since, most of them originating in the United States. Early American radiologists took few precautions against exposure to the rays with which they were working, and some of them paid the price in terms of leukemia. Later, it was also shown that among patients who had been treated with large doses of x-rays, there was an increased incidence of leukemia.[47]

Clearly, therefore, ionizing radiation can cause leukemia. The only exception is the chronic lymphatic form, which has never been recorded after radiation exposure. However, it is not known to what extent radiation is implicated in the causation of the leukemias that occur sporadically in the general population. In Hiroshima and in the professionally exposed radiologists and the therapeutically irradiated patients, the doses of radiation were very high, and large parts or the whole of the body were exposed. Such exposures do not occur in ordinary circumstances, and it has, so far, been impossible to determine if the relatively tiny doses of radiation to which

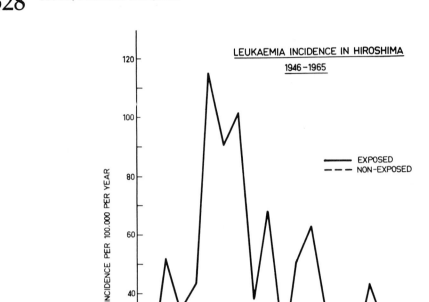

Figure 15-3 The leukemia incidence in Hiroshima, 1946–1965, in individuals exposed and nonexposed to atomic radiation.

ordinary people are exposed can also cause leukemia. It is obviously wise to control as strictly as possible all sources of man-made radiation and, thus, to diminish any possible risk. In peace time, medical radiation is by far the greatest source of exposure, and, ideally, its use should be limited to circumstances where it is likely to benefit the patient. However, the effect—if any—that such restrictions might exert on the incidence of leukemia is at best doubtful. It would certainly be unrealistic to attribute past changes in leukemia rates to changes in radiation exposure, or to expect that leukemia would decline substantially if there were less radiation.

Exposure to many *chemicals* can trigger the onset of leukemia in experimental conditions, but in humans only one substance has been shown beyond reasonable doubt to have induced the disease. This is benzol (or benzene), an industrial solvent.[48] Small groups of cases of leukemia have been reported among workers in industries where there was heavy exposure to benzol.

Numerous other chemicals and pharmaceuticals are capable of damaging the blood-forming cells and may be able to cause leukemia in exceptional circumstances. But because human beings today are constantly exposed to a great variety of such substances, it has so far been impossible to identify any one of them as being clearly responsible for leukemia. There are many suggestive case reports, but solid statistical evidence is lacking and will obviously be hard to get.

One of the most vexing aspects of leukemia is its *genetic basis*. Patients and their relatives worry more about the possibility of the disease being heritable than almost anything else. Fortunately, it is possible to reassure them on this point, for none of the leukemias are inherited in the same sense as, for instance, hemophilia, that is, through a single mutant gene (Mendelian inheritance). On the other hand, as already indicated, indirect evidence points to an increased susceptibility to leukemia in some people. Such susceptibility also exists in other forms of cancer, the occurrence of the disease being determined by the interaction of a number of inherited genes with factors such as the triggers that have just been discussed.

The occurrence of more than one case in a family is termed *familial* leukemia. This was first reported as long ago as 1861, but those particular cases were probably incorrectly diagnosed.[49] Among many subsequent publications, some evidently dealt with multiple familial cases of genuine leukemia, others with misdiagnosed or poorly documented cases. The whole literature was reviewed in 1947 by Aage Videbaek of Denmark in a major monograph.[50] He accepted 26 "apparently incontrovertible instances of familial occurrence of leukemia," and to them he added another 17 of his own. These figures are not very meaningful as they stand, for by the laws of chance alone, more than one case of leukemia must at times occur in a family. In order to demonstrate a real increase in susceptibility, it must be shown that the disease is more common among relatives of patients with leukemia than among properly matched control patients, or in the general population. The first attempt to do this was made by Videbaek, who reported that hereditary factors appeared indeed to play a part in the production of the disease and concluded that the predisposition to the disease was probably inherited. The techniques used in this study left something to be desired, and the results were not universally accepted. However, further work over the past 20 years by the present author and his associates has confirmed Videbaek's findings (Figure 15-4) and leaves little doubt that familial occurrence of leukemia is a genuine phenomenon. It was estimated[51] that among first-degree relatives of patients with either acute leukemia or chronic lymphatic leukemia (but *not* chronic myeloid leukemia), the incidence of leukemia was 2.8 to 3 times higher than expected and in more distant relatives, 2.3 times higher. The evidence suggested that the excess incidence was chiefly due to genetic predisposition in these families but that the disease was not inherited by a Mendelian mechanism. The predisposition

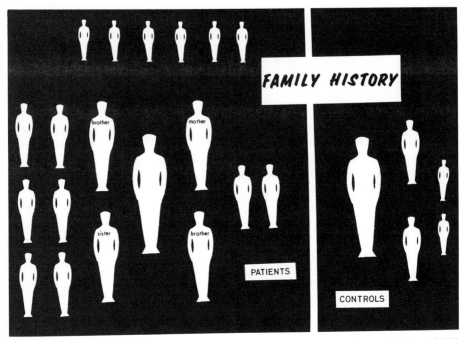

Figure 15-4 Results of a family survey of 251 patients with leukemia (left) and 251 control subjects (right). The large central figure on each side denotes the patient (or control). Each of the other figures shows a relative with leukemia, their size indicating the degree of relationship. Thus, the leukemia patient had four first-degree, eight second-degree, and six more distant relatives with leukemia. The control subject had no first-degree, two second-degree, and two more distant relatives with leukemia.

to the development of leukemia did not extend to other forms of cancer. A similar specificity has also been found in other cancers with a familial background.

Conclusions concerning the genetic basis of human leukemia drawn from family studies are reinforced by a number of other findings.[52] In identical twins, there is a 25 percent chance of leukemia occurring in the second member of the pair if the first has it. In children with some constitutional diseases—notably Down's syndrome or mongolism—leukemia is very much more frequent than in unaffected children (15 to 50 times),[53] and there are rarer familial diseases in which those affected—and possibly their close relatives—have an increased risk of developing leukemia.[54] It thus seems reasonably well established that in humans, as in the mouse, leukemia can arise on a genetic basis because of a raised level of personal susceptibility.

Thus, in the genetic background, and in the occasional activity of trigger factors, there are striking similarities in the cause of human and experimental leukemias. However, one major discrepancy remains; although it has been clearly shown that tumor viruses are involved in the cause of all leukemias in mice, similar evidence has not been obtained for human leukemia. Highly specialized and sophisticated techniques have given hints, but nothing more. It has been argued that by analogy with nearly every class of animal that has been investigated, humans too should show evidence of virus activity in the etiology of leukemia, but proof of such activity so far is lacking.

Failure to demonstrate human leukemia viruses has not resulted from want of trying. Almost as soon as Ellermann and Bang[41] first showed that fowl leukemia must be virus-induced, interest arose among those studying the disease in humans. Extracts of human leukemic tissues were injected into a variety of experimental animals, and many claims were made that leukemia had thereby been produced. Each time, however, it turned out that either the extracts had contained leukemic cells, which had multiplied in the injected animals, or that the leukemia that had been induced was not of human origin. In extensive electron microscopic studies of human leukemic tissues, very occasional particles resembling the viruses in animals were seen,[55] but these were not positively identified. All attempts to isolate or demonstrate viruses in human material have failed so far; no doubt they will continue to be made, and perhaps one day they may be successful.

The situation is different with the many studies that have been designed to show not viruses themselves but what have been termed their "footprints" in human leukemia. This phase began less than 10 years ago with the discovery[56,57] that tumor-inducing (i.e., oncogenic) viruses in animals possess a special enzyme, reverse transcriptase, which enables the viruses to reproduce themselves and is not present in normal tissues or in most other viruses. Reverse transcriptase has been found in human leukemic cells and has been shown in some cases to be closely related to similar enzymes in animal oncogenic viruses, notably that of a primate, the gibbon ape.[58] Nearly all known viruses causing leukemia in animals contain, among other substances, ribonucleic acids (RNA) of a characteristic physicochemical composition. Human leukemic cells also have been found to harbor such an RNA.[59] Finally, deoxyribonucleic acid (DNA), the principal constituent of cell nuclei, when isolated from leukemic cells in animals like baboons, has been shown by subtle chemical probing to contain constituents that are characteristic of certain oncogenic viruses. Constituents apparently related to those in the baboon have also been discovered in the DNA of some human leukemic cells.[60]

In some patients with leukemia, there may, therefore, be viruses present that are closely related to others known to be concerned in the induction of leukemia in higher animals. However, even if this is true, the part—if any— that such viruses play in the cause of human leukemia remains unknown. Conceivably they may be among the factors that interact and finally cause the transformation of normal blood-forming cells to leukemic ones. However, the viruses, if present, might be of a different nature altogether and might be acting, as it were, as mere bystanders that only become involved in the leukemic process once the basic transformation has taken place. As long as the viruses cannot be isolated or tested experimentally, an answer to this fundamental question will not be obtained easily.

Care and Cure of Leukemia and Lymphoma

In 1854, Virchow[12] treated a patient suffering from advanced leukemia with a nourishing diet, ferric iodide, embrocations to the abdomen, and foot baths. Not surprisingly, she died within a few days. The case is typical of many others in the contemporary literature and illustrates the physician's impotence in the face of this grave disease. If his twin aims were to relieve symptoms and prolong life, he had few means of achieving the first while the second was quite unattainable.

EARLY TREATMENTS

Chance took a hand in the introduction of the first agent effective for the treatment of the chronic leukemias. This was arsenic, a heavy metal and a favorite means for the quiet dispatch of unwanted persons (*aqua Toffana*, a solution of arsenious oxide, was named after Toffa, a female poisoner executed in Naples in 1709). In 1786, Thomas Fowler, of York, England, introduced a 1% solution of arsenic trioxide for "the cure of agues, remittent fevers, and periodic headaches," and Fowler's solution became a popular standby as a general tonic for domestic animals as well as their owners. It was in that capacity that Lissauer,[61] a German physician so obscure that even his initials are unknown, used it in 1865 in the treatment of a woman with chronic myeloid leukemia. Horses, one of his colleagues remembered, "look better, have a smoother skin and better digestion" after prolonged use of Fowler's solution. To his surprise, Lissauer found that when similarly treated, his apparently moribund patient became remarkably well and remained so for some months. Others soon obtained equally happy results both in leukemias and lymphomas. Not only did the enlarged organs, such as the spleen and lymph nodes, become smaller but the white blood cells diminished greatly in number while the red ones increased, so that the anemia was relieved. Arsenic thus became the first agent clearly beneficial in some leukemias, and its use was the first example of what would much later be called chemotherapy. After being used in leukemia therapy for over 30 years, arsenic was almost entirely superseded by the newly discovered x-rays, although later it enjoyed a brief renaissance. Two facts detracted from its general success: it was useless in the acute leukemias and was only temporarily effective in the chronic leukemias and lymphomas, for these diseases would inevitably recur and eventually prove to be fatal in spite of continued treatment.

X-RAYS

Röntgen discovered x-rays in 1895, and soon they were used enthusiastically for many medical purposes, including the treatment of lymphomas and leukemias.[62,63] Their effects curiously were similar to those which arsenic produced but were more predictable. When the x-rays were directed against enlarged organs, such as the spleen in chronic leukemia or a mass of lymph nodes in Hodgkin's disease, these organs rapidly began to shrink and often returned to their normal size. In addition, in many chronic leukemias, the blood also became less abnormal and the patient's general well-being improved beyond anticipation. It was soon found in the laboratory that x-rays had the power of preventing the division of many kinds of cells. Therefore, their effect on the organs exposed to them could be readily explained as the result of inhibition of cell growth and of cell destruction. The improvement in the blood and in the patient's general health was more difficult to understand,

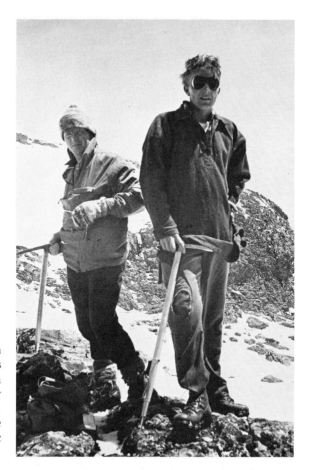

Figure 15-5 By definition, a complete remission permits the patient with leukemia to lead a normal life. This may include strenuous exercise, as in the mountaineer in the foreground, who has chronic myeloid leukemia.

but was believed to come about because the irradiated organs liberated substances capable of inhibiting cells growing at a distance. Because x-rays destroyed cells that were dividing, it was clear that their activity would be most pronounced in those tissues that had the highest proportion of dividing cells, and these included the blood-forming organs.

The course of events following irradiation of patients (radiotherapy) with leukemia was characteristic. In a high proportion of patients, the condition improved to the extent that the symptoms disappeared and normal activities could be resumed. This state became known as a remission of the disease; such remissions might be of varying duration, from weeks to years (Figure 15-5). Almost inevitably, however, remissions eventually gave way to relapses, in which the disease reasserted itself with recurrence of the original symptoms or the addition of new ones. Further treatment might lead to renewed remissions, but in the end patients became resistant to the x-rays, with a fatal outcome. Such was the usual course in many chronic leukemias and some lymphomas. All acute leukemias, a few chronic ones, and a proportion of the lymphomas proved completely resistant to treatment with x-rays.

For at least 40 years, x-rays or, later, other forms of irradiation, such as the administration of radioactive phosphorus,[64] remained the treatment of choice. These agents were certainly a great boon to patients for they relieved their symptoms without causing many unpleasant side effects in the process. After the first course of treatment, these people could often return to their usual occupations and live a normal life, and this might continue for some time. But there was a sinister side to this comparatively serene picture, for while the quality of life was greatly improved after treatment, its quantity was not; in 1924, George Minot, of Boston (Chapter 10), showed[65] that patients with chronic leukemia survived no longer after radiotherapy than those who had not been so treated. Even today, this picture is essentially unchanged in the chronic leukemias.

CHEMOTHERAPY

In 1938, Forkner[33] began his chapter on the treatment of leukemia with two significant sentences: "Although leukemia is a fatal disease much can be done to add to the comfort, and promote the general health of sufferers from the chronic forms of the disease. Unfortunately acute leukemia does not respond satisfactorily to any form of therapy." Happily, this somber picture has changed for the better since these words were written. Many patients with acute leukemia do respond to modern therapy, and, indeed, some have better prospects for long-term survival than the victims of chronic leukemia. Much has also been learned about the treatment of the lymphomas, especially Hodgkin's disease. These changes have come about largely because of remarkable developments in chemotherapy, initially as a by-product of secret research on the techniques for waging chemical warfare.

The poisonous "mustard gas" had been one of the many barbaric innovations introduced during World War I. Certain classified research during World War II was concerned with the study of the nitrogen mustards, which were chemical analogues of the gas. Given by injection, they caused unpleasant gastrointestinal upsets and, in large doses, destruction of the bone marrow. This was the clue to their possible usefulness in clinical medicine, and in 1946, the first two papers appeared in which the results were summarized.[66,67] As predicted from the laboratory experiments, it was found that nitrogen mustard (known then by the code name HN2) could cause profound depression of the blood cells, but, surprisingly, its most beneficial clinical effect occurred in the lymphomas rather than the leukemias. Most importantly, some patients were found to respond to treatment with HN2 even though they were—or had become—resistant to x-ray therapy. Thus, there was now an alternative to radiotherapy, at least in some cases. The chronic leukemias responded variably to this form of chemotherapy, but the acute ones were still entirely resistant to treatment.

Over the next 10 to 20 years, intense efforts were made to find new agents that would be more specific than HN2 and, if possible, less toxic. A large crop of such drugs gradually came into use, some very useful for treating chronic leukemia, with the principal advantage of easier administration compared with the cumbersome techniques of radiotherapy. Most of these agents were related to each other, either directly by virtue of their chemical structure, or indirectly by means of similar mechanisms of activity. Collectively, they were known as *alkylating* agents, and to a varying degree, they were effective in the treatment of the lymphomas, chronic leukemias, and some other cancers but not in the 60 or more percent of leukemia cases that belonged to the acute types. For these an altogether different approach was eventually found to be necessary. This consisted in the use of *antimetabolites*, compounds which are similar in structure to vitamins or other substances of physiologic importance but antagonists to them in their biologic activity.

One of the vitamins known to be important for the formation of blood cells is folic acid (Chapter 10). Lack of folic acid in the diet of experimental animals causes, among other disturbances, anemia and a decrease in the number of white cells. Toward the end of World War II, reports appeared that some preparations containing folic acid inhibited the growth of experimental tumors, and other observations purported to show that folic acid itself might stimulate the growth of leukemic cells. Although much of this work was later shown to be of doubtful validity, it encouraged a group at the Lederle Laboratories led by Subbarow to synthesize a series of new drugs that were deliberately designed as antagonists of folic acid for trial in the therapy of human cancer. One of these agents, Aminopterin, turned out to be a winner, not in the treatment of solid cancers, but of acute leukemia. The first report on its activity came from the Boston Children's Hospital in a paper that proved to be the herald of a new era.[68] A group headed by Sidney Farber, a pathologist, found that of 16 infants and children treated with Aminopterin, 10 "showed clinical, hematologic, and pathologic evidences of improvement of important nature"; and while stressing that such improvement was only temporary and did not amount to a cure, they concluded conservatively that a promising direction for further research appeared to have been established.

The Boston group had demonstrated for the first time that it was possible to produce temporary remissions in a sizable proportion of patients with acute leukemia. Their findings, which were rapidly confirmed, created a sensation and gave a very powerful stimulus to research on the possibilities of creating antagonists to many of the substances necessary for the building of cells, especially the nucleic acids (DNA and RNA). An enormous number of such compounds were synthesized in the years that followed,[69] but only a few of them turned out to be effective therapeutic agents, either when given alone or in combination with others. This small group of antimetabolites has become one of the mainstays of the management of acute leukemia. Other groups of drugs were also gradually added to the arsenal for combating acute leukemia. Among them were naturally occurring or synthetic steroids,[70] plant extracts,[71] and antibiotics.[72] The effort concentrated on this field grew enormously, as did the expenditure lavished on it. The result has been a revolutionary improvement in the outlook for children with acute leukemia, and a less dramatic one for adults.

REMISSIONS AND RELAPSES

To understand remissions, it is necessary to appreciate the events that lead to them. Underlying all approaches to the treatment of leukemia is the concept of a struggle between two "populations" of cells in the blood-forming organs— the abnormal and the normal cells. These two populations can usually be told apart by their appearance, and often also by a study of their chromosomes (cytogenetics). In patients with untreated leukemia, there is a massive predominance of the abnormal cell population, so much so that in some forms no normal cells can be recognized. After appropriate treatment, a remarkable reversal occurs, the normal blood-forming cells being now in ascendancy, with an apparent absence of their leukemic counterparts. This is the sign of remission and without it, there is no response to treatment. Originally it was thought that remissions happened because leukemic cells were more sensitive to the drugs used than were the normal ones. We now know that both populations are attacked by the antileukemic drugs but that in favorable cases, the normal cells show a greater recuperative power than the leukemic ones and, thus, outgrow them. They repopulate the marrow, which is then said to be "in remission."

Relapses of the disease eventuate because the remnants of leukemic cells that survived the original therapy revive. Unfortunately, there is no way of ensuring that all leukemic cells have been destroyed at the time the patient appears to have entered remission. The *total quantity* of such remaining cells may not be considerable, but they are widely dispersed among the normal population and are difficult to discover when present in small numbers.[73] Efforts are therefore usually made to consolidate remissions by continuing treatment, and in most cases, *maintenance* therapy is given—often for long periods—so as to prevent or, should that be impossible, to delay the regrowth of leukemic cells.

The length of the remissions testifies to the degree of success of these maneuvers. In chronic myeloid leukemia, for instance, a study of the chromosomes has shown that leukemic cells nearly always still dominate the marrow, even in apparently excellent remissions, so that relapses are certain to take place sooner or later. The outlook for patients with this form of the disease has, in fact, not greatly improved when compared with 50 years ago. In children, on the other hand, the predominant form of leukemia is acute lymphatic leukemia, and here, adequate treatment causes a profound depression of leukemic cells in most cases. Therefore, an extraordinary improvement in the outlook has occurred, as has been mentioned already. About 90 percent of the children with this type experience remissions, and of these, nearly half now live 5 years or longer, some of them for so long that they may be regarded as probably cured of their disease. Adults with acute leukemia respond much less favorably; only about 50 percent enter remission, and in those who do, survival is likely to be less than 2 years. In the nonresponders, death occurs after only a few weeks or months at best.

It would be a mistake to attribute the improved outlook solely to the use of the new chemotherapeutic agents, however. Part at least is due to the development of *supportive therapy,* that is, the new methods for combating the immediate and often very dangerous symptoms of the disease or, in some instances, those produced by the powerful specific agents used for destroying leukemic cells. The transfusion of blood or its components (red cells, platelets, and, recently, normal white cells), protection against infections or their treatment by antibiotics, and the management of kidney or liver failure are all essential in the therapy of patients with leukemia; nor should the support given by psychological services be forgotten. Farber used the term *total care* for the leukemic patient 30 years ago; it has become increasingly important ever since.

THE LYMPHOMAS

The lymphomas share with the leukemias a history of considerable therapeutic achievement since the end of World War II, but the picture is not uniform. In a number of the so-called non-Hodgkin's lymphomas, most patients either remain resistant to treatment or relapse after unpredictable periods of time, although for some life is greatly prolonged. Some patients may live for so long that cure is probable. These results have been achieved by the use of combinations of drugs, with and without the addition of radiotherapy; new treatment regimens are constantly appearing.[74] Much, however, remains to be done.

By contrast, the therapy of Hodgkin's disease—formerly very often fatal—has taken enormous strides forward, largely because the nature of the disease and, especially, its mode of spread have become well understood. Compared with the other lymphomas, Hodgkin's disease is often confined to local groups of lymph nodes when the patient first comes to see the physician; and by means of extensive clinical and laboratory studies ("staging"), it is usually possible to pinpoint its seat quite accurately. For this reason, very precise treatment can be given, usually by means of x-rays. For more widespread disease, the use of drugs, either by themselves or with radiotherapy, may be required. The therapy of Hodgkin's disease thus demands a multidisciplinary approach, in which internists, radiotherapists, surgeons, and pathologists are all involved. Its results are such that a very high proportion of the patients achieve remissions. Permanent cures can now be achieved in 90 percent or more of patients in the earlier stages of the disease, and even those with the advanced forms have a substantial chance of cure. Further, because it is known that most relapses occur within the first 5 years after treatment, it can be predicted that "anyone who survives the first five years has a 95 percent chance of cure."[75] Here, indeed, is success beyond the dreams of those treating the lymphomas and leukemias even 20 years ago.

Leukemia: An Interim Summary and a Look at the Future

The history of leukemia, in the 13 or 14 decades since its first positive recognition, mirrors the development of the medical sciences during the same period. Its early exploration as an entity occurred in the heyday of German pathology. Its clinical description and the hopelessness of its outlook were fit subjects for the rising Viennese school, with its cult of therapeutic nihilism. The search for causes involved the whole gamut of the life sciences and, later, the physical sciences as they entered their period of explosive growth. In time, medical statistics became available and gave studies on mortality and incidence a more solid base. Modern therapy of acute leukemia is almost entirely an outcome of the postwar flowering of American medicine.

Today, in parts of the world where there are good medical services, much is known about the distribution of the leukemias and the risk of acquiring the disease. It is also clear that what seemed a rather frightening increase in incidence during the first half of the present century can be largely, though perhaps not entirely, accounted for by a progressive deployment of greatly improved diagnostic facilities to which access has become easier over the years. Most workers in the field now accept the leukemias and lymphomas as specialized forms of cancer.

Certain factors—notably ionizing radiations—are known to have been concerned in the causation of leukemia in well-defined circumstances. There is evidence in favor of a genetic predisposition, and almost certainly, genetic and extraneous factors interact to produce the disease in individual patients. The role of tumor viruses is being actively studied, but no positive proof exists as yet that such viruses are implicated in the cause of human, as opposed to animal, leukemias. Clearly there are gaping voids in our knowledge of what causes any of the diseases in this group, but the chances probably are improving that these will gradually be filled as a result of epidemiologic and laboratory research. The well-studied animal leukemias form a useful model for comparison with those in human beings.

But it is the treatment of the leukemias and lymphomas on which the most intense effort has been concentrated. Here the story is a mixed one. It includes what may be fairly described as therapeutic triumphs, notably in childhood leukemia and in Hodgkin's disease, but also many bitter disappointments. The early successes of radiotherapy gave hopes that the chronic leukemias would be instantly cured, but these hopes were soon dashed. Three-quarters of a century later, there are more ways of treating chronic leukemia, but the results are not significantly better. Half or more of all adults with acute leukemia still cannot be offered any prospect of great improvement, and when such patients first consult their physician, he usually cannot predict whether they will or will not respond to treatment.

It is not even possible to say precisely why some modes of treatment did succeed, for often therapy was given for reasons which we now know to be spurious. Lissauer gave arsenic because it was reputed to be a tonic which might do his weary patient good; but for unknown reasons, his horse cure did more than that—it caused a remission in human leukemia, probably the first in history. The original trials of folic acid antagonists in acute leukemia were conducted because of the doubtful observation that folic acid, a natural vitamin, caused an acceleration of the leukemic process. No one has been able to confirm this, but the folate antagonists still have a useful place in therapy.

In general terms, almost all drugs were first employed because they were found to have an inhibitory or destructive effect on cells that were dividing or preparing to do so. The rationale of such therapy was the assumption that leukemic cells, being cancerous, divide faster than normal ones and must, therefore, succumb more rapidly if division is interfered with. Modern studies, as discussed elsewhere (Chapter 13), have revealed that this basic assumption is unsound; leukemic and many other cancerous cells actually multiply more slowly than their normal counterparts,[76] and when drugs are effective, this is so in spite of and not because of the growth potential of these cells. Again, when leukemia relapses after an initial remission, it is often impossible to pinpoint the mechanism responsible for this event.[77]

Investigation of a great range of problems is being continued on a vast scale in the field of the leukemias and lymphomas. The activity is so intense that it may well be wondered why a group of comparatively rare diseases has usurped such a central place in scientific and public interest. The subject of leukemia arouses strong emotions in many who are not directly concerned with patients. The nexus of atomic energy and the wartime bombing, with its sequel of leukemia "epidemics," is well established in the public conscience, and the known fatality of the disease adds a feeling of urgency. Appeals for funds in support of leukemia research have, thus, a strong likelihood of being successful, and additional workers are attracted as a result.

At the same time, there has long been a feeling among scientists that the efforts in the leukemia field may well pay dividends in the wider area of cancer research as a whole. The leukemic cell, being free-floating in the bloodstream, is relatively easy to obtain and study. Its chemical and physical properties, as well as its reactions to other cells, are commonly regarded as prototypes of the properties and reactions of all cancer cells. Experimental leukemias often serve as models in the search for better anticancer drugs.

These studies are being pursued with constantly increasing sophistication. As new methods become available, they are adapted to the leukemia field. Both the quantity and the quality of research are steadily increasing, as is, of course, its cost. Whether such efforts have always been well directed can be questioned. There may, for instance, be more than one opinion on the chances of the large so-called task forces discovering the ultimate causes or therapy of leukemia by the use of methods analogous to those that led to the successful moon landings. The breakthroughs that are so frequently demanded have proved elusive in leukemia research. Advances usually come as the climax of many small steps taken by workers in many disciplines and diverse places.

As to the future, uncertainty still dominates many of the most important questions. To take therapy as an example, the need for altogether novel approaches is being increasingly considered by many workers in the leukemia field. At present, the basic tendency still is to search for new and more effective drugs or combinations of drugs, and for improved methods of administering them, the philosophy being "more of the same." It is argued that the complete eradication of the malignant cells must remain the ultimate goal and that there is a chance of achieving this if only present-day techniques can be further improved. This may conceivably be correct, but there are clear limits; all drugs that have yet been studied damage normal as well as cancerous cells, and excessive therapy may damage normal cells beyond recovery. This danger imposes constraints on the therapist, for even if extermination of all leukemic cells were feasible, this would not benefit the patient if there were no normal cells left to sustain life.

Transplantation Therapy

Consideration of this dilemma has led to the suggestion that transplantation of the normal bone marrow might have a role to play in the therapy of acute leukemia. The argument is that if there were no need to worry about the survival of the patient's normal cells because they could be replenished by transplantation from another individual, then much more drastic measures could be taken to eliminate the leukemic cells. In practice, it has turned out that the transplantation of bone marrow is a relatively simple procedure, but, unfortunately, there are enormous other difficulties. The first is the choice of a suitable donor, for the marrow cells must be compatible with the patient's. So far, this has meant a search among the patient's close relatives, nearly always his or her siblings, fewer than half of whom can be expected to be compatible. Secondly, even after extensive laboratory testing, it is impossible to guarantee that the cells from an apparently compatible donor will in fact be fully compatible; if they are not, the transplant may fail or damage may be caused to the patient's normal tissues (graft-versus-host reaction). Thirdly, the most drastic attempts to destroy all leukemic cells may be unavailing, so that relapses can occur even after transplantation. Because of these various problems, the care of patients undergoing marrow transplantation requires extensive and costly facilities. For these reasons, such patients have been concentrated in a few highly specialized units, which are gradually acquiring experience in evaluating what is still an experimental procedure. A number of successful transplantations have, in fact, been carried out on patients with acute leukemia, and a few of these patients have survived without relapses for up to five years so far.[78] Time will be needed to assess the place of marrow transplantation in the treatment of acute leukemia.

Immunotherapy

There have been other proposals for supplementary treatment. One of the most interesting is the use of what has been termed immunotherapy. This consists of attempts to stimulate the body's defenses against its own tumor and, thereby, to aid other therapeutic measures in eliminating the cancerous cells. It is known that some cancers act like grafted foreign tissues and cause the patient's body to mount an immunologic attack on them. Such cancers may respond particularly well to small doses of chemotherapy. An example is the so-called Burkitt tumor in African children. Claims have been made that in some leukemias, and lymphomas as well, the body is capable of reacting immunologically against the cancerous cells. In such cases it would be logical to try to boost these natural reactions, but considerable uncertainty still persists in this area. Nevertheless, some attempts at immunotherapy have been made, and occasional successes have been reported;[79] these still need confirmation. Two means of stimulating the immune system are currently under trial. The first is by means of a group of nonspecific agents, the best-known of which is the antituberculosis vaccine BCG, while the second, more specifically, comprises killed leukemic cells. Both are given repeatedly over long periods to patients in remission after chemotherapy in an effort to extend the remission for as long as possible. Whether this can be achieved regularly remains yet to be seen.

Concluding Remarks

When we turn our thoughts back to the situation even 20 years ago, we are entitled to some gratification at the progress that has been made in the treatment of certain leukemias and lymphomas. But much remains to be done, for we still cannot provide relief, let alone long-term survival, for a very substantial proportion of patients. Whether current therapeutic methods, even if greatly refined and amplified, are capable eventually of subjugating the presently resistant forms is still uncertain. In addition, it is only realistic to consider the constantly escalating cost of treatment. Several years ago, the total expense of caring for a patient with acute leukemia in an American hospital was estimated as \$40,000.[80] Addition of newer and much more expensive techniques would add greatly to this large sum. Perhaps the time will come when communities will be unwilling to incur what appear to be extravagant costs for either the study or treatment of relatively rare diseases. Some may wish to reallocate medical priorities. Such changes in public policy would enforce fundamental changes in the approach to the leukemia problem.

Meanwhile, it seems prudent to look for alternatives. Indeed, concern has been expressed lately about whether the concept of the leukemic process as a kind of handicap race between "good" and "bad" cells is an oversimplification.[81] What is basically wrong, at least with some types of leukemic cells, is their inability to develop into mature forms; they do not grow excessively, as had long been thought, but they remain immature and, therefore, cannot carry out the functions of normal cells. Perhaps rather than trying harder and harder knockout blows against them, it might be more sensible to look for ways of rendering them mature and of thus "reeducating" them. Much work is now going on in attempts to define those factors that make normal cells grow and develop. The results of these studies might well be of considerable help in designing new strategies for the conquest of the leukemias and lymphomas.

References

1   Virchow R: Weisses Blut und Milztumoren. *Med Z* 16:9–15, 1847.
2   Sigerist HE: *Great Doctors: A Biographical History of Medicine.* London, George Allen and Unwin, 1933, 436 pp, pp 335–346.
3   Gunz FW, Baikie AG (eds): *Leukemia,* 3d ed. New York, Grune and Stratton, 1974, 841 pp.
4   Virchow R: Weisses Blut. *Froriep's Notizen* 36:151–156, 1845.
5   Bennett JH: Two cases of disease and enlargement of the spleen in which death took place from the presence of purulent matter in the blood. *Edinburgh Med Surg J* 64:413–423, 1845.
6   Donné A: *Cours de Microscopie Complémentaire des Études Médicales.* Paris, Balliere, 1844, 552 pp.
7   Craigie D: Case of disease of the spleen, in which death took place in consequence of the presence of purulent matter in the blood. *Edinburgh Med Surg J* 64:400–412, 1845.
8   King LS: The blood-letting controversy: a study in the scientific method. *Bull Hist Med* 35:1–13, 1961.
9   McKendrick JG: Obituary: John Hughes Bennett. *Edinburgh Med J* 21:466–474, 1875.
10 Bennett JH: *Leucocythaemia or White Cell Blood.* Edinburgh, Sutherland and Knox, 1852, 133 pp.
11 Virchow R: Die farblosen Blutkörperchen, in: *Gesammelte Abhandlungen zur wissenschaftlichen Medizin.* Frankfurt, Meidinger, 1856, 1038 pp, pp 212–218.
12 Virchow R: Die Leukämie, in: *Gesammelte Abhandlungen zur wissenschaftlichen Medizin.* Frankfurt, Meidinger, 1856, 1038 pp, pp 190–211.
13 Donné A: De l'origine des globules du sang, de leur mode de formation et de leur fin. *Compt Rend Acad Sci (Paris)* 14:366–368, 1842.
14 Neumann E: Ein Fall von Leukämie mit Erkrankung des Knochenmarkes. *Arch Heilk* 11:1–14, 1870.
15 Ebstein W: Ueber die acute Leukämie und Pseudoleukämie. *Dtsch Arch Klin Med* 44:343–396, 1888–1889.
16 Gowers WR: Splenic leucocythaemia, in Reynolds JR (ed): *System of Medicine.* New York, Macmillan, 1879, vol 5, 1064 pp, pp 216–305.
17 Ehrlich P: *Farbenanalytische Untersuchungen zur Histologie und Klinik des Blutes.* Berlin, Hirschwald, 1891, 141 pp.
18 Cohnheim J: Ein Fall von Pseudoleukämie. *Arch Pathol Anat* 33:451–454, 1865.
19 Pel PK: Zur Symptomatologie der sog. Pseudo-Leukämie. *Berl Klin Wochenschr* 22:3–7, 1885.
20 Hodgkin T: On some morbid appearances of the absorbent glands and spleen. *Med Chir Trans* 17:68–114, 1832.
21 Wilks S: Cases of a peculiar enlargement of the lymphatic glands frequently associated with disease of the spleen. *Guy's Hosp Rep* 2:114–132, 1856.
22 Wilks S: Cases of enlargement of the lymphatic glands and spleen (or, Hodgkin's disease). *Guy's Hosp Rep* 11:56–67, 1865.
23 Naegeli O: Der Symptomenkomplex Pseudoleukämie, in *Blutkrankheiten und*

Blutdiagnostik. Lehrbuch der Klinischen Hämatologie, 5th ed. Berlin, Springer, 1931, 721 pp, pp 531–534.

24 Sternberg C: Über eine eigenartige unter dem Bilde der Pseudoleukämie verlaufende Tuberculose des lymphatischen Apparates. *Z Heilk* 19:21–90, 1898.

25 Lumb G: Hodgkin's disease, in *Tumours of Lymphoid Tissue.* Edinburgh, Livingstone, 1954, 204 pp, pp 71–99.

26 Smithers D: *Hodgkin's Disease.* Edinburgh and London, Churchill, 1973, 258 pp.

27 Virchow R: *Die Krankhaften Geschwülste.* Berlin, Hirschwald, 1863, vol 2, 756 pp, pp 728–738.

28 Kundrat H: Ueber Lympho-Sarkomatosis. *Wien Klin Wochenschr* 6:211–213, 234–239, 1893.

29 Türk W: Ein System der Lymphomatosen. *Wien Klin Wochenschr* 16:1073–1085, 1903.

30 Symmers D: The relationship of the toxic lymphoid hyperplasias to lymphosarcoma and allied diseases. *Arch Intern Med* 21:237–251, 1918.

31 Virchow R, quoted in Ackerknecht EH: *Rudolf Virchow: Doctor, Statesman, Anthropologist.* Madison, University of Wisconsin Press, 1953, 319 pp, p 270.

32 Statistics on Cancer, *CA.* New York, American Cancer Society, 1968, vol 18, p 16.

33 Forkner CE: Etiology of leukemia, in: *Leukemia and Allied Disorders.* New York, Macmillan, 1938, 334 pp, pp 9–27.

34 Craver LF: Clinical manifestations and treatment of leukemia. *Am J Cancer* 26:124–136, 1936.

35 Whitby L: Whither clinical pathology? Trends and opportunities. *J Clin Pathol* 4:129–136, 1951.

36 *Blakiston's Gould Medical Dictionary*, 3d ed. New York, McGraw-Hill, 1972.

37 Langhans T: Das maligne Lymphosarkom (Pseudoleukämie). *Virchow's Arch* 54:509–537, 1872.

38 Symmers D: Follicular lymphadenopathy with splenomegaly. A newly recognized disease of the lymphatic system. *Arch Pathol Lab Med* 3:816–820, 1927.

39 Burns A: *Observations on the Surgical Anatomy of the Head and Neck.* Edinburgh, Bryce, 1811, 415 pp, p 369. (Quoted in Rolleston H: The history of haematology. *Proc R Soc Med* 27:1161–1178, 1934.)

40 Solly S: Remarks on the pathology of mollities ossium, with cases. *Med Chir Trans* 27:435–461, 1844.

41 Ellermann V, Bang O: Experimentelle Leukämie bei Hühnern. *Zentralbl Bakteriol* 46:595–609, 1908.

42 Gross L: "Spontaneous" leukemia developing in C3H mice following inoculation in infancy with AK leukemic extracts of AK embryos. *Proc Soc Exp Biol Med* 76:27–32, 1951.

43 Hanes B, Gardner MB, Loosli CG, Heidbreder G, Kogan B, Marylander H, Huebner RJ: Pet associations with selected human cancers: A household questionnaire survey. *J Natl Cancer Inst* 45:1155–1162, 1970.

44 Kaplan HS: Leukemia and lymphoma in experimental and domestic animals. *Ser Haematol* 7:94–163, 1974.

45 Bizzozzero OJ Jr, Johnson KG, Ciocco A: Radiation-related leukemia in Hiroshima and Nagasaki, 1946–64. I. Distribution, incidence and appearance time. *N Engl J Med* 274:1095–1101, 1966.

46 Jagić N, Schwarz G, Siebenrock L von: Blutbefunde bei Röntgenologen. *Berl Klin Wochenschr* 48:1220–1222, 1911.
47 Court-Brown W, Doll R: *Leukaemia and Aplastic Anaemia in Patients Irradiated for Ankylosing Spondylitis.* London, H.M. Stationery Office, 1957, 135 pp.
48 Forni A, Vigliani EC: Chemical leukemogenesis in man. *Ser Haematol* 7:211–223, 1974.
49 Biermer: Ein Fall von Leukämie, *Arch Pathol Anat Physiol* 20:552–554, 1861. (Quoted in Videbaek A: *Heredity in Human Leukemia, and its Relation to Cancer.* Copenhagen, Munksgaard, 1947, 279 pp.)
50 Videbaek A: *Heredity in Human Leukemia and its Relation to Cancer.* Copenhagen, Munksgaard, 1947, 279 pp.
51 Gunz FW, Gunz JP, Veale AMO, Chapman CJ, Houston IB: Familial leukaemia: A study of 909 families. *Scand J Haematol* 15:117–131, 1975.
52 Gunz FW: Genetics of human leukemia. *Ser Haematol* 7:164–191, 1974.
53 Stewart A, Webb J, Hewitt D: A survey of childhood malignancies. *Br Med J* 1:1495–1511, 1958.
54 Swift M: Fanconi's anaemia in the genetics of neoplasia. *Nature* 230:370–373, 1971.
55 Dmochowski L: Ultrastructural studies in leukemia, in Dameshek W, Dutcher RM (eds): *Perspectives in Leukemia.* New York, Grune and Stratton, 1968, 302 pp, pp 34–62.
56 Baltimore D: RNA-dependent DNA polymerase in virions of RNA tumour viruses. *Nature* 226:1209–1211, 1970.
57 Temin HM, Mizutani S: RNA-dependent polymerase in virions of Rous sarcoma virus. *Nature* 226:1211–1213, 1970.
58 Todaro GJ, Gallo RC: Immunological relationship of DNA polymerase from human acute leukaemia cells and primate and mouse leukaemia virus reverse transcriptase. *Nature* 244:206–209, 1973.
59 Mak TW, Kurtz S, Manaster J, Housman D: Viral-related information in oncorna-virus-like particles isolated from cultures of marrow cells from leukemic patients in relapse and remission. *Proc Natl Acad Sci USA* 72:623–627, 1975.
60 Reitz MS, Miller NR, Wong-Staal F, Gallagher RE, Gallo RC, Gillespie DN: Primate type-C virus nucleic acid sequences (woolly monkey and baboon types) in tissues from a patient with acute myelogenous leukemia and in viruses isolated from cultured cells of the same patient. *Proc Natl Acad Sci USA* 73:2113–2117, 1976.
61 Lissauer: Zwei Fälle von Leucaemie. *Berl Klin Wochenschr* 2:403–404, 1865.
62 Pusey WA: Report of cases treated with Roentgen rays. *JAMA* 38:911–919, 1902.
63 Senn N: Case of splenomedullary leukemia successfully treated by the use of Röntgen Ray. *Med Rec (NY)* 64:281, 1903.
64 Lawrence JH: Nuclear physics and therapy: Preliminary report on a new method for the treatment of leukemia and polycythemia. *Radiology* 35:51–60, 1940.
65 Minot GR, Buckman TE, Isaacs R: Chronic myelogenous leukemia: Age incidence, duration and benefit derived from irradiation. *JAMA* 82:1489–1494, 1924.
66 Goodman LS, Wintrobe MM, Dameshek W, Goodman MJ, Gilman A, McLennan MT: Nitrogen mustard therapy. *JAMA* 132:126–132, 1946.
67 Jacobson LO, Spurr CL, Barron ESG, Smith T, Lushbaugh C, Dick GF: Nitrogen mustard therapy. *JAMA* 132:263–271, 1946.
68 Farber S, Diamond LK, Mercer RD, Sylvester RF, Wolff JA: Temporary remissions in

acute leukemia in children produced by folic acid antagonist, 4-aminopteroyl-glutamic acid (Aminopterin). *N Engl J Med* 238:787–793, 1948.

69   Burchenal JH, Murphy ML, Ellison RR, Sykes MP, Tan TC, Leone LA, Karnofsky DA, Craver LF, Dargeon HW, Rhoads CP: Clinical evaluation of a new antimetab-olite, 6-mercaptopurine, in the treatment of leukemia and allied diseases. *Blood* 8:965–999, 1953.

70   Pearson OH, Eliel LP, Rawson RW, Dobriner K, Rhoads CP: ACTH- and corti-sone-induced regression of lymphoid tumors in man. A preliminary report. *Cancer* 4:943–945, 1949.

71   Hodes ME, Rohn RJ, Bond WH: Vincaleukoblastine. I. Preliminary clinical studies. *Cancer Res* 20:1041–1049, 1960.

72   Holton CP, Vietti TJ, Nora AH, Donaldson MH, Stuckey WJ, Watkins WL, Lane DM: Daunomycin and prednisone for induction of remission in advanced leukemia. *N Engl J Med* 280:171–174, 1969.

73   Skipper HE, Schabel FM, Wilcox WS: Experimental evaluation of anti-cancer agents. XIII. On the criteria and kinetics associated with "curability" of experi-mental leukemia. *Cancer Chemother Rep* 35:1–111, 1964.

74   De Vita VT: Summary of symposium on non-Hodgkin's lymphomas. *Cancer Treat Rep* 61:1223–1227, 1977.

75   Kaplan HS: Hodgkin's disease: multidisciplinary contributions to the conquest of a neoplasm. *Radiology* 123:551–558, 1977.

76   Vincent PC: Cell kinetics of the leukemias, in Gunz F, Baikie AG (eds): *Leukemia,* 3d ed. New York, Grune and Stratton, 1974, 841 pp, pp 189–221.

77   Gunz FW, Vincent PC: Towards a cure of acute granulocytic leukemia? *Leukemia Res* 1:51–66, 1977.

78   Thomas ED, Fefer A, Buckner CD, Storb R: Current status of bone marrow transplantation for aplastic anemia and acute leukemia. *Blood* 49:671–681, 1977.

79   Mathé G, Amiel JL, Schwarzenberg L, Hayat M, Pouillart P, Schneider M, Cattan A, Jasmin C, Belpomme D, Schlumberger JR, De Vassal F, Musset M, Misset JL: Immunothérapie active des leucémies aiguës et des lymphosarcomes leucémi-ques. Bilan de 10 ans—étude de 200 cas. *Nouv Presse Méd* 4:1337–1342, 1975.

80   Esterhay RJ Jr, Vogel VG, Fortner CL, Shapiro HM, Wiernik PH: Cost analysis of leukemia treatment. *Cancer* 37:646–652, 1976.

81   Metcalf D: Human leukaemia: recent tissue culture studies on the nature of myeloid leukaemia. *Br J Cancer* 27:191–202, 1973.

CHAPTER 16

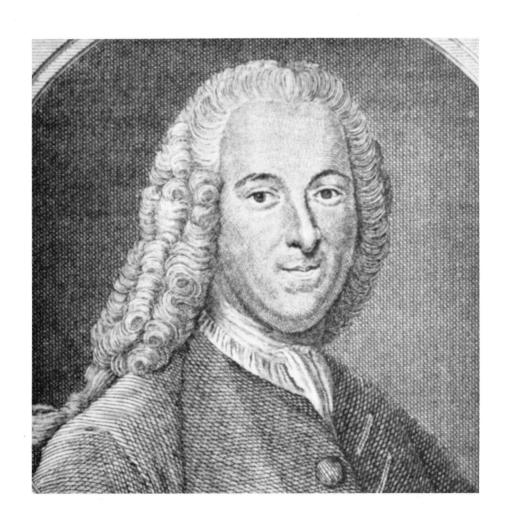

PLATELETS: THE BLOOD DUST
Theodore H. Spaet

Platelets are elusive.

When van Leeuwenhoek[1] first put blood under his homemade microscope, he had little difficulty in identifying erythrocytes; within the next century, leukocytes were established[2] as a respectable component of blood. These cells were readily viewed with the crude optics of the time. They are large enough to be seen easily, and their morphological behavior is respectably consistent. In contrast, platelets are tiny, with a diameter about one-fourth that of erythrocytes. Moreover, they may assume many forms, depending upon the conditions that precede examination of the blood.

Nevertheless, an important manifestation of platelets had been recognized previously, without an inkling of its basis. Clot retraction (shrinking) was observed and recorded as the separation of blood after coagulation into a solid clot and a liquid phase (serum). This phenomenon had been noted and used diagnostically by Hewson in the late eighteenth century; reasonable methods for its quantification were in use shortly thereafter.[3] In fact, Thackrah, in 1819, found that clotted blood could express about 40 percent of its serum by weight,

Chapter Opening Photo Paul G. Werlhof (1699–1767): morbus maculosis Werlhofi.

549

a figure that would elicit no major disagreement today. However, it was not until the middle of the nineteenth century that steps were taken to admit platelets as bona fide members of the hematological community.

Platelets: The New Blood Cell

The early history of platelet identification has been detailed in the admirable reviews by Tocantins[4] and by Robb-Smith.[5] The technical advance that allowed these tiny cells to be seen was the development of the compound microscope in about 1826 or 1830.[1] Because platelets usually have a diameter less than 2 μm, their resolution awaited the availability of these optics, which were capable of demonstrating particles over 1 μm in diameter. After a 15-year latent period, three men are credited with the first description of platelets as morphological entities. Alfred Donné was a French physician, who is also remembered for having first used a microscopic projector as a teaching aid for biology students.[6] Donné reported, "There exist in the blood 3 types of particles. . . ." The erythrocytes and leukocytes were clearly defined. But the third was more elusive. "These globules are the product of chyle, and show incessant diversity in the blood. They group into triplets and quartets, are enveloped by an albuminous coat while circulating in the blood, and in this manner constitute the white cells." He concluded that the entire mixture is similar "to milk."[7] Donné's brief report suggests that he was looking at platelets, but it would not pass muster with a contemporary editor. There are no illustrations, his methodology is barely given, and the reader must take much on faith. Nevertheless, hindsight would suggest that he was on the right track.

In a similarly suggestive but also far from conclusive report, these Lilliputian cells may have been recognized by the British physician George Gulliver and simultaneously by his colleague William Addison (no relation to the more famous Thomas). Addison stated that ". . . minute particles or granules are abundant in all animal and vegetable structures. . . . I am not, however, aware that similar molecules have ever before been noticed in human blood."[8]

Preliminary and groping as these studies were, they gave a glimmering of events to come. Soon the platelet field was characterized by the serendipity which accompanies new technological breakthroughs. The availability of suitable microscopy enabled numerous biological knights to explore the kingdom of the previously unseen, to describe the hitherto unknown flora and fauna, and to generate hypotheses according to their leanings. Many names are associated with such activities, but more than 20 years elapsed before the modern concepts of platelet biology began to emerge.

Then, within an 8-year period, three outstanding investigators, each making his contributions independently, supplied observations that established the foundation for our present knowledge. With our hindsight polished, it is possible to be amused at some of the false starts and unsteady steps that characterized this early work. Thus, the 24-year-old William Osler (Figure 16-1) noted the presence of bacterialike particles which were often ("manchmal") found in the blood of normal humans and animals.[9] A year later, in 1874, although still in complete darkness as to their nature or function, he reported a series of observations, supplemented with illustrations, that provided a relatively modern picture of blood platelets.[10] He noted that these structures were "pale round disks" which were "$\frac{1}{8}$–$\frac{1}{2}$ the size of a red corpuscle." In comments that could well be most instructive to many investigators of today, he added that ". . . in the vessels . . . they were always present as separate elements, showing no tendency to adhere to one another." However, ". . . in a drop of blood taken from one of these young animals [rats], the corpuscles were always to be found accumulated together. . . ." In this early

Figure 16-1 William Osler (1849–1919) in 1887.

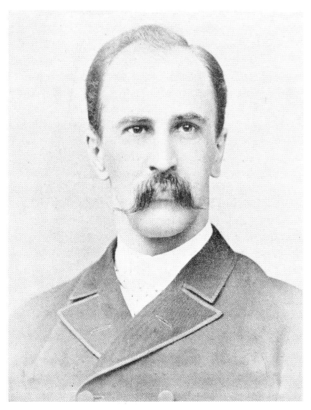

paper, there follows a description of events in the drawn blood which would appear to represent a combination of fibrin, the final product of coagulation, and associated platelet reactions, the details of which remained for the future to unravel. Dr. Osler concluded, "As there is no evidence that these bodies are in organic continuity with any other recognized animal or vegetable form, or possess the power of reproduction, nothing can at present be said of their nature or of their relation to *Bacteria*." At this point, Osler moved on to other matters and added only an occasional commentary in subsequent years—which may have reflected a certain degree of nostalgia for a field which was proving to have more significance than he had suspected.

William Osler was one of the great physicians of all time, and his encounter with platelets represents a minor incident in his distinguished career. He performed the work during a period of European postgraduate training, most of which was in London but did include a stay in Vienna and Berlin as well. Perhaps as a gesture to Dr. E.A. Schäfer, a London colleague from Germany, the original observations were published in a German journal. Although these studies were perhaps among Osler's most significant scientific contributions, they are not generally given much attention by Osler's various biographers. Indeed, in a massive memorial volume published in 1926,[11] they are barely mentioned! Osler's contributions ranged far and wide; perhaps he is best known as a medical teacher and philosopher. This diversity must preclude the type of depth required to pursue a scientific problem to its conclusion. It remained for more single-minded investigators to work out the platelet story.

Georges Hayem (Chapter 1) is credited by many with launching the platelet on its journey, a journey which is to this day one of the great sagas of adventure and discovery. The biography of Hayem is written lovingly and reverently by Dreyfus,[6] and a strong case is made for designating Hayem as the father of modern hematology. In fact, by the time Hayem turned his full attention to platelets, he was already well known for a host of medical contributions, including the first effective treatment for cholera, the intravenous administration of saline solution. In 1878, at the age of 37, he was already a full professor and was shortly to be elected to the prestigious French Academy of Medicine. Evidently, his meteoric career was accompanied by a comparable degree of self-reliance, which may have made him overly refractory to the observations of others, as we shall see.

Hayem's first major contribution on platelets begins, "There exist in the blood of all vertebrates tiny structures which are not erythrocytes, and not leukocytes; destined in their ultimate development to become erythrocytes, they represent a very young form of these elements, and are a varied precursor of the red blood cell. Thus, we have proposed to name these cells hématoblastes."[12] There follows an account of studies on these "hématoblastes," which provides some of the basis of the enthusiasm of Dreyfus for this scientist. Platelets are shown to be biconvex discs, to separate in freshly drawn blood, and to have a great tendency to change their form, to aggregate, and to interact with fibrin strands when blood is removed from the animal. He counted these "hématoblastes" with an accuracy that any laboratory director would envy today and indicated their role in clotting and clot retraction. And yet in 1923, when the evidence was overwhelming that platelets were an independent cell line derived from megakaryocytes, Hayem still (perhaps nostalgically) clung to his original view at least in part, naming an extensive monograph L'Hématoblaste, Troisième Element du Sang.[13]

Although Hayem's fixation on the ultimately untenable relationship between platelets and erythrocytes could be understood in the early days of discovery, his adherence to it subsequently requires an explanation. Hayem was obviously a brilliant and creative investigator of impeccable integrity and complete thoroughness. One can only speculate as to the basis of the problem. One major possibility is that a driving and ambitious individual may egotistically go his own way, rejecting the contributions of others if they are not in conformity with his own. Although Hayem may have had some characteristics of this type, they may have been emphasized greatly by cultural factors. In Europe, in the past and to a great extent to this day, a professor holds an exalted position, his word is law, and it is not to be challenged by those of lesser rank. Although such a condition may favor social stability, the search for scientific truth requires that every concept be subjected to the most careful scrutiny. This is best accomplished by input from the scientist's immediate colleagues on a day-to-day basis. Hayem was evidently insulated from this experience.

Julius Bizzozero also was a hematologist. In 1868, he had reported that blood cells originated in the bone marrow (Chapter 3), and by 1882, he had generated sufficient data to publish a monograph on platelets,[14] which could serve as the basis for an introduction on the subject to this day. As did Osler, he worked with preparations from living animals and applied direct microscopy with the aid of an apparatus of his own design to visualize by transillumination the mammalian microcirculation. Among the specimens that he used were the bat wing and the rodent mesentery, which still today serve as experimental models.

Bizzozero was able to define and distinguish leukocytes and erythrocytes from the smaller, discoid cells which he designated "Blutplättchen" and then "Plättchen," taking great pains to point out that these "new" cells represented an independent line with a specialized function and that this function was hemostasis, the arrest of the flow of blood. In blood vessels either severed or damaged, these "Plättchen" rapidly accumulated to form the mass that finally became the effective hemostatic plug. The change in shape of the individual platelets that had been described by previous workers was confirmed, and it was determined that clotting was a subsequent and independent event, thereby indicating that hemostasis and blood coagulation were not synonymous, a message that ever requires repeating. Bizzozero demonstrated that the reactions of normal hemostasis and early thrombosis—the formation of a clot of blood—were parallel and, in a leap of insight that anticipated the work of the next 75 years, stated that ". . . die Plättchen eine Substanz entsenden, welche mikroskopisch unsichtbar ist."* This is evidently the first formulation of the now all-important release reaction.

This initial monograph by Bizzozero contains a massive amount of substantial experimental and theoretical material. Thrombosis and normal hemostasis are shown to represent quite analogous processes; blood cells are shown to release activity which accelerates clotting; the early friability of the hemostatic deposit and its subsequently increased tensile strength are noted; the nonthrombogenic properties of normal blood vessels are recognized. A broad outline was accurately drawn, leaving details for the future. Yet evidently Bizzozero did not present the "omniscient professor syndrome." He carefully recognized the studies of others and gave them the respect they deserve; he acknowledged his debt to the past.

Soon after, Eberth (Figure 16-2) and Schimmelbusch[15] undertook studies that supplemented earlier data with most interesting additions. They also carried out direct studies on the blood vessels of living mammals and showed that with normal blood flow the cells assumed an orderly relationship in which

*Platelets liberate a substance that is not visible microscopically.

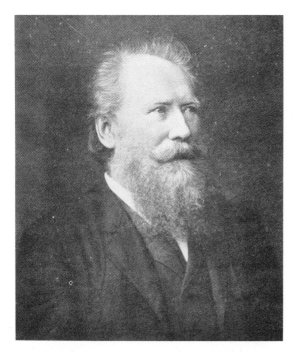

Figure 16-2   Karl J. Eberth (1835–1926) illuminated the hemostatic process.

a plasma space normally intervened between them and the vessel wall. Occasional leukocytes were seen to be rolling along the wall, a reaction which was subsequently shown by Chambers and Zweifach[16] to represent one of the earliest signs of vessel trauma. On the other hand, when normal conditions were disrupted, the axial flow of cells no longer prevailed, and leukocytes and especially platelets were brought into contact with the vessel wall; ultimately these came to form a thrombotic deposit. Certain of the findings in these studies raised questions that have not been resolved to this day. When the animal preparation was excessively traumatized in certain ways, such as by the application of excessive heat ("starkes Erwärmen"), the major cell deposit at the vessel wall was composed of leukocytes. We know that certain types of tissue injury are associated with thrombotic deposits; others produce a typical inflammatory response. Did this early study foreshadow the possibility of an effect governed by local thermal conditions? Eberth and Schimmelbusch demonstrated the effects of flow on the thrombotic deposit and noted that stagnation favored the formation of a "red" thrombus. They also coined the term "viscose Umwandlung" (viscous metamorphosis) of platelets, which has only recently been superseded by more precise biochemical terminology.

Perhaps the curtain may be closed upon the first act of the platelet drama after noting how the origin of these cells was definitively identified. We have seen how Osler had problems distinguishing them from bacteria, how Hayem related them to erythrocyte formation. Others pictured them as arising from leukocytes, and as recently as 1976, one investigator still held them to be derived from erythrocytes.[17] In fact, however, the matter was settled in 1906 by the great pathologist James Homer Wright.[18] He had just perfected his famous stain for blood cells and had applied it to the study not only of blood but also of the morphology of bone marrow. In the blood, he noted that the platelets ("plates") had staining properties whereby he could distinguish a central granular area from a marginal hyalin zone. In addition, he examined "Wright-stained" tissues of cats, including the bone marrow, where his study target was the already identified megakaryocyte. He showed that these huge cells shed their cytoplasm to form clearly identifiable platelets but that there was no good correlation between the number of megakaryocytes in the bone marrow of patients and the number of blood platelets.

The twentieth century thus begins with platelets identified as a unique hemostatic cell (or cell fragment) which is produced in the bone marrow, among other sites, from megakaryocytes.

The Platelets Demonstrate a Multiplicity of Functions

The early workers in the platelet field promptly recognized the hemostatic potential of these cells: how they adhered to damaged vascular surfaces, and how they aggregated subsequently to form an obstructive hemostatic mass. It shortly became evident that they possess many additional properties, which indicates an amazing degree of versatility.

CLOT RETRACTION

We noted earlier that the description of clot retraction preceded by a long time the recognition of platelets. How platelets were found to participate in this process is thoroughly reviewed by Budtz-Olsen,[3] and here again the contribution of Hayem[19] is preeminent. He demonstrated that horse blood, when prevented from clotting by cooling, sedimented into three major fractions: the top was cell-poor, the middle platelet-rich, and the bottom mainly red cells. Upon warming, although all clotted, only the middle layer gave optimal clot retraction. Moreover, removal of the platelets from the middle layer by filtration greatly reduced the retraction. It remained for Le Sourd and Pagniez[20] to establish the unique ability of platelets to produce clot retraction and to show that "living" functional platelets were required.

How do platelets accomplish this feat? It had already been noted that fibrin strands are present in close association with altered platelets when blood clots,[11,12] but many tortuous avenues of investigation had to be traversed before the picture developed with reasonable clarity. The first distinction that had to be made was between true retraction of the fibrin strands and a loss of fibrin itself because of proteolytic activity generated within the system. Although the possibility of lysis never had a major group of adherents, it was finally put to rest by Budtz-Olsen, who traveled with his family by automobile from South Africa to join Professor A. G. Macfarlane at Oxford. This intrepid investigator recorded no loss of weight in retracted as compared to non-retracted clots.

Next, an important relationship was established: the efficiency of clot retraction is proportional to platelet concentration within the limits of methodological precision. Moreover, several blood components can interfere with this efficiency. Hayem had noted that retraction was greatly diminished in the red cell fraction of his sedimented horse blood, a finding that was subsequently confirmed repeatedly in comparable studies by others, and Budtz-Olsen showed a similar inhibitory effect of leukocytes. In fact, an unexpected relationship emerged; not only was retraction inhibited by cells but fibrinogen, the soluble precursor of fibrin, itself retarded the process; the optimal response was found to occur with merely concentrated platelets and minimal fibrinogen concentrations.[21] There had been considerable speculation as to what the physiological function could be of the sluggish process of clot retraction. Hemostasis requires prompt sealing of a severed blood vessel, and clot retraction in clotted whole blood is well under way only after a delay of 15 minutes or more. It has become clear that clot retraction is a derivative reaction and that the essential process is platelet retraction of the hemostatic deposits, as demonstrated long before by Eberth and Schimmelbusch.[15]

How platelets perform their function of retraction, whether it be by pulling together strands of fibrin or converting a platelet clump into a more compact mass, leads us from the domain of morphology to that of biochemistry. Intimations of the direction the work would take were provided by several studies that showed platelets to be active metabolic units despite their anuclear structure.[22] A major breakthrough was achieved by Professor Ernst F. Lüscher at the University of Berne, in Switzerland. Lüscher had been studying at the California Institute of Technology when he received an urgent letter to return to Switzerland. His assignment was to isolate and prepare a hypothetical enzyme that had been described in platelet-depleted plasma and that produced clot retraction. To his dismay, Lüscher found that this "enzyme" was actually residual platelets and merely reflected inadequate centrifugation of the specimens. It is now known that some platelets sediment extremely slowly even at high centrifugal speeds (hence, the term "platelet-poor" plasma) unless rigorous techniques are used to remove platelets. Science is full of such pitfalls. Lüscher had been sent on a wild goose chase, and his shamefaced superiors made it up to him by allowing him a period of undisturbed research. He threw himself into the problem of clot retraction and promptly demonstrated that the reaction depended upon active glycolysis.[23] Shortly thereafter, in association with his colleague Bettex-Galland,[24] the punch line was revealed—platelets are richly endowed with a contractile protein; clot retraction and platelet retraction are manifestations of this contractile activity. It is now generally accepted that all cell motility from amoeboid motion to mitotic division depends upon some variety of contractile response; Lüscher and his colleagues opened the window to this monumental generality.

ADHESION

The early studies of Bizzozero and of Eberth and Schimmelbusch on platelet accumulation at the site of vessel damage were concerned with identifying the phenomenon, and for almost a century, the reaction was vaguely considered as an interaction between platelets and damaged "endothelium." It was not until the late 1950s that the biochemical basis of this process came under investigation. The pioneering work responsible for this advance was initiated by two Belgian scientists working in the laboratory of Professor Jacques Roskam in Liege. Bounameaux[25] had noted the unique ability of platelets to stick to certain nonbiological surfaces and found that the reaction of rabbit platelets with the connective tissue of ground-up aorta was virtually instantaneous. In the same laboratory, Hugues, who had followed with interest the in vivo studies on rat mesentery hemostasis by Marjorie Zucker,[26] demonstrated that normal rabbit mesentery was nonreactive with platelets but that when this tissue was traumatized, platelets adhered to its collagen fibers.[27] Hugues postulated that the thrombogenic surface of the damaged vessel was exposed collagen, a conclusion that has been abundantly confirmed in recent years, during which an explosion has occurred in the understanding of collagen biochemistry. Hugues went on to demonstrate that the adhesion reaction between platelets and collagen could be dissociated from the subsequent aggregation of platelets with each other because even the platelets from patients with Glanzmann's thrombasthenia, a disorder which will be described shortly, underwent normal adhesion, although they were incapable of aggregating.[28]

AGGREGATION

Again, Bizzozero's experiments serve as an historical reference point. In the damaged vessel, not only do the platelets form an adherent layer; they also heap up to produce an effective hemostatic plug; i.e., they aggregate. The basis of the aggregation response was unsuspected until a most curious observation was made. Professor Paul A. Owren had organized the Institute for Thrombosis Research in Oslo, which had developed into an Athens for its time and subject. In 1960, Dr. Arvid J. Hellem was involved in studies on platelet "adhesiveness," by which he meant, ". . . the property of platelets to adhere to foreign surfaces." He measured this property by the reduction in platelet number when blood or platelet-rich plasma was passed through a column of glass beads. Since that time, variations of the glass bead column test have been called tests of adhesiveness, although the mechanism of count reduction is complex and is affected perhaps more by the retention of aggregated platelet masses than by the adhesion of platelets directly to the glass. The term, *platelet retention* is more appropriate, and, as we shall see, Hellem himself was misled by his own terminology.

The observation that set the ball rolling was that platelet retention in the glass bead columns was a function of the quantity of red cells—the more red cells, the greater the retention. It is now known that the effect of red cells is largely to increase platelet convection, thereby bringing more of them into contact with the beads and their already deposited material. In any event, Hellem found that an activity was present in red cell hemolysate that increased platelet retention in glass bead columns and clumped the platelets when it was mixed with platelet-rich plasma. This new aggregating agent was named "factor R" after its presumed cell of origin (the red cell), although Ollgard[29] in neighboring Denmark had independently found a similar material in platelets. Preliminary tests of its properties showed it to be dialyzable through semipermeable membranes and stable to boiling. It was clearly a compound of low molecular weight.[30] What could it be? The answer was quickly forthcoming. A group from the Institute for Thrombosis Research was led by a brilliant young investigator, A. Gaarder, whose career was tragically cut short by a fatal automobile accident. She subjected an extract of boiled red cells to column chromatography and definitively identified the platelet aggregating fraction as adenosine diphosphate.[31] An entire new dimension was thereby created, which has kept plateletologists busy to this day elaborating the details and working out the implications of a humoral mechanism of platelet aggregation.

ACCELERATION OF BLOOD COAGULATION BY PLATELETS

We return again and again to the fundamental observations made by the nineteenth century biologists. They had noted that fibrin filament formation was typically associated with platelets, from which these filaments evidently originated; this suggested that platelets were somehow involved in the process of blood coagulation. However, demonstration of an activity in platelets that affects the coagulation process did not come easily. In fact, it was readily observed that blood appeared to clot with equal facility whether or not platelets were abundant. Convincing evidence for platelet coagulant activity was finally provided in 1947 by Dr. Kenneth Brinkhous, himself the founder of a United States "Athens" of hemostasis at the University of North Carolina. Brinkhous made use of the newly developed silicone-coated glassware to sensitize clotting tests so that more subtle abnormalities of clotting could be revealed. He was able to demonstrate that low-temperature, high-speed centrifugation produced plasma that showed a progressively longer clotting time which was proportional to the reduction in platelets, and the phenomenon was further amplified when hemophilic blood was used.[32] This topic was fresh and new when there was initiated a series of meetings, the Josiah Macy Jr. Foundation Conferences on "Blood Clotting and Allied Problems"[33] (Figure 16-3). The proceedings make delightful reading because they represent virtually unedited transcriptions of most lively interactions between outstanding scientists. Dr. Brinkhous presented his findings at this conference, but the discussion that followed provided few clues as to what the relationship between platelets and clotting would actually turn out to be.

Nevertheless, the basis for our present concepts had been available more than a decade earlier. Dr. Edwin Chargaff and his associates at Columbia University[34] had prepared a lipid extract from horse platelets that accelerated clotting in cell-free chicken plasma. The activity was found to reside in the phospholipid fraction. Perhaps it was this curious mixing of species that dampened the immediate impact of Chargaff's findings upon the Macy Conference participants. In any event, the key observation was soon forthcoming when Professor van Creveld in Amsterdam separated from platelet extracts a fraction with an antiheparin (i.e., a procoagulant) effect that he named "platelet factor."[35] Many subsequent investigators contributed data to the present concept that *platelet factor 3* derives its activity from a phospholipid that platelets make available and that is central to the process of blood coagulation. Moreover, platelets have a special role in providing this reactant, although all cells contain it.

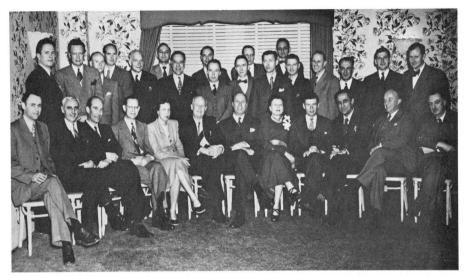

Figure 16-3 Participants at a Macy Conference. Front Row: John D. Ferry, John H. Ferguson, Paul A. Owren, Nelson W. Barker, Jessica H. Lewis, Frank Fremont-Smith, Irving S. Wright, Janet Freed, Joseph E. Flynn, Karl Paul Link, Charles H. Best, Hans F. Jensen. Second Row: J. Garrott Allen, Walter H. Seegers, Frank D. Mann, Hardin Jones, John T. Edsall, Benjamin Alexander, L. M. Tocantins, Ralph S. Overman, Kenneth M. Brinkhous, Eugene Loomis, John H. Olwin, Pietro de Nicola, Leonard S. Sommer, Eugene P. Cronkite. Back Row: Ancel C. Blaustein, Louis B. Jacques, Emory D. Warner, Charles E. Brambel.

PLATELETS AND VASCULAR FRAGILITY

When platelets are reduced in number to a sufficient degree and for a great enough period of time, patients and experimental animals develop increased vascular fragility and purpura, i.e., hemorrhages in the skin, mucous membranes, and elsewhere. I shall deal with platelet diseases later in this essay, but the subject now is how this phenomenon was interpreted and explored experimentally.

The clinical clue that such a relationship exists was provided by Hayem, who noted the marked paucity of his "hématoblastes" in a patient with purpura.[36] The development of techniques for preparing potent heteroantibodies against platelets[37] initiated a series of studies in animals to determine the mechanism of purpura that is associated with reduced platelet counts (thrombocytopenia). Early in this century, two British investigators, Ledingham and Bedson, prepared such antibodies against the platelets of rabbits, guinea pigs, and rats and also antibodies against other blood cells.[38-40] Only the antiplatelet reagents produced thrombocytopenic purpura. In experiments that continued over a decade, they further showed that thrombocytopenia alone was not sufficient because platelet reduction produced by intravenous agar was not accompanied by hemorrhagic lesions. However, thrombocytopenia was necessary. When the platelet count was elevated by splenectomy, antiplatelet serum failed to produce purpura when the count similarly dropped numerically but not to levels below normal values. These early studies are crude indeed in light of modern immunological wisdom. The antibodies were certainly broad spectrum, and their administration to animals may have produced many complex systemic effects unsuspected by their users. Nevertheless it is now generally agreed that they did produce conclusions about the contribution of platelets to microvascular integrity which are even now generally accepted. How the platelets perform the "vascular supporting" function, whether they are continuously repairing minute areas of damage, as the famous Dutch boy with his finger in the dike, or are supplying some essential product that becomes incorporated into the vessels is still a total mystery. Some of our most capable researchers have attempted to get a handle on the problem only to give up in frustration. Nevertheless, these early investigators defined the problem, which is the first step in its solution.

PLATELET AS A SPONGE

As we have seen, the platelet is tiny as compared to other mammalian cells. Yet its versatility is out of proportion to its size. It performs functions that range all the way from producing the plug that mechanically seals defects in ruptured vessels to providing procoagulant activity for the complex reactions of blood coagulation. The presence of circulating platelets seems even to have a role in maintaining the health of the small blood vessels. Indeed, the list of platelet activities continues to expand into unexpected areas, as evidenced by the recent studies of Russell Ross and his colleagues,[41] which establish for platelets the task of delivering to the damaged blood vessel wall a humoral agent that causes its smooth muscle cells to proliferate. Over the years, a picture has evolved that underlines the concept, formulated by Adelson et al.,[42] that the platelet is a sponge. It is loaded with diverse and biologically active compounds, some of which it can soak up during its voyage through the circulation and all of which it can discharge where they are needed. The term sponge is used in the sense of a functional item rather than a description of the marine animal. In fact, this spongelike property of platelets would appear to serve as a focus whereby many other properties can be brought into a unified perspective.

Serotonin is a compound that well illustrates the point being made. It had been known in the nineteenth century that the infusion of serum into living vessels causes them to constrict and to impede the flow of blood. In 1918, a paper was published in the *Archives of Internal Medicine* by Hirose,[43] which showed that this vasoconstrictor activity was proportional to the platelet count of the blood used to prepare the serum; almost simultaneously and in the same journal, Janeway[44] and his colleagues showed that a platelet extract was evidently the most potent source of the vasoconstrictor. The substance proved to have all the properties of a relatively low molecular weight compound. It was some 30 years later that Rappaport published his classical work establishing the active compound as 5-hydroxytryptamine (serotonin).[45] Platelets do not have the synthetic mechanisms to manufacture this compound; they must collect it from other tissues, i.e., sponge it up. In fact, it was found that when serotonin was added to platelet-rich plasma, the platelets collected almost all of it.[46] Moreover, when platelets are exposed to the stimuli that initiate the hemostatic response, such as thrombin or collagen, the serotonin is released[47]—the sponge is squeezed—and the transported material is delivered to its consumer at the site of hemostasis. The importance of this serotonin-mediated vasoconstrictor response may not be great; drugs that deplete platelets of their serotonin have little demonstrable effect upon the animal's ability to mount a hemostatic response. However, clarification of the phenomenon opened up an entirely new area, in which many loose pieces of the jigsaw puzzle fell into place.

Again we look to the Oslo group, where Kristian Grette was bathed in its creative atmosphere. Grette found that when platelets were exposed to thrombin, an enzyme elaborated in shed blood from the inactive precursor prothrombin (Chapter 17), there was a massive release from their cytoplasm of multiple constituents, including adenosine diphosphate.[48] He coined the term *release reaction*. The anatomical basis of this release reaction was promptly forthcoming from Oslo when Kjaerheim and Hovig[49] applied electron microscopic techniques to platelet preparations in vitro and to platelets participating in hemostatic reactions in animals. From van Leeuwenhoek to electron microscopy represents perhaps a ten-thousandfold improvement in resolving power. The platelets proved to have a complexity (known in electron microscopy as ultrastructure) that was in conformity with their diverse responsibilities. In this particular study, only a preliminary inventory was taken of the platelet ultrastructural components, but it was evident that intact platelets contained granules which were lost when the platelets did their job; i.e., they were released. Ultimately, the contractile components of the platelet were defined morphologically by others, and the physiological-anatomical-biochemical circle was joined.

The contributions of this basic biology to the activities of the practicing physician were considerable.

The Patient

Long before there was any possible concept of platelets, in fact before cells had been recognized at all, diseases were described that can now be attributed to platelet problems.

Physicians from the Ancients through the Renaissance recognized diseases that were accompanied by "purpura," large discolored areas resulting from bleeding into the skin. This word is related etymologically to the color (purple) of a dye produced by the mollusk *Purpura lapillus*.[50] Undoubtedly, the whole spectrum of hemorrhagic diseases was included among the purpuras, and many of the unfortunates so afflicted no doubt suffered from platelet disorders. It was in the eighteenth century that perspective was focused by the observations of Paul Gottlieb Werlhof, Court Physician to King George II of England (Chapter Opening Photo), who described a young woman's acute and reversible purpura.[51] Until 20 or 30 years ago, what is now termed *idiopathic thrombocytopenic purpura* or *ITP* went by the name of Werlhof's disease.

More than 100 years elapsed between Werlhof's clinical description and Hayem's report of thrombocytopenia as a basis for the disease,[36] an interval beyond comprehension today; the physician who now is two years behind in his professional understanding is hopelessly out of date. In any event, the link between reduced circulating platelets and hemorrhagic problems which Hayem's brief paper proposed showed the relationship of basic biology and practical clinical medicine. It was evident that if hemostatic integrity depended upon effective platelet reactions, loss of platelets meant the development of a bleeding disorder. However, things are never as simple as is first hoped, and it soon became evident that additional factors had to be considered. Some early clinical tests ultimately yielded hints of what was to come.

THE BLEEDING TIME

The first formal test of hemostasis was attributed by Jones and Tocantins to an 1823 report by Stoker, who used a skin bleeding time to obtain normal values of about 5 minutes. This test came to be a measure of platelet defects when it was popularized by the work of William W. Duke, a Kansas pathologist,[52] in 1910. Duke showed that there was a relatively constant interval between the onset and the cessation of bleeding in normal people when a small incision was made in the earlobe; there was a progressive prolongation of this interval in patients with reduced circulating platelets, an interval which was roughly proportional to the magnitude of the platelet loss. Although this test has been modified in its details and in many ways over the years, it remains a useful measure of hemostasis for the modern physician.[53]

When a dark room is suddenly flooded with bright light, many details are unseen, and the view appears to be less complex than it is shown to be after adaptation to the light occurs. So it is with new discoveries and so it was with the bleeding time. Professor Roskam in Belgium[54] was disturbed by the many instances in which there was a poor correlation between the bleeding time and the platelet count. He agonized over this paradox for many years, and he performed numerous animal experiments and made many observations on bleeding patients. The problems that worried Professor Roskam are at least partly resolved, and his concern for them stimulated others to recognize them as problems and, thereby, to bring fresh approaches to their solution. We now know that not all platelets are equal. Their effectiveness as hemostatic bodies may be influenced by their age, their plasma environment, the state of the tissue with which they react, and the associated diseases and treatment.

DEFECTS IN PLATELET FUNCTION

Edward Glanzmann (Figure 16-4), a Swiss pediatrician, noted in 1918 that some of his patients had many symptoms of thrombocytopenic purpura[55] but had normal platelet counts. Typically, their bleeding times were prolonged, and their blood failed to undergo the expected degree of clot retraction. Glanzmann was familiar with the platelet functions characterized by the biologists and appropriately concluded that his patients had defective platelets; the prevalence of the disease in families and its presence early in life suggested that it had a hereditary basis. It is now probable that Glanzmann's

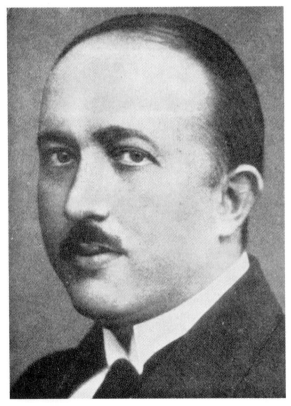

Figure 16-4 Edward Glanzmann (1887–1959): the weak platelet.

patients had several types of platelet abnormality, but the point was established that the platelet factory could turn out a shoddy product, a familiar analogy to much of modern life in general. Patients with Glanzmann's disease, now usually called *thrombasthenia*, are extremely rare, but their abnormality set subsequent researchers to work to define the problem. An entire branch of platelet research has grown from this quest, and various measures of platelet function have been applied to these and related patients.

In thrombasthenia, the platelets fail to aggregate in response to reagents that produce this reaction in normal platelets, and the thrombasthenic platelets, as noted, do not normally produce clot retraction. Moreover, it has turned out that for each platelet function, there are diseases in which each is respectively abnormal. In addition, although the congenital and inherited examples of this group of defects are relatively uncommon, such is not the case with patients who have been born with normal platelets but who acquire abnormalities for some reason. Certainly the most frequent basis for functionally abnormal platelets is the response to the administration of certain drugs. Possibly the most prevalent hemostatic defect in the world is the platelet functional defect produced by aspirin.

Perhaps the first observation made about this relationship was that of Beaumont and his colleagues,[56] who reported in 1955 that patients with inherited defects of blood coagulation developed prolonged bleeding times when they took the usual therapeutic doses of this drug. As is so often the case, understanding of the way aspirin produced this effect was facilitated by a technological development. Working independently in England, Drs. John R. O'Brien and Gustave V.R. Born had devised a technique for measuring platelet aggregation by the changes of optical density in platelet-rich plasma.[57,58] O'Brien had already noted the inhibition of platelet aggregation by a variety of drugs; a report by Hardisty and Hutton[59] described patients with a long bleeding time and what seemed to be a reduced platelet release reaction in response to collagen stimulation. Dr. Marjorie Zucker, whose prolific contributions to the understanding of hemostasis have continued for some three decades as a supplement to the raising of four demanding children, demonstrated convincingly that aspirin produces exactly this effect when used in doses commonly recommended to treat headache.[60] The defect in platelets that fail to release their normal hemostatic constituents is now known as *thrombocytopathy*. This defect can be produced by a variety of drugs and also by increased blood levels of products which accumulate in the course of liver or kidney disease. The ability to perform platelet function tests as well as to enumerate these cells has made possible the identification of many varieties of thrombocytopathy, most of which are acquired, a few of which are seen in patients with hereditary and congenital diseases. It has also generated a new branch of pharmacology in which deliberate platelet inhibition is being explored as a means of preventing thrombotic disease.

TREATMENT

Medical research is ultimately aimed at achieving health benefits for the patient. Although this end has been served by a spectrum of routes, ranging from the accidental observation to the reasoned conclusion derived from a basic understanding of the disease process, the approach to the latter ideal must be the most effective way. In the case of thrombocytopenia, the evolution of an effective treatment well illustrates this principle. A review by Jones and Tocantins[50] indicates that many false starts and misplaced enthusiasms characterized the attempts to treat purpura in the pre-Hayem period, and these serve as a lesson to present-day enthusiasts who may allow their euphoria to color their judgment in the treatment of diseases that are still poorly understood.

In 1916, Kaznelson effectively treated a patient with thrombocytopenic purpura by splenectomy.[61] Because the spleen had already been established as a graveyard for blood cells that had completed their life span, Kaznelson reasoned that under certain circumstances, thrombocytopenia might be the consequence of an excessive platelet trap. Since that time, splenectomy has become a standard form of treatment for certain patients with thrombocytopenic purpura, and the refinement of diagnostic techniques has progressively increased the accuracy of predicting which are likely to benefit from this form of treatment.

In 1950, the field of hematology was shaken by a development that was characterized by Dr. William Dameshek, the founder and editor of the journal *Blood*, as follows: "Although new therapeutic methods follow one another in bewildering succession these days, it is probably safe to say that nothing more startling than ACTH will enter the medical horizon for a long time to come."[62] As if to supply confirmation of this prediction, there appeared a report in the same issue of the same journal by Wintrobe and his associates on the effects of ACTH on various diseases of the blood. In it, a patient with idiopathic thrombocytopenic purpura was described who responded to injections of ACTH with an increase in platelets and amelioration of symptoms.[63] Management of the disease by endocrine manipulation was thereby launched and, with much refinement, is used to this day. In fact, this development indicated that nonsurgical treatment was a promising possibility, and the succeeding years have seen the emergence of a whole host of medications that can control the symptoms of idiopathic thrombocytopenic purpura (ITP) and restore platelets to the blood.

Some of these have been applied because there was increasing evidence of an immunological basis for ITP. The disease resembled that produced in experimental animals given antiplatelet serum, and William J. Harrington, a budding hematologist in St. Louis, had performed a spectacular experiment. He gave himself plasma from an ITP patient and showed that this produced a replica of the donor's disease. Although Dr. Harrington's resulting symptoms were considerable, he fortunately recovered and was able to characterize the ingredient in the patient's plasma that was responsible for the effect.[64] It proved to be immunological in nature, a gamma globulin, and this suggested therapeutic possibilities from drugs that moderated the immune response. In fact, immunosuppressive therapy by a variety of agents is an additional weapon available to fight the manifestations of ITP.

There are other such weapons, and each has its roots in a diversity of soils. Thus, selective transfusion of platelets has emerged from the growing field of blood banking, as has the clarification of basic platelet biology. Platelet transfusion is valuable for patients who require a temporary restoration of platelet functions, as in the thrombocytopenia that accompanies leukemia treatment or when surgery is performed upon a patient with thrombocyto-pathy.

Conclusions

It would be tempting to summarize the material that has been presented in the preceding pages by stating that from ancient times there were diseases which were accompanied by abnormal bleeding and that when platelets were dis-covered to be a blood component necessary for normal hemostasis, the basis for these symptoms became evident. Further, it might be stated that bleeding symptoms resulted from reduced numbers of platelets, or their abnormal function, and that surgical or medical methods were devised to correct these defects.

Such a summary, although reasonably accurate, would miss a major message that is perhaps considerably more important than the practical end that has been outlined. The writer should like to propose that the prime conclusion to be drawn is that the final product, that which is of practical application, represents an interdependency of many disciplines and that the potential contribution of one to another is not obvious or predictable. Thus, the physician who is confronted with a puzzling illness defines a problem to be investigated. The biologist provides information as to the normal functions of various organs and tissues, but his ability to obtain such information is limited by his tools, which are, in turn, a function of the contributions of physics and chemistry; the practitioners of these sciences are stimulated by the needs of the biologists and the problems that their findings pose. With improved tools, the biologist perceives unexpected phenomena, which are applicable in novel ways to the practitioner. The permutations on this theme are inexhaustible. But above all, they are unpredictable. Little did Werlhof suspect that van Leeuwenhoek had an instrument which would clarify his new disease, and the Dutch microscopist was equally unaware of these implications.

The conclusion that appears to be inevitable from these considerations is that the most certain path to improved health care is the careful cultivation of basic science without respect to its apparent applications. There are times when planned attacks on specific problems are appropriate, but the progress that represents a true quantum leap must derive from the free exploration by the creative scientist, whatever his specific area may be.

Many features of platelets are still elusive but, thanks to the fertile interchange among the sciences, many of their properties have been perceived and harnessed for the benefit of humanity.

References

1   Singer C, Holmyard EJ, Hall AR, William TI (eds): *A History of Technology.* New York, Oxford University Press, 1957, vol III, pp 229–233.

2   Dittrich H: Physiology of neutrophiles, in Braunsteiner H, Zucker-Franklin D (eds): *The Physiology and Pathology of Leukocytes.* New York, Grune and Stratton, 1962, 293 pp, pp 130–131.

3   Budtz-Olsen OE: *Clot Retraction.* Oxford, Oxford University Press, 1951, 149 pp, pp 1–2.

4   Tocantins LM: Historical notes on blood platelets, in Dameshek W, Taylor FHL (eds): *George R. Minot Symposium of Hematology.* New York, Grune and Stratton, 1949, 984 pp, pp 553–562.

5   Robb-Smith AHT: Why the platelets were discovered. *Br J Haematol* 13:618–637, 1967.

6   Dreyfus C: *Some Milestones in the History of Hematology.* New York, Grune and Stratton, 1957, 87 pp, pp 38–40.

7   Donné A: De l'origine des globules du sang, de leur mode de formation et de leur fin. *C R Se Acad Sci (Paris)* 14:366–368, 1842.

8   Addison W: On the colorless corpuscles and on the molecules and cytoblasts in the blood. *Lond Med Gaz* 30:144–146, 1841–1842.

9   Osler W, Schafer A: Ueber einige im Blute vorhandene Bacterienbildende Massen. *Zentralbl Med Wissensch* 11:577–578, 1873.

10   Osler W: An account of certain organisms occurring in the liquor sanguinis. *Proc R Soc Lond* 22:391–398, 1874.

11   Sir William Osler in Memorial Volume, *Appreciations and Reminiscences,* Abbott ME (ed), Bull IX. Montreal and Washington, Int Assoc Med Museums, 1926, 633 pp.

12   Hayem G: Recherches sur l'évolution des hématies dans le sang de l'homme et des vertébrès. *Arch Physiol Norm Pathol* 5:692–734, 1878.

13   Hayem G: *L'Hématoblaste, Troisième Element du Sang.* Paris, Presse Universitaires de France, 1923, 295 pp.

14   Bizzozero J: Ueber einen neuen Formbestandtheil des Blutes und dessen Rolle bei der Thrombose und der Blutgerinnung. *Virchows Arch Pathol Anat Physiol* 90:261–332, 1882.

15   Eberth JC, Schimmelbusch C: Experimentelle Untersuchungen über Thrombose. *Fortschr Med* 3:379–389, 1885.

16   Chambers R, Zweifach BW: Intercellular cement and capillary permeability. *Physiol Rev* 27:436–463, 1947.

17 Leiter SS: The human blood platelet: its derivation from the red blood cell. A morphological study. *Folia Haematol* (Leipz) 103:878–882, 1976.

18 Wright JH: The origin and nature of the blood plates. *Boston Med Surg J* 154:643–645, 1906.

19 Hayem G: Cited by Budtz-Olsen OE: *Clot Retraction.* Oxford, Oxford University Press, 1951, 149 pp, pp 36–37.

20 Le Sourd L, Pagniez P: Du rôle des hématoblastes dans la retraction du caillot. *C R Soc Biol (Paris)* 61:109–111, 1906.

21 Ballerini G, Seegers WH: A description of clot retraction as a visual experience. *Thromb Diath Haemor* 3:147–164, 1959.

22 Born GVR, Esnouf MP: The breakdown of adenosine triphosphate in blood platelets during clotting. *J Physiol* 133:61P–62P, 1956.

23 Lüscher EF: Glukose als Cofaktor bei der Retraktion des Blutgerinnsels. *Experientia* 12:294–295, 1956.

24 Bettex-Galland M, Lüscher EF: Extraction of an actomyosin-like protein from human thrombocytes. *Nature* 184:276–277, 1959.

25 Bounameaux Y: L'accolement des plaquettes aux fibres sous-endotheliales. *C R Soc Biol (Paris)* 153:865–867, 1959.

26 Zucker MB: Platelet agglutination and vasoconstriction as factors in spontaneous in normal, thrombocytopenic, heparinized and hypoprothrombinemic rats. *Am J Physiol* 148:275–288, 1947.

27 Hugues J: Accolement des plaquettes au collagène. *C R Soc Biol (Paris)* 154:866–868, 1960.

28 Hugues J, Lapiere CM: Nouvelle recherches sur l'accolement des plaquettes aux fibres de collagène. *Thromb Diath Haemor* 11:327–354, 1964.

29 Ollgard E: Macroscopic studies of platelet aggregation. Nature of an aggregating factor in red cells and platelets. *Thromb Diath Haemor* 6:86–97, 1964.

30 Hellem AJ: The adhesiveness of human blood platelets in vitro. *Scand J Clin Lab Invest* 12(suppl 51): 1960, 117 pp.

31 Gaarder A, Jonsen J, Laland S, Hellem A, Owren PA: Adenosine diphosphate in red cells as a factor in the adhesiveness of human blood platelets. *Nature* 192:531–532, 1961.

32 Brinkhous KM: Clotting defect in hemophilia; deficiency in a plasma factor required for platelet utilization. *Proc Soc Exp Biol Med* 66:117–120, 1947.

33 Brinkhous KM: Initiation and acceleration factors in thrombosis, in Flynn JE (ed): *Blood Clotting and Allied Problems.* New York, Josiah Macy Jr Foundation, 1948, vol 1, 179 pp, pp 39–48.

34 Chargaff E, Bancroft FW, Stanley-Brown M: Studies on the chemistry of blood coagulation. III. The chemical constituents of blood platelets and their role in blood clotting, with remarks on the activation of clotting by lipids. *J Biol Chem* 116:237–251, 1936.

35 Creveld S van, Paulssen MMP: Significance of clotting factors in blood platelets, in normal and pathological conditions. *Lancet* 2:242–244, 1951.

36 Hayem G: Sur un cas de diathèse hémorragique. *Bull Mem Soc Med Hop Paris* 8:389–394, 1891.

37 Cole RI: Note on the production of an agglutinating serum for blood platelets. *Bull Johns Hopkins Hosp* 18:261–262, 1907.

38 Ledingham JCG, Bedson SP: Experimental purpura. *Lancet* 1:311–316, 1916.
39 Bedson SP: Blood platelet anti-serum, its specificity and rôle in the experimental production of purpura. *J Pathol Bacteriol* 24:469–476, 1921.
40 Bedson SP: Blood-platelet anti-serum, its specificity and role in the experimental production of purpura. Part II. *J Pathol Bacteriol* 25:94–104, 1922.
41 Ross R, Glomset J, Kariya B, Harker L: A platelet-dependent serum factor that stimulates the proliferation of arterial smooth muscle cells in vitro. *Proc Natl Acad Sci* (USA) 71:1207–1211, 1974.
42 Adelson E, Rheingold JJ, Crosby WH: The platelet as a sponge: a review. *Blood* 17:767–774, 1961.
43 Hirose K: Relation between platelet count of human blood and its vasoconstrictor action after clotting. *Arch Intern Med* 21:604–612, 1918.
44 Janeway TC, Richardson HB, Park EA: Experiments on the vasoconstrictor action of blood serum. *Arch Intern Med* 26:565–603, 1918.
45 Rappaport MM, Green AA, Page IH: Serum vasoconstrictor (serotonin). IV. Isolation and characterization. *J Biol Chem* 176:1243–1251, 1948.
46 Humphrey JH, Toh CC: Absorption of serotonin (5-HT) and histamine by dog platelets. *J Physiol* 124:300–304, 1954.
47 Zucker MB, Borrelli J: Relationship of some blood clotting factors to serotonin release from washed platelets. *J Appl Physiol* 7:432–442, 1955.
48 Grette K: Studies on the mechanism of thrombin-catalyzed hemostatic reactions in blood platelets. *Acta Physiol Scand* (suppl 195): 1962, 93 pp.
49 Kjaerheim Ä, Hovig T: The ultrastructure of haemostatic blood platelet plugs in rabbit mesenterium. *Thromb Diath Haemor* 7:1–15, 1962.
50 Jones HW, Tocantins LM: The history of purpura hemorrhagica. *Ann Med Hist* 5:349–364, 1933.
51 Werlhof PG, Wichmann JE: *Opera Medica.* Hannoverae, imp fratorem Helwingiorum, 1775–1776, 830 pp, p 748.
52 Duke WW: The relation of blood platelets to hemorrhagic disease. Description of a method for determining the bleeding time and the coagulation time. *JAMA* 55:1185–1192, 1910.
53 Bowie EJW, Owen CA: The bleeding time. *Prog Hemostasis Thromb* 2:249–271, 1974.
54 Roskam J, Nolf P: Globulins et temps de saignment. *C R Soc Biol (Paris)* 84:484–487, 1921.
55 Glanzmann E: Hereditäre haemorrhagische Thrombasthenie. Ein Beitrag zur Pathologie der Blutplättchen. *Jahrb Kinderheilk* 88:113–141, 1918.
56 Beaumont JL, Caen J, Bernard J: Action hémorragique de l'acid acétylsalicylique au cours des maladies de sang. *Bull Mem Soc Med Hop Paris* 71:1087–1092, 1955.
57 O'Brien J: Platelet aggregation. II. Some results from a new method of study. *J Clin Pathol* 15:452–481, 1962.
58 Born GVR: Aggregation of blood platelets by adenosine diphosphate and its reversal. *Nature* 194:927–929, 1962.
59 Hardisty RM, Hutton RA: Bleeding tendency associated with "new" abnormality of platelet behaviour. *Lancet* 1:983–985, 1967.
60 Zucker MB, Peterson J: Inhibition of adenosine diphosphate-induced secondary aggregation and other platelet functions by acetylsalicylic acid ingestion. *Proc Soc Exp Biol Med* 127:547–551, 1968.

61 Kaznelson P: Verschwinden den haemorrhagischen Diathese bei einem Fallen von essentieller Thrombopenie (Frank) nach Milz Extirpation. Splenogene thrombolitische Purpura. *Wien Klin Wochenschr* 29:1451–1454, 1916.
62 Dameshek W: ACTH and its hematologic impact. *Blood* 5:779–780, 1950.
63 Wintrobe MM, Cartwright GE, Kuhns WJ, Palmer JG, Lahey ME: The effects of ACTH on the hematopoietic system. *Blood* 5:789–790, 1950.
64 Harrington J, Minnich V, Hollingsworth JW, Moore CV: Demonstration of a thrombocytopenic factor in the blood of patients with thrombocytopenic purpura. *J Lab Clin Med* 38:1–10, 1951.

CHAPTER 17

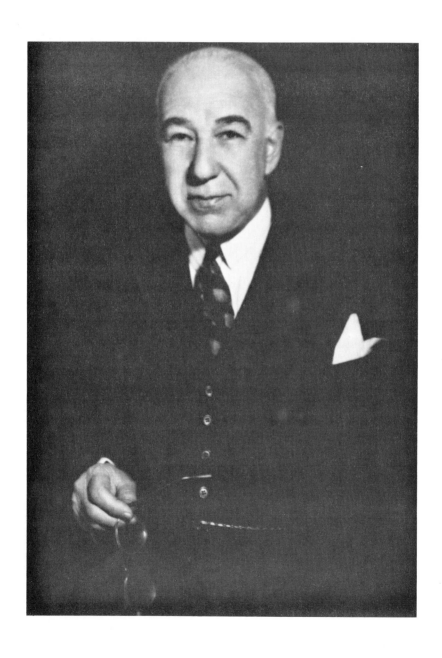

PLASMA, THE TRANSPORT FLUID FOR BLOOD CELLS AND HUMORS

Charles A. Janeway

Although plasma, the complex aqueous solution in which blood cells and platelets are suspended and transported throughout the body, actually accounts for 50 to 80 percent of the volume of the blood circulating in different parts of the vascular system, its true importance was not fully appreciated until recently. The discovery of the nature and functions of its many other components is a comparatively late development in the history of medicine.

Vesalius, Harvey, Malpighi, and Hewson

The need for an understanding of the role played by the plasma was initiated by publication of William Harvey's great book in 1628,[1] in which he convincingly described the circulation of the blood, as discussed in Chapter 1. Harvey's *De Motu Cordis* substitued a dynamic role for the heart and blood vessels for more static concepts—he described a true circulatory system always

Chapter Opening Photo   Edwin J. Cohn in a characteristic pose in his laboratory during the plasma fractionation program.

in motion, one in which the blood, ejected by the force of the beating heart, passed into the great arteries and the branching arterial system and ultimately flowed into a system of coalescing veins, through which it returned to the heart to begin another cycle.

The basis for this new physiologic concept was the work of another great pioneer, Andreas Vesalius (1514–1564),[2] whose anatomical studies were founded on careful dissection of human cadavers and on meticulous observations and drawings. Vesalius' drawings of his dissections provided accurate information about the structural organization of the circulatory system. However, the demonstration of how the blood could actually pass from the arteries into the veins required the closer observations of the celebrated microscopist Malpighi (1628–1694), whose instruments enabled him in 1660 to describe the tiny capillaries which form the connecting links joining the two different types of blood vessels.[3] We now know that the thin-walled capillaries provide the conditions under which exchanges of chemical substances may take place between the circulating plasma and the surrounding fluids that bathe the tissues.

These discoveries laid the foundation during the next two centuries for a steady accumulation of knowledge about the circulation, with its ramifying vessels, and provided a clear anatomical basis for the role of the blood in transporting blood cells, nutriments, and waste products to and from the different organs of the body. However, in contrast to the gradual progress in the study of the blood cells that was made with the improvement of the microscope, as described in preceding chapters, the study of the blood plasma was difficult for several reasons: (1) blood clots rapidly after it is shed; (2) it is very opaque because of the large mass of red cells that account for most of the blood's cellular constituents; and, above all, (3) the lack of appropriate methods and instruments. The last ultimately became available as the result of advances in physics and chemistry during the eighteenth and nineteenth centuries.

For a systematic investigation of the plasma's myriad but microscopically invisible chemical constituents, two technical developments had to take place. First, a system was needed for overcoming the spontaneous coagulation that occurs when blood is removed from the blood vessels; second, a convenient means for separating the plasma from the blood cells had to be devised. Effective anticoagulant chemicals to maintain the fluidity of the blood after shedding and satisfactory centrifuges to permit mechanical separation of the plasma and cells did not become readily available until the twentieth century.

As mentioned earlier (Chapter 1), scientific investigation in hematology began with a remarkable young man, William Hewson (1739–1774). Like a true clinical investigator, Hewson took full advantage of the opportunities his clinical work provided for scientific study. He made careful observations on the behavior of the blood as it flowed into basins during the process of "cupping," a therapeutic measure widely and often unwisely performed by eighteenth century physicians.[4,5] He measured rates of flow and observed the differences in the manner of coagulation when he bled patients with different conditions under various circumstances. He speculated, developed theories to explain his clinical observations, and put them to experimental test in both patients and animals. In so doing, he identified fibrinogen as the agent responsible for the clotting of blood (Chapter 18), collecting it in solid form as fibrin as he beat the blood with glass rods.[6]

Scientific Advances That Laid the Foundations for the Study of the Blood Plasma

PHYSIOLOGY AND THE CONCEPT OF THE INTERNAL ENVIRONMENT

The nineteenth century was a period of tremendous scientific progress in Europe, a period characterized by great activity in the medical sciences. Physiology, the study of how the living body functions, and pathology, the study of disease processes, became predominant fields of investigation, replacing anatomy and the microscopic study of normal tissues (histology). Two figures towered over others in midcentury. First, Rudolph Virchow (1821–1902), the astute German observer of disease, founded scientific pathology[7] by his gross dissection of diseased tissues at the autopsy table and careful study of the microscopic changes accompanying various diseases. Second, Claude Bernard (1813–1878), working in his Paris laboratory, firmly established well-controlled experiments in animals as the preferred method for studies in physiology.[8] The techniques and concepts introduced by these two men still form the basis of many fundamental principles of modern scientific medicine. Claude Bernard's concept of the constancy of the "milieu internal," was later elaborated by Walter B. Cannon (1871–1945)[9] under the term *homeostasis*. It still exerts a strong influence upon medical thinking and provides the theoretical foundation for the whole field of resuscitation and supportive treatment, so essential to the care of seriously ill patients, to modern surgery, and to the rapidly developing field of emergency medicine.

Cannon, who was brought up in rural Wisconsin and Minnesota, became George Higginson Professor of Physiology at the Harvard Medical School in 1906, only 6 years after his graduation from that institution. He pursued a consistent career of teaching and research upon the sympathetic nervous system and its control of emotional and glandular responses, except for a brief hiatus in 1917–1918, when he was in France and England to investigate traumatic shock. The title of his book *The Wisdom of the Body*[9] was borrowed from Professor E.H. Starling (1866–1927), who used it as the title for his Harveian Oration before the Royal College of Physicians in 1923 to express his "admiration for the marvelous and beautiful adjustments in the organism that had been revealed by following Harvey's injunction to study out the secrets of nature by way of experiment." "Only by understanding the wisdom of the body," Starling declared, "shall we attain that mastery of disease and pain which will enable us to relieve the burden of mankind."[10]

IMMUNOLOGY AND INFECTIOUS DISEASE

Bacteriology, with its closely related subject immunology, grew out of the brilliant work of Pasteur (1822–1895)[11,12] on plant diseases, fermentation, and infection and became the next exciting frontier. Pasteur, Robert Koch (1843–1910),[13,14] and many others identified the various microbial agents that cause specific infections, and they began to experiment with ways to prevent and treat the many epidemics and infectious diseases of animals[15] and humans. As described in Chapter 13, Ilya Metchnikov (1845–1916) discovered phagocytosis as a means of defense in infectious disease and received the Nobel Prize in 1908 for his work on specific antibacterial immunity.[16] Most of these studies flourished in the laboratories of the growing universities of Europe, particularly in Germany, France, Austria, and the British Isles.

Meanwhile, less dramatic but steady progress was being made in the methodical development of chemistry and its application to the study of biological and clinical problems; this work did not reach its full fruition until the twentieth century. As discussed in Chapter 1, Ehrlich's (1854–1915) success in the staining of blood cells and tissues[17,18] was a direct application of progress in the German chemical industry. It was Ehrlich's understanding of chemistry and his way of approaching scientific problems that helped to develop modern immunology as a science that obeys laws analogous to those governing all chemical reactions.

EPIDEMIOLOGY, HYGIENE, AND ANTIMICROBIAL CHEMOTHERAPY

It is well to recall, however, that while these results of growing prosperity, intellectual activity, and systematic investigation were being accumulated in the laboratories of Europe, keen clinical observation, with careful reasoning and deduction, particularly by certain British physicians, had led to the solution of a number of major medical problems even before their scientific rationales could be fully understood. Thus, William Withering (1741–1799),[19] having learned from an old *grande dame* of Shropshire of the value of foxglove as a remedy for dropsy, gave cardiologists their basic drug for the treatment of heart failure (digitalis).

Jenner's (1749–1823)[20] introduction of vaccination with cowpox virus in England provided the first effective and safe method for the prevention of smallpox. A half-century later in Boston, Oliver Wendell Holmes (1809–1894) began publishing his observations on the role of childbirth attendants, including doctors, in transmitting puerperal fever from one woman to another;[21,22] his views were confirmed by the studies of Semmelweiss in Vienna, thus opening the way to ridding lying-in hospitals of their high mortality by strict sanitary measures[23] before the causative microorganisms had been clearly identified. John Snow's (1813–1858)[24] careful study of cholera outbreaks led to formulation of his hypothesis of the waterborne nature of its spread. Ultimate proof of the correctness of this theory was established by the termination of a cholera epidemic after the closing of the Broad Street pump.

The explosion of information about infectious diseases, which had until then been the principal causes of morbidity and mortality, came from advances in bacteriology and focused attention once more upon the blood. But this time, attention was drawn to the serum, the clear straw-colored fluid which separates from the coagulum as the blood clots. Von Behring (1854–1917) and Kitasato (1856–1931) were the first to show that serum from the blood of animals that had been actively immunized by serial injections of the toxins (sterile culture filtrates) of diphtheria or tetanus bacilli contained antitoxins.[25] These sera, they found, when injected into experimental animals, conferred passive protection against the effects of the poisons which these disease organisms produce during growth.[26] Thus, the precedent was established for a specific therapeutic use of a plasma derivative.

This work was later elaborated into a variety of studies upon *active* immunizing agents (i.e., vaccines, toxoids, etc.) for establishing protection against specific infections; the search began for other agents, such as specific antibodies in the serum after convalescence, which might be used for temporary protection (*passive immunization*) by transferring immunity from one animal to another or even for treatment of the active disease itself. The bacteriological era and its immunological extensions, initiated by the work of Pasteur, was the dominant field of medical endeavor for over 50 years; it certainly represented the greatest scientific and medical revolution in our time until the development of the antimicrobial drugs. This latter discovery, too, grew out of the German chemical industry with Gerard Domagk's (1895–1964) demonstration in 1935 that Prontosil,[27] a red dye and a conjugated sulfonamide, could arrest the multiplication of virulent bacteria in an animal host, thus bringing about a chemical cure of experimental streptococcal infection in mice. This exciting finding was confirmed by Colebrook and Kenny in 1936[28] in patients with severe and often fatal puerperal sepsis (childbed fever) caused by hemolytic streptococci.

A personal reminiscence will serve to emphasize the revolutionary nature of these publications. As a medical student, I recall a distinguished lecturer discussing the possibilities of antibacterial chemotherapy in 1932 and concluding that, in view of the simplicity of bacteria compared to the biochemical complexities of animals and humans, it was probable that any chemical which was toxic to bacteria would be far more toxic to humans. The irony of this was that in the next few years, he became the pioneer in working out methods for the measurement of sulfonamide drugs in body fluids and the leader in rationalizing their use.[29] In the light of what he had taught me, I remember my intense excitement upon coming upon the contradiction of his prediction in Colebrook and Kenny's report in *The Lancet* in the summer of 1936 and in watching the clinical success of the beginnings of the revolutionary antimicrobial chemotherapeutic era that was taking place in hospitals in Boston and Baltimore during the next year.

STUDIES OF OSMOTIC PRESSURE, ELECTROLYTES AND THE BEHAVIOR OF SOLUTIONS

During the nineteenth century, other less spectacular but more sophisticated lines of chemical investigation that ultimately became important for the future of medicine were quietly being pursued in other laboratories; these were usually separated from most medical research because of their more theoretical nature. Between 1827 and 1835, Dutrochet (1776–1847)[30] published the first papers on the passage of water across a membrane from one solution to another and initiated studies of osmosis (as he called this phenomenon). In 1861, Graham's[31,32] (1805–1869) experiments upon osmosis and dialysis (the process of equilibrating solutions across membranes) made the all-important distinction between colloids (large molecules restrained by the membrane) and crystalloids (small molecules that are freely diffusible). Ultimately, the work of van t'Hoff (1852–1911) clarified the laws governing osmotic pressure,[33,34] while Arrhenius (1859–1927)[35] described the behavior of solutions and the dissociation of electrolytes (simple salts, such as sodium chloride) into positively (Na^+) and negatively (Cl^-) charged ions, which affects their osmotic behavior and interactions.

As a branch of chemistry based on mathematical and physical principles, the science of physical chemistry was established. It was destined to have a strong influence upon the studies of the plasma because of the unusual properties of the protein molecules. Their large size (Starling described them as "monstrous"), their organic constituents, and their varied net charges marked them as unique components that distinguished plasma from simple salt solutions.

These fundamental studies of osmotic pressure, of electrolytes, and of the forces controlling the behavior of solutions began to have an influence on the physiologists whose experimental work toward the end of the century was beginning to unravel the complex functions of the kidney and other internal organs. Richard Bright (1789–1858) had described the pathology of glomerulonephritis (chronic inflammation of the kidneys, often referred to as Bright's disease) and was aware of the fact, even in 1836, that the disease was characterized by the abnormal presence in the urine of albuminous material like that in blood serum.[36] However, it took many years of work, largely in the physiological laboratories of Europe, before the modern concept of the role of the "corpuscles" first described by Malpighi (the glomeruli) was established. It was shown that they serve as filters, normally restraining the passage of the large plasma protein molecules while permitting the diffusion of fluid, salts and their ions, and small organic molecules into Bowman's capsule. From this cuplike collecting receptacle surrounding each glomerulus, the filtrate passes through the kidney's tubular system and is modified during its passage by the cells lining these tubules to emerge as urine in the excretory system of the ureters and bladder.

All this information had to be acquired before an understanding could be reached about the role of the plasma. For the circulation of the blood—a form of perpetual motion lasting throughout life—mechanisms are required to sustain the volume of the contents of the vascular system because great alterations in blood volume could seriously impair its function. As the study of physiology developed, it became apparent that a major role of the circulatory system is to transport essential substances, such as oxygen from the lungs and glucose from the liver to the tissue cells and to carry the waste products of cellular activities, e.g., carbon dioxide from the oxidation of nutriments to the lungs for exhalation, and urea and other nitrogenous wastes derived from the breakdown of foods and tissues to the kidneys for excretion in the urine. These substances leave the circulation and return to it at the level of the capillaries, whose thin membranes permit the relatively free diffusion of water, salts, and other small organic molecules.

Ernest H. Starling (1866–1927), the great British physiologist, devoted much of his active professional life to the study of the circulation and its adjustment to the needs of the body. Because his textbook *Principles of Human Physiology* went through a number of editions, as his own work and those of others advanced, one may trace the evolution of his ideas over a period of years in sections devoted to "the absorption of lymph and tissue fluids" and to the relationship of the circulation to the nutritional and metabolic needs of the tissue cells.

Since his own words are the best, the following quotations have been excerpted from the fourth and last edition, published in 1926.[37]

> Nowhere in the body does the blood come in actual contact with the living cells of the tissues. In all parts the blood flows in capillaries with definite walls consisting of a single layer of cells and is thus separated from the tissue elements by these walls and varying thickness of tissue.

(Capillaries in various parts of the body vary greatly in permeability, those of the liver and lung being most permeable.)

> The lymph may be looked upon as part of the plasma which exudes through the capillary wall, bathes all the tissue elements, passes between the endothelial cells of the capillaries into the peripheral lymphatic network, whence it is carried by

lymphatic trunks into the thoracic duct, by which it is returned again to the blood. . . . The lymph is . . . truly a middleman; as any substance, oxygen or foodstuff, is taken up by a tissue cell from the lymph surrounding it, the latter recoups itself at once at the expense of the blood. Thus there would seem to be no need for lymphatics to drain the limb, were it not that under many conditions . . . the exudation of lymph from the blood vessels is so excessive that if it were not carried off at once and restored to the blood it would accumulate in the tissue spaces, give rise to dropsy, and by pressure on the cells and blood vessels affect them injuriously.

With water leaving the circulation through the walls of the capillaries, the question became, what counterbalancing force could bring fluid back into the circulation to sustain its volume and maintain its pressure? In 1896, Starling suggested that it was the osmotic pressure exerted by the plasma proteins at the venular end of the capillary bed that balanced the forces of diffusion at its arteriolar end.[38] Although there have been modifications in the details of Starling's theory, this general concept about the maintenance of capillary volume in equilibrium with the tissue fluids and the cells that they bathe still stands. Without such a balancing of forces, life would probably not be possible, for neither the red cells that carry oxygen from the lungs, so essential to cell survival, nor the sources of chemical energy like glucose, from the liver, could be transported throughout the body for metabolic use by the tissue cells.

The Impact of the Two World Wars

Wars have always had a major impact upon medicine. One of the principal characteristics of war wounds is the loss of blood and oozing of plasma from injured tissues. These are major factors in the production of "shock." Their loss decreases blood volume and results in a diminished blood flow of oxygen and nutriments, and, hence, failure of the circulation to supply the needs of the tissues for oxygen and essential chemical substances. Reversal of shock requires restoration of circulating blood volume. During World War I, the practical difficulties of performing blood transfusions at the front were too great to permit their wide use for this purpose. Although based on the concept of the role of the plasma proteins as natural colloids that exert osmotic pressure to maintain blood volume, artificial colloids such as gum acacia proved rather unsatisfactory.[39] During World War II, transfusions of blood, plasma, and albumin solutions (see below) saved hundreds of thousands of lives and now are recognized as essential for support in the care of patients with severe injuries or of those undergoing major operations (see Chapter 19).

During the 1930s, technical advances created new possibilities. The introduction of *sodium citrate* as an anticoagulant (Chapter 19) meant that blood could be collected in fluid form from a compatible donor for immediate use or its cellular components could be sedimented in a large centrifuge and the supernatant plasma saved for use to combat shock when needed at a later date. A second advance, the process of *lyophilization*, developed by Flosdorf and Mudd,[40] made it possible to freeze the freshly collected plasma and to remove the water under high vacuum, leaving a dry powder that is stable enough to be kept at room temperature. This powder could then be reconstituted for use by adding sterile water weeks or even months later, thus yielding a plasma solution that contained most of its original protein constituents undamaged.

The third development stimulated by the war was *plasma fractionation.*[41] The principal practical problems envisaged by those preparing the United States medically for a war that might be fought anywhere in the world were: (1) the collection of sufficient quantities of blood; (2) the necessity for its transport to processing and storage facilities in varied climates in many parts of the world; (3) the need for reducing the bulk of the package of dried plasma and its sterile water, which preempted valuable cargo and storage space; and (4) the importance of shortening the interval between the injury and the restoration of osmotic pressure and plasma volume.

The suggestion was made by Wangensteen, then professor of surgery at the University of Minnesota, that cattle, slaughtered in large numbers for meat, could provide a tremendous supply of bovine plasma. Wangensteen showed that bovine plasma could be used in humans and actually gave some to a few of his surgical patients.[42,43] There were many reactions, but by first mixing the bovine plasma with human red blood cells, most of the factors giving rise to immediate reactions could be absorbed and removed by centrifugation and separation of the cells. However, delayed reactions, characterized by the onset of fever, rashes, joint pains, retention of fluid, and swelling of the lymph nodes (serum sickness) after 5 to 7 days, still occurred. This phenomenon had first been encountered and studied by von Pirquet (1879–1929) and Schick (1877–1967)[44] when they used the serum of immunized horses as a specific antitoxin for the treatment of diphtheria in Vienna in the early days of the twentieth century. Subsequently, such patients proved to have been sensitized by the foreign proteins of the horse serum; they would react more rapidly or more violently to a second much smaller dose. This posed a difficult and potentially dangerous problem for the clinical use of plasma proteins from animal sources, but, since such delayed reactions had occurred in only a few patients, Edwin J. Cohn, professor of physical chemistry at the Harvard Medical School, was asked by the National Research Council to see what could be done to render bovine plasma more suitable for clinical use. Cohn had previously worked on a liver extract for pernicious anemia (as detailed in Chapter 10), and his laboratory, which was systematically investigating the solubility of proteins, was studying methods for their separation from mixtures in biological fluids.[45]

THE HARVARD PROTEIN LABORATORY AND THE BEGINNINGS
OF THE PLASMA FRACTIONATION PROGRAM

Cohn was an unusual man, a cultured scientist who knew most of his fellow
chemists in Europe and America (Chapter Opening Photo). He also possessed
the driving force and organizing ability that one might expect to find in an
American corporation executive. His laboratory was quickly organized for the
task he had accepted, and it became one of the major group efforts in medical
research in this country. A multidisciplinary team of chemists, medical scientists, physicians, and public health workers was organized. Obviously directed
and run by Cohn, who seemed to think of every detail as he devoted his
enormous energies to this program, he, nevertheless, created the opportunity
for all involved to participate and contribute their ideas to this group effort. His
first step was to separate the major proteins in bovine plasma on the theory
that these components might differ markedly in their effects.

The successful development of a system for separating the proteins of the
plasma into fractions that could be applied on a scale sufficient for their
production for chemical study and therapeutic use arose from Professor
Cohn's ability to synthesize the basic knowledge arising from previous research, his shrewdness in visualizing practical production problems on a large
scale, and his ability to lead a team of diversely trained individuals. This is
graphically illustrated in the basic paper of a series presented to the American
College of Physicians in May 1947.[46] The system depended upon the ability to
control five variables—pH (hydrogen ion concentration), ionic strength,
alcohol (ethanol) concentration, protein concentration, and temperature—all
variables that influence the solubility of proteins. These had to be controlled
within limits tolerated by the protein molecules in order to avoid damage to
the structure upon which their physiological properties depend.

Knowledge of the structure and molecular properties of the plasma
proteins and information concerning their molecular size, shape, and electrical
charges had come from the introduction of the technique of electrophoresis by
Tiselius[47] and the development of the ultracentrifuge by Svedberg and Pedersen.[48] These new research tools, of Scandinavian origin and principally
developed in Uppsala, provided Cohn the means he needed to characterize the
different fractions of plasma and to establish the purity and molecular characteristics of the different fractions.[49] Subsequent characterization of isolated
proteins, accomplished by immunochemical methods of identification and
measurement (Figure 17-1), was carried out in France, Switzerland, Germany,
and the United States. For even greater precision, combinations of physical
and immunological methods were used (Figure 17-2).

Within a few months, the earlier work of the laboratory on the solubility of
proteins paid off. It became clear that the tendency for bovine plasma to induce
delayed reactions was associated with some of the globulins rather than with

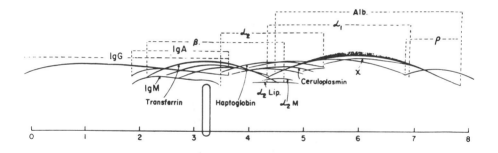

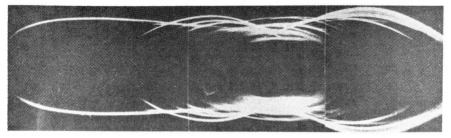

Figure 17-1 Typical immunoelectrophoretic analysis of whole human serum with a horse antiserum to normal human serum. The diagram above identifies the components. (*From Putnam FW [ed]: The Plasma Proteins. Structure, Function and Genetic Control, 2d ed. New York, Academic Press, 1975, vol 1, p 15.*)

the albumin fraction. Furthermore, existing data, reinforced by a few experiments in animals, indicated that the albumin fraction, with its smaller molecular size and greater net charge, should exert the greater osmotic effect. This was quickly proven by Dunphy and Gibson in studies upon animals in experimental shock.[50] Moreover, skin tests of preparations of bovine serum albumin gave rise to few reactions, in contrast with bovine globulin fractions similarly tested in humans. Solutions of bovine albumin, crystallized for maximum purity, seemed to have ideal physical properties for use as a blood substitute to be given intravenously. They were administered intravenously to human volunteers, with few difficulties. The results looked hopeful, but it was never possible to rid these bovine albumin solutions of their tendency to produce delayed serum sickness in a small percentage of human recipients.[41,51]

Meanwhile, Dr. Cohn, with his characteristic foresight, had surmised that even if the preparatory work were successful, it might be exceedingly difficult to persuade physicians, with their traditional conservatism, to take two bold new steps simultaneously in the treatment of the severely wounded. First, they would have to use an animal protein derivative; second, the use of a fraction rather than whole plasma to replace lost blood was also novel. So he arranged to obtain blood from human volunteers through a neighboring hospital's blood bank and initiated a study of its fractionation by methods

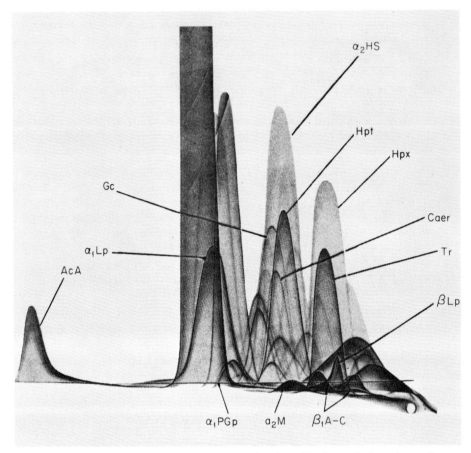

Figure 17-2 Crossed immunoelectrophoresis developed by Laurell gives three-dimensional effect. *(From Clarke and Freeman in Putnam FW [ed]: The Plasma Proteins. Structure, Function and Genetic Control, 2d ed. New York, Academic Press, 1975, vol 1, p 17.)*

similar to those used for animal blood. In a short time, a comparable fraction of human plasma albumin was available for trial. Its physiological effects and chemical properties were very similar to those of bovine albumin, but it was immunologically different, being a protein native to human beings. In human subjects, its injection was not followed by the delayed reactions that had been seen with the bovine preparations.

Human Serum Albumin

The work on human serum albumin was pushed ahead rapidly with the support of the United States Office of Scientific Research and Development on the advice of its Committee on Medical Research. Part of Cohn's laboratory was turned into a small-scale manufacturing plant staffed by its members. This pilot plant, which operated 7 days a week, 24 hours a day throughout the war, continued to produce human serum albumin and other fractions from the plasma collected in Boston by the American Red Cross for research purposes (Figure 17-3). Standards were established and bottling, sterility, and safety testing were carried out by the federally licensed biological laboratories of the Massachusetts Department of Public Health, while the clinical effectiveness and safety of human serum albumin were tested in various teaching hospitals.

This unusual effort in a university laboratory was already in full swing when news of the bombing of Pearl Harbor reached Boston. All the finished preparations of human serum albumin in the pilot plant (about a dozen bottles!) were hastily packed for a flight to Hawaii with Dr. I.F. Ravdin, then professor of surgery at the University of Pennsylvania, who was a member of the National Research Council's Committee on Blood and Blood Derivatives. He administered them to a few wounded and burned patients and satisfied himself of the effectiveness of albumin administration as a safe antishock measure. With the considerable experience gained from previous clinical trials in civilian hospitals and with this limited but rather dramatic experience at

Figure 17-3 Plasma processing. Compare the scale of operations in the Harvard pilot plant and in an industrial plasma fractionation plant. (*From Cohn EJ: The history of plasma fractionation, in Advances in Military Medicine. Boston, Little, Brown, 1948, vol 1, 472 pp, p 368.*)

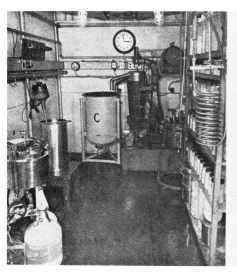
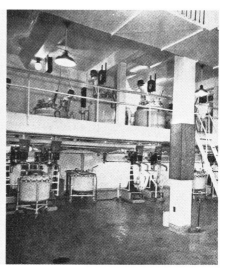

Harvard pilot plant.   *Industrial plant.*

Pearl Harbor, a unit of 100 ml of a 25% solution of human serum albumin was recommended by the National Research Council to the armed forces for the emergency treatment of shock; this was roughly equivalent in osmotic effect to the standard 500-ml infusion of human blood plasma reconstituted from the frozen and dried state.

Steps were immediately undertaken to organize production of albumin on an industrial scale in a number of pharmaceutical laboratories under contracts with the U.S. Navy, in addition to production of dried plasma under previously negotiated Army contracts. Before the war ended, 13,326,242 voluntary donations of blood had been made to the Red Cross Blood Donor Service by U.S. citizens. Some 10,299,470 of these donations were processed to dried plasma, while 2,239,175 were used for the preparation of human serum albumin by certain biological laboratories.

But before this massive production feat could be accomplished, much had to be done—the assurance of adequate supplies of donor blood and its collection and allocation for different purposes (e.g., fresh blood, plasma, and albumin, as well as whole blood for research). All this was accomplished through the network of Red Cross Blood Donor Centers. Health standards for donor acceptance had to be established by the U.S. Public Health Service, together with standardization of the methods of preparation and specifications and proper safety controls for the testing of each preparation, based on the pilot plant's experience. Chemists and production technicians from those pharmaceutical firms with contracts were brought to Boston for instruction in the new methods of fractionation developed in the pilot plant while their pharmaceutical laboratories were being equipped for this new task. Dr. Cohn was given full authority by the Navy to see to it that contracts were fulfilled, that the technical personnel were properly trained, and that adequate control of the chemical processing, sterility, and safety standards was maintained so that no product would be released that did not conform to the standards established by research. In fact, only with Dr. Cohn's express approval was any preparation of albumin to be delivered to the Navy for distribution. This was made possible by having the pilot plant technicians work closely with the research group and by insistence upon careful clinical trials by our group in Boston before release.

Close collaboration with the armed forces was very important to the success of the albumin program. Representatives of the Army Medical Corps (Lt. Col., later Col., Douglas Kendrick) and of the Navy Medical Corps (Lt. Comdr., later Capt., Lloyd Neuhouser) worked very closely with Dr. Cohn's group. The latter was principally responsible for the design and production of the package to meet the Navy's special needs. It occupied approximately one-fifth of the space and weighed about one-sixth as much as the standard dried plasma package. The solution was placed in a double-ended bottle with

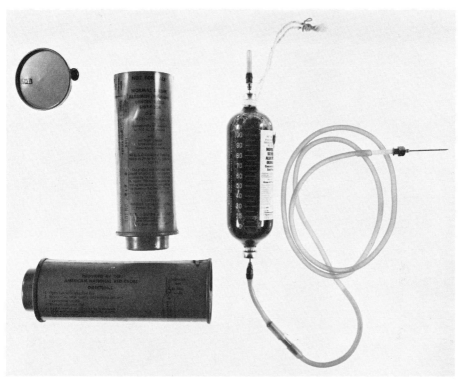

Figure 17-4 A single unit of 100 ml of concentrated human (25%) serum albumin assembled for clinical use. The whole unit was packaged in a cylindrical can; three cans in a box occupied very little space. (*Courtesy of Dr. Lloyd Neuhouser, MC, USN Ret.*)

a rubber stopper at each end, one at the top to permit insertion of an airway needle and one at the bottom for insertion of the administration line leading to the patient. This made it possible to start an infusion with a minimum of maneuvers and time (Figure 17-4). The upper stopper permitted the insertion of a needle through which other parenteral fluids, such as saline, glucose, or whole blood, all of which were freely miscible with the albumin solution, could be administered.

Clinical investigation led to the choice of package size and dosage. Moving from animal experiments, physiological investigators studied the hemodynamic changes following removal of measured amounts of blood from volunteers and their rates of recovery under different conditions (Figure 17-5).[52,53] These experiments provided an excellent baseline for studies of the effects of the administration of concentrated human serum albumin upon plasma

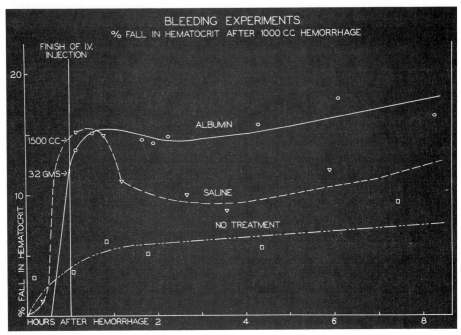

Figure 17-5 The type of experiment carried out in human volunteers by Ebert, Stead, and Gibson[53] to establish the osmotic activity of concentrated human albumin following acute blood loss. (*From Cohn EJ: The history of plasma fractionation, in Andrus EC, Bronk DW, Carden GA Jr, Keefer CS, Lockwood JS, Wearn JT, Winternitz MC [eds]: Advances in Military Medicine. Boston, Little, Brown, 1948, p 787.*)

volume and the circulation (Figure 17-6). Prof. George Scatchard, of the Massachusetts Institute of Technology, who was in charge of studies of osmotic pressure, developed a theoretical figure indicating that each gram of albumin administered should increase the plasma volume of a normal person by approximately 18 ml if equilibration were prompt following the removal of blood and the infusion of concentrated albumin.[54] With the usual variation inherent in physiological studies, there was remarkably good agreement between the expected results and those actually obtained in a series of clinical experiments with volunteers.

Considerable controversy arose over the wisdom of using a concentrated protein solution to increase osmotic pressure and plasma volume in the wounded, who were often already dehydrated. This question had been studied in volunteer experiments, but was raised again as a result of clinical studies made by the Army on the Italian front.[55] Consequently, Dr. Dickinson Richards, professor of medicine at the Columbia College of Physicians and Surgeons, and a collaborating group of investigators did a series of studies on

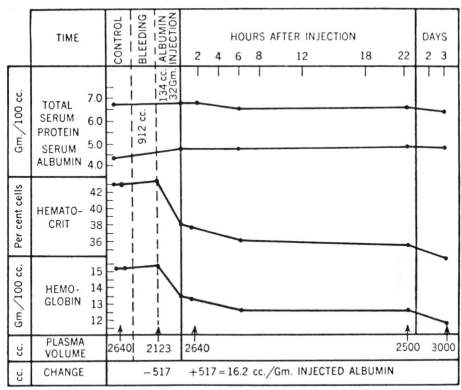

INCREASE PREDICTED FROM OSMOTIC PRESSURE MEASUREMENTS: 18 cc./Gm. albumin

Figure 17-6 A similar experiment showing the quantitative data obtained. *(From Cohn EJ: The history of plasma fractionation, in Andrus EC, Bronk DW, Carden GA Jr, Keefer CS, Lockwood JS, Wearn JT, Winternitz MC [eds]: Advances in Military Medicine. Boston, Little, Brown, 1948, p 788.)*

shock patients in hospitals in this country under the auspices of the National Research Council. Their data showed marked variations in the response to albumin because of the varied nature of the injuries and consequent differences in the amount and duration of the fluid losses in different patients. Nevertheless, careful study of the data did suggest that the average increment of plasma volume in the whole group studied was close to that expected on the basis of the figures derived from studies under much more controlled conditions.[56] This work justified the recommendation of 100 ml of 25% serum albumin solution as the standard unit, which ideally should increase plasma volume by approximately 500 ml in the absence of continuing plasma loss or dehydration. Naturally, dehydration as well as loss of blood or plasma needed to be corrected, but over the years there has been no evidence of harm from the use of the concentrated albumin solution except in a few instances where it was due to misunderstanding of the quantitative factors, particularly when albumin was administered to small infants by those without previous experience in its use.

Other Achievements of the Plasma Fractionation Program

There were several important consequences of the human albumin program, in addition to the provision of ample supplies of a safe, effective, stable, compact kit for the immediate resuscitation of the wounded at the front. First was the experimental confirmation in humans of Starling's work on the role of osmotic pressure in maintaining plasma volume and adequate perfusion of the tissues. Second was the demonstration that a fraction of the plasma, the one most responsible for its osmotic properties, could be separated and administered for that particular purpose. This information led the way to blood component therapy, i.e., the separation of each blood component in a form that could be concentrated, preserved in a stable form, and used at a time when it was specifically needed for therapy. This meant, in turn, a more economical use of each blood donation and better results because the specific protein needed could be given in a purer and more potent form.

Dr. Cohn felt a personal sense of responsibility for the careful stewardship of every voluntary blood donation. In the preparation of albumin, he took great care to see to it that all other fractions were processed to a stable state and preserved as well as possible for future study. Because the Navy only wanted the albumin, the American Red Cross, as trustee for the public, who had supplied the blood, was asked to arrange for the storage and processing of those products that might possibly have a further clinical use.

HUMAN ANTIBODIES

Using other funds, Dr. Cohn turned to study of the other plasma proteins. Dr. Joseph Stokes, Jr., professor of pediatrics at the University of Pennsylvania, had foreseen the possibility of using the crude gamma globulin fractions, fractions II and III, as a source of pooled human antibodies. By starting with pools of plasma from a large group of human adults (100 to 10,000), differences in antibody titer due to individual variations were likely to be minimized. Further purification of these two fractions by a group under J.L. Oncley separated the prothrombin in fraction III for use in coagulation studies from the major antibodies in fraction II, thereby obtaining immune serum globulins in a pooled product that represented an approximately 20- to 25-times concentration of human antibodies against diseases to which the donors of the plasma were immune. Standards for the chemical purity of this preparation, a clear 16.5% solution of 95% pure human serum gamma globulins, were established. The preparations were tested for their content of certain common antibodies by Dr. John Enders.[57] Finally, serum gamma globulin was used for the prevention and modification of measles in exposed, susceptible children. At that time, no direct laboratory measurement of measles antibody was possible, but analysis of the effects in exposed children of over 1000 injections of fraction II gamma globulin (immune serum globulin [human]) prepared from the plasma of healthy adult donors clearly proved two points: first, the results observed were predictably dose-related (Figure 17-7);[58] second, the product was safe, with a minimum of reactions following intramuscular injection and with no instances of subsequent serum hepatitis, a safety feature which had already been demonstrated for serum albumin. This observation led Stokes and Neefe[59] to test the protective effect of gamma globulin in individuals who had been exposed to epidemic hepatitis (now known as hepatitis A) from a contaminated well, and here again it was shown to have a modifying influence or even to prevent this disease. Gamma globulin has since been widely used to protect troops, Peace Corps volunteers, and travelers in tropical areas where hepatitis A is endemic. However, a modifying effect on serum hepatitis (hepatitis B) or on infection caused by more recently discovered viruses has not yet been established; the work of Krugman and others has attempted to unravel the complexity of immunity to the hepatitis viruses.[60] The development of sensitive methods for detection of hepatitis B antigens and antibodies in the serum of possible blood donors and the exclusion of those with positive tests has diminished the risk of hepatitis in recipients of blood and its derivatives in recent years.

It is possible to enhance the usefulness of human gamma globulin for specific purposes by using only the plasma of selected donors, such as those convalescent from recent infections who have been bled when high titers of specific antibody appear in the plasma or of those adults who have been actively immunized against certain specific infections. Thus, convalescent gamma globulin made from plasma of donors after *herpes zoster* (a recurrence of chicken pox virus infection in previously immune individuals) is used to protect children with leukemia or with certain types of immunodeficiencies against chicken pox infection, which may be very severe or even fatal in them. Hyperimmunization of adult donors with tetanus toxoid has provided plasma rich in human tetanus antitoxin as an alternative to that made from horse serum; it is more effective in protection and eliminates serum sickness, which was a frequent complication in the past. Krugman's group has tested high-titer convalescent gamma globulin for protection of individuals known to have been exposed to hepatitis B. This field of convalescent or hyperimmune gamma globulin prophylaxis and therapy is open for still further exploration.

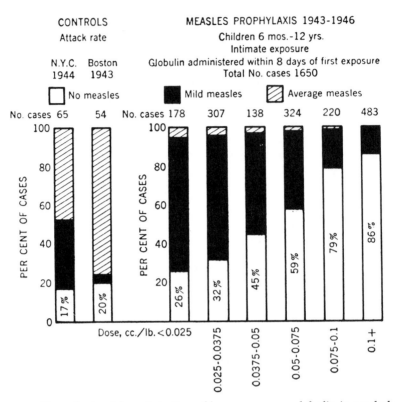

Figure 17-7 Data obtained from injection of human gamma globulin in graded doses during an 8-day period between first known exposure to active measles in a sibling at home and the appearance of clinical signs of measles in two epidemics that were carefully studied. Controls were similarly exposed and susceptible. Note linear relationship between the dose of gamma globulin injected and clinical results. (*From Janeway CA: Plasma fractionation, in Advances in Internal Medicine. New York, Interscience, 1949, vol III, 444 pp, p 328.*)

PROTEINS OF THE COAGULATION SYSTEM

While human serum albumin and human serum gamma globulin remain as standard derivatives of human plasma in general clinical use, a number of other derivatives have influenced the development of therapeutic agents from pooled human plasma. Fraction I, the fibrinogen fraction, originally was used to provide fibrinogen in instances where it was needed, for example, in certain obstetrical emergencies in which the blood becomes incoagulable because of in vivo formation of fibrinolysins or in those in whom synthesis of fibrinogen is depressed, as it may be in severe liver disease or in congenital afibrinogenemia

(Chapter 18).[61] The main drawback to its general therapeutic use has been the high frequency of serum hepatitis in its recipients. Fraction I, although principally fibrinogen, also contains the antihemophilic factor, as first demonstrated by Minot and Taylor;[62] it is capable of restoring normal coagulability to hemophilic plasma in vitro or in vivo to patients bleeding from this disease. However, a better preparation for this purpose from normal plasma, cryoprecipitate,[63] is now available, as discussed by Dr. Ratnoff in Chapter 18. Some fractions of human plasma may provide starting material for further research on newly described proteins or for the discovery of new proteins. In some cases, special precautions may be necessary to preserve the delicate molecular structure of a protein upon which its functional properties depend; knowledge of these relationships may require special preparative techniques. As research advanced during the 15 years between publication of the first and second editions of Putnam's comprehensive book on the plasma proteins, the list of known plasma proteins has expanded from albumin and the α, β, and γ globulins to an ever growing list, "limited only by the sensitivity of the methods of detection and the zeal of the investigator."[64]

Still Other Proteins

There are proteins for the specific binding and transport of certain substances, for example, *haptoglobin*, which combines so specifically and firmly with free hemoglobin that their combination can be used for measurement of its concentration in blood. *Transferrin* combines specifically with iron for its transport from the intestinal tract to the bone marrow for use in hemoglobin synthesis. *Ceruloplasmin* is a normal copper-containing protein with oxidase enzyme activity. Its solutions are sky blue in color. Ceruloplasmin is known to be involved in the metabolism of copper but in ways that are still not fully understood. Wilson's disease is a hereditary disease which progressively affects the function of the liver and brain with gradual copper accumulation in abnormally large amounts in these tissues, resulting in the development of symptoms in affected older children or young adults. Diagnosis may be confirmed by measurement of the serum level of ceruloplasmin. By limiting copper intake and enhancing its excretion, progress of the disease can be slowed and symptoms prevented.

The fatty substances absorbed from foods and the cholesterol synthesized in the tissues are rendered water-soluble for transport by combining them with special peptides as *lipoproteins*. Many of the hormones that regulate metabolism have special transport proteins. Although hormones are often present in trace amounts, the development of sensitive radioactive assay techniques has made it possible to readily measure the function of most of the endocrine glands.[65]

Tissue damage or overactivity of certain enzyme systems results in the liberation of those enzymes into the plasma.[66] These can be measured and may serve, for example, as indicators of heart muscle injury in heart attacks or as evidence of the growth of certain tumors. These "passenger proteins" represent an overflow of tissue proteins into the circulation.

In addition, several groups of proteins in the plasma represent important functional systems that are normally in balance, but these, once triggered by an appropriate stimulus, set off a chain of reactions, which manifest themselves in various ways. Thus, the coagulation system (see Chapter 18) is triggered by the escape of blood; contact with a foreign surface initiates a sequence of reactions, ending with a clot, which ultimately may dissolve by the subsequent activation of an inert protein, plasminogen, to a potent fibrinolysin. The complement system, consisting of some nine interacting proteins and at least three inhibitors of certain components, accounts for many of the phenomena of inflammation and plays a role in resistance to infectious disease.

Proteins, synthesized for specific functions, may be deficient and, thus, can give rise to symptoms due to such deficiency. These may arise in several ways. Thus, a genetic defect may result either in the absence of a specific protein or in the synthesis of a functionally inadequate molecule or "nonsense" protein. For example, hereditary angioneurotic edema is due to the lack of an inhibitor of the enzymatic activity of the activated first component of the complement system (C1 esterase). The majority of affected individuals lack this inhibitor, but in a few families, normal amounts of inhibitor are demonstrable when measured by the use of specific immune serum. However, the esterase activity is not neutralized by this inhibitor; thus, a nonfunctional protein is produced by such persons.

Certain general properties of the plasma proteins are important in relation to their functional role. By and large, those protein molecules with high net charge and lower molecular weight are responsible for osmotic pressure and, hence, for the maintenance of blood volume and for the binding and transport of various ions and drugs. In this role, albumin is predominant. It is synthesized by the liver cells; its level tends to fall in protein malnutrition or with chronic loss of protein, as in the case of nephritis or burns.

The immunoglobulins or antibodies are the one large group of plasma proteins not formed in the liver but by cells of the lymphoid tissues (Chapter 14) in response to antigenic stimuli to the reticuloendothelial system. Of all the groups of plasma proteins, specific immunoglobulins may increase to very high levels, either from the stimulus of chronic infection or the synthetic activities of clones of cells of specific lymphoid tumors.

The synthesis of the different individual proteins is under genetic control, both as to amount and structure of the protein. Most of the blood proteins have polymorphisms (different structures in terms of the sequence of the amino acids that account for their properties that do not necessarily affect their major functional role). Analysis of the inheritance of these polymorphisms has been a very useful tool in studies of human heredity.

Conclusion

Thus, the plasma fractionation program clearly established the principle that specific proteins can be purified, stored under conditions best adapted to each, and administered to patients to restore the missing components and the function which each subserves, thereby ensuring the most economical use of each blood donation. It also led to the establishment of high standards for the processing and purification of proteins from biological mixtures based on an exact knowledge of their chemical properties and to improvements in standards for the acceptance of biological products and their control by the Public Health Service. The methods of fractionation were designed for ease in production on an industrial scale, for the production of the major fractions (albumin and gamma globulin) in large quantities, and also as a means of salvaging these useful therapeutic agents from outdated blood and plasma in blood banks and even from the blood contained in placentas properly stored after delivery.

Dr. Cohn emphasized that it is a *medical* responsibility to select donors so as to avoid harm to them and to avoid the transmission of disease to recipients of the blood and blood derivatives, but it is a *technical* responsibility of chemists and engineers to protect the properties of the biological materials throughout the processes of blood collection, processing, and storage. Then, it once more becomes a *medical* responsibility to use the final product in those for whom it is indicated, without waste of a valuable material or danger to the patient. From these early beginnings, and as the result of the contributions of investigators throughout the world, the significance of the main transport fluid of the body, the plasma, and, particularly, the nature and functions of its numerous components has begun to be appreciated.

References

1   Harvey W: *Exercitatio Anatomica de Motu Cordis et Sanguinis in Animalibus*. London, Leach, 1653, 86 pp.
2   Vesalius A: *De Humani Corporis Fabrica Libri Septem*. Basileae, Ioannis Oporini, 1543, 663 pp.
3   Malpighi M: *De Pulmonibus Observationes Anatomicae*. Bononiae, Baptistae Ferronj, 1661, 24 pp.

4   Hewson W: An experimental inquiry into the properties of the blood, 1771.

5   Gulliver G (ed): *The Works of William Hewson.* London, Sydenham Society, 1846, 360 pp.

6   Hewson W: *An Experimental Inquiry into the Properties of the Blood. Part III. A Description of the Red Particles of the Blood.* London, T. Cadell, 1771, 204 pp.

7   Virchow R: *Die Cellular Pathologie in ihre Begründung auf Physiologische und Pathologische Gewebelehre.* Berlin, A. Hirschwald, 1858, 440 pp.

8   Bernard, C: *Lecons de Physiologie Expérimentale Appliqué à la Médicine.* 2 vols, Paris, J.B. Baillère, 1855, 1856, vol 1, 520 pp; vol 2, 510 pp.

9   Cannon WB: *The Wisdom of the Body.* New York, Norton, 1932, 312 pp.

10 Starling EH: The wisdom of the body: the Harveian Oration. *Br Med J* 2:685–690, 1923.

11 Pasteur L: *Oeuvres de Pasteur, réunies par Pasteur Vallery-Radot.* 7 vols, Paris, Masson, 1922–1939, vol 1, 480 pp; vol 2, 664 pp; vol 3, 519 pp; vol 4, 761 pp; vol 5, 361 pp; vol 6, 906 pp; vol 7, 666 pp.

12 Vallery-Radot P: *Life of Pasteur, 1902,* Devonshire RL (trans). New York, Doubleday, 1928, 484 pp.

13 Koch R: *Untersuchungen Über die Aetiologie der Wundinfectionskrankheiten.* Leipzig, F.C.W. Vogen, 1878, 80 pp.

14 Koch R: Die Aetiologie der Nützbrand-Krankheit, begründet auf die Entwicklungs-Geschichte des Bacillus anthracis. *Beitr Biol Pflanzen,* 2:277–310, 1876.

15 Pasteur L: Méthode pour prévenir la rage après morsure. *C R Acad Sci (Paris)* 101:765–774, 1885; 102:459–469, 1886; 102:835–838, 1886; 103:777–785, 1887.

16 Metchnikoff E: *L'immunité dans les Maladies Infectieuses.* Paris, Masson, 1901, 600 pp.

17 Ehrlich P: Uber die methylenblaureaciton der lebenden nervensubstanz. *Dtsch Med Wochenschr* 12:49–52, 1886.

18 Ehrlich P: Beitrag zur Kenntnis der Anilin farbung und ihre Verwendung in der mikrosckopischen Technik. *Arch Mikr Anat* 13:263–277, 1877.

19 Withering W: *An Account of the Foxglove and Some of Its Medical Uses.* Birmingham, Swinney, 1785, 207 pp.

20 Jenner E: *An Inquiry into the Causes and Effects of Variolae Vaccinae.* London, S. Low, 1798, 207 pp.

21 Holmes OW: The contagiousness of puerperal fever. *N Engl Q J Med Surg* 1:503–530, 1842–1843.

22 Holmes OW: *Puerperal Fever, as a Private Pestilence.* Boston, Ticknor and Fields, 1855, 60 pp.

23 Semmelweiss I: *Die Aetiologie, der Begriff und die Prophylaxis des Kindbettfiebers.* Pest, Wien, und Leipzig, C.A. Hartleben, 1861, 543 pp.

24 Snow J: On the pathology and mode of communication of the cholera. *Lond Med Gaz* 44:730–732, 745–752, 923–929, 1849.

25 Von Behring E, Kitasato SB: Ueber das Zustandikommen der Diphtheria-Immunitäts und der Tetanus-Immunitat bei Thieren. *Dtsch Med Wochenschr* 16:1113–1114; 1145–1148, 1890.

26 Von Behring E: Die Behandling der Diphtherie mit Diphtherie-heilserum. *Dtsch Med Wochenschr* 19:543–547, 1893; 20:645–646, 1894.

27 Domagk G: Ein Beitrag zur Chemotherapie der bakteriellen Infektionen. *Dtsch Med Wochenschr* 61:250–253, 1935.

28 Colebrook L, Kenny M: Treatment of human puerperal infections and of experimental infections in mice, with Prontosil. *Lancet* 1:1279–1286, 1936.

29 Marshall EK: Bacterial chemotherapy; pharmacology of sulfanilamide. *Physiol Rev* 19:240–269, 1939.

30 Dutrochet RJH: Nouvelles observations sur l'endosmose et l'exosmose. *Ann Chim Phys* 35:393–400, 1827; 37:191–201, 1828; 49:411–437, 1832; 51:159–166,; 60:337–368, 1835.

31 Graham T: On osmotic force. *Philos Trans* 144:177–228, 1854.

32 Graham T: Liquid diffusion applied to analysis. *Philos Trans* 151:183–224, 1861.

33 t'Hoff JH van: Lois d'équilibre chimique dans l'état dilué, gazeuse, ou dissous. *K Svenska Vetensk Akad Handl Stockholm* 21:1–41, 1885.

34 t'Hoff JH van: Die Rolle des osmotischen Druckes in der analogie zwischen Lösungen und Gasen. *Z Physikel Chem* 1:481–508, 1887.

35 Arrhenius SA: Ueber die Dissociation der in Wassergelösten Stoffe. *Z Physikel Chem* 1:631–648, 1887.

36 Bright R: Cases and observations; illustrative of renal disease, accompanied with the secretion of albuminous urine. *Guy's Hosp Rep* 1:338–400, 1836.

37 Starling EH: *Principles of Human Physiology*, 4th ed. London, Churchill, 1926, 1074 pp.

38 Starling EH: On the absorption of fluids from the connective tissue spaces. *J Physiol (Lond)* 19:312–326, 1896.

39 Janeway CA, Oncley JL: Blood substitutes, in Andrus EC, Bronk DW, Carden GA Jr, Keefer CS, Lockwood JS, Wearn JT, Winternitz MC (eds): *Advances in Military Medicine. I. History of the Office of Scientific Research and Development under Sponsorship of the Committee on Medical Research.* Boston, Little, Brown, 1948, 472 pp, pp 444–461.

40 Flosdorf EW, Mudd S: Procedure and apparatus for preservation in "lyophile" form of serum and other biological substances. *J Immunol* 29:389–425, 1935.

41 Cohn EJ: The history of plasma fractionation, in Andrus EC, Bronk DW, Carden GA Jr, Keefer CS, Lockwood JS, Wearn JT, Winternite MC (eds): *Advances in Military Medicine. I. History of the Office of Scientific Research and Development under Sponsorship of the Committee on Medical Research.* Boston, Little, Brown, 1948, 472 pp, pp 364–443. (This chapter on the history of plasma fractionation is complete and fully referenced by the man who not only directed this plasma fractionation program throughout the war years, but was so familiar with all its details that only a few other references are given where special emphasis is needed.)

42 Wangensteen OH, Hall H, Kremen A, Stevens B: Intravenous administration of bovine and human plasma to man: proof of utilization. *Proc Soc Exp Biol Med* 43:616–621, 1940.

43 Kremen AJ, Hall H, Koschnitzke HK, Stevens B, Wangensteen OH: Studies on the intravenous administration of whole bovine plasma and serum to man. *Surgery* 11:333–355, 1942.

44 Pirquet C von, Schick B: *Die SerumKrankheit.* Leipzig und Wein, Franz Deuticke 1905. Schick B (trans): Baltimore, Williams and Wilkins, 1951, 130 pp.

45 Cohn EJ, Edsall JT: *Proteins, Amino Acids and Peptides.* New York, Reinhold, 1943, 686 pp.

46   Cohn EJ: The separation of blood into fractions of therapeutic value. *Ann Intern Med* 26:341–352, 1947.

47   Tiselius A: A new apparatus for electrophoretic analysis of colloidal mixtures. *Trans Farad Soc* 33:524–531, 1937.

48   Svedberg T, Pedersen K: *The Ultracentrifuge.* Oxford, Clarendon, 1940, 478 pp.

49   Pedersen KO: *Ultracentrifugal Studies on Serum and Serum Fractions.* Uppsala, Sweden, Almquist und Viksells Boktryckeri A.B., 1945, 178 pp.

50   Dunphy JE, Gibson JG II: Effect of infusions of bovine serum albumin in experimental shock. *Surgery* 14:509–518, 1943.

51   Material presented on studies on bovine plasma albumin will be found in part in reference 40 and also in chapter XXIX of *Advances in Military Medicine,* vol I on Blood Substitutes, pp 444–461. Little, Brown & Co., Boston, 472 pp.

52   The Use of Human Albumin in Military Medicine. Part I. Heyl JT, Janeway CA: The theoretical and experimental basis for its use, pp 785–790; Part II. Woodruff L, Gibson ST: The clinical evaluation of human albumin, pp 791–796; Part III. Neuhouser LR, Lozner EL: The standard Army-Navy package of serum albumin human (concentrated), pp 796–799. *US Naval Med Bull* 40:785–799, 1942.

53   Ebert RV, Stead EA Jr, Gibson JG II: Response of normal subjects to acute blood loss. *Arch Intern Med* 68:578–590, 1941.

54   Scatchard G, Batchelder AC, Brown A: Chemical, clinical and immunological studies on the products of human plasma fractionation. VI. The osmotic pressure of plasma and of serum albumin. *J Clin Invest* 23:458–464, 1944.

55   Beecher HK: The preparation of battle casualties for surgery. *Ann Surg* 121:769–792, 1945.

56   Cournand A, Noble RP, Breed ES, Lauson HD, Baldwin ED, Pinchot GB, Richards DW Jr: Chemical, clinical and immunological studies on the products of human plasma fractionation. VIII. Clinical use of concentrated human serum albumin in shock and comparison with whole blood and rapid saline infusion. *J Clin Invest* 23:491–505, 1944.

57   Enders JF: Chemical, clinical and immunological studies on the products of human plasma fractionation. X. The concentrations of certain antibodies in globulin fractions derived from human blood plasma. *J Clin Invest* 23:510–530, 1944.

58   Janeway CA: Plasma fractionation, in *Advances in Internal Medicine.* New York, Interscience, 1949, vol III, 444 pp, p 328.

59   Stokes JW, Neefe JF: The prevention and attenuation of infectious hepatitis by gamma globulin. *JAMA* 127:144–145, 1945.

60   Krugman S: Viral hepatitis: Recent developments and prospects for prevention. *J Pediatr* 87:1067–1077, 1975.

61   Gitlin D, Borges WH: Studies on the metabolism of fibrinogen in two patients with congenital afibrinogenemia. *Blood* XIII:679–686, 1953.

62   Minot GR, Taylor FHL: Hemophilia. The clinical use of antihemophilic globulin. *Ann Intern Med* 26:363–367, 1947.

63   Pool JG, Shannon AE: Production of high-potency concentrates of antihemophilic globulin in a closed bag system. *N Engl J Med* 273:1443–1447, 1965.

64   Putnam FW (ed): *The Plasma Proteins. Structure, Function and Genetic Control,* 2d ed. New York, Academic, 1975, vol I, 481 pp, p XIII.

65 Antoniades H: *Hormones in Human Blood: Detection and Assay.* Cambridge and London, Harvard University Press, 1976, 810 pp.
66 Fishman WH, Doellgast GJ: Tissue derived plasma enzymes, in Putnam FW(ed): *The Plasma Proteins. Structure, Function and Genetic Control,* 2d ed. New York, Academic, 1975, vol II, 436 pp, pp 214–261.

CHAPTER 18

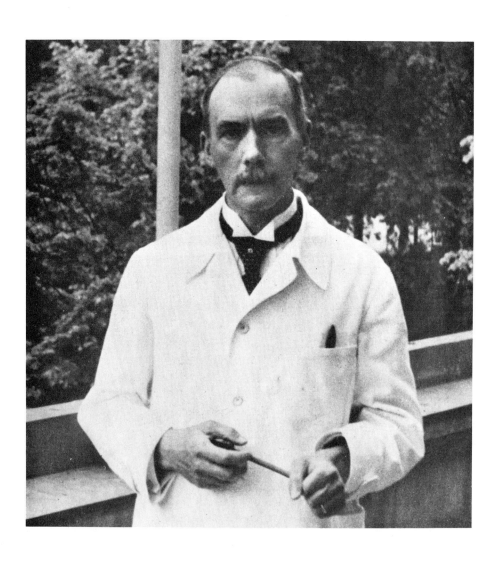

WHY DO PEOPLE BLEED?

Oscar D. Ratnoff

"One of the most striking properties of blood," William Henry Howell,[1] professor of physiology at the new Johns Hopkins University, wrote in 1900, "is its power of clotting or coagulating shortly after it escapes from the blood vessels." That hemorrhage might be stanched by the coagulation of blood was realized only at the beginning of the eighteenth century, when Jean Louis Petit,[2] the leading French surgeon of the time, recognized that bleeding would stop if blood clotted within and around a severed artery, plugging the wound. This observation was contrary to a prevalent view, that constriction and retraction of the injured vessel closed the wound mechanically.[3] Only at the end of the last century, with the studies of Bizzozero,[4] Eberth and Schimmelbusch,[5] and others, was it appreciated that platelets, the last of the blood cells to be discovered, provided an additional force to hemostasis, that is, the arrest of bleeding, by adhering to the walls of injured blood vessels.

Until the nineteenth century, progress toward an understanding of the nature of blood coagulation was necessarily slow and reflected the crudity of

Chapter Opening Photo   Paul Morawitz (1879–1936). (*Courtesy of M.M. Wintrobe.*)

601

biochemical knowledge. Now we are in an era in which each day seems to bring new insights into the intimate nature of the many reactions that change fluid plasma into the gellike state we call a clot. These advances have been spurred by a continual cross-fertilization of ideas and techniques between clinic and laboratory; studies of individuals with defective coagulation have led to the unanticipated discovery of one or another "clotting factor" participating in the sequence of events that brings about formation of a clot.

The earliest speculations about clotting are found in the writings of the Greek philosophers of the fourth century B.C. Plato,[6] in the *Timaeus*, thought that blood contained fibers which caused it to congeal when it left the warmth of the body and became cooled, a view that held until the end of the eighteenth century. Aristotle[7] added that the fibers were composed of earth and were solid and that blood from which the fibers were removed did not solidify. Two thousand years later, in 1666, the pioneer anatomist Marcello Malpighi[8] washed clotted blood so as to "dislodge the incorporated red particles," and in this way, he separated from it white fibrous strands. "If you enjoy a pretty sight," he said, "examine this blood with a microscope. You will see a fibrous texture, and a network of nerve-like threads." This experiment was repeated in a variety of ways by his successors, but no substantial progress was made until the 1770s, when William Hewson[9] localized the source of the fibers to the "coagulable lymph," that is, the liquid part of blood we now call plasma.

Hewson came as close as anyone to fathering the study of coagulation. Born in Hexam, England, in 1739, Hewson, like his father before him, became a surgeon and was, for a time, a partner of the great British surgeon William Hunter.[10] He married Mary Stevenson, whose mother Margaret was a close friend of Benjamin Franklin, a lodger at her home in London. During his brief life, as mentioned in Chapter 1, Hewson made many extraordinary observations, not only about coagulation but also about the red blood cells (erythrocytes) and the lymphatic system. He died at 34, the victim of an infection acquired in the dissecting room. His biographer George Gulliver[10] wrote of him, "If his works are not weighty and comprehensive enough to place him in the first class of physiologists, he is certainly entitled to the most exalted rank in the second," an understatement that reminds us that perspective about scientific contributions changes with time.

Hewson[9] observed that, contrary to the teachings of Plato, cooling blood slowed the clotting process. Other investigators soon found that coagulation took place most rapidly at or near body temperature, disposing of the view that clotting was comparable to gelling. Hewson had another explanation for the initiation of coagulation, believing that it was due to the exposure of blood to air when it was withdrawn from the body. This hypothesis was rejected by John Hunter[11] when he showed that blood clotted rapidly in a vacuum. John Hunter, William's brother, was one of the first clinical investigators, and his influence is still felt, although seldom appreciated. John's views on clotting, however, have not stood the test of two centuries. He thought, for example, that coagulation was due to some "vital principle" in blood. This nebulous theory found support in the writings of Thackrah,[12] Ernst Brücke,[13] and others, who refined it by stating that a vital or nervous influence provided by blood vessels kept blood from clotting.

Charles Turner Thackrah,[12] in his Astley P. Cooper prize essay, confirmed Hewson's[9] basic observation that blood clotted very slowly in a segment of vein isolated between ligatures, an experiment repeated ever since at frequent intervals. Thackrah wrote, "The inference is obvious, that the loss of motion is not the cause of coagulation," thus countering another popular view; Thackrah had been anticipated by Hewson,[9] who had concluded that "rest does not of itself in the least assist the coagulation of the blood." Another possibility, that the roughness of surfaces foreign to the blood vessels brings about coagulation, was shown to be incorrect by Rudolf Virchow,[14] the great German pathologist, when he found that a drop of mercury introduced into a blood vessel induced coagulation. Still another hypothesis suggested that the fluidity of blood during life was sustained by the continual removal of fibrin (as "citoyen" Chaptel[15] had named the fibers of the blood in 1797) from the circulation; perhaps fibrin was a source of nutrition.[16] This speculation has its modern counterpart in the probably incorrect hypothesis that clotting normally occurs continually throughout the vascular tree, a process later described as disseminated intravascular coagulation (see below), and that the fibrin that forms is continually degraded.

Hewson[9] and others of his time were aware that high concentrations of various salts kept blood fluid but that clots would form when blood was diluted with water. Such experiments brought about the view that alkalis might be therapeutically useful in preventing the deposition of clots. Conversely, carbonic acid impaired coagulation, as well it might because the enzymatic reactions of the clotting process and the formation of fibrin proceed optimally at the neutral pH of normal blood. Indeed, it was thought that carbonic acid was always being given off by blood during its coagulation, and the more quickly this occurred, the more quickly clotting ensued. A relatively modern expression of this erroneous view is Stuber's[17] suggestion that clotting results from the acidity induced in shed blood by glycolysis, the digestion of sugars. Bad ideas die hard.

The Conversion of Fibrinogen to Fibrin

Early investigators of the clotting process were unable to free themselves from the platonian view that fibrin, the insoluble protein that forms the structure of the clot, was present as such in circulating blood and that coagulation was, in effect, a precipitation or gelation of this preexisting substance. Early challenges were provided by Babington[18] and Richardson,[16] who believed that fibrin was formed during coagulation from a precursor, nowadays called *fibrinogen* (factor I),* a term popularized by Virchow.[19]

The source of fibrinogen was the subject of much debate, some believing, for example, that it originated within the red blood cells (erythrocytes) or within the white blood cells (leukocytes) while others localized its origin to the *liquor sanguinis,* that is, the plasma, and particularly to "albumin," the name then given to the bulk of the plasma proteins. Reflecting the primitiveness of early thoughts about plasma proteins Thackrah[12], in 1819, wrote that fibrin "is well known to form the basis of muscle," one of many similar speculations. Its synthesis in the liver was first suggested by the experiments of Corin and Ansiaux[20] at the beginning of this century and some years later was clearly localized to the cells of the liver.

Fibrinogen was first isolated from plasma in a crude way by Denis de Commercy,[21] who confused matters by calling it *plasmine* and later more completely by Olaf Hammarsten,[22] professor of medical and physiological chemistry at the University of Uppsala (Figure 18-1). It has been highly purified by many modern investigators and its structure almost completely elucidated.

How fibrinogen is converted into strands of fibrin is certainly not yet fully understood. The first clue was provided in 1845 by Buchanan,[23] professor of physiology at the University of Glasgow. Buchanan found that the addition of fresh serum induced the coagulation of hydrocele fluid, an abnormal collection of liquid within the coverings of the testis. Thus, he recorded, it takes two agents to bring about coagulation, what we now call fibrinogen and another substance that transforms this protein into an insoluble form (Figure 18-2). The substance in fresh serum that clots fibrinogen was rediscovered and intensively studied in the last century by Alexander Schmidt,[24] of Dorpat, in Estonia, who first named it *fibrin ferment* (that is, an enzyme that forms fibrin from fibrinogen) and, later, *thrombin.* Schmidt was a pupil of Felix Hoppe-Seyler, Rudolf Virchow's biochemical associate at the Pathologische Institut in Berlin. Jorpes[25] tells us that Schmidt's grandfather had fled from Prussia to Estonia to avoid military duty. After many years as a student in Germany, Schmidt returned in 1862 to the University of Dorpat (or Tartu), whose faculty was largely German. Schmidt was an imaginative investigator, unafraid to change his views as new data emerged. He was one of the giants of our heritage.

---

* Beginning in 1954, a group of investigators under the leadership of Dr. Irving Wright in New York tried to bring order out of the chaotic nomenclature that confused the scientific literature concerning blood coagulation. They formed an "International Committee of Blood Clotting Factors," now part of the International Society of Thrombosis and Haemostasis. Each clotting factor was assigned a Roman numeral, and authors were urged to use this nomenclature in parallel with the terms they preferred. Now the numerical nomenclature has largely displaced the use of trivial names. Although this has provided much clarity, misprints abound in the literature, and diagnostic and therapeutic errors have resulted from misinterpretation or misapplication of the Roman numerals. Wherever possible, trivial names are used to avoid these problems.

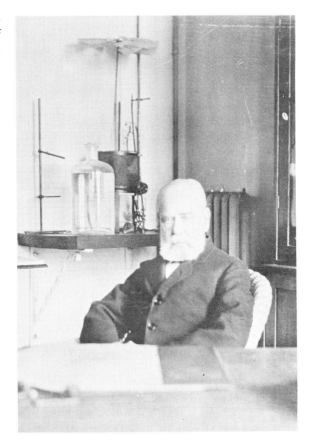

Figure 18-1 Olaf Hammarsten (1841–1912). *(Courtesy of the National Library of Medicine, Bethesda, Md.)*

Schmidt realized that thrombin could not exist in circulating blood without inducing coagulation. He therefore postulated that it evolved only during clotting from a precursor that Pekelharing[26] named *prothrombin* (Figure 18-3).

The source of Schmidt's proposed prothrombin was long a puzzle. Early investigators localized its origin to platelets, to leukocytes, or to other cells, views that only relatively recently have been shown to be incorrect by Harry Eagle[27] and others. Studies of Warner, Brinkhous, and Smith,[28] members of a potent team of investigators assembled by H.P. Smith at the University of Iowa, determined that the site of synthesis of prothrombin was the liver. Both prothrombin and thrombin have now been highly purified, current methods stemming from the monumental work of Seegers,[29] originally based on experiments of Jules Bordet.[30] Brinkhous and Seegers, Smith's students at the

Figure 18-2 Andrew Buchanan's (1798–1882) theory of clotting in modern terms.

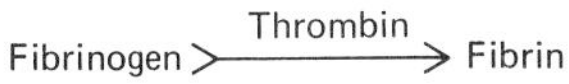

$$\text{Fibrinogen} \xrightarrow{\text{Thrombin}} \text{Fibrin}$$

University of Iowa, established schools of their own at the University of North Carolina and Wayne State University, respectively, where they have made almost innumerable notable contributions to our understanding of the clotting process. An early view expressed by Bordet[30] and by Quick,[26] that prothrombin exists in plasma in the form of a precursor, proserozyme or prothrombinogen, is no longer tenable.

Just how thrombin converts fibrinogen to fibrin was a puzzle. Before he appreciated the role of thrombin, Schmidt[31] thought that fibrinogen combined with another plasma agent, to which he gave the name *fibrinoplastin*, to form fibrin. Hammarsten,[22] however, could not confirm a role for Schmidt's hypothetical fibrinoplastin, and Schmidt dropped the idea. Rather, he accepted Hammarsten's view that fibrin ferment would clot fibrinogen in the absence of other recognized substances. Hammarsten[22] and Schmidt[24] believed that in this interaction thrombin behaved like an enzyme that partially digested fibrinogen. This concept had its adherents, notably John Mellanby,[32] but it was by no means universally accepted. The contrary view, that the reaction between thrombin and fibrinogen was stoichiometric, that is, nonenzymatic, had many supporters, among them Howell,[33] who was undoubtedly confused because the natural inhibitors of thrombin in plasma disguised its enzymatic properties. Acceptance of the proteolytic (protein-digesting) nature of thrombin has come only relatively recently with the studies of Eagle,[34] Bailey and his associates,[35] and Sherry and Troll.[36]

In its action upon fibrinogen, thrombin severs several small fragments of protein called *fibrinopeptides* from each molecule. What remains, the bulk of the original fibrinogen, is referred to as fibrin monomer. These fibrin monomers join one with another to form the insoluble fibers of the clot. That this process of *polymerization* occurs in stages was first proposed by Schmidt[24] and Hammarsten[22] and then revived by Apitz,[37] who called the soluble, as yet unclotted, intermediate forms *profibrin.*

One current view suggests that the first fibrin monomers that are generated form loose complexes with the surrounding unaltered fibrinogen molecules and are held together by electrical rather than chemical bonds. When sufficient fibrin monomers have evolved, these complexes break up, and fibrin monomers adhere to each other to form the visible fibrin clot, a process called *aggregation.* Contrary to early teachings,[38,39] calcium ions are not needed for the coagulation of fibrinogen by thrombin. Still, such ions greatly accelerate fibrin formation by speeding the aggregation of the fibrin monomers, so that the common discreditation of the earlier view seems harsh.

In 1858, Richardson[16] noted that once blood had coagulated, rapid re-

Figure 18-3 Alexander Schmidt's (1831–1894) concept of the origin of thrombin.

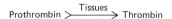

Prothrombin >——Tissues——> Thrombin

solution was extremely difficult. If, however, he immersed freshly prepared fibrin in a solution of ammonium hydroxide, the fibrin dissolved and could then be recoagulated by the addition of calcium or potassium hydroxide. Similarly, Gamgee[40] could dissolve freshly prepared fibrin in strong salt solutions, but he also called attention to earlier studies of Denis, in which *arterial blood* clots did not dissolve under similar conditions. These observations are consistent with our current knowledge that fibrin prepared from purified fibrinogen and thrombin lacks tensile strength and dissolves in solutions of urea or other "dispersing agents," as if it were held together only loosely. In contrast, fibrin formed in normal plasma has high tensile strength and is insoluble in dispersing agents. Robbins[41] and Laki and Lorand[42] attributed these properties of the fibrin formed in plasma to the formation of tight chemical bonds among the fibrin monomers brought about by the action of a plasma enzyme, *fibrin-stabilizing factor (fibrinoligase, factor XIII)*. Inert in circulating plasma, plasma fibrin-stabilizing factor is converted by thrombin to a form that can build these chemical links (Figure 18-4).

DISORDERED FIBRIN FORMATION

In normal individuals, the concentration of fibrinogen averages about 270 to 300 mg per 100 ml, values accurately stated in the early nineteenth century by Thackrah[43] and by Gabriel Andral.[44] At various times professor of hygiene and professor of medicine at the University of Paris, as mentioned in Chapter 1, Andral was the author of one of the first textbooks on hematology, and one of the first to amass systematic hematologic data. Andral considered himself a "neohumorist," raising clinical chemistry to a position of importance.

Elevation of the concentration of fibrinogen during pregnancy and in inflammatory conditions such as pneumonia and "rheumatism" was clearly recognized in the early 1800s.[44] The increased concentration of fibrinogen in these conditions was correctly believed to be responsible for the rapid settling of erythrocytes that can be observed when unclotted blood is allowed to stand undisturbed within an appropriate container. This phenomenon, the basis for modern tests of the erythrocyte sedimentation rate, was observed at least as far back as the time of Hippocrates[16] and was one intellectual foundation for the clinical practice of bloodletting, which dominated therapeutics for more than 2000 years. This topic was discussed in Chapter 1.

That hemorrhage might result because the fibrinogen in plasma was decreased in concentration (hypofibrinogenemia) or altogether absent (afibrinogenemia) was first proposed by Andral[44] in the early nineteenth century,

Figure 18-4 A modern view of fibrin formation.

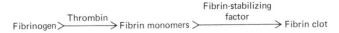

but his case histories lack conviction to current day readers. In more recent times, both hereditary and acquired hypofibrinogenemic and afibrinogenemic states have been described. *Congenital afibrinogenemia* was first recognized by Rabe and Salomon,[45] and, somewhat later, *congenital hypofibrinogenemia* was described by Risak.[46] These hereditary disorders must be distinguished from *congenital dysfibrinogenemia*, originally reported by Imperato and Dettori,[47] a condition in which fibrinogen, although present in plasma in normal or near-normal concentration, is functionally incapable of clotting in a normal manner. Dysfibrinogenemia is one of many coagulative disorders that are analogous to sickle-cell anemia and similar diseases in which the hemoglobin molecule has an apparently trivial defect that profoundly interferes with its function. (See Chapter 11.)

Acquired dysfibrinogenemia has been observed, too, primarily in patients with diseases of the liver. In the manner of biblical scholarship, one can always find prescient writers. In the early 1800s, Babington[48] wrote that "fibrine" may undergo alterations in quality in disease, while Rokitansky[49] provided a more universal hypothesis, that *all* disease was due to variations in the types of fibrin from situation to situation.

Hereditary deficiency of fibrin-stabilizing factor, a disorder associated with a severe bleeding tendency, was recognized first by Duckert.[50] In most instances, a nonfunctional variant of fibrin-stabilizing factor can be found in the patient's plasma, another example of synthesis of an aberrant protein.

The Formation of Thrombin via the Extrinsic Pathway of Coagulation

In 1832, during the course of a medical meeting, de Blainville[51] reported the astonishing observation that the intravenous injection of a suspension of brain tissue was immediately lethal, occluding the animal's blood vessels with clots. Thackrah,[43] too, was aware of the clot-promoting properties of tissues, noting that "if (blood) trickle from a wound or flow over an extensive surface, concretion almost immediately ensues, but if . . . it issue in a full stream and be received into a proper vessel, several minutes elapse before this process commences."

The clot-promoting effects of tissues was confirmed by Buchanan[23] and extensively studied during the last century. The major contributor to our understanding of their role was Alexander Schmidt. Tissues, said Schmidt,[24] provide a "zymoplastic," that is, an enzyme-forming, substance that can convert prothrombin to thrombin, the enzyme that changes fibrinogen to fibrin (Figure 18-4). Schmidt's experiments were repeated at the beginning of the present century by Fuld and Spiro[52] and Morawitz,[53] who confirmed that tissue extracts did not clot fibrinogen directly; rather, as Schmidt had said, they had the property of changing prothrombin to thrombin. Morawitz renamed the zymoplastic substance *thrombokinase*; later, Nolf[54] used the term *thromboplastin,* and Howell,[33] *tissue factor,* currently popular names. The action of tissue thromboplastin depended upon the presence of calcium salts, as had been proposed by Hammarsten;[22] this was in agreement with earlier observations that clotting was inhibited by the addition of oxalate[38] or citrate[55] solutions that made calcium unavailable for use.

Schmidt recognized that the "zymoplastic substance" he had extracted from tissues contained phospholipids (i.e., fatty substances combined with phosphorus). Much later, Mills,[56] Chargaff,[57] and others found that the procoagulant properties of tissue thromboplastin were associated with phospholipoproteins (complexes of protein and phospholipid); two components, both required for clot-promoting activity could be separated; one, a heat-stable phospholipid and the other, a heat-labile protein. Thromboplastic activity can be demonstrated in most tissues. Despite earlier views,[58] platelets are a notable exception.[59]

How the prothrombin that Schmidt had postulated was converted to thrombin has been the subject of almost as many theories as there have been investigators in this field. In 1905, Paul Morawitz[53] (Chapter Opening Photo), then an assistant physician at the Medical Clinic at Strassburg, proposed his now classical synthesis of the information then available, in which he described what is now called the *extrinsic pathway* of coagulation.* Clotting, he believed, took place in two steps. In the first, tissue thromboplastin changed prothrombin to thrombin; next, the thrombin that evolved converted fibrinogen to fibrin. Calcium was needed for the first but not the second step (Figure 18-5).

Innumerable other explanations for the clot-promoting properties of tissue thromboplastin were offered, probably the most influential being those of Wooldridge[58] and of Howell.[33] Wooldridge thought that tissues furnished a thrombin-like agent that brought about clotting through a direct action upon fibrinogen. Blood, he said, contained two components, each composed of protein and a fatty substance, lecithin, and to these he gave the names A-fibrinogen and B-fibrinogen. Tissues, instead, contained only A-fibrinogen.

---

* That is, a pathway of coagulation that requires tissue factor. Coagulation, we now know, is initiated by two fundamentally different mechanisms, by the action of tissue factor (extrinsic pathway) and by contact activation (intrinsic pathway). These ultimately converge by activating a third common pathway, as will be described below.

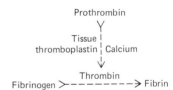

Figure 18-5 Morawitz's classic theory of clotting.

Clotting was brought about by a reaction between A-fibrinogen and B-fibrinogen; Schmidt's thrombin was viewed, cart before horse, as a product of coagulation rather than as a prime mover. Thus, Wooldridge denied Schmidt's explanation of the action of tissue thromboplastin—and this he did, rather characteristically, in the most acrimonious terms.

Wooldridge, an assistant physician to Guy's Hospital, in London, was apparently a contentious figure, and his heterodox ideas were such that some of his papers, even his Croonian lectures, were rejected for publication "with comments . . . more forcible than polite." In Morawitz's[53] words, "Wooldridge consistently interpreted his own accurate data incorrectly," not exactly a unique phenomenon. His views, however, had a wide circulation and a lingering life and were echoed as late as 1921 by Mills and Guest,[60] who suggested that clotting took place when "tissue fibrinogen" was linked directly to plasma fibrinogen by calcium ions. And, more recently, Murray[61] claimed that extracts of aorta contained a thrombin-like substance, to which he gave the name "vasculokinase."

Howell's ideas were similarly both ingenious and unorthodox. He[33] thought that circulating blood did not clot because it contained inhibitors that were normally joined to prothrombin. When tissue thromboplastin was added to plasma, its phospholipid portion detached the inhibitors from prothrombin. In this way thrombin was separated from the prothrombin inhibitor complex and was now available for clotting. Undoubtedly in part because Howell was the first professor of physiology at the Johns Hopkins University School of Medicine, his ideas carried great weight. Variants of his construct were provided by the distinguished Belgian immunologist Jules Bordet[30] and by John Ferguson,[62] a South African physiologist transplanted to the United States. These investigators suggested that thrombin resulted from the formation of a complex of tissue thromboplastin (cytozyme), or its phospholipid portion, and prothrombin (i.e., serozyme). Another Belgian, Nolf,[54] thought much along the same vein: fibrin, he said, was a complex of fibrinogen and thrombin, the latter derived from the union of thrombogen (i.e., prothrombin) and thrombozyme (i.e., thromboplastin); in turn, thrombozyme was a proteolytic enzyme derived from white blood cells or from the vascular endothelium, the cells lining blood vessels. And Pickering[63] saw the action of tissue thromboplastin as disturbing a colloidal complex of prothrombin and fibrinogen so that the latter gelled.

The times were not ripe. An explanation for the role of tissue thromboplastin had to await the discovery of the additional agents in plasma that are required for the formation of thrombin via the extrinsic pathway.

PROACCELERIN, FACTOR VII, AND STUART FACTOR

Despite many challenges, for many years Morawitz's classic theory provided the best explanation for the events that take place when blood coagulates.

Largely overlooked were the disturbing experiments at the beginning of the century of Nolf[54] and Bordet[30] that suggested that substances in addition to tissue thromboplastin, prothrombin, and calcium ions were needed for the evolution of thrombin. Then, during the 1930s, observations by the Iowa group of investigators[64] and by Armand J. Quick[65] (Figure 18-6) provided the impetus needed for a reexamination of Morawitz's views, for the new data could not be fitted into the earlier paradigm.

As is often the case, the new insights were made possible by improvements in technology. Warner, Brinkhous, and Smith[28] devised a two-stage assay for measuring prothrombin in plasma. In the first step, prothrombin was converted to thrombin by the addition (in vitro) of tissue thromboplastin and calcium ions, and, in the second step, the thrombin that was generated in this way was quantified. At almost the same time, Quick[66] introduced a one-stage assay for prothrombin in which the clotting time of decalcified plasma was measured upon the addition of thromboplastin and calcium, so that the two stages envisioned by Morawitz were not separated. This test, the one-stage

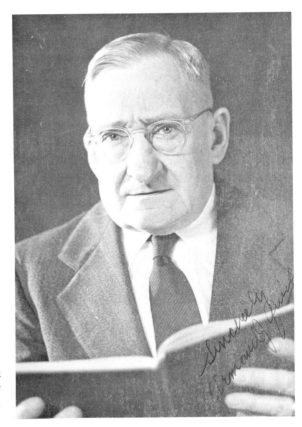

Figure 18-6 Armand J. Quick (1894–1977). (*Courtesy of the National Library of Medicine, Bethesda, Md.*)

prothrombin time, quickly became one of the commonest of laboratory procedures. It provided clinicians with a ready diagnostic tool for uncovering any defects of the extrinsic pathway of clotting (Figure 18-7) and provided indispensible aid in the treatment of patients with oral anticoagulant agents. Quick, working first in New York and later in Milwaukee, was a contributor of the first magnitude to our understanding of the clotting mechanism, but his simple prothrombin time towers over his other achievements because of its extraordinary everyday utility.

Soon after the one-stage and two-stage techniques for measuring pro-thrombin were devised, it became apparent that the results obtained by the two methods were discordant in some situations, such as in early infancy and when blood was stored at 4°C. These discrepancies led to the assumption that the conversion of prothrombin to thrombin by tissue thromboplastin was dependent upon the presence of additional plasma agents. During the suc-ceeding years, three such additional clotting factors were found, proaccelerin (factor V), factor VII, and Stuart factor (factor X).

Proaccelerin, the first of the new factors to be discovered, was described independently by Quick and Owren. Quick[65] reported that an agent in plasma corrected the prolonged prothrombin time of oxalated plasma that had been stored at refrigerator temperatures. At first he believed that the agent that was depleted by storage was a component of prothrombin, but later, recognizing that this was not the case, he renamed it *labile factor*.[26] Meanwhile, unbe-knownst to Quick, Paul Owren,[67] while a physician of the Norwegian under-ground during World War II, studied the plasma of a woman with a lifelong bleeding tendency. The one-stage prothrombin time was abnormally long, a defect that was corrected by prothrombin-depleted plasma. Owren concluded that prothrombin-depleted plasma contained a substance, lacking in his

Figure 18-7 The extrinsic pathway of thrombin formation.

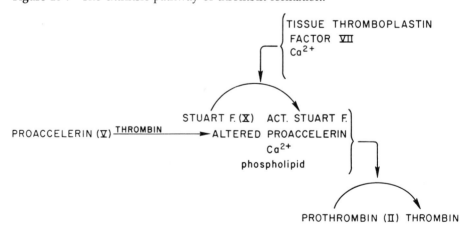

patient, to which he gave the name factor V (fibrinogen, prothrombin, tissue thromboplastin, and calcium ions being the other four factors). Factor V has been assigned many names, most happily Tage Astrup's[68] invention *proaccelerin*.

Two additional factors were soon found that seemed to be needed for the optimal conversion of prothrombin to thrombin. Their properties were such that at first they could not be distinguished one from another. Thus, in 1947, Owren[69] showed that something in plasma besides proaccelerin was necessary for tissue thromboplastin to change prothrombin to thrombin; similar observations were reported by several other groups of investigators. The usual congeries of names were applied to this newly discovered "factor," among which only factor VII survives. The importance of factor VII seemed established when Benjamin Alexander,[70] of Boston, reported studies of a patient with a bleeding disorder associated with a long one-stage prothrombin time. The prothrombin time was shortened by addition of serum, which was presumably deficient both in prothrombin and proaccelerin but contained the new agent.

A few years later, Hougie[71] and Telfer[72] proved that matters were more complicated. They described two additional patients, a lay preacher named Mr. Stuart and a young woman, one Miss Prower. Like Alexander's patients, these individuals had a long one-stage prothrombin time, corrected by the addition of serum. They were readily distinguished, however, because the defect in their plasmas was corrected by the addition to these plasmas of plasma known to be deficient in factor VII. Further, unlike the case of factor VII deficiency, their clotting defect was also corrected by the addition of the venom of Russell's viper, earlier recognized by Macfarlane[73] to have procoagulant properties. These patients appeared to be deficient in a distinctive clotting agent, to which the names Stuart factor[71] and Prower factor[72] were applied.

Factor VII and Stuart factor (factor X) have now been highly purified from bovine and human plasma. The possibility that activity originally attributed to factor VII might be due to two separate substances had been predicted earlier by Duckert.[74] Looking farther back, we can now understand some of Bordet's[30] (Figure 18-8) experiments demonstrating that fresh serum accelerated the generation of thrombin in plasma. And Nolf's[54] "thrombozyme," a constituent of plasma needed for the formation of thrombin, had characteristics suggestive of Stuart factor.

The early failure to distinguish between factor VII and Stuart factor was due not only to their similar properties but also to the fact that both need vitamin K for their synthesis. These similarities led Seegers and his colleagues[29] to a unifying hypothesis, that factor VII (autoprothrombin I), Christmas factor (factor IX, autoprothrombin II), and Stuart factor (autoprothrombin III) were all derivatives of prothrombin. This exciting view, based on

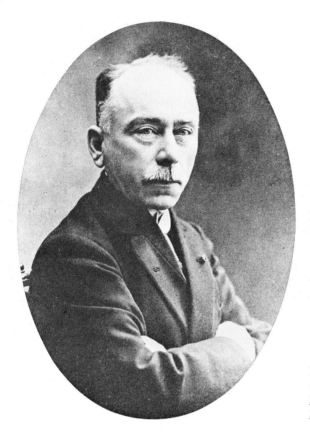

Figure 18-8 Jules Borde (1870–1961). (*Courtesy of the National Library of Medicine, Bethesda, Md.*)

meticulous experimental observation, did not gain general acceptance. One support for Seeger's theory was that certain preparations of prothrombin converted spontaneously to thrombin when dissolved in concentrated solutions of sodium citrate.[29] Mellanby,[75] too, had observed—and puzzled about—spontaneous thrombin formation in his prothrombin concentrates. Other investigators attributed this phenomenon to contamination of prothrombin with other clotting factors. At times, the debate concerning the nature of prothrombin took on an atmosphere of unseemly contentiousness, which was to a large extent subdued by the friendly atmosphere of the meetings of the International Committee of Blood Clotting Factors mentioned earlier. Now, Seegers, too, rejects his own earlier views.

THE ROLE OF VITAMIN K

To understand the development of modern ideas about the extrinsic pathway requires a diversionary glimpse at the part that vitamin K plays in the synthesis of clotting factors. The discovery of this vitamin is an example of the capitalization by keen investigators of accidental observations. In an attempt to study cholesterol metabolism, Henrik Dam,[76] of Copenhagen, fed chicks an ether-extracted diet. The chicks became anemic and developed a severe tendency to bleed; in at least one chick, the clotting time was abnormally long. Similar observations were reported by McFarlane[77] at Ontario Agricultural College, in Guelph, and by Almquist and Stokstad[78] at the University of California at Berkeley. Dam found that he could prevent bleeding by administering agents in cereals or seeds, to which he gave the name vitamin K, the "Koagulations-Vitamin."[79] The nature of the defect in vitamin K–deficient chicks was soon localized to a deficiency of prothrombin[80] that could be corrected by alfalfa;[78] only much later did it become clear that vitamin K was also needed for the synthesis of factor VII, Stuart factor, and Christmas factor. A role for vitamin K in human physiology was established by demonstrating that this agent corrected the deficiency of prothrombin in patients suffering from obstructive jaundice,[81–83] a situation in which bile salts, needed for the absorption of vitamin K, cannot reach the gut from the liver.[84] Isolation of vitamin K from alfalfa was achieved by Dam and his associates; its synthesis was announced simultaneously by several investigators.[85–87]

Meanwhile, Schofield,[88] a Canadian veterinarian, had investigated "a somewhat mysterious" hemorrhagic disease of cattle that had appeared in numerous herds during the winter of 1921–1922. He associated the disorder with the feeding of spoiled sweet clover. Schofield attributed the bleeding to impaired blood clotting.[89] The cause of this impairment was localized by Roderick to a profound deficiency of prothrombin; his treatment of the affected cattle by transfusion of normal blood is now one accepted practice for an overdose of oral anticoagulant drugs.

During the Great Depression of the 1930s, a farmer named Ed Carlson became desperate about the financial devastation brought about by the loss of his cattle, which he had been forced by necessity to feed spoiled sweet clover. He loaded his truck with a dead heifer, a milk can containing incoagulable blood, and about 100 pounds of spoiled sweet clover, and he drove some 190 miles to the University of Wisconsin looking for help.[90] Fortuitously, he interested Karl Paul Link, a biochemist at the University's Agricultural Experiment Station, in his plight, and Link identified the toxic component in the clover as bishydroxycoumarin (Dicumarol). This agent and its congeners, notably warfarin (named for the Wisconsin Agricultural Research Foundation), have found wide use as an effective rat poison and in anticoagulant prophylaxis and therapy for thrombotic states, the latter introduced by Butt,[91] Bingham,[92] and their coworkers. The coumarin anticoagulants have structural similarities to compounds with vitamin K–like properties and probably exert their effect by the competitive inhibition of the action of vitamin K in the cells of the liver.

How vitamin K brings about the synthesis of prothrombin and the other vitamin K–dependent proteins has recently been clarified. Vitamin K is not a constituent of those proteins that require its presence for their synthesis. Rather, as Quick[26] suggested, it appears to be an integral part of an enzyme that is needed for the synthetic process. The plasma of patients under treatment with coumarin-like drugs contains agents that are related to the vitamin K–dependent factors,[93] but these agents cannot bind calcium ions[94] and lack procoagulant properties. Studies by Olson[95] and others have shown that the synthesis of the vitamin K–dependent factors by the liver takes place in two steps. In the first, a nonfunctional protein is synthesized, a process that does not require the participation of vitamin K. In the second step, vitamin K directs the creation of an unusual amino acid through alteration of glutamic acid, one of the amino-acid building blocks of the protein molecule.[96] Ordinary glutamic acid has a carboxyl group, composed of carbon and oxygen, at one end of its structure. Vitamin K brings about the insertion of a second carboxyl group into certain of these glutamic acid components of the vitamin K–dependent factors. These uniquely altered *dicarboxylic* glutamic acids are necessary for procoagulant activity.

THE EXTRINSIC PATHWAY OF THROMBIN FORMATION

With the discovery of the three additional factors needed for the action of tissue thromboplastin, and of the way in which vitamin K brings about the synthesis of the factors dependent upon its presence, a new formulation of Morawitz's classic theory became possible (Figure 18-7). In the presence of calcium ions, a stoichiometric reaction occurs between tissue thromboplastin and factor VII.[97,98] Factor VII, treated in this way, then converts Stuart factor to an activated proteolytic state.

How tissue thromboplastin brings about the alteration in factor VII that is needed for its activity is not yet certain. Morawitz[53] believed that thromboplastin was an enzyme, a view that was later bolstered by observations that enzymes such as pancreatic trypsin could convert prothrombin to thrombin.[99] Now we know that these enzymes act at steps subsequent to the participation of tissue thromboplastin, and that Morawitz's view is untenable in its original form. Tissue thromboplastin also furnishes the phospholipids that are necessary but insufficient in themselves for the conversion of prothrombin to thrombin.

As Haskell Milstone,[100] a quiet and underappreciated physiologist at Yale, and Seegers[101] proposed, Stuart factor, once it has been activated, behaves like a proteolytic enzyme that slowly liberates thrombin from its precursor, prothrombin. The first small amounts of thrombin that form change proaccelerin (factor V) to a new, procoagulant state, a process first recognized by Ware and Seegers.[29] Proaccelerin, altered in this way, then binds through phospholipid and calcium links to the unique dicarboxylic acid components of as yet unaffected prothrombin molecules. These are then swiftly severed by activated Stuart factor, thus bringing about an explosive release of thrombin.

A review of earlier work reveals some insights that could not be exploited at the time. For example, many years ago, Arthus[102] recognized that thrombin was generated very slowly at first and then with dramatic rapidity in shed blood; Bordet[30] found that the addition of fresh serum, undoubtedly containing activated Stuart factor and thrombin, accelerated the formation of thrombin in plasma; and Bordet,[30] Wooldridge,[58] and Howell[33] were aware of the importance of phospholipids in the formation of thrombin. The possibility that calcium ions form a complex with phospholipids was the basis of Wadsworth's[103] theory of clotting. And the linkage of calcium ions to prothrombin that is currently envisioned is reminiscent of Pekelharing's[39] early proposal that prothrombin combines with calcium to form thrombin; this idea found a different expression in Quick's[104] view that prothrombin was normally combined in plasma with calcium ions and Mills'[60] and Ferguson's[62] hypothesis that the generation of thrombin followed formation of a complex of prothrombin, phospholipid, and calcium ions.

DISORDERS OF THE EXTRINSIC PATHWAY

Hereditary deficiencies of prothrombin,[26] factor VII,[70] Stuart factor,[71,72] and proaccelerin[67] have all been described. These familial deficiencies are inherited as autosomal, that is, as non-sex-linked, traits, in which homozygotes (individuals who have inherited the tendency from both parents) have a bleeding tendency. In some individuals, the factors that appear to be deficient in clotting tests can be detected by other means, giving us additional examples of the heterogeneity of inherited disorders.

Acquired deficiencies of prothrombin, factor VII, Stuart factor, and Christmas factor, which will be described later, are found in combination when there is a deficiency of vitamin K, that is, when this vitamin is available but is not absorbed by the gut or when it cannot be utilized because of the presence of liver disease or because vitamin K antagonists have been administered.

Hemorrhagic disease of the newborn is the principal example of a deficiency of the vitamin K–dependent factors secondary to an inadequate supply of this vitamin. It is unclear how long ago this disorder was first recognized, but Quick[104] reminds us that ritual circumcision among Jews is not performed until the eighth day of life, when any bleeding symptoms resulting from vitamin K deficiency have waned; this time may have been selected on the basis of empiric observation. Cases of neonatal bleeding that may have been due to hemorrhagic disease of the newborn were reported from time to time beginning in 1682,[104] but confusion with other causes of bleeding, for example, hemophilia, persisted until relatively recently. In a daring experiment for the time, Lambert,[105] in 1908, induced a prompt cure of hemorrhagic disease of the newborn by transfusion of blood by end-to-end anastomosis of the father's radial artery to the infant's left popliteal vein; we now know how this would correct the deficiency of clotting factors. A few years later, George Whipple[107] recorded that the plasma of an affected baby was deficient in prothrombin. By modern standards, Whipple's observations are easily faulted, but some years later Kenneth Brinkhous (Figure 18-9),[108] whom we have already seen as a major contributor to the understanding of hemostasis, firmly established that prothrombin was deficient in hemorrhagic disease of the newborn. Almost immediately thereafter, Waddell[109] introduced the use of vitamin K to treat this disease; untreated, hemorrhagic disease of the newborn is soon cured if the infant survives, as it acquires a supply of the missing vitamin both from its diet and from synthesis by bacteria in the gut.

Deficiencies of the vitamin K–dependent clotting factors are also a primary cause of bleeding in cases of diseases of the liver. Wedelius[110] is said to have described fatal hemorrhage in a patient with severe jaundice at the end of the seventeenth century, but it is not possible to know whether in this instance this symptom was attributable to liver disease. Little was written about the association of bleeding with liver affections until more than a century later, when Budd[111] recorded that there was likely to be "a tendency to hemorrhage

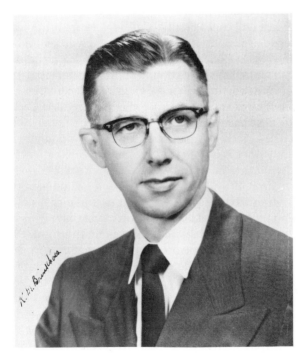

Figure 18-9   Kenneth M. Brinkhous (1908–   ). *(Courtesy of the National Library of Medicine, Bethesda, Md.)*

from the nose and other parts" in jaundiced patients. Trousseau,[112] in making similar observations, recalled that Galen had described epistaxis from the *right* nostril in hepatic disease.

Thackrah[12] may have been the first to observe delayed blood coagulation in patients with disorders of the liver. Many years elapsed until Morawitz[113] ascribed this delay to the decreased generation of thrombin, presumably because thrombin's precursor, prothrombin, was in short supply. And it was only relatively recently that the concomitant deficiencies of other vitamin K–dependent clotting factors became evident. These abnormalities are usually not corrected by treatment with vitamin K, in part because the diseased liver cannot utilize this vitamin and in part because other abnormalities of hemostasis are almost always present, including deficiencies of proaccelerin and other clotting factors as well as a decrease in the number of platelets in the circulating blood.

Bleeding is also frequent in patients with obstructive jaundice, a condition in which the flow of bile from the liver to the gut is blocked. The earliest reported cases of bleeding in jaundiced patients are as likely to have been due to an unrecognized obstruction of the bile duct as to intrinsic disease of the liver. It was only toward the end of the last century that Sims[114] and Murchison[115] associated hemorrhage with biliary obstruction. As physicians learned to operate upon patients with obstructive jaundice, bleeding during and after surgery was a major cause of morbidity and mortality.

In 1913, George Whipple[116] described a patient with obstructive jaundice in whom, he believed, the concentration of prothrombin was depressed. This observation was confirmed by Quick[66] and was consistent with experimental findings made during the 1930s that bile salts were needed for the transportation of vitamin K across the wall of the bowel.[117,118] Understanding of this phenomenon soon led to the use of vitamin K to correct the clotting defect of patients with obstructive jaundice,[81-83] and, by and large, this hazard of surgery for this condition has disappeared.

The Intrinsic Pathway of Thrombin Formation

"Why does the blood circulating in the vessels not coagulate?" asked T.W. Jones[119] in 1842, a question that today still has no satisfactory answer. Before the role of tissue thromboplastin was appreciated, no one doubted that clotting was an intrinsic property of blood. Rather, the focus of attention was upon how clotting was held in check within the blood vessels and was only brought into play when blood was shed.

When John Hunter[11] reported that blood clotted most readily "round the edge of the dish which it contained," he clearly did not grasp the implications of this observation. In 1863, Lister[120] embarked upon experiments that were designed to examine the idea that clotting was due to the liberation of ammonia. Almost incidentally, he made the important discovery that blood remained partially fluid for several hours in a vulcanized India-rubber tube but clotted promptly in an ordinary cup. He concluded that coagulation came about from the contact of blood with some—but not all—foreign surfaces and that blood remained fluid within our vessels as the passive consequence of the noncoagulant nature of their linings. Lister's conclusions were supported by Freund,[121] who found that clotting was retarded when blood flowing from an artery was collected in tubes lined with oil or vaseline, results similar to earlier experiments by Babington.[18] Thus, a century after Hewson had begun the scientific study of coagulation, the thesis seemed well established that circulating blood was fluid because it did not come into contact with agents that could initiate the clotting process.

Morawitz apparently believed that tissue thromboplastin was a sine qua non for coagulation. Nonetheless, he was aware that Wooldridge,[58] Barrier,[122] Bordet,[30] and Nolf[54] all had demonstrated that mammalian *plasma* remained liquid in paraffin-lined tubes but clotted when it came into contact with glass. With the exception that these experimenters took more pains to remove blood cells, their results were in agreement with the studies of Petit,[2] Hewson,[9] and Babington,[48] all of whom had appreciated that clotting occurred in plasma that had spontaneously separated from blood cells. These newer studies of cell-depleted plasma flew in the face of dogmas, probably first proposed by Hayem[123] and Bizzozero[4] and persisting to this day, that platelets must be present for blood to clot. Georges Hayem's ideas were particularly influential as he was probably the greatest French hematologist of his time. Morawitz[53] assumed that clotting occurred because plasma contained thromboplastic substances that constantly escaped into the plasma from tissues, particularly from extravascular platelets. Later, this view was modified by Collingwood and MacMahon,[124] who held that such platelet-derived thromboplastin was ordinarily in an inactive form in plasma and had to be activated for clotting to occur. Only a few investigators—Bordet,[30] Nolf,[54] Lenggenhager,[125] and Lozner[126]—championed the view that plasma itself contained all the factors needed for coagulation and could provide a "thromboplastin" that would initiate clotting.

The concept that plasma would clot in the absence of tissue thromboplastin languished until C. Lockard Conley's[127] decisive experiments, reported in 1949. Conley took advantage of Jaques'[128] technique of retarding surface-mediated clotting by coating the surfaces with which blood came into contact with silicone. He demonstrated that normal "native" plasma, separated from blood cells without the addition of anticoagulants, remained liquid indefinitely in silicone-coated tubes but quickly clotted when exposed to glass. The idea that plasma contained an activator of prothrombin that was in an inert state was the basis of Milstone's[129] seminal views on blood clotting, summarized in 1952. He envisioned that the conversion of prothrombin to thrombin was brought about by a "thrombokinase complex" derived during clotting from a "prothrombokinase complex." The latter, he thought, was composed of tissue, platelet factors, and the plasma agents that were then recognized, including phospholipids, antihemophilic factor (factor VIII), proaccelerin, and proconvertin (i.e., factor VII and the as yet undescribed factor X).

The course of events through which glass initiates coagulation in plasma is now described as the *intrinsic pathway* of thrombin formation (Figure 18-10). A modern paradigm for the steps of the intrinsic pathway, defined as the "cascade"[130] or "waterfall"[131] hypothesis, envisions that clotting is brought about by a sequential series of enzymatic steps; the details of this sequence have had to be modified as new knowledge has accumulated, but the general framework has remained unchanged until the present time.

Two techniques devised a quarter of a century ago greatly accelerated the study of the coagulation of plasma in the absence of tissue thromboplastin. The earlier of these, the thromboplastin generation test of Biggs and Douglas,[132] in Oxford, attempted to separate the clotting process into two steps: the generation of an agent that could convert prothrombin to thrombin and the measurement of the coagulant effect of this agent on normal plasma. Appropriate manipulation of the reagents used in the first step localized the defect in abnormal blood to the platelets, the serum, or a fraction of plasma that was depleted of the vitamin K–dependent clotting factors. Phospholipid

Figure 18-10 The intrinsic pathway of thrombin formation.

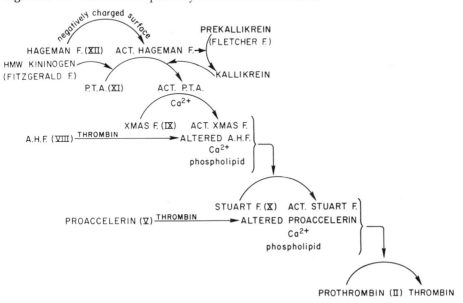

suspensions could be substituted for platelets in the reaction mixtures, supporting the view that these cells were not required for clotting. Although the theoretic basis of the thromboplastin generation test has gradually eroded, this procedure represented a major step in the evolution of current knowledge and, in modified form, still finds many uses.

The second method, described by Langdell, Wagner, and Brinkhous,[133] was the measurement of what they called the *partial thromboplastin time*. In essence, plasma was clotted by the addition of calcium ions and a source of phospholipid. Either the deficiency of a clotting factor or the presence of an abnormal inhibitor of clotting resulted in a delayed partial thromboplastin time. Later, this test was modified by the addition of a glasslike activator of clotting, such as kaolin, diatomaceous earth (Celite), or ellagic acid. The sensitivity of measurement is such that all but the mildest defects in the intrinsic pathway can be recognized.

THE EARLY STEPS OF THE INTRINSIC PATHWAY

Resolution of the question of which factor in plasma was activated by contact with glass waited for more than 50 years after the studies of Bordet, when a railroad brakeman, one John Hageman, came to Cleveland seeking surgery for his peptic ulcer (Figure 18-11). Although Mr. Hageman had no symptoms

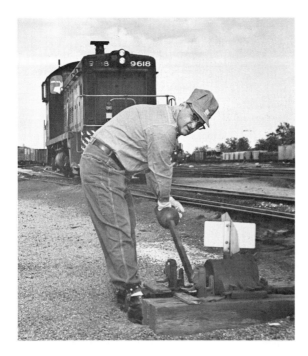

Figure 18-11 Mr. John Hageman, a patient whose clotting defect opened a new field of investigation. (*Courtesy of Robert Packo, Toledo, Ohio.*)

suggestive of a bleeding tendency, his blood clotted abnormally slowly. The defect was localized to the intrinsic pathway and could be corrected by the addition of a fraction of normal plasma which was devoid of the then recognized clotting factors.[134] The agent deficient in his plasma, to which the name Hageman factor (factor XII) was applied, had properties suggesting that it might have been responsible for phenomena that had been described earlier. For example, Bordet[30] was aware that plasma filtered through clay (kaolin) accelerated clotting, and Conley, Hartmann, and I[135] had observed that a crude fraction of plasma depleted of all the then known clotting factors nevertheless had clot-promoting properties. Hageman trait is a familial disorder that occurs in both sexes; protein resembling Hageman factor cannot be demonstrated in the plasma of affected individuals. Human Hageman factor has now been highly purified; its site of synthesis is unknown, but one likely candidate site is the liver.

Over the years, as "new" clotting factors were discovered, the site of action of glasslike agents in the initiation of clotting was assigned now to one and now to another. By 1956, Margolis,[136] at Oxford, and Shafrir and deVries,[137] in Israel, were able to show that glass did not act upon any of a number of clotting factors. In experiments borrowing their methodology, the clot-promoting properties of glass were localized to an action upon Hageman factor,[138] the shape of which was later shown to be warped as a result of the action.

An extraordinary number of insoluble substances besides glass can bring about the change of Hageman factor to a clot-promoting form. Physiologically, sebum, the oily film on skin, and some forms of collagen, a protein found in the connective tissues of the body, may play this role.[139] Common to all insoluble activators of Hageman factor is a negative surface charge.

Most clot-enhancing agents are solids. Tannins have long been known for their hemostatic properties; the barks of plants are said to have been used by the ancient Egyptians and Greeks for this purpose, and Richardson,[16] in 1858, remarked that coagulation "is favored in drawn blood" by the addition of tannin. A chance observation led to the discovery that solutions of an oxidation product of tannic acid could activate Hageman factor.[139] This agent, ellagic acid, was the major constituent of the bezoar stone, a concretion found in the fourth stomach of certain Middle Eastern mountain goats. During the Middle Ages, the bezoar stone was highly prized as an antidote against poisons and as a cure for depression; a search for a new, cheaper source was one of the motives that led to the discovery of the Americas. Indeed, the llamas of Peru furnished bezoar stones. Alas, the author has not been able to uncover any claim that the bezoar stone was used to halt bleeding.

The clot-promoting properties of Hageman factor, once it has been altered by glasslike agents, are mediated by its activation of plasma thromboplastin antecedent (PTA, factor XI), as first proposed by Margolis,[136] at Oxford, and

Vroman,[140] a native of the Dutch East Indies but now in Brooklyn, New York. PTA was described by Rosenthal[141] as a substance deficient in the plasma of two sisters with a relatively benign hemorrhagic tendency. Its deficiency has been observed with special frequency in Ashkenazi Jews and in Japanese in whom it is an autosomal trait that must be inherited from both parents.[142]

In early studies with relatively crude materials, the activation of PTA by Hageman factor appeared to be an enzymatic reaction. Unexpectedly, when purified preparations of Hageman factor and PTA became available, no activation of PTA could be detected. Clearly, some other agent or agents were needed for the activation of PTA. The nature of these reagents was learned in an unusual way.

Shortly after Hageman factor was recognized as the agent upon which glass acted to promote clotting, other reactions mediated by surface-activated Hageman factor were discovered. In brief, plasma that has been exposed to glass enhances the permeability of small blood vessels (thus allowing local leakage of plasma into extravascular tissues), induces pain, dilates small blood vessels, lowers arterial blood pressure, and stimulates the contraction of certain smooth muscles.[139] These effects are attributable to the release of certain small fragments of protein, known as *kinins*, from their precursors in plasma, appropriately called the *kininogens* (that is, the originators of kinins). Margolis[143] proposed that the release of kinins was brought about by the activation of Hageman factor and that this agent in turn changed a plasma enzyme, *plasma kallikrein*, to an active form that could bring about the release of kinins from the kininogens, a conjecture that was indeed correct.[139] There are several kininogens in plasma, and Jacobsen[144] reported that those of relatively high molecular weight were peculiarly susceptible to the action of plasma kallikrein (Figure 18-12).

In 1965, members of a family named Fletcher were brought to the University of Kentucky Medical Center Hospital for treatment of exposure to cold after the mountain cabin in which they lived had been destroyed by fire. Through this chance, Hathaway and his associates[145] found that four small children in this family had an abnormality of blood clotting that could be distinguished from other known disorders. Nonetheless, these children, said to have Fletcher trait, had no clinical evidence of a bleeding tendency. Hathaway separated a fraction of normal plasma that appeared to contain a hitherto unknown clotting factor that corrected the clotting defect of the affected children and to this agent they applied the name Fletcher factor. In parallel

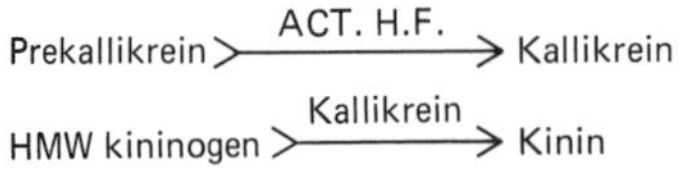

$$\text{Prekallikrein} \xrightarrow{\text{ACT. H.F.}} \text{Kallikrein}$$

$$\text{HMW kininogen} \xrightarrow{\text{Kallikrein}} \text{Kinin}$$

Figure 18-12 The evolution of kinins.

manner, in 1975, Waldmann and his coworkers[146] found a similar abnormality of clotting in a 71-year-old man, Mr. Fitzgerald, who was under treatment for a gun-shot wound but was otherwise asymptomatic. Again, a "new" clotting factor, lacking in Mr. Fitzgerald's plasma, was found in normal plasma, to which the name Fitzgerald factor was given. Almost at the same time, similar patients were found, some described as having Williams trait,[147] Flaujeac trait,[148] and Reid trait.[149] Both Fletcher factor and Fitzgerald factor appeared to function early during the course of the intrinsic pathway, before the participation of PTA.

At first, the nature of Fletcher factor and Fitzgerald factor was uncertain. Then, in an extraordinary series of studies, Wuepper[148,150] made the astonishing discovery that Fletcher factor was none other than plasma prekallikrein, the precursor of plasma kallikrein and that Fitzgerald factor was the same as high molecular weight kininogen. How these two agents bring about activation of PTA is uncertain and is now the subject of a healthy debate. No explanation is as yet available why patients lacking Hageman factor, prekallikrein, or high molecular weight kininogen are asymptomatic.

ANTIHEMOPHILIC FACTOR, CLASSIC HEMOPHILIA, AND VON WILLEBRAND'S DISEASE

To understand the subsequent steps of the intrinsic pathway, we must take another detour and review the evolution of knowledge about two closely related hereditary hemorrhagic disorders, classic hemophilia and von Willebrand's disease.

The disorder now called classic hemophilia was probably recognized as early as the second century. The Babylonian Talmud,[151] written several hundred years later, describes the decision of Rabbi Judah, a distinguished scholar, that the son of a woman whose three previous sons had bled to death after circumcision be excused from this rite. Thereafter, sporadic descriptions of individuals with severe bleeding tendencies appeared, notably those of an Arabian physician, Abu-'l'Qāsim Khalif ibn 'Abbis al-Zarāwi, otherwise known as Alsaharavius or Albucasis,[152] who died at Córdoba in 1107, and those of an anonymous author assumed to be G.W. Consbruch. In 1793, Consbruch described what Bulloch and Fildes[153] believed to be the first "classic instance of the disease . . . in the history of hemophilia," and recognized that only males were affected.

Appreciation of the sex-linked inheritance of hemophilia was one of the first American contributions to science; McKusick[154,155] has provided much information about this early history. In 1791, a newspaper account reported the story of a man named Zoll who had hemophilic sons by one wife and normal sons by another. A more penetrating analysis was soon provided by John Conrad Otto, a Philadelphia physician whose grandfather had been in charge of the hospital at Valley Forge during the bitter winter of 1778. Otto was apprenticed to Benjamin Rush, whom he succeeded as attending physician at the Pennsylvania Hospital. In 1803, Otto[156] recorded the "hemorrhagic disposition" that a "woman named Smith, settled in the vicinity of Plymouth, New Hampshire," transmitted to her descendants. "It is a surprising circumstance," he wrote, "that males only are subject to this affliction and that all of them are not liable to it. Although females are exempt, they are still capable of transmitting it to their male children." Otto may have been the first to use the English term "bleeders" to describe affected individuals, a word he ascribed to common parlance; perhaps the bleeders of Tenna, in Switzerland, who have Christmas disease, may have used the word "Bluter" earlier.[157]

During the last century, many attempts were made to unravel the hereditary nature of the disease that Johann Lucas Schönlein, the first professor of internal medicine at Zurich, is said to have named hemophilia.[158] The confusion that may have been posed because the many hereditary bleeding disorders were not yet distinguished was lessened by the happy coincidence that the two most common, classic hemophilia and Christmas disease, are inherited in the same way. That hemophilia was transmitted by apparently normal women, as Otto had pointed out, was soon elevated to the status of Nasse's law.[159] Reports that women might have hemophilia were largely due to an understandable confusion with other disorders. Grandidier,[160] for example, believed that the ratio of male to female hemophiliacs was 14 to 1, but Bulloch and Fildes,[153] in their massive review of the heredity of hemophilia, published in 1911, could not find a single authentic case of hemophilia in a female. That the normal males in hemophilic families cannot transmit the disease was not clearly recognized as late as 1909.[160a]

The key to understanding the inheritance of hemophilia was provided by John Hay,[161] an American physician. In 1813, he reported that the daughter of a hemophiliac could transmit the disorder to her sons, a personal worry as his own son had married a carrier of the disease. This clue was ignored until half a century later, when Wickham Legg[162] made the same observation. Father-to-son inheritance, repeatedly described in the early literature, never occurs in hemophilia. The sex-linked inheritance of a hemophilia-like disease in Queen Victoria's descendants, sometimes misnamed the curse of the Hapsburgs, has been a subject of great fascination to both physicians and nonphysicians. Whether these regal bleeders had classic hemophilia or Christmas disease is not known to the author.

An explanation for the pattern of inheritance of hemophilia came about through the insights of Thomas Hunt Morgan,[163] an American biologist, who, at the beginning of this century, proposed the gene theory of heredity, as the result of studies with fruit flies. The genes, individual packets of hereditary material, are carried on structures called chromosomes. Human beings have 46 chromosomes. The chromosomes are present in pairs, one of each pair inherited from each parent. Twenty-two of the pairs are autosomal; that is, grossly similar in both sexes. The twenty-third pair consists of morphologically dissimilar structures, the X and Y chromosomes. A female has two X chromosomes, one inherited from each parent. A male, instead, has an X chromosome inherited from his mother and a Y chromosome inherited from his father. Each ovum or sperm contains, at random, one chromosome of each pair. Thus, each ovum contains one or the other of the two X chromosomes of the mother, and each sperm contains either an X or a Y chromosome of the father; fertilization restores the normal complement of chromosomes.

The abnormal gene responsible for classic hemophilia is located on an X chromosome (Figure 18-13). A woman who has one abnormal X chromosome and one normal X chromosome is a carrier and is said to be heterozygous for

Figure 18-13 The pattern of inheritance of classic hemophilia and other sex-linked syndromes. (*From Ratnoff OD: Hereditary defects in clotting mechanisms, in Dock W, Snapper I [eds]: Advances in Internal Medicine. Chicago, Year Book Medical Publishers, 1958, vol IX. Used by permission.*)

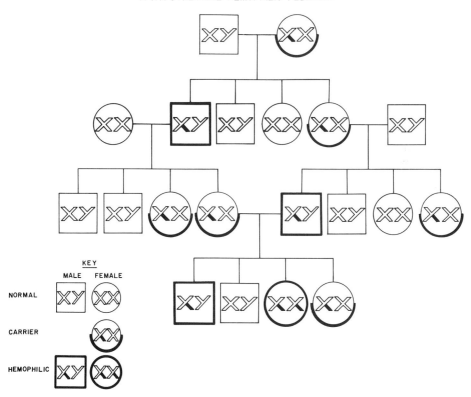

A HYPOTHETICAL HEMOPHILIC PEDIGREE

the abnormal gene. Mated to a normal male, she has an even chance of having a daughter or son, depending on whether one of her X chromosomes is paired with a paternal X or Y chromosome, respectively. Further, her sons have an even chance of inheriting her normal X chromosome, and are, therefore, normal, or of inheriting her abnormal X chromosome, and, therefore, have hemophilia, a condition described as the hemizygous state. Similarly, a carrier's daughters have an even chance of being normal or being carriers themselves. When a male with classic hemophilia mates with a normal woman, all his sons must be normal, as they necessarily inherit only his Y chromosome, and all his daughters must be carriers, as they must inherit his abnormal X chromosomes.

In 1819, a surgeon, one Mr. Ward,[164] suggested that hemophilia was due to a defect in blood clotting. Toward the end of the century, Georges Hayem,[181] too, held the same view. Because no satisfactory method had yet been devised to measure the time that elapsed until blood clotted, these reports were ignored, and many alternative hypotheses were proposed to explain why hemophiliacs had a bleeding tendency. William Koch,[53] for example, looked upon hemophilia as a manifestation of scurvy, while others viewed it as one of the rheumatic disorders, undoubtedly because of the accompanying damage to muscles and joints.[152] Yet another view was that hemophilia was an affliction of the blood vessels[40] and that bleeding was the consequence of an abnormal thinness of the arterial walls, possibly the results of an increase in the volume of circulating blood.[152] Alternatively, because hemophilia occurred only in males, perhaps it was a form of vicarious menstruation. Only in 1878 was a primitive clinical method for measuring the clotting time introduced.[165] Fifteen more years elapsed before Sir Almroth Wright,[166] whose ideas about immunology were reflected by Sir Colenso Rigeon in Shaw's The Doctor's Dilemma, reported that the clotting time of whole blood was abnormally long in hemophilia. Wright provided a variety of explanations that now seem bizarre.

Progress toward an understanding of the nature of the defective coagulation of hemophilic blood was necessarily slow. The same year that Wright localized the abnormality in hemophilia to blood, Manteuffel,[167] Alexander Schmidt's pupil, found that tissue extracts—Schmidt's zymoplastic substance—shortened the clotting time of hemophilic blood, an observation repeatedly confirmed. Thus, the prothrombin time—that is, the clotting time of recalcified plasma in the presence of tissue thromboplastin—is normal in this disease. In modern terms, then, the defect in hemophilia resides in the early steps of the intrinsic pathway of thrombin formation, as the extrinsic pathway is normal. Thomas Addis[168] added to Manteuffel's insight through studies that suggested that the conversion of prothrombin to thrombin was impaired in hemophilia; in retrospect, it is not clear whether the patient he studied had classic hemophilia or Christmas disease. Addis believed his experiments showed that the prothrombin of hemophilic plasma was functionally impaired, a view that Howell[33] showed was erroneous.

During the early years of this century, the issue whether the abnormality of hemophilic blood was localized to the plasma or to the platelets[169] remained unsettled. The idea that defective platelets represented the basic flaw in hemophilia (a reflection of the difficulty with which platelets are freed from the surrounding plasma), gained influential adherents, among them George Minot, of Harvard University.[170] In one form or another, the platelet hypothesis prevailed for some years after Frank and Hartmann,[171] Govaertz and Gratia,[172] and Patek and Stetson[173] demonstrated that the addition of normal plasma corrected the clotting defect of hemophilic plasma. Patek[174] localized the corrective effect of plasma to a crude fraction of plasma; the analogous fraction of hemophilic plasma lacked this property. The agent in normal plasma is now referred to as antihemophilic factor (AHF, factor VIII).

Patek expressed uncertainty whether the plasma of patients with classic hemophilia was deficient in antihemophilic factor or whether this agent was present in a nonfunctional form. Soon the prevailing view was that hemophilia was associated with the deficient synthesis of antihemophilic factor. Alternatively, some investigators, notably Frank and Hartmann[171] and Leandro Tocantins,[175] believed that hemophilic plasma contained an excess of a normal inhibitory agent. The solution to the problem appeared in a little-noted abstract that was submitted to the Central Society for Clinical Research by Shanberge and Gore:[176] the plasma of patients with classic hemophilia contained an agent immunologically similar to normal antihemophilic factor. (Those who select papers for the programs of scientific societies should keep in mind that this abstract was not chosen for presentation!) Because Shanberge's observation was antithetical to contemporary dogma, his experiments were ignored for some years. Finally, improved technology made it possible to demonstrate that the plasma of all patients with classic hemophilia contained normal amounts of a variant of the antihemophilic molecule that did not sustain blood clotting.[177,178] An unexpected result of this newer understanding was the discovery of a practical test for recognizing which of the female relatives of a hemophiliac were carriers. In a high proportion of carriers, the titer of antihemophilic factor as assayed in clotting tests is significantly less than the concentration of this agent measured immunologically.[177,179]

Classic hemophilia is only one of several hereditary diseases in which a functional deficiency of antihemophilic factor is present. The most important besides hemophilia is von Willebrand's disease, sometimes called vascular hemophilia or pseudohemophilia type B. In 1926, von Willebrand[180] described a hemorrhagic disorder present in both sexes and appearing in successive generations of a family living in the Finnish Åland Islands, in the Gulf of Bothnia. In contrast to patients with classic hemophilia, von Willebrand's patients had a long bleeding time—a test measuring the duration of bleeding from a deliberately incised wound, first introduced into medicine by Hayem[181] and later standardized by Duke.[182] Similar patients were described independently by Minot[183] and others. Von Willebrand thought that the bleeding tendency reflected a defect in the platelets, but in fact no *intrinsic* abnormality of these cells has been demonstrated. A contrary view, expressed by Macfarlane[184] and by Quick,[104] that the disorder was due to a vascular abnormality, has not been corroborated.

The pathogenesis of von Willebrand's disease became clearer only after some years, when Alexander,[185] Larrieu,[186] and Quick,[187] in 1953, described similar patients in whom the titer of antihemophilic factor, as measured in clotting tests, was deficient. Other characteristics distinguishing von Willebrand's disease from classic hemophilia gradually emerged. When normal blood is trickled through a column of glass beads, a substantial proportion of the platelets are retained within the column, a property often impaired in von Willebrand's disease.[188,189] Further, an antibiotic, ristocetin, brings about the clumping of platelets; this aggregation of platelets is impaired in von Willebrand's disease.[190] And astonishingly, the transfusion of normal plasma—or even that of hemophiliacs—is followed after several hours by an increase in the titer of antihemophilic factor, as measured by clotting assays, to levels substantially higher than would have been predicted.[191] In contrast to classic hemophilia, the plasma of patients with von Willebrand's disease usually is deficient in a protein related to the antihemophilic factor,[177] and at least some of the features of the disorder have been attributed to this deficiency. A large number of variants of von Willebrand's disease have now been described, the significance of which is still uncertain.

This newer knowledge about the nature of classic hemophilia and von Willebrand's disease has intensified the efforts being made to understand the chemical structure of antihemophilic factor. Briefly, it appears to be a giant molecule composed of two readily dissociated parts. One sustains blood clotting (and is, therefore, presumably synthesized under the direction of a gene located on an X chromosome); the other contains the bulk of the protein and supports the platelet-related functions deficient in von Willebrand's disease (and is apparently synthesized under the direction of an autosomal gene).[192,193] Synthesis of the noncoagulant part of antihemophilic factor has been localized to the "endothelial" cells that line blood vessels.[194]

The treatment of classic hemophilia and von Willebrand's disease has undergone as remarkable an evolution as our understanding about these disorders. In 1840, Samuel Lane[195] reported that he was able to stem bleeding by a transfusion of blood into a boy with a hemorrhagic disease which was in all likelihood hemophilia. The times were not ready for the use of this procedure, and it was not until 1905 that Paul Émile-Weil[196] again attempted transfusing small amounts of serum, which we now know is devoid of antihemophilic factor. Weil observed sporadic shortening of the clotting time; perhaps some of his patients really had Christmas disease, which does respond to infusions of serum. Some years later, Feissly[197] demonstrated that the transfusion of normal plasma shortened the clotting time of hemophiliacs, but this mode of therapy did not come into general use until the 1940s. Attempts to use fractions of plasma rich in antihemophilic factor began with Patek's[174] demonstration that this agent could be separated in a crude way. When World War II stimulated E.J. Cohn's group at Harvard to fractionate plasma with ethanol (Chapter 17), antihemophilic factor was found in the fibrinogen-rich "fraction I."[198] Therapy with this fraction was attempted, but the results obtained were often erratic because the content of antihemophilic factor varied from lot to lot. Two striking advances then made transfusion therapy feasible. Wagner and his associates,[199] in Kenneth Brinkhous's productive laboratory at the University of North Carolina, learned to separate antihemophilic factor from plasma by precipitating it with neutral amino acids. And Judith Graham Pool and her colleagues[200] found that a large proportion of the antihemophilic factor in plasma was present in "cryoprecipitates," that is, in the fraction that remained insoluble after fresh, quick-frozen plasma was allowed to thaw at 4°C. Both these preparations could be dried (a process called lyophilization), thus making possible the self-administration of these materials by patients at a distance from the hospital, thereby often greatly improving the quality of their lives. Therapy of von Willebrand's disease with these plasma fractions has also been used widely, though often with less satisfactory results. It is entertaining to note that Wooldridge[58] and Mills[201] had detected unusual clot-promoting properties in cryoprecipitates long ago; what Pool provided was insight.

Unfortunately, sooner or later, as many as one-fifth of severely affected hemophiliacs become refractory to therapy. This complication was first described by Lawrence,[202] who suggested that it was due to the appearance of antibodies against antihemophilic factor. This view was soon corroborated by Munro,[203] tragically himself the patient under study. Perhaps more excitingly, such "circulating anticoagulants" also occasionally arise in otherwise normal women after delivery,[204] or in individuals of either sex with a wide variety of diseases, or after therapy with penicillin or other drugs.[205] What induces the formation of these strange antibodies remains a puzzle.

CHRISTMAS FACTOR AND CHRISTMAS DISEASE

In 1944, Castex, Pavlovsky, and Simonetti,[206] in Argentina, reported the results of studies that represented a turning point in our understanding of hemostasis. Pavlovsky and his collaborators observed, in their words, a paradoxical fact. Occasionally, the blood of two hemophiliacs seemed to be mutually corrective in the test tube, and, in at least one instance, transfusion of plasma from one hemophiliac to another dramatically shortened the clotting time of the recipient.

The significance of these striking effects soon became clear with the appearance in 1952 of two papers that were submitted for publication within a week of each other. Paul Aggeler[207] and Irving Schulman[208] described patients with a hemophilia-like syndrome that was attributable to a functional deficiency of a plasma protein other than antihemophilic factor. Aggeler called the newly identified agent *plasma thromboplastin component* and Schulman, *plasma factor X*, a misfortune in retrospect because factor X was later designated as a synonym for Stuart factor. The trivial name most often used for the new substance is Christmas factor, after the patronym of one of six additional patients described in the Christmas issue of the British Medical Journal later the same year by Biggs and her associates.[209]

Like classic hemophilia, Christmas disease, the hereditary deficiency of Christmas factor, is an X chromosome–linked disorder. Indeed, one of the earliest families thought to have hemophilia, the "bleeders of Tenna" in Switzerland, was found to have Christmas disease instead.[157] In some families, the plasma of patients with Christmas disease contains little or no Christmas factor. In others, a nonfunctional variant of Christmas factor can be detected in plasma, as first reported by Fantl in Australia.[210]

Christmas factor is one of the clotting factors that requires vitamin K for its synthesis, which takes place in the liver. It has been highly purified, permitting studies of its mode of action. Christmas factor, unlike antihemophilic factor, is present in normal serum. As mentioned earlier, in 1905 Émile-Weil[196] reported that human or bovine serum corrected the defective clotting of several patients with "hemophilia."

THE LATER STEPS OF THE INTRINSIC PATHWAY

After PTA has been changed by activated Hageman factor to its activated state, it converts Christmas factor to an active form that, in concert with antihemophilic factor, phospholipid, and calcium ions, in turn activates Stuart factor.[211,212] In this process, both activated Christmas factor and antihemophilic factor are adsorbed to phospholipids.[213–215] The enzymatic groups responsible for activation of Stuart factor are almost certainly localized to the Christmas factor molecule, as originally hinted at by Spurling[216] in 1954.

The roles of antihemophilic factor and of calcium ions in the activation of Stuart factor are not yet clear. Thrombin greatly enhances the functional activity of antihemophilic factor.[217,218] Thus, thrombin seems to activate two factors that participate in clotting before the conversion of prothrombin to thrombin, antihemophilic factor and proaccelerin. Thrombin also brings about the clumping of platelets with the release of various components into the surrounding milieu. Quick[219] was an early proponent of the view that in this way platelets furnished the agents needed for the coagulation of plasma once some thrombin had formed. Indeed, although plasma phospholipids will support clotting, their effect is minimal, as Conley's[127] studies had implied; platelets probably furnish the bulk of the phospholipids required for the intrinsic pathway[30]—a property often called *platelet factor 3*.

Once activated, Stuart factor forms through the reactions of the intrinsic pathway, it brings about the formation of fibrin through the same series of steps traversed by the extrinsic pathway.

Plasma Inhibitors of Clotting

Alexander Schmidt[24] was probably the first student of blood coagulation to suggest that the fluidity of blood was sustained by the presence of inhibitors of clotting; he believed these were derived from tissues. Later investigators, notably Nolf,[54] Fuchs,[220] Howell,[33] and Tocantins,[175] expanded upon this base by hypothesizing that clotting was a consequence of the removal of this inhibition. Their conception, however appealing, has not stood the test of time, although plasma indeed contains many substances that retard clotting by inhibiting clotting factors that have been activated during the process of coagulation. From an evolutionary point of view, limitation of the clotting process may well have survival value by preventing the spread of thrombosis.

Diverse mechanisms have been elucidated over the years through which the effects of thrombin, the enzyme ultimately responsible for the formation of a clot, are limited. That thrombin gradually lost its activity once clotting had taken place was recognized early in this century by Fuld[221] and by Morawitz.[53] One possible mechanism for this phenomenon was described by Morawitz[53] and by Foà,[222] who observed that fibrin itself removed thrombin from the surrounding plasma, curtailing this enzyme's action. Morawitz[53] assumed that, additionally, plasma itself had antithrombic properties, and this possibility was later studied more thoroughly by Rettger.[223] At first this inhibition was attributed to albumin[59] or to some closely related constituent of plasma.[104] Instead, later investigators found that the principal inhibitor of thrombin in plasma was a specific protein to which the name antithrombin III has been applied.[29]

In 1889, Schmidt-Mülheim[224] reported that the blood of dogs injected with a crude mixture of protein fragments, Witte peptone, was incoagulable. This phenomenon was ascribed to the appearance in the dogs' plasma of antithrombic agents, named "antithrombosin" by Nolf.[54] The nature of antithrombosin waited for the discovery of heparin by Jay McLean, a medical student at the Johns Hopkins University. McLean was a remarkable youth, overcoming not only financial handicaps but his temporary rejection for admission to the school. He was compelled by an urge to be a "physiology-based" rather than an "anatomy-based" surgeon. He therefore sought the opportunity to study with William Howell, who put him to the task of purifying clot-promoting phospholipid cephalin from various tissues. An incidental result of these studies was the isolation of a crude fraction of hepatic tissue that "showed a marked power to inhibit coagulation."[225] Howell[33] (Figure 18-14) named the inhibitor *heparin* and demonstrated that it was apparently the agent responsible for the incoagulable state of dogs' blood after

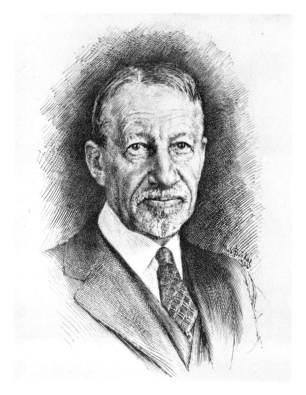

Figure 18-14 William H. Howell (1860–1945).

the injection of Witte peptone. Heparin is a complex sugar; its chemistry was elucidated by Erik Jorpes[226] and others. Recently, Jaques[227] has suggested that McLean's heparin was in fact a different agent than the heparin we know today.

In agreement with the earlier studies of Howell and Holt,[33] Quick,[104] and others, the inhibition of clotting by heparin has been found to depend upon its combination with the agent in plasma now called antithrombin III;[228] in the absence of antithrombin III, heparin does not inhibit thrombin.[33] Antithrombin III is an even more potent inhibitor of the *formation* of thrombin than of thrombin itself,[229,230] a view anticipated by Howell and Holt[33] and by Brinkhous and his associates.[231] This effect of heparin led Howell[33] to the erroneous view recounted earlier, that the action of tissue thromboplastin was to free prothrombin from inhibition, in this way liberating thrombin.

That heparin might be useful clinically in preventing an occurrence or the extension of thrombosis derives from the studies of Mason[232] in 1924, who used this substance to inhibit intravascular clotting in rabbits that were injected with tissue thromboplastin. A year later, he[233] also infused heparin into human subjects; the blood clotting time was prolonged as a result, but the material he used was too crude, and the patients suffered reactions. Heparin suitable for clinical use was prepared by Scott and Charles[234] in Charles Best's laboratory in Toronto and by Jorpes[226] in Stockholm; its first use in patients was by Murray[235] and Crafoord[236] in 1937.

Antithrombin III is only one of several inhibitors of clotting found in plasma. Among other such agents are C$\bar{1}$ inactivator, first described as an inhibitor of the first component of complement[237] but also effective against activated Hageman factor, activated PTA, and plasma kallikrein; α_2-macroglobulin, probably responsible for about one-fourth the thrombin-inhibitory properties of plasma;[238] α_1-antitrypsin, which inhibits both thrombin[239] and activated PTA;[240] one or more plasma inhibitors of the activation of Hageman factor, probably nonspecific in character;[241] and α_2-plasmin inhibitor, which blocks the activity of several clotting factors.[242] Parenthetically, functional deficiency of C$\bar{1}$ inactivator in the plasma of patients with hereditary angioneurotic edema was the first example described of the inherited deficiency of the inhibitor of an enzyme;[243] subsequently, deficiencies of α_1-antitrypsin and antithrombin III have been discovered.

When activated clotting factors are infused into animals, they are rapidly inactivated. In part, this phenomenon is undoubtedly due to their neutralization by these various plasma inhibitors. Additionally, as Delezenne[244] determined at the end of the last century, the activated clotting factors may be altered or destroyed by their passage through the liver.

Plasmin and Fibrinolysis

That the blood of individuals who die suddenly may be fluid was probably appreciated by the Hippocratic school.[245] Andral,[44] writing in the 1840s, tells us that the ancients ranked dissolution of the blood among the causes of hemorrhage, and he anticipated that under these conditions the plasma would contain less fibrinogen than normally. The fluidity of some postmortem blood was recognized by John Hunter,[11] who observed that this was more likely to occur in individuals who died as the result of "fits, anger, electricity, or lightening." Characteristically, Hunter attempted to study the mechanisms responsible. He found that the blood of two deer that he "had run till they dropped down and died" did not appear to coagulate. Some time later, the dissolution of clotted blood after death was noted by Andral[44] and was attributed by Morawitz[246] to the plasma's intrinsic proteolytic activity. It is as likely that in some cases the failure of postmortem blood to clot is the consequence of defibrination during the course of disseminated intravascular coagulation, which will be discussed later.

That clots may liquefy was first demonstrated in 1838 by Denis,[247] who described the dissolution of fibrin in solutions of neutral salts; such reliquefied clots could not be clotted again.[248] In 1893, Dastre[249] made the important additional observation that fibrin was digested when it was incubated with serum, a process he named *fibrinolysis*. Fibrinolysis was especially prominent in the blood of dogs that had been poisoned with phosphorus.[250] Soon the proteolytic property was localized by Hedin[251] to a crude fraction of serum. Another crude fraction inhibited the proteolytic process.

Somewhat earlier than Dastre and Hedin, Denys and Marbaix[252] found that the addition of chloroform to serum enhanced its fibrinolytic activity, an effect ascribed by them and by Delezenne and Pozerski[253] to the development of proteolytic properties. How chloroform brings about an increase in plasma proteolytic activity is still not certain, but Ogston[254] has proposed that under these conditions, proteolytic activity evolves via mechanisms that involve the participation of Hageman factor. Still, these observations do not tell us how the activation of proteolytic activity comes about.

In recent years, the agent responsible for proteolysis has been named *plasmin* or *fibrinolysin* (Figure 18-15). Despite lingering reports that still appear, plasmin can be sharply differentiated from trypsin, a pancreatic digestive enzyme not found in normal plasma. Plasminogen, the precursor of plasmin, has been highly purified by many methods, the most ingenious perhaps being Deutsch and Mertz's[255] technique of adsorbing this protein onto an insoluble complex of the amino acid lysine and the insoluble carbohydrate agarose.

In experiments whose implications were ignored, Gratia[256] in 1921 noted that staphylococcal extracts induced the lysis of a clot. Some years later, in 1933, Tillett and Garner[257] reported that bacteria-free filtrates of cultures of beta hemolytic streptococci contained a substance that rapidly dissolved clotted plasma or fibrin; this agent was called streptoccal fibrinolysin. Milstone[258] soon found that streptoccal fibrinolysin's activity depended upon the presence of a substance in the euglobulin fraction of plasma that was later identified by Kaplan[259] as none other than plasminogen, the agent converted by chloroform to plasmin. Believing that the active agent in streptococcal filtrates was an enzyme, Christensen and MacLeod[260] renamed it streptokinase. Later studies suggested instead that streptokinase reacted stoichiometrically (that is, nonenzymatically) with plasminogen,[261] a view that has since been confirmed.

Plasminogen can be activated in many other ways. For example, in 1902, Conradi[262] demonstrated that the "press juice" extracted from various organs erratically induced fibrinolysis of dog or rabbit blood clots. A few years later, Fleisher and Loeb[263] dissolved clots by the addition of tissue particles, a process that was realized only some years later to be due to the activation of

Plasminogen $\longrightarrow$ Plasmin   **Figure 18-15** The formation of plasmin, the enzyme in plasma that digests fibrinogen.

plasminogen. The nature of these tissue agents has been elaborated particularly carefully by Astrup and his associates.[264] Urine, too, contains a potent activator of plasminogen,[265] now called *urokinase;* agents in human milk, tears, saliva, and seminal fluid also bring about the formation of plasmin.

Of much greater clinical interest is the fact that plasminogen can be converted to plasmin "spontaneously" in clots formed from plasma or its euglobulin fraction. This spontaneous fibrinolysis was found by Goodpasture[266] to be greatly exaggerated in the clotted blood of patients with cirrhosis of the liver. Increased fibrinolytic activity has since been described in the plasma of individuals undergoing various types of stress or strenuous physical activity.[267,268]

Several mechanisms have been proposed to explain spontaneous fibrinolysis. Sherry, Fletcher, and Alkjaersig[269] thought that this phenomenon was due to the appearance in plasma of an activator of plasminogen, and Kwaan[270] suggested further that this activator might be derived from venous endothelium, as Nolf[271] and Todd[272] had earlier reported; such an activator has now been partially purified.[273]

An intrinsic mechanism in plasma that might bring about the activation of plasminogen also has been delineated. Thus, clots formed from human plasma may undergo spontaneous fibrinolysis upon exposure to glass. This phenomenon was found by Niewiarowski and Prou-Wartelle[274] to depend upon the presence of Hageman factor. Activation of plasminogen by Hageman factor requires the presence of an additional enzyme that, upon conversion to an active form by activated Hageman factor, in turn changes plasminogen to plasmin.[275] The nature of this intermediate has been the subject of controversy.

Plasmin is an enzyme of broad specificity, digesting not only fibrin but other plasma proteins as well, including fibrinogen and other clotting factors and components of the complement and kallikrein-kinin systems. An early view,[271] that plasmin can induce clotting, is without support.

From a teleological point of view, the existence of a means of dissolving clots has broad implication. Much effort has therefore been expended to understand the course of events when fibrin clots are dissolved. In 1961, Nussenzweig and his collaborators[276] observed that fibrinogen was degraded into progressively smaller fragments; the sequential steps have since been studied in great detail, beginning with the important studies of Marder.[277] The "degradation" products that result from the digestion of fibrinogen and fibrin inhibit clotting in several ways.[278] Demonstration of these degradation products in plasma or urine has been extensively studied as a clue to processes involved in both disseminated and localized thrombosis.

As might be expected, plasma possesses complex devices to limit the proteolytic action of plasmin. As early as 1903, Delezenne and Pozerski[279] recognized that plasma contained inhibitors of plasmin, and since then a number of distinct agents that possess this property have been found. Inhibitors of the activation of plasminogen by various substances also have been described.

The possibility that the fibrinolytic activity of plasmin might be put to good use has intrigued investigators for many years. Probably the first attempt to do this was made by Meneghini[280] in 1949; he injected vaccines intravenously in an effort to induce fibrinolysis of thrombi in the vena cava. More promising have been studies of the effects of the injection of activators of plasminogen, principally streptokinase and urokinase; these were first attempted in human subjects with experimentally induced thrombi by Johnson,[281] and then were thoroughly studied over many years by Sherry and his colleagues.[269]

Thrombosis

This chapter would be incomplete without a brief glance at the growth of knowledge about thrombosis. That blood can coagulate within the vascular system during life is an old idea. Twenty-five hundred or more years ago in China, Huang Ti wrote, "When it coagulates within the pulse, the blood ceases to circulate beneficially; when the blood coagulates within the foot, it causes pain and chills."[282] There are, however, few early references to the process of thrombosis, a term that may have been used by Galen.[49] Diocles[283] in the fourth century B.C. noted that obstruction of the lumen of blood vessels may occur in the course of inflammatory processes. A disorder reminiscent of septic thrombophlebitis of the leg was said to have been cured miraculously by the intervention of Saint Louis in A.D. 1217, but of course the diagnosis is inferential.[283a] During the renaissance of medicine, pathologists were familiar with the presence at autopsy of clotted blood within the heart,[8] within aneurysms,[284] and within blood vessels,[2,285] but they did not at first distinguish among *thrombosis*, the process of clotting within the heart or vessels during life; *embolism*, the process through which thrombi break off and are carried down stream to obstruct the flow of blood at a point removed from the site of thrombosis; and *postmortem coagulation*. That thrombi formed during life might obstruct the flow of blood with disastrous results was propounded by John Hunter,[11] who described gangrene distal to a clot in the iliac artery. By the 1830s, the reality of thrombosis was still only grudgingly admitted.[48]

Richard Wiseman,[286] in 1686, described the coagulation of blood within varicose veins and ascribed the varices "either to the coagulation of the serum or the grumousness of the blood, or to the obstruction of the vein somewhere in its passage by some angustation [i.e., narrowing] upon it by part of the tumor [swelling], from whence it will often happen that the vein beyond it hath its current stopped and is forced to swell. . . ." It is unclear whether Wiseman meant to infer that stasis (i.e., slowing of blood flow) and an alteration in blood were factors that induce coagulation within veins, but by the middle of the nineteenth century, Richardson,[16] in England, attributed thrombosis to the impairment of blood flow and "a peculiar kind of coagulation." Virchow[287] added that inflammation of the walls of veins, arteries, or the heart might bring about thrombosis. He minimized this possibility, arguing strongly that Cruveilhier's earlier view that thrombosis and inflammation were intimately related was based on misconstrued evidence. Virchow also introduced the revolutionary idea that intravascular clots might fragment and then be carried along by the current of the blood into remote vessels, the phenomenon of embolism.

The three possible factors in the genesis of thrombosis outlined by early investigators, that is, alterations in blood flow, in the intrinsic propensity of blood to clot, and in the integrity of the blood vessel wall, remain the central themes of modern views about thrombosis. Experimental support for the importance of each of these factors has accumulated in a steady—and, alas, often repetitive—fashion over the last century. Probably the first recorded induction of experimental thrombosis was performed by Franciscus de la Boë, or Sylvius,[288] of Leyden, in the middle of the seventeenth century. Sylvius found that injection of acid substances into the veins of a living animal resulted in instantaneous coagulation of blood. Welch[289] tells us that the first systematic experimental examination of the pathogenesis of thrombosis was made by Zahn,[290] who concluded that the process was brought about by the accumulation of leukocytes (white blood cells), which, by their disintegration, gave rise to granular detritus. This was quickly followed by the appearance of fibrin, clotting having been initiated by thromboplastic substances derived from the disintegrated leukocytes. Beginning in 1882 with Giulio Bizzozero, of Turin,[4] later workers pointed instead to the platelets as the cells most concerned with thrombosis. In experiments with guinea pigs, Bizzozero observed that platelets adhered to the cut edges of an injured blood vessel, where they formed the nidus for a thrombus. Studies of Hayem,[123] Lubnitzky,[291] Eberth and Schimmelbusch,[5] and Osler[292] reinforced Bizzozero's ideas. Particularly important were Eberth and Schimmelbusch's experiments in which they observed that platelets adhered to the site of vascular injury induced by chemical or physical means. The aggregates of platelets gradually occluded the vessels, and, thereafter, the stagnant blood clotted. Welch[289] subsequently suggested a role in this localized formation of fibrin for white blood cells, primarily polymorphonuclear leukocytes, which collect at the margins of the platelet masses and between platelets. Thus, these experimental models seem to mimic the initial stages of clinical thrombosis, in which a mass of white blood cells, platelets, and fibrin—the so-called white thrombus or white head—adheres to the wall of the affected blood vessel. Once this has taken place, an ordinary clot forms at the margins of the white thrombus. This *red thrombus*, or *tail*, usually grows in the direction of the current of blood, but sometimes it may form in the opposite direction. The thrombus seems to be crossed with lamellae of platelets and fibrin that project upon the surface of the thrombus as the so-called lines of Zahn, as if the clot were laid down in successive layers. The importance of platelets as the structural basis of white thrombi was stressed early by Osler.[292]

Hewson,[9] it will be recalled, had noted that the stagnation of blood within a vessel isolated between ligatures was a poor stimulus to clotting. A wealth of subsequent experimental evidence, however, has emphasized that the combination of stasis and vascular injury is a potent initiator of thrombosis. Eberth's[5] experiments were particularly pertinent. In rapidly flowing blood, the blood elements appeared to flow in the central portion of the vascular cavity (the lumen) while the peripheral area of the blood vessels seemed to contain no leukocytes. When flow in a blood vessel was slowed, the platelets appeared to detach from the central stream of cells and wander toward the vessel walls. When the vascular endothelium was then damaged, the detached platelets aggregated at and adhered to the injured site, forming the white head. Stasis is also a requisite for the formation of intravascular clots by injection of *activated* plasma clotting factors, first described by Hayem[293] in 1886, reexamined by Feissly,[294] and, later, exquisitely studied by Wessler.[295]

Clinical observation confirms the importance of vascular injury and stasis in the genesis of thrombosis in arteries and veins except in the phenomenon described as disseminated intravascular coagulation. No clear-cut support has yet appeared for the hypothetical role of a "hypercoagulable" change in circulating clotting factors, which was propounded by Carl Rokitansky.[296] A brief calendar of some clinical situations that are commonly complicated by thrombosis emphasizes the paucity of our current understanding. Thus, neoplasms, as first recorded by Trousseau,[112] the strange metabolic abnormality known as homocystinuria, and the regular ingestion of oral contraceptive agents may be associated with thrombosis; in addition, individuals with blood group A are more likely to sustain thrombosis than those of group O. In none of the situations is there a satisfactory explanation for thrombosis, and even less why this process is expressed for so brief a time. Any hypothesis that is to explain the pathogenesis of thrombosis under conditions such as these must also account for the episodic nature of the process.

DISSEMINATED INTRAVASCULAR COAGULATION

Perhaps more satisfying has been evolution of knowledge about what has been called disseminated (or diffuse) intravascular coagulation or consumption coagulopathy, the last an ungainly but perhaps more accurate term. What may have been the earliest attempt to study disseminated intravascular coagulation was made by Sylvius,[288] who tried to explain the fluidity of blood in malignant fevers and in the plague by the presence of an excess of alkaline substances.

De Blainville's[51] dramatic demonstration that the intravenous injection of brain tissue led immediately to lethal massive intravascular clotting was mentioned earlier. About 50 years later, Wooldridge[58] modified de Blainville's experiment by infusing tissue extracts more slowly. Animals treated in this way survived, but their blood was incoagulable and, under these conditions, further infusions of tissue were harmless. Unexpectedly, relatively little evidence of thrombosis was found in these animals. An explanation for Wooldridge's experiments came from the much later observation of Mills[297] that the blood of animals which had been infused slowly with tissue extracts was depleted of fibrinogen. A reasonable conclusion is that the infused tissues furnished tissue thromboplastin, which induced clotting within the animals' blood vessels via the extrinsic pathway of thrombin formation (Figure 18-7). Innumerable variations of Wooldridge's experiments have been described, as though their repetition were a *rite de passage* for coagulationists. Intravascular coagulation and depletion of fibrinogen have been accomplished not only by infusion of tissue thromboplastin but also of thrombin[32] or various procoagulant snake venoms.[298–300] In most experimental models, few or no thrombi can be found despite depletion of the animal's fibrinogen; perhaps fibrin, formed diffusely throughout the circulation, is removed from the bloodstream, either before or after its polymerization is complete. Alternatively, fibrin may be dissolved by plasma or cellular proteases activated during the clotting process.

The laboratory models that have been described above have obvious clinical implications. Perhaps some instances of acute hypo- or afibrinogenemia are due to the inadvertent activation of the clotting process within the bloodstream, the human counterpart of Wooldridge's experiments. The clearest examples of this postulated syndrome are amniotic fluid embolism, in which the amniotic fluid that surrounds the baby in the uterus enters the bloodstream during childbirth, and envenomation by the bite of snakes whose venoms contain coagulant agents. John Hunter[11] long ago reported that the blood of a woman who died suddenly during childbirth was incoagulable. A modern guess is that she had sustained disseminated intravascular coagulation induced by infusion into her circulation of thromboplastic amniotic fluid and its contaminants; evidence supporting this was first obtained only about a quarter of a century ago. The hemorrhagic nature of certain snake venoms has long been appreciated[298] and their procoagulant properties repeatedly studied. One such venom, that of the Malayan pit viper *Ankistrodon rhodostoma*, clots fibrinogen directly, and Reid[301] related the bleeding tendency of individuals bitten by this snake to the resultant hypofibrinogenemia.

Many additional examples of hypo- or afibrinogenemia have been recorded, although evidence for the mechanisms involved is not always secure. Premature separation of the placenta was recognized as a cause of systemic bleeding by De Lee[302] early in this century and later related by Dieckmann[303] to hypofibrinogenemia. Extensive studies by Charles Schneider,[304] a Detroit obstetrician, suggested that thromboplastic placental tissue gained access to the maternal circulation and in this way induced disseminated intravascular coagulation. Similar mechanisms may explain the depletion of circulating fibrinogen after a transfusion of incompatible blood, brain injury, burns, and neoplasms, although earlier writers tended to emphasize fibrinolysis as a cause for the patients' difficulties. Not as readily explicable is the pathogenesis of the depletion of fibrinogen in such disorders as sepsis and heat stroke. Almost innumerable syndromes have now been reported in which a decreased concentration of plasma fibrinogen has been attributed to disseminated intravascular coagulation. In most cases, the patient's serum, normally free of fibrinogen, contains material that can be related to this protein.[305] Identification of this fibrinogen-like material is now an important diagnostic clue to the presence of disseminated intravascular coagulation.

Demonstration of such fibrinogen-related agents in the serum during the course of many diseases usually unassociated with decreased plasma fibrinogen has led to the assumption that disseminated intravascular coagulation may have taken place. The degree to which this inference is correct varies from situation to situation.

PURPURA FULMINANS

Depletion of plasma fibrinogen also has been observed in situations in which localized, rather than disseminated, intravascular coagulation appears to be present. An important advance came about from studies of one such disorder, purpura fulminans, a peculiarly terrifying syndrome characterized by superficial gangrene that results from thrombosis of small blood vessels. Little[306] found that he could stay the progression of thrombosis by administration of the anticoagulant heparin. This success led to the use of heparin in selected cases of hypo- or afibrinogenemia, although an attack on the primary cause is usually more effective and safer. It has also brought about therapy with heparin for patients thought to have disseminated intravascular coagulation in the absence of recognized depletion of plasma fibrinogen, but the results obtained are often disappointing.

Conclusion

In 1921, Bordet[30] wrote, "Coagulation has been studied for years and years by many investigators; none of them can presume that the problem is yet solved; every one of them merely indulges in the hope of gathering some complementary data; a little more information." We act at a more sophisticated level these days, but Bordet's statement remains true. The prevalence of hemorrhagic and thrombotic states tells us there is much unfinished business. Were we the Merlin of T.E. White's *The Sword in the Stone* and, therefore, lived backwards, we would know the nature of what remains to be done. Perhaps we will be happier to be surprised.

Acknowledgment

A note of thanks is due to Ms. Virginia Bullock of the Allen Memorial Library of Cleveland for help to me above and beyond the call of duty.

References*

1 Howell WH: Blood and lymph, in Howell WH (ed): *An American Textbook of Physiology*. Philadelphia, Saunders, 1901, 553 pp, pp 54–63.

2 Petit JL: Dissertation sur la manniere d'arrester le sang dans les hémorrhagies. *Mem Acad Roy Sci* 1:85–102, 1731.

3 Harvey SC: The history of hemostasis. *Ann Med Hist* n.s. 1:127–154, 1929.

4 Bizzozero G: Ueber eine neuen Formbestandtheil des Blutes und desen Rolle bei der Thrombose und der Blutgerinnung. *Virchows Arch (Pathol Anat)* 90:261–332, 1882.

5 Eberth JC, Schimmelbusch C: Experimentalle Untersuchungen über Thrombose. *Virchows Arch (Pathol Anat)* 103:39–87, 1886.

6 Plato: Timaeus, in Jewett B (ed): *The Dialogues of Plato,* 3d ed. New York, Macmillan, 1892, vol 3, pp 339–543, p 508.

7 Aristotle: *Meteorologica,* Lee HDP (trans), Loeb Classical Library. Cambridge, Harvard University Press, 1952, 432 pp.

8 Malpighi M: *De Polypo Cordis, 1686,* Forester JM (trans). Uppsala, Almqvist and Wiksels, 1956, 12 pp.

9 Hewson W: *The Works of William Hewson, F.R.S.,* Gulliver G (ed). London, The Sydenham Society, 1846, 360 pp.

10 Gulliver G: *Introduction to the Works of William Hewson, F.R.S.* London, The Sydenham Society, 1846, 360 pp.

11 Hunter J: *A Treatise on the Blood, Inflammation, and Gun-Shot Wounds.* Philadelphia, Webster, 1817, 514 pp.

12 Thackrah CT: *An Inquiry into the Nature and Properties of the Blood.* London, Cox, 1819, 132 pp.

13 Brücke E: Ueber die Ursache der Gerinnung des Blutes. *Arch Pathol Anat* 12:81–100; 172–196, 1857.

14 Virchow R: Ueber die akute Entzüdung der Arterien. *Arch Pathol Anat* 1:272–378, 1847.

15 Chaptal HA: Des observations sur les sens de quelques végétaux, et sur les

---

*The list of references provided is, of course, selective rather than exhaustive. It has two characteristics. When an investigator has written reviews of his work, these have been used rather than listing his individual papers, a concession needed to keep this account within reasonable bounds. References to many modern papers have been consciously omitted as there are innumerable current reviews on hemostasis; the writer offers his apologies to the authors who have been in this way slighted.

moyens dont le carbone circule dan le végétal et s'y dépose pour servir à la nutrition. *Ann Chim* 21:284–293, 1797.

16 Richardson BW: *The Cause of the Coagulation of the Blood.* London, Churchill, 1858, 466 pp.

17 Stuber B, Lang K: *Die Physiologie und Pathologie des Blutgerinung.* Berlin, Urban und Schwarzenberg, 1930, 91 pp.

18 Babington BG: Some considerations with respect to the blood founded on one or two very simple experiments on that fluid. *Med Chir Trans* 16:293–319, 1830.

19 Virchow R: *Gesammette Abdhandlungen zur Wissenschaftlischen Medicin.* Frankfurt, M Meidinger Sohn, 1856, 1024 pp.

20 Corin G, Ansiaux G: Untersuchungen über Phosphorvergiftung. *Vierteljahrsch. Gerichtl Med öffenlt Sanitätswesen* (3 folge) 7:80–95, 1894.

21 Denis de Commercy: Sur le sang considéré quand il est fluide, pendant qu'il se coagulé et lorsqu'il est coagulé. *C R Acad Sci (Paris)* 47:996–997, 1858.

22 Hammarsten O: *A Textbook of Physiological Chemistry,* 6th ed, Mandel JA (trans). New York, Wiley, 1911, 964 pp.

23 Buchanan A: On the coagulation of the blood and other fibriniferous liquids. *Lond Med Gaz* 1(n.s.):617, 1845; reprinted in *J Physiol* 2:158–168, 1879–1880.

24 Schmidt A: *Zur Blutlehre.* Leipzig, Vogel, 1892, 270 pp.

25 Jorpes JE: One hundred years of research on blood coagulation, leading to the present day anticoagulant therapy of thrombosis, in Koller T, Merz WR (eds): *Thrombosis and Embolism.* Basel, Benno Schwabe, 1955, pp 23–30.

26 Quick AJ: *Hemorrhagic Diseases.* Philadelphia, Lea and Febiger, 1957, 451 pp.

27 Eagle H: Studies on blood coagulation. I. The role of prothrombin and of platelets in the formation of thrombin. *J Gen Physiol* 18:531–545, 1935.

28 Warner ED, Brinkhous KM, Smith HP: A quantitative study on blood clotting: prothrombin fluctuations under experimental conditions. *Am J Physiol* 114:667–675, 1936.

29 Seegers WH: *Prothrombin.* Cambridge, Harvard University Press, 1962, 728 pp.

30 Bordet J: The theories of blood coagulation. *Bull Johns Hopkins Hosp* 32:213–218, 1921.

31 Schmidt A: Ueber den Faserstoff und die Ursachen seiner Gerinnung. *Arch Anat Physiol Wissensch Med* 28:545–587, 1861.

32 Mellanby J: Thrombase—its preparation and properties. *Proc R Soc Lond Sect B* 113:93–106, 1933.

33 Howell WH: Theories of blood coagulation. *Physiol Rev* 15:435–470, 1935.

34 Eagle H: Studies on blood coagulation. II. The formation of fibrin from thrombin and fibrinogen. *J Gen Physiol* 18:547–555, 1935.

35 Bailey K, Bettleheim FR, Lorand L, Middlebrook WR: Action of thrombin in the clotting of fibrinogen. *Nature* 167:233–234, 1951.

36 Sherry S, Troll W: The action of thrombin on synthetic substrates. *J Biol Chem* 208:95–105, 1954.

37 Apitz K: Über Profibrin. I. Die Entstehung und Bedeutung des Profibrins in Gerinnungsverlauf. *Z Gesamte Exp Med* 101:552–584, 1937.

38 Arthus M, Pagès C: Nouvelle théorie chimique de la coagulation du sang. *Arch Physiol Norm Pathol* (5s) 2:739–746, 1890.

39 Pekelharing CA: Über die Bedeutung dee Kalksalze für die Gerinnung. *Internat*

Beitr Z Wissensch Med (Festschrift, Rudolf Virchow) August Hirschwald, Berlin, 1:433–456, 1891.

40 Gamgee A: *A Text-Book of Physiological Chemistry of the Animal Body,* etc., London, Macmillan, 1880, 487 pp.

41 Robbins KD: A study on the conversion of fibrinogen to fibrin. *Am J Physiol* 142:581–588, 1944.

42 Laki K, Lorand L: On the solubility of fibrin clots. *Science* 108:280, 1948.

43 Thackrah CT: *An Inquiry into the Nature and Properties of the Blood.* London, Cox, 1834, 246 pp.

44 Andral G: *Practical Haematology. An Essay on the Blood in Disease,* Meigs JF, Stillé A (trans). Philadelphia, Lea and Blanchard, 1844, 129 pp.

45 Rabe F, Salomon E: Uber Faserstoffmangel im Blute bei einem Falle von Hämophilie. *Dtsch Arch Klin Med* 132:240–244, 1920.

46 Risak E: Die Fibrinopenie. *Z Klin Med* 128:605–629, 1935.

47 Imperato C, Dettori AG: Ipofibrinogenemia congenita con fibrinoastenia. *Helv Paediatr Acta* 13:380–399, 1958.

48 Babington B: On the morbid condition of the blood, in *Medical and Surgical Monographs.* Philadelphia, Dunglison's American Medical Library, A. Waldie, 1838, 31 pp.

49 Robb-Smith AHT: The growth of knowledge of the functions of the blood, in Macfarlane RG, Robb-Smith AHT (eds): *Functions of the Blood.* New York, Academic Press, 1961, 635 pp, pp xv–liv.

50 Duckert F, Jung E, Schmerling DH: A hitherto undescribed congenital haemorrhagic diathesis probably due to fibrin stabilizing factor deficiency. *Thromb Diath Haemorr* 5:179–186, 1961.

51 De Blainville HMD: Injection de matiere cerebrale dans les veins. *Gaz Med Paris* (ser. 2) 2:524, 1834.

52 Fuld E, Spiro K: Der Einfluss einiger gerinnungshemender Agentien auf das Vogelplasma. *Beitr Chem Phys Pathol* 5:171–190, 1904.

53 Morawitz P: The chemistry of blood coagulation. *Ergebn Physiol* 4:307–422, 1905. Reprinted in Hartmann RC, Guenther PF (trans), Springfield, Ill, Charles C Thomas, 1958, 194 pp.

54 Nolf P: The coagulation of the blood. *Medicine* (*Baltimore*) 17:381–411, 1938.

55 Sabbatini L: Le calcium-ion dans la coagulation du sang. *C R Soc Biol* (*Paris*) 54:716–718, 1902.

56 Mills CA: Chemical nature of tissue coagulins. *J Biol Chem* 46:135–165, 1921.

57 Chargaff E, Bendich A, Cohen SS: The thromboplastic protein: structure, properties, disintegration. *J Biol Chem* 156:161–178, 1944.

58 Wooldridge LD, in Horsley V, Starling E (eds): *On the Chemistry of the Blood and other Scientific Papers.* London, Kegan, Paul, Trench, Trübner, and Co, 1893, 354 pp.

59 Lenggenhager K: Neue Ergebnisse der Blutgerinnungsforschung. *Helv Med Acta* 1:527–542, 1935.

60 Mills CA, Guest GM: The rôle of tissue fibrinogen (thrombokinase) in fibrin formation and normal clotting. *Am J Physiol* 57:395–419, 1921.

61 Murray M: Vasculokinase: A clotting substance from arteries. *Am J Clin Pathol* 36:500–504, 1961.

62   Ferguson JH: An experimental analysis of coagulation activation. *Am J Physiol* 117:587–595, 1936.
63   Pickering JW: *Blood Plasma in Health and Disease.* London, Heinemann, 1928, 247 pp.
64   Warner ED, Brinkhous KM, Smith HP: The prothrombin conversion rate in various species. *Proc Soc Exp Biol Med* 40:197–200, 1939.
65   Quick AJ: On the constitution of prothrombin. *Am J Physiol* 140:212–220, 1943.
66   Quick AJ, Stanley-Brown M, Bancroft FW: A study of the coagulation defect in hemophilia and in jaundice. *Am J Med Sci* 190:501–511, 1935.
67   Owren PA: The coagulation of blood. Investigations on a new clotting factor. *Acta Med Scand* Suppl 194:1–327, 1947.
68   Astrup T: Blood clotting and related processes, in Nord FF (ed): *Advances in Enzymology and Related Subjects of Biochemistry.* New York, Interscience, 1950, vol 10, pp 1–49.
69   Owren PA, Bjerkelund C: A new, previously unknown clotting factor. *Scand J Clin Lab Invest* 1:162–163, 1949 (letter).
70   Alexander B, Goldstein R, Landwehr G, Cook CD: Congenital SPCA deficiency: A hitherto unrecognized coagulation defect with hemorrhage rectified by serum and serum fractions. *J Clin Invest* 30:596–608, 1951.
71   Hougie C, Barrow EM, Graham JB: Stuart clotting defect. I. Segregation of an hereditary hemorrhagic state from the heterogenous group heretofore called "stable factor" (SPCA, proconvertin, factor VII) deficiency. *J Clin Invest* 36:485–496, 1957.
72   Telfer TP, Denson KW, Wright DR: A "new" coagulation defect. *Br J Haematol* 2:308–316, 1956.
73   Macfarlane RG, Barnett B: The haemostatic possibilities of snake venom. *Lancet* 2:985–987, 1934.
74   Duckert F, Flückiger P, Koller F: Le role du facteur X dans la formation de la thromboplastine sanguine. *Rev Hematol* 9:489–492, 1954.
75   Mellanby J, Pratt CLG: Calcium and blood coagulation. *Proc R Soc Med Sect B* 128:201–213, 1940.
76   Dam H: Cholesterinstoffwechsel in Hühnereiern und Hühnchen. *Biochem Z* 215:475–492, 1929.
77   McFarlane WD, Graham WR Jr, Richardson F: The fat soluble vitamin requirement of the chick. I. The vitamin A and vitamin D contents of fish meal and meat meal. *Biochem J* 25:358–366, 1931.
78   Almquist HJ, Stokstad ELR: Hemorrhagic chick disease of dietary origin. *J Biol Chem* 111:105–113, 1935.
79   Dam H: The antihaemorrhagic vitamin of the chick. *Biochem J* 29:1273–1285, 1935.
80   Dam H, Schønheyder F, Tage-Hansen E: Studies on the mode of action of vitamin K. *Biochem J* 30:1075–1079, 1936.
81   Butt HR, Snell AM, Osterberg AE: The use of vitamin K and bile in treatment of the hemorrhagic diathesis in cases of jaundice. *Proc Staff Meet Mayo Clinic* 13:74–77, 1938.
82   Warner ED, Brinkhous KM, Smith HP: Bleeding tendency of obstructive jaundice: prothrombin deficiency and dietary factors. *Proc Soc Exp Biol Med* 37:628–630, 1938.
83   Dam H, Glavind J: Vitamin K in human pathology. *Lancet* 1:720–721, 1938.

84 Hawkins WB, Brinkhous KM: Prothrombin deficiency the cause of bleeding in bile fistula dogs. *J Exp Med* 63:795–801, 1936.

85 Almquist HJ, Close AA: Synthetic and natural antihemorrhagic compounds. *J Am Chem Soc* 61:2557–2558, 1939.

86 Binkley SB, Cheney LC, Holcomb WF, McKee RW, Thayer SA, MacCorquodale DW, Doisy EA: The constitution and synthesis of vitamin K. *J Am Chem Soc* 61:2558–2559, 1939.

87 Feiser LF: Synthesis of 2-methyl-3-phytyl-1, 4-naphthoquinine. *J Am Chem Soc* 61:2559–2560, 1939.

88 Schofield FW: Damaged sweet clover: The cause of a new disease in cattle simulating hemorrhagic septicemia and black leg. *J Am Vet Med Assoc* 64:(n.s. 17):553–575, 1924.

89 Roderick LM: A problem in the coagulation of the blood. "Sweet clover disease of cattle." *Am J Physiol* 96:413–425, 1931.

90 Link KP: The discovery of Dicumarol and its sequels. *Circulation* 19:97–107, 1959.

91 Butt HR, Allen EV, Bollman JL: A preparation from spoiled sweet clover [3,3'-methylene-bis-(4-hydroxycoumarin)] which prolongs coagulation and prothrombin time of the blood: preliminary report of experimental and clinical studies. *Proc Staff Meet Mayo Clinic* 16:388–395, 1941.

92 Bingham JB, Meyer OO, Pohle FJ: Studies on the hemorrhagic agent 3,3'-methylenebis (4-hydroxycoumarin). I. The effect on the prothrombin and coagulation time of the blood of dogs and humans. *Am J Med Sci* 202:563–578, 1941.

93 Goodknight SH Jr, Feinstein DI, Østerud B, Rapaport SI: Factor VII antibody-neutralizing material in hereditary and acquired factor VII deficiency. *Blood* 38:1–8, 1971.

94 Suttie JW: Cellular biochemistry of prothrombin synthesis. 21st Wayne State Symposium on Blood. Detroit. Jan. 18–19, 1973, in Hammen EF, Anderson GF, Barnhart MI (eds): *Thromb Diath Haemorr, Suppl 57*. Stuttgart, New York, Schattauer, 1974, 340 pp, pp 6–7.

95 Olson JP, Miller LL, Troup SB: Synthesis of clotting factors by the isolated perfused rat liver. *J Clin Invest* 45:690–701, 1966.

96 Stenflo J, Fernlund P, Egan W, Roepstorff P: Vitamin K dependent modifications of glutamic acid residues in prothrombin. *Proc Natl Acad Sci USA* 71:2730–2733, 1974.

97 Williams WJ, Norris DG: Purification of a bovine plasma protein (factor VII) which is required for the activity of lung microsomes in blood coagulation. *J Biol Chem* 241:1847–1856, 1966.

98 Nemerson Y: The reaction between bovine brain tissue factor and factors VII and X. *Biochemistry* 5:601–608, 1966.

99 Eagle H, Harris TN: Studies in blood coagulation. V. The coagulation of blood by proteolytic enzymes (trypsin, papain). *J Gen Physiol* 20:543–560, 1937.

100 Milstone JH: Thrombokinase of the blood as trypsin-like enzyme. *J Gen Physiol* 45(suppl):103–113, 1962.

101 Seegers WH: Enzyme theory of blood clotting. *Fed Proc* 23:749–756, 1964.

102 Arthus M: Étude sur la production de fibrinferment dans le sang extrait de vaisseaux. *C R Soc Biol (Paris)* 53:1024–1027, 1901.

103 Wadsworth A, Maltaner F, Maltaner E: A study of the coagulation of the blood; the chemical reactions underlying the process. *Am J Physiol* 80:502–521, 1927.

104 Quick AJ: *The Hemorrhagic Diseases and the Physiology of Hemostasis.* Springfield, Ill., Charles C Thomas, 1942, 340 pp.

105 Lambert SW: Melaena neonatorum with report of a case cured by transfusion. *Med Record* 73:885–887, 1908.

106 Townsend CW: The haemorrhagic disease of the new-born. *Arch Pediatr* 11:559–565, 1894.

107 Whipple GH: Hemorrhagic disease—septicemia, melena neonatorum and hepatic cirrhosis. *Arch Intern Med* 9:363–399, 1912.

108 Brinkhous KM, Smith HP, Warner ED: Plasma protein level in normal infancy and in hemorrhagic disease of the newborn. *Am J Med Sci* 193:475–480, 1937.

109 Waddell WW Jr, Guerry DuP III, Bray WE, Kelley OR: Possible effects of vitamin K on prothrombin and clotting time in newly-born infants. *Proc Soc Exp Biol Med* 40:432–434, 1939.

110 Wedelius GW: *De haemorrhagia universali, ex ictero nigro lethali,* 1683, quoted by Butt HR, Snell AM, Osterberg AE: The preoperative and postoperative administration of vitamin K to patients having jaundice. *JAMA* 113:383–390, 1939.

111 Budd G *On Diseases of the Liver.* Philadelphia, Lea and Blanchard, 1846, 401 pp.

112 Trousseau A: *Lectures on Clinical Medicine Delivered at the Hotel Dieu, Paris,* 3d ed, Cormack JR (trans). London, New Sydenham Soc, 1872, vol 4, p 313; vol 5, p 287.

113 Morawitz P, Bierich R: Ueber die Pathogenese der cholämischen Blutungen. *Arch Exp Pathol Pharm* 56:115–129, 1907.

114 Sims JM: Remarks on cholecystotomy in dropsy of the gall-bladder. *Br Med J* 1:811–815, 1878.

115 Murchison C: *Clinical Lectures on Diseases of the Liver,* 3d ed. London, Longmans Green, 1885, 702 pp.

116 Whipple GH: Hemorrhagic disease. Antithrombin and prothrombin factors. *Arch Intern Med* 12:637–659, 1913.

117 Greaves JD, Schmidt CLA: Nature of the factor concerned in loss of blood coagulability of bile fistula rats. *Proc Soc Exp Biol Med* 37:43–45, 1937.

118 Smith HP, Warner ED, Brinkhous KM, Seegers WH: Bleeding tendency and prothrombin deficiency in biliary fistula dogs: effect of feeding bile and vitamin K. *J Exp Med* 67:911–920, 1938.

119 Jones TW: Observations on some points in the anatomy, physiology, and pathology of the blood. *Br Foreign Med Rev* 14:585–600, 1842.

120 Lister J: On the coagulation of the blood. *Proc R Soc Lond* 12:580–611, 1863.

121 Freund E: Ein Beitrag zur Kenntniss der Blutgerinnung. *Med Jahrb (Wien)* n.s. (3) 1:46–48, 1886.

122 Barrier: quoted by Hayem G: *Du sang et des alterations anatomiques.* Paris, Masson, 1889, 1035 pp, pp 219–220.

123 Hayem G: *Du sang et des alterations anatomiques.* Paris, Masson, 1889, 1035 pp.

124 Collingwood BJ, MacMahon MT: The anti-coagulants in blood and serum. *J Physiol* 45:119–145, 1912.

125 Lenggenhager K: Irrwege der Blutgerinnungsforschung. *Klin Wochenschr* 15:1835–1838, 1936.

126 Lozner E, Taylor FHL: The effect of foreign surfaces on blood coagulation. *J Clin Invest* 21:241–245, 1942.

127 Conley CL, Hartmann RC, Morse WI II: The clotting behavior of human "plate-

let-free'' plasma: Evidence for the existence of a "plasma thromboplastin." *J Clin Invest* 28:340–352, 1949.

128 Jaques LB, Fidlar E, Feldsted ET, Macdonald AG: Silicones and blood coagulation. *Can Med Assoc J* 55:26–31, 1946.

129 Milstone JH: On the evolution of blood clotting theory. *Medicine (Baltimore)* 31:411–447, 1952.

130 Macfarlane RG: An enzyme cascade in the blood clotting mechanism, and its function as a biochemical amplifier. *Nature* 202:498–499, 1964.

131 Davie EW, Ratnoff OD: Waterfall sequence for intrinsic blood clotting. *Science* 145:1310–1311, 1964.

132 Biggs R, Douglas AS: The thromboplastin generation test. *J Clin Pathol* 6:23–29, 1953.

133 Langdell RD, Wagner RH, Brinkhous KM: Effect of antihemophilic factor on one-stage clotting tests: A presumptive test for hemophilia and a simple one-stage antihemophilic factor assay procedure. *J Lab Clin Med* 41:637–647, 1953.

134 Ratnoff OD, Colopy JE: A familial hemorrhagic trait associated with a deficiency of a clot-promoting fraction of plasma. *J Clin Invest* 34:602–613, 1955.

135 Ratnoff OD, Hartmann RC, Conley CL: Studies on a proteolytic enzyme in human plasma. V. The relationship between the proteolytic activity of plasma and blood coagulation. *J Exp Med* 91:123–133, 1950.

136 Margolis J: Glass surface and blood coagulation. *Nature* 178:805–806, 1956.

137 Shafrir E, deVries A: Studies on the clot-promoting activity of glass. *J Clin Invest* 35:1183–1190, 1956.

138 Ratnoff OD, Rosenblum JM: Role of Hageman factor in the initiation of clotting by glass. Evidence that glass frees Hageman factor from inhibition. *Am J Med* 25:160–168, 1958.

139 Ratnoff OD: Some relationships among hemostasis, fibrinolytic phenomena, immunity, and the inflammatory response, in Dixon FJ Jr, Kunkel HG (eds): *Advances in Immunology*. New York, Academic Press, 1969, vol 10, pp 145–227.

140 Vroman L: Surface contact and thromboplastin formation. Thesis, U. of Utrecht, 1958, Druckkerij Elinkwijk, Utrecht.

141 Rosenthal RL, Dreskin OH, Rosenthal N: New hemophilia-like disease caused by deficiency of a third plasma thromboplastin factor. *Proc Soc Exp Biol Med* 82:171–174, 1953.

142 Rapaport SI, Proctor RR, Patch MJ, Yettra M: The mode of inheritance of PTA deficiency: evidence for the existence of major PTA deficiency and minor PTA deficiency. *Blood* 18:149–165, 1961.

143 Margolis J: Activation of plasma by contact with glass: evidence for a common reaction which releases plasma kinin and initiates coagulation. *J Physiol* 144:1–22, 1958.

144 Jacobsen S, Kriz M: Some data on two purified kininogens from human plasma. *Br J Pharmacol Chemother* 29:25–36, 1967.

145 Hathaway WE, Belhasen LP, Hathaway HS: Evidence for a new plasma thromboplastin factor. I. Case report, coagulation studies and physicochemical properties. *Blood* 26:521–532, 1965.

146 Waldmann R, Abraham JP, Rebuck JW, Caldwell J, Saito H, Ratnoff OD: Fitzgerald factor: A hitherto unrecognized clotting factor. *Lancet* 1:949–950, 1975.

147 Colman RW, Bagdasarian A, Talamo RC, Scott CF, Seavey M, Guimares JA, Pierce JV, Kaplan AP: Williams trait: human kininogen deficiency with diminished levels of plasminogen proactivator and prekallikrein associated with abnormalities of the Hageman factor–dependent pathways. *J Clin Invest* 56:1650–1662, 1975.

148 Wuepper KD, Miller DR, Lacombe MJ: Flaujeac trait: deficiency of human plasma kininogen. *J Clin Invest* 56:1663–1672, 1975.

149 Lutcher CL: Reid trait: A new expression of high molecular weight kininogen (HMW-kininogen) deficiency. *Clin Res* 24:47A, 1976.

150 Wuepper KD: Biochemistry and biology of components of the plasma kinin-forming system, in Lepow IH, Ward PA (eds): *Inflammation, Mechanisms and Control*. New York, Academic Press, 1972, 409 pp, pp 93–117.

151 Epstein I (ed): *The Babylonian Talmud, Yebamoth. Sect. 64B*, Slotki WI (trans). London, Soncino Press, 1936, 34 vols, vol 1, p 431.

152 Immerman NH: Hemophilia, scurvy and morbus maculosus, in Ziemssen H von (ed): *Cyclopedia of the Practice of Medicine*. American Edition, New York, Wm Wood, 1878, vol 17, pp 1–104.

153 Bulloch W, Fildes P: Hemophilia, in *Treasury of Human Inheritance*, Galton Lab., U. London, Parts V and VI, Sect. XIVa, pp. 169–347. London, Cambridge University Press, 1911, 591 pp.

154 McKusick VA: Hemophilia in early New England. A follow-up of four kindreds in which hemophilia occurred in the pre-revolutionary period. *J Hist Med* 17:342–365, 1962.

155 McKusick VA: The earliest record of hemophilia in America? *Blood* 19:243–244, 1962.

156 Otto JC: An account of an hemorrhagic disposition existing in certain families. *Med Repository* 6:1–4, 1803.

157 Moor-Jankowski JK, Huser HJ, Rosin S, Truog G, Schneeberger J, Geiger M: *Haemophilie B: Genetische, klinische und gerinnungsphysiologische Aspekte (Untersuchungen an einem weitverbreiteten Bluterstamm)*. Basel, S Karger, 1958, 234 pp.

158 Brinkhous KM: Chairman's comments, in Brinkhous KM, de Nicola P (eds): *Hemophilia and Other Hemorrhagic States*. Chapel Hill, University of North Carolina Press, 1959, 266 pp, pp xix–xx.

159 Nasse CF: Vor einer erblichen Neigung zu tödtlichen Blutungen. *Arch Med Erfahr* 1:385–434, 1820.

160 Grandidier L: *Die Haemophilie oder die Bluterkrankheit*. Leipzig, O. Wigand, 1855, 158 pp (quoted by Bulloch and Fildes[153]).

160a Crile GW: *Hemorrhage and Transfusion. An Experimental and Clinical Research*. New York, D. Appleton, 1909, 560 pp.

161 Hay J: Account of a remarkable haemorrhagic disposition, existing in many individuals of the same family. *N Engl J Med Surg* 2:221–225, 1813.

162 Legg JW: Report on haemophilia with a note on the hereditary descent of colour-blindness. *St Bartholomew's Hosp Rep* 17:303–320, 1881.

163 Morgan TH: *The Theory of the Gene*. New York, Haffner, 1964, 351 pp (reprint of 1929 edition, second printing).

164 Mr. Ward, quoted by Wardrop J: *On the Curative Effects of the Abstraction of Blood*. Philadelphia, A. Waldie, 1837, 73 pp, pp 9–10.

165 Vierordt CH: Die Gerinnungszeit des Blutes in gesunden und kranken Zustände. *Arch Heilk* 19:193–221, 1878.

166 Wright AE: On the method of determining the condition of blood coagulability for clinical and experimental purposes, and on the effect of the administration of calcium salts in haemophilia and actual or threatened hemorrhage. *Br Med J* 2:223–225, 1893.

167 Manteuffel Z v: Bermerkungen zur Blutstillung bei Häemophilie. *Dtsch Med Wochenschr* 19:665–667, 1893.

168 Addis T: The pathogenesis of hereditary hemophilia. *J Pathol Bacteriol* 15:427–452, 1911.

169 Fonio A: Über die Gerinnungsfaktoren des hämophilien Blutes. Eine Studie über die Gerinnungsvorgänge. *Mitt Grenz Geb Med Chir* 28:313–348, 1915.

170 Minot GR, Lee RI: The blood platelet in hemophilia. *Arch Intern Med* 18:474–495, 1916.

171 Frank E, Hartmann E: Über das Wesen und die therapeutische Korrektur der Hämophilen Gerinnungsstörung. *Klin Wochenschr* 6:435–439, 1927.

172 Govaertz P, Gratia A: Contribution á l'étude de l'hémophilie. *Rev Belge Sci Med* 3:689–696, 1931.

173 Patek AJ Jr, Stetson RH: Hemophilia. I. The abnormal coagulation of the blood and its relation to the blood platelets. *J Clin Invest* 15:531–542, 1936.

174 Patek AJ Jr, Taylor FHL: Hemophilia. II. Some properties of a substance obtained from normal plasma effective in accelerating the clotting of hemophilic blood. *J Clin Invest* 16:113–124, 1937.

175 Tocantins L: Hemophilic syndromes and hemophilia. *Blood* 9:281–285, 1954.

176 Shanberge JN, Gore I: Studies on the immunologic and physiologic activities of antihemophilic factor (AHF). *J Lab Clin Med* 50:954, 1957 (abstract).

177 Bennett E, Heuhns ER: Immunologic differentiation of three types of haemophilia and identification of some female carriers. *Lancet* 2:956–958, 1970.

178 Zimmerman TS, Ratnoff OD, Powell AE: Immunologic differentiation of classic hemophilia (factor VIII deficiency) and von Willebrand's disease, with observations on combined deficiencies of antihemophilic factor and proaccelerin (factor V) and on an acquired circulating anticoagulant against antihemophilic factor. *J Clin Invest* 50:244–254, 1971.

179 Zimmerman TS, Ratnoff OD, Littell AS: Detection of carriers of classic hemophilia using an immunologic assay for antihemophilic factor (factor VIII). *J Clin Invest* 50:255–258, 1971.

180 Willebrand EA von: Über hereditare Pseudohämophilie. *Acta Med Scand* 76:521–549, 1931.

181 Hayem G, quoted by Dreyfuss C: *Some Milestones in the History of Hematology.* New York, Grune and Stratton, 1956, 87 pp.

182 Duke WW: The relation of blood platelets to hemorrhagic disease. Description of a method for determining the bleeding time and coagulation time and report of three cases of hemorrhagic disease relieved by transfusion. *JAMA* 55:1185–1192, 1910.

183 Minot GR: A familial hemorrhagic condition associated with prolongation of the bleeding time. *Am J Med Sci* 175:301–306, 1928.

184 Macfarlane RG: Critical review: The mechanism of hemostasis. *Q J Med* n.s. 10:1–29, 1941.

185 Alexander B, Goldstein R: Dual hemostatic defect in pseudohemophilia. *J Clin Invest* 32:55, 1953 (abstract).

186   Larrieu M-J, Soulier JP: Deficit en factuer anti-hemophilique a chez une fille associé à un trouble de saignement. *Rev Hematol* 8:361–370, 1953.

187   Quick AJ, Hussey CV: Hemophilic condition in the female. *J Lab Clin Med* 42:929–930, 1953 (abstract).

188   Salzman EW: Measurement of platelet adhesiveness: a simple *in vitro* technique demonstrating an abnormality in von Willebrand's disease. *J Lab Clin Med* 62:724–735, 1963.

189   Zucker MB: *In vitro* abnormality of the blood in von Willebrand's disease correctable by normal plasma. *Nature* 197:601–602, 1963.

190   Howard MA, Firkin BG: Ristocetin—a new tool in the investigation of platelet aggregation. *Thromb Diath Haemor* 26:362–369, 1971.

191   Nilsson IM, Blombäck M, Blombäck B: The use of antihaemophilic globulin (fraction I-O) in haemophilia A and in von Willebrand's disease. *Acta Haematol (Basel)* 24:116–123, 1960.

192   Owen WG, Wagner RH: Antihemophilic factor: separation of an active fragment following dissociation by salts and detergents. *Thromb Diath Haemor* 27:502–515, 1972.

193   Weiss HJ, Phillips LL, Rosner W: Separation of subunits of antihemophilic factor (AHF) by agarose gel chromatography. *Thromb Diath Haemor* 27:212–219, 1972.

194   Jaffe EA, Hoyer LW, Bachman RL: Synthesis of antihemophilic factor antigen by cultured human endothelial cells. *J Clin Invest* 52:2757–2764, 1973.

195   Lane S: Hemorrhagic diathesis. Successful transfusion of blood. *Lancet* 1:185–188, 1840.

196   Émile-Weil P: L'hemophilie. Pathogénie et sérothérapie. *Presse Méd* 2:673–676, 1905.

197   Feissly R: Beiträge zur Wesen und zur Therapie der Hämophilie. *Jahrb Kinderheilk* 110:297–308, 1925.

198   Edsall JT, Ferry RM, Armstrong SH Jr: Chemical, clinical and immunological studies on the products of human plasma fractionation. XV. The proteins concerned in the blood coagulation mechanism. *J Clin Invest* 23:557–565, 1944.

199   Wagner RH, McLester WD, Smith M, Brinkhous KM: Purification of antihemophilic factor (factor VIII) by amino acid precipitation. *Thromb Diath Haemor* 11:67–74, 1964.

200   Pool JG, Hershgold EJ, Pappenhagen AR: High-potency antihaemophilic factor concentrate prepared from cryoglobulin precipitate. *Nature* 203:312, 1964.

201   Mills CA: The clotting properties of pure blood and of pure plasma. *Chin J Physiol* 1:249–262, 1927.

202   Lawrence JS, Johnson JB: The presence of a circulating anticoagulant in a male member of a hemophiliac family. *Trans Am Clin Clim Assoc* 57:223–231, 1942.

203   Munro FL, Munro MP: Electrophoretic isolation of a circulating anticoagulant. *J Clin Invest* 25:814–815, 1946.

204   Chargaff E, West R: The biological significant of the thromboplastic protein of blood. *J Biol Chem* 166:189–197, 1946.

205   Shapiro SS, Hultin M: Acquired inhibitors to the blood coagulation factors. *Semin Thromb Hemostas* 1:336–385, 1975.

206   Pavlovsky A: Contribution to the pathogenesis of hemophilia. *Blood* 2:185–191, 1947.

207 Aggeler PM, White SG, Glendenning MB, Page EW, Leake TB, Bates G: Plasma thromboplastin component (PTC) deficiency: a new disease resembling hemophilia. *Proc Soc Exp Biol Med* 79:692–694, 1952.

208 Schulman I, Smith CH: Hemorrhagic disease in an infant due to deficiency of a previously undescribed clotting factor. *Blood* 7:794–807, 1952.

209 Biggs R, Douglas AS, Macfarlane RG, Dacie JV, Pitney WR, Merskey C, O'Brien JR: Christmas disease: a condition previously mistaken for haemophilia. *Br Med J* 2:1378–1382, 1952.

210 Fantl P, Sawers RJ, Marr AG: Investigation of a haemorrhagic disease due to beta-prothromboplastin deficiency complicated by a specific inhibitor of thromboplastin formation. *Australas Ann Med* 5:163–176, 1956.

211 Bachman F, Duckert F, Fisch U, Streuli F, Gerber D, Koller F: Der Gerinnungsdefekt beim konigenitalen PTA-mangel. *Schweiz Med Wochenschr* 88:1037–1044, 1958.

212 Soulier JP, Wartelle O, Ménaché D: Caractères differentiels des facteurs Hageman et P.T.A. Rôle du contact dans la phase initiale de la coagulation. *Rev Fr Etudes Clin Biol* 3:263–267, 1958.

213 Barton PG: Sequence theories of blood coagulation re-evaluated with reference to lipid-protein interactions. *Nature* 215:1508–1509, 1967.

214 Hemker HC, Kahn MJP: Reaction sequence of blood coagulation. *Nature* 215:1201–1202, 1967.

215 Hougie C, Denson KWE, Biggs R: A study of the reaction product of factor VIII and factor IX by gel filtration. *Thromb Diath Haemor* 18:211–222, 1967.

216 Spurling CL, King PDW: Studies on thromboplastin generation. *J Lab Clin Med* 44:336–348, 1954.

217 Quick AJ, Hussey CV, Epstein E: Activation of thromboplastinogen by thrombin. *Am J Physiol* 174:123–126, 1953.

218 Rapaport SI, Schiffman S, Patch MJ, Ames SB: The importance of activation of antihemophilic globulin and proaccelerin by traces of thrombin in the generation of intrinsic prothrombinase activity. *Blood* 21:221–236, 1963.

219 Quick AJ: Discussion, in Flynn JE (ed): *Trans. Fourth Conference on Blood Clotting and Allied Problems.* New York, Josiah Macy, J., Foundation, 1951, 272 pp, pp 68–69.

220 Fuchs HJ, Falkenhausen MV, Small V, Hartmann E: Uber die Beteiligung des Komplements bei Blutgerinnung. Eines neue Theorie über den Ablauf der Blutgerinnung. *Z Gesamte Exp Med* 64:227–238, 1929.

221 Fuld E: Über die Vorbedingungen der Blutgerennung sowie über die Gerinnbarkeit des Fluorplasmas. *Zentralbl Physiol* 17:529–533, 1903.

222 Foà C: Sulle leggi d'azione dell thrombina. *Arch Fisiol* 10:479–500, 1912.

223 Rettger LA: The coagulation of blood. *Am J Physiol* 24:406–435, 1909.

224 Schmidt-Mülheim A: Beiträge zur Kentniss des Peptons und seiner physiologischen Bedeutung. *Arch Anat Physiol: Phys Abth* 38–56, 1880.

225 McLean J: The discovery of heparin. *Circulation* 19:75–78, 1959.

226 Jorpes E: *Heparin in the Treatment of Thrombosis. An Account of its Chemistry, Physiology and Application in Medicine,* 2d ed. New York, Oxford University Press, 1946, 260 pp.

227 Jaques LB: Addendum: The discovery of heparin. *Semin Thromb Hemostas* 4:350–353, 1978.

228 Monkhouse FC, France ES, Seegers WH: Studies on the antithrombic and heparin cofactor activities of a fraction absorbed from plasma by aluminum hydroxide. *Circ Res* 3:397–402, 1955.

229 Seegers WH, Marciniak E: Inhibition of autoprothrombin C activity with plasma. *Nature* 193:1188–1190, 1962.

230 Yin ET, Wessler S, Stoll PJ: Biological properties of the naturally occurring plasma inhibitor to activated factor X. *J Biol Chem* 246:3703–3711, 1971.

231 Brinkhous KM, Smith HP, Warner ED, Seegers WH: The inhibition of blood clotting: an unidentified substance which acts in conjunction with heparin to prevent the conversion of prothrombin into thrombin. *Am J Physiol* 125:683–687, 1939.

232 Mason EC: Blood coagulation. The production and prevention of thrombosis and pulmonary embolism. *Surg Gynecol Obstet* 39:421–428, 1924.

233 Mason EC: A note on the use of heparin in blood transfusion. *J Lab Clin Med* 10:203–206, 1924.

234 Scott D, Charles AF: Studies on heparin III. The purification of heparin. *J Biol Chem* 102:437–448, 1933.

235 Murray DWG, Jacques LB, Perrett TS, Best CH: Heparin and the thrombosis of veins following injury. *Surgery* 2:163–187, 1937.

236 Craoford C: Preliminary report on post-operative treatment with heparin as a preventive of thrombosis. *Acta Chir Scand* 79:407–426, 1937.

237 Ratnoff OD, Lepow IH: Some properties of an esterase derived from preparations of the first component of complement. *J Exp Med* 106:327–343, 1957.

238 Lanchantin JF, Plesset ML, Friedman JA, Hart DW: Dissociation of esterolytic and clotting activities of thrombin by trypsin-binding macroglobulin. *Proc Soc Exp Biol Med* 121:444–449, 1966.

239 Rimon A, Shamash Y, Shapiro B: The plasmin inhibitor of human plasma. IV. Its action on plasmin, trypsin, chymotrypsin, and thrombin. *J Biol Chem* 241:5102–5107, 1966.

240 Heck LW, Kaplan AP: Substrates of Hageman factor. I. Isolation and characterization of human factor XI (PTA) and inhibition of the activated enzyme by α_1-antitrypsin. *J Exp Med* 140:1615–1630, 1974.

241 Saito H, Ratnoff OD, Donaldson VH, Haney G, Pensky J: Inhibition of the adsorption of Hageman factor (factor XII) to glass by normal human plasma. *J Lab Clin Med* 84:62–73, 1974.

242 Saito H, Goldsmith GH, Moroi M, Aoki N: The spectrum of α_2-plasmin inhibitor. *Blood* 50 (suppl 1):232, 1977 (abstract).

243 Donaldson VH, Evans RR: A biochemical abnormality in hereditary angioneurotic edema. Absence of serum inhibitor of C'1 esterase. *Am J Med* 35:37–44, 1963.

244 Delezenne C: *Travaux de Physiologie.* U. de Montpellier, 1898, quoted by Howell (1).

245 Konttinen YP: *Fibrinolysis: Chemistry, Physiology, Pathology and Clinics.* Finland, Cy. Star. Ab., 1968, 643 pp.

246 Morawitz P: Uber einege postmortale Blutveranderungen. *Beitr Chem Physiol Pathol Brunschweig* 8:1–14, 1906.

247 Denis PS: *Essai sur l'Application de la Chemie à l'Étude Physiologique du Sang de l'Homme et à l'Étude Physio-pathologique, Hygiéneque et Thérapeutique des Maladies de Cette Humeur.* Paris, Béchet Jeune, 1838, 366 pp.

248 Green JR: Note on the action of sodium chloride in dissolving fibrin. *J Physiol* 8:372–377, 1887.
249 Dastre A: Fibrinolyse dans le sang. *Arch Physiol Norm Pathol* 5:661–663, 1893.
250 Jacoby M: Ueber die Beziehungen der Leber—und Blutveränderungen bie Phosphovergiftung zume Autolyse. *Z Physiol Chem* 30:174–181, 1900.
251 Hedin SG: On the presence of a proteolytic enzyme in the normal serum of the ox. *J Physiol* 30:195–201, 1904.
252 Denys J, de Marbaix H: Sur les peptonisations provoqueés par le chloroforme et quelques autre substances. *Cellule* 5:197–251, 1889.
253 Delezenne C, Pozerski E: Action du sérum sanguin sur la gélatine en présence du chloroforme. *C R Soc Biol (Paris)* 55:327–329, 1903.
254 Ogston D, Ogston CM, Ratnoff OD, Forbes CD: Studies on a complex mechanism for the activation of plasminogen by kaolin and by chloroform: The participation of Hageman factor and additional cofactors. *J Clin Invest* 48:1786–1801, 1969.
255 Deutsch DG, Mertz ET: Plasminogen: purification from human plasma by affinity chromatography. *Science* 170:1095–1096, 1970.
256 Gratia A: Quoted by Kontinnen YP, in *Fibrinolysis: Chemistry, Physiology, Pathology and Clinics*. Finland, Cy. Star. Ab., 1968, 643 pp.
257 Tillett WS, Garner RL: The fibrinolytic activity of hemolytic streptococci. *J Exp Med* 58:485–502, 1933.
258 Milstone JH: A factor in normal human blood which participates in streptococcal fibrinolysis. *J Immunol* 42:109–116, 1941.
259 Kaplan MH: Nature and role of the lytic factor in hemolytic streptococcal fibrinolysis. *Proc Soc Exp Biol Med* 57:40–43, 1944.
260 Christensen LR, MacLeod CM: Proteolytic enzyme of serum: characterization, activation and reaction with inhibitors. *J Gen Physiol* 28:559–583, 1945.
261 Ratnoff OD: Studies on a proteolytic enzyme in human plasma. II. Some factors influencing the enzymes activated by chloroform and by streptococcal fibrinolysin. *J Exp Med* 87:211–228, 1948.
262 Conradi H: Über die Beziehung der Autolyse zur Blutgerrinung. *Beitr Chem Physiol Pathol* 1:136–182, 1902.
263 Fleisher MS, Loeb R: On tissue fibrinolysins. *J Biol Chem* 21:477–501, 1915.
264 Astrup T, Permin PM: Fibrinolysis in the animal organism. *Nature* 159:681–682, 1947.
265 Williams JRB: The fibrinolytic activity of urine. *Br J Exp Pathol* 32:530–537, 1951.
266 Goodpasture EW: Fibrinolysis in chronic hepatic insufficiency. *Bull Johns Hopkins Hosp* 25:330–336, 1914.
267 Biggs R, Macfarlane RG, Pilling J: Observations on fibrinolysis: experimental activity produced by exercise or adrenaline. *Lancet* 1:402–405, 1947.
268 Tagnon HJ, Levenson SM, Davidson CS, Taylor FHL: The occurrence of fibrinolysis in shock, with observations on the prothrombin time and the plasma fibrinogen during hemorrhagic shock. *Am J Med* 211:88–96, 1946.
269 Sherry S, Fletcher A, Alkjaersig N: Fibrinolysis and fibrinolytic activity in man. *Physiol Rev* 39:343–381, 1959.
270 Kwaan HC, Lo R, McFadzean AJS: On the production of plasma fibrinolytic activity within veins. *Clin Sci* 16:242–253, 1957.
271 Nolf P: De la nature de l'hypoleucocytose propeptonique. *Arch Int Physiol* 1:242–260, 1904.

272   Todd AS: The histological localisation of fibrinolysin activator. *J Pathol Bacteriol* 78:281–283, 1959.
273   Ogston D, Bennett B, Mackie M: Properties of a partially purified preparation of a circulating plasminogen activator. *Thromb Res* 8:275–284, 1976.
274   Niewiarowski S, Prou-Wartelle O: Rôle du facteur contact (facteur Hageman) dans la fibrinolyse. *Thromb Diath Haemor* 3:593–603, 1959.
275   Iatridis SG, Ferguson JH: Active Hageman factor: a plasma lysokinase of the human fibrinolytic system. *J Clin Invest* 41:1277–1287, 1962.
276   Nussenzweig V, Seligmann M, Pelmont J, Grabar P: Les produits de dégradation du fibrinogène humain par la plasmine. I. Séparation et proprietes physico-chemiques. *Ann Inst Pasteur (Paris)* 100:377–389, 1961.
277   Marder VJ, Shulman NR, Carroll WR: The importance of intermediate degradation products of fibrinogen in fibrinolytic hemorrhage. *Trans Assoc Am Physicians* 80:156–167, 1967.
278   Niewiarowski S, Kowalski E: Un nouvel anticoagulant dérivé du fibrinogène. *Rev Hematol* 13:320–328, 1958.
279   Delezenne C, Pozerski E: Action proteolytique du sérum sanguin préalablement traité par le chloroforme. *C R Soc Biol (Paris)* 55:690–692, 1903.
280   Meneghini P: The development of thrombolytic activity, in *Thrombolytic Activity and Related Phenomena. Thromb Diath Haemor* (suppl), 1961, pp 217–226.
281   Johnson AJ, McCarty WR: The lysis of artificially induced intravascular clots in man by intravenous infusions of streptokinase. *J Clin Invest* 38:1627–1643, 1959.
282   Anning ST: The historical aspects of venous thrombosis. *Med Hist* 1:28–37, 1957.
283   Silberberg M: The causes and mechanisms of thrombosis. *Physiol Rev* 18:197–228, 1938.
283a   Dexter L, Folch-Pi W: Venous thrombosis: an account of the first documented case. *JAMA* 228:195–196, 1974.
284   Stehbens WE: History of aneurysms. *Med Hist* 2:274–280, 1958.
285   Benivieni A, quoted by Long ER: *A History of Pathology.* Baltimore, Williams and Wilkins, 1928, 291 pp.
286   Wiseman R: *Several Chirurgical Treatises,* 2d ed. London, R. Norton and J. Macock, 1686, book 1, 577 pp, 64.
287   Virchow R: *Cellular Pathology as Based Upon Physiological and Pathological Histology.* 2d ed, (trans) by Chance F. Philadelphia, J.B. Lippincott, 1863, 511 pp.
288   Sylvius, Deleboe: *Praxis medica,* quoted by Andral G: *Practical Hematology. An Essay on the Blood in Disease.* Meigs JF, Stillé A (trans). Philadelphià, Lea and Blanchard, 1844, 129 pp.
289   Welch WH: Thrombosis, in *Papers and Addresses by William Welch.* Baltimore, The Johns Hopkins Press, 1920, vol 3, pp 110–192.
290   Zahn FW: Untersuchungen über Thrombose Bildung der Thromben. *Virchows Arch Pathol Anat* 62:81–124, 1875.
291   Lubnitzky S: Die Zusammensetzung des Thrombus in Arterienwunden in den ersten funf Tagen. *Arch Exp Pathol Pharm* 19:185–208, 1885.
292   Osler W: On certain problems in the physiology of the blood corpuscles. Lecture III. The relation of the corpuscles to coagulation and thrombosis. *Med News* 48:421–425, 1886.
293   Hayem G: Correspondence, *L'Union Médicale,* Jan 7, 1886, pp 32–33.

294 Feissly R: La stabilité du fibrinogène *in vivo*. *C R Soc Biol* (*Paris*) 92:319–320, 1925.
295 Wessler S: Studies in intravascular coagulation. III. The pathogenesis of serum-induced thrombosis. *J Clin Invest* 34:647–651, 1955.
296 Rokitansky, quoted by Silberberg M: The causes and mechanism of thrombosis. *Physiol Rev* 18:197–228, 1938.
297 Mills CA: The action of tissue extracts in the coagulation of blood. *J Biol Chem* 46:167–192, 1921.
298 Fontana F: *Traité sur le Vénin de la Vipere sur les Poisons Americains sur le Laurier cerise et sur quelques autres Poisons végetaux.* Florence, 1781, vol 2, 373 pp.
299 Martin CJ: On some effects upon the blood produced by injection of the Australian black snake (Pseudoechis porphyriacus). *J Physiol* (*Lond*) 15:380–400, 1893.
300 Mellanby J: The coagulation of blood. Part II. The action of snake venom, peptone and leech extract. *J Physiol* (*Lond*) 38:441–503, 1909.
301 Reid HA, Chan Ke, Thean PC: Prolonged coagulation defect (defibrination syndrome) in Malayan viper bite. *Lancet* 1:621–626, 1963.
302 De Lee JB: A case of a fatal hemorrhagic diathesis with premature detachment of the placenta. *Am J Obstet* 44:785–792, 1901.
303 Dieckmann WJ: Blood chemistry and renal function in abruptio placentae. *Am J Obstet Gynecol* 31:734–745, 1936.
304 Schneider C: Etiology of fibrinopenia: fibrination defibrination. *Ann NY Acad Sci* 75:634–675, 1959.
305 Mersky C, Kleiner GJ, Johnson AJ: Quantitative estimation of split products of fibrinogen in human serum, relation to diagnosis and treatment. *Blood* 28:1–18, 1966.
306 Little JR: Purpura fulminans treated successfully with anticoagulation. Report of a case. *JAMA* 169:36–40, 1959.

CHAPTER 19

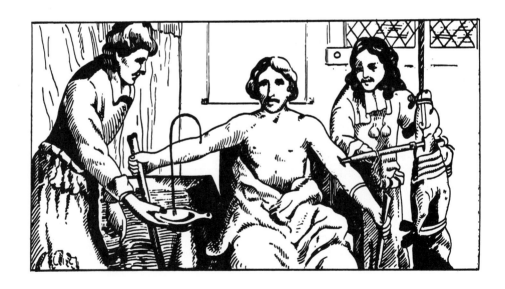

A HISTORY OF BLOOD TRANSFUSION
Louis K. Diamond

The life of the flesh is in the blood.

T he above pronouncement in the Bible (Leviticus 17:11) places blood in a prime position from time immemorial. It took thousands of years, however, before the true therapeutic value of blood was appreciated and exploited, years of fanciful theories, of trial and error, daring experimentation by a few, and their censure by many. Only in the last century has the lifesaving potential of blood and its component parts been truly appreciated. Now, the use of blood transfusion ranks as one of the foremost therapeutic advances for the restoration of health. It may outstrip drugs, antibiotics, and chemicals in helping millions to overcome disease, debility, and disastrous injury.

Blood, in one form or another, was mentioned as a possible therapeutic measure throughout ancient times. The Egyptians were said to advocate blood baths for purposes of recuperation and rejuvenation. Roman gladiators com-

Chapter Opening Photo   Blood transfusion from animal to human as supposedly practiced in 1672 (Lamswerde). (*Drawn after Scultiti. Courtesy of Dr. Michael E. DeBakey; from Kilduffe RA, DeBakey ME: The Blood Bank and the Technique and Therapeutics of Transfusion. St. Louis, Mosby, 1943, 558 pp, p 24.*)

peting in the arena were encouraged to drink the blood of fallen adversaries in order to acquire some of the foe's courage and strength. Even the spectators were permitted to rush down and participate in occasional orgies of this kind. In the Bible, blood is mentioned more than 500 times, beginning, appropriately, with Genesis 9:4; however, there is no suggestion here that blood has any health-promoting value. On the contrary, the *eating* of blood is absolutely forbidden in Leviticus 7:26, and several times thereafter. Members of the fundamentalist sect known as Jehovah's Witnesses interpret this so rigidly that they absolutely refuse even lifesaving blood transfusions not only for themselves but also for their children.

> This prohibition against eating blood may have been the basis for the Judaic dietary law of preparing fresh meat for consumption by draining off all the blood, washing, salting heavily, and allowing to set for thirty minutes, then again washing and draining well. As was rediscovered centuries later by Hewson (1774), concentrated salt keeps blood from clotting. Much of the fluid blood in the meat is thereby gotten rid of. Like other of these dietary laws (e.g., against eating pork and shellfish), there probably were sound preventive medical principles behind this taboo if it was believed, as may have been noted by keen observers, that the blood carried diseases passed on by the much later discovered parasites and microorganisms.

As late as the fifteenth century, blood was recommended to remedy a variety of ailments, such as lunacy, fits, palsy, melancholia, and bad disposition, but not for blood loss or anemia, as would have seemed more logical. It was even prescribed for the revival and rejuvenation of the aged. This, too, harks back to ancient times, for in Ovid's *Metamorphosis* (43 B.C.) it is told that the witch Medea restored Jason's aged father Aeson to vigorous adulthood by slitting his throat to let out his wornout blood and replacing it with a magic brew she concocted. Through the ages the idea of possible rejuvenation has had great appeal. Ponce de Leon sought the fountain of youth in Florida. The search still goes on for the *elixir vitae* in drugs, hormones, foods, and vitamins, as well as in blood.

Returning to the Middle Ages, there is the apocryphal story that when Pope Innocent VIII was on his deathbed in 1492, a last desperate attempt at his revival was made on the recommendation of an unknown physician. He received the blood of three youths supposedly by transfusion, though more likely as a draught. The fact is that shortly thereafter he passed on, to Heaven doubtlessly. So did the three youths, one hopes. And the prescribing physician wisely and quickly disappeared, in which direction is not recorded.

Throughout this period the concept existed that ill health, insanity, depressions, manias, and mood changes were due to "bad humors" or poisons in the blood, and, therefore, purging and bleeding seemed appropriate. Bloodletting was practiced freely. Certainly it was a quick and simple procedure to puncture a prominent forearm vein and just let the blood drain into a measuring bowl. It could be and was repeated ad extremum. It did not even require the ministrations of a physician, merely a barber-surgeon. To watch the "bad blood" pouring out may have truly benefited the plethoric hypertensive carnivore. It may have made the sufferer from other spiritual and humoral ailments also feel better.

Early Suggestions for Transfusions

Up to the seventeenth century, blood must have been given only by mouth. Direct transfusion into the circulation had to await the discovery that there was a circulation. There were vague suggestions of such a procedure early in the sixteenth century, but no evidence of effectual transfer is recorded, probably because of blood loss, blood clotting, and many technical difficulties during such attempts, if indeed any were made. Most likely they were speculations or armchair experiments. An oft-quoted example of one such is the priority claim attached to the name of Andreas Libavius,[1] a celebrated German chemist. In 1615 he described how a transfusion could be done by using silver tubes fitted into each other to connect the blood vessels of "a strong, healthy youth rich in spirited blood and a powerless cachectic old man." But he recommended placing the tubes in arteries of each, an unlikely practical approach. He made no claim that he had tried this. Indeed, there is a suggestion that he was ridiculing the whole idea.

A Florentine physician, Francesco Folli,[2] claimed he had "invented" blood transfusion in 1654 and, in his book published in 1680, illustrated his apparatus of funnels, tubes, and metal cannulas with instructions for their operation. But in the end, he confessed, he had yet to do the experiment.

The beginnings of transfusion therapy date from the mid-seventeenth century following Harvey's momentous discovery of the circulation of the blood. William Harvey[3] learned to acquire knowledge by direct observation in Padua, Italy, where science flourished in the sixteenth century. He brought back to England this investigational approach. Concentrating his attention on the blood, he announced in a monumental treatise, De Motu Cordis, that blood circulated within the body in a closed system, maintained by the heart acting as a pump, and that the blood was sent to the limbs through the arteries and returned through the veins, whose valves did not oppose its course that way. Harvey was a shrewd observer and tireless investigator. In addition, he was a superb teacher and a highly successful practitioner. He had only one fault professionally and "even that became a cherished tradition. His handwriting was appalling."[3] He first announced his observations on the circulation in his lectures in 1616, published in 1628. This stimulated actual experimentation with injections into the blood stream.

The famous architect Christopher Wren, originally known as an astronomer and an anatomist, in 1656 assembled quills and silver tubes as cannulas and employed animal bladders for injectors, as syringes are now used. He showed that dogs could be given drugs, and even liquor, intravenously more effectively than by mouth. This suggested the method and the needed tools for the transfer of fluids from one body into another. In a short time, intravenous infusions of everything including blood were being tried by a few other innovative scientists.

One who is known to have attempted experimental transfusions about 1652 was Francis Potter, of Kilmington, Somerset, an eccentric rector but also an inventive genius. However, he used pullets, with small fragile veins, as subjects and quills and bladders as instruments. He admitted that he was unsuccessful in completing any transfusions. Nevertheless, his claim to recognition as a first transfusionist was repeatedly and strongly urged on the Royal Society by a friend and contemporary, John Aubrey.[4]

The First Transfusions: English or French?

The first well-documented successful human transfusions took place in 1667 and involved two widely separated investigators, one English, the other French. Both individual and national priorities being at stake, considerable controversy was engendered. Numerous publications resulted as to who should be accredited with doing the first transfusion in humans.[5-8]

In England, a young physiologist and physician, Richard Lower, of Oxford, excited by the work of Wren, participated in experiments of injecting opiates, emetics, and other medicines into the veins of living animals. As he stated in letters then and in a book published later, this stimulated ideas about injecting large quantities of blood from different animals. In February 1665, after several attempts, he developed the needed surgical skill and performed his first successful transfusion, from the cervical artery of one dog into the jugular vein of another, previously almost agonally exsanguinated. The recipient animal was promptly restored to a healthy active state. There was no untoward reaction, for dogs do not have natural isoagglutinins although they do vary in blood group antigens. Lower was thus encouraged to consider blood transfusions in humans. He may have been prodded toward this by a report from Paris that a sheep-to-man transfusion had been successfully performed there in the summer of 1667. Curiously, the obvious indication for transfusion, i.e., blood loss or blood want, which his dog experiments involved, was not stressed by Lower. He does at least mention it in his famous book *Treatise on the Heart* published in 1669 (in Latin).[6] In one paragraph he states:

> . . . when simple hemorrhage results in such a great loss of blood that succor from some source is demanded in the emergency, there is no doubt but that the blood of an animal could be allowed to slip in and substitute in its place to advantage.

This is hardly a strong recommendation, but Lower should receive credit for recognizing this most important indication for blood transfusion more than 100 years before it was stressed by others. The possible emotional and psychic benefits of blood, which had long been the only consideration, continued to be the *idée fixe* of the medical profession.

The subject of blood infusion had been brought to the attention of the Fellows of the Royal Society in London by the famous Robert Boyle (Boyle's law) and other members. Following a number of discussions of the idea of transfusion, as recorded in the Journal Book of the Society during 1665–1666, an invitation was given to Lower in October 1667 to demonstrate his procedure to the membership. This lapse of more than 2 years after the successful dog transfusions by Lower may have been due to an epidemic of the plague, which claimed more than 100,000 lives in 1665–1666, and the great fire in London in September 1666. At the meeting of October 24, 1667, it was proposed that transfusion should first be tried on "some mad person in Bedlam," but the physician in charge "scrupled" and could not be induced to consent. "On November 21, Dr. Lower acquainted the company that one Arthur Coga was willing to suffer the experiment of transfusion to be tryed upon himself for a guiny."

On November 23, then, Lower and his skilled associate Edmund King performed their first human transfusion before the Royal Society. The patient was this 22-year-old member of the clergy, Arthur Coga, "somewhat unbalanced, whose brain was considered a little too warm." It was hoped the operation would alter his character. Accordingly, he was bled from his antecubital vein for 6 to 7 ounces. He was then connected via silver tubes and quills to a sheep's carotid artery. It was surmised that during 2 minutes, 9 to 10 ounces of blood were so transferred. The patient afterward "found himself very well" and 6 days later gave the society a talk in Latin telling how much better he felt. This was mentioned in *Pepys' Diary*.[9]* With a prestigious audience of scientists and men of letters like Samuel Pepys, word of this innovative procedure spread surprisingly rapidly, even to the continent, where it stirred up the long-lasting priority debate.

It is not mentioned in most histories of blood transfusion and even in detailed accounts of the priority controversy or of Lower's experiments, but the Register Books of the Royal Society, although not its published Transactions, record that on December 12, 1667 (or December 14), a second transfusion

---

* The attitude of the general public toward such experiments is shown in a popular play of 1676 by Thomas Shadwell, the Poet Laureate of England.[10] It was a satire on contemporary science, in which he lampooned the Royal Society and its activities. The play was called *The Virtuoso*, which was a complimentary name applied to members of the Royal Society and of the comparable French Academy. The public often used it in a derogatory sense as meaning an "antiquarian, a dabbler or collector" who carried his hobby to absurd excesses. In one short scene there is a discussion of a supposed cross-transfusion between a mangy spaniel and a healthy bulldog resulting in the spaniel becoming a bulldog and the bulldog a spaniel.

was done by Dr. King on the same Arthur Coga. This time, 8 ounces of blood were taken from his arm vein into "a porenger and about 2 oz spilt." Then, about 14 ounces of arterial blood from a sheep were allowed to run in during 7 minutes. "On December 19, Mr. Coga came in and gave an account of the operation repeated upon him. He found himself very well at present though he had been at first somewhat feverish which was imputed to the excess of drinking wine he committed soon after the operation." Nowhere is there any comment about the effect of these transfusions upon Coga's temperament or his "too warm brain." He must have had a strong cool body to withstand two sheep's blood transfusions with so little obvious reaction.

To revert to the happenings on the Continent, a French philosopher-mathematician and physician, Jean-Baptiste Denis,[5] on June 15, 1667, after experimenting and perfecting his technique on dogs, proceeded to transfuse a boy of 15, a sufferer from a prolonged febrile illness and profound lethargy. He had been subjected to, and had somehow managed to survive, 20 phlebotomies. Denis succeeded in transfusing him with about 9 ounces of sheep's blood and actually "cured" him of his ailment. Encouraged by this success, Denis tried his good fortune again. This time he used a healthy paid volunteer, who received 20 ounces of sheep's blood without recorded difficulties except for feeling "very great heat" along the vein in his arm and later voiding "black urine." It is stated he was so little disturbed that he proceeded to butcher the sheep and then went off on a drinking bout with companions.

A third subject, a Swedish nobleman already moribund, did not fare so well and died soon after an attempted transfusion. Although Denis had encountered opposition from numerous physicians in Paris, possibly from jealousy and fear of being criticized for their practice of purging and bleeding, he was undaunted and allowed himself to be persuaded by the wife of a lunatic to treat him by transfusion. The man was subject to episodes of violent maniacal behavior. Denis transfused him on December 19, 1667,[11] with 5 or 6 ounces of blood from the femoral artery of a "gentle calf," which "might dampen his spirits." The patient seemed to improve. A few days later, the procedure was repeated. This time, there developed all the signs now recognized as typical of a severe transfusion reaction: a burning sensation traveling up the arm, pain in the kidney regions, an oppressive feeling in his chest, sweating, vomiting, and diarrhea and, later, repeated voiding of urine "black as soot." After recovery from all this, he remained well for 2 months. When he relapsed and again became maniacal, his wife insisted on yet another transfusion. Denis attempted this but without success because the man was violent and would not cooperate. He died the following night.

It was later suggested that Denis' enemies persuaded the wife to bring suit charging the transfusion had killed her husband. Considerable furor was raised among Parisian physicians, but at the trial the defense was successful in proving that the man had been poisoned with arsenic by his wife. Although Denis was thus exonerated, the Paris Society of Physicians declared itself against such experiments and persuaded the criminal court in Paris on April 17, 1668, to forbid further transfusions without approval from the Faculty of Medicine of Paris, known to be bitterly opposed to the procedure. Ten years later, an edict of Parliament prohibited transfusion experiments on humans. Soon thereafter, the Royal Society in England disapproved transfusion practices, as did the magistrates in Rome. This eclipse of overt interest in transfusion therapy lasted 150 years.

In the meantime, an international debate had been initiated as to who and which country should be credited with the first transfusion. England's claim was based on Lower's thoroughly documented dog-to-dog transfusions in 1665. The French claimed that the idea had been proposed 10 years earlier and that the actual human transfusions were first done by Denis. National prestige seemed to be at stake even though the treatment was admittedly less than uniformly successful. A considerable exchange of letters between Denis and Henry Oldenburg,[12] the secretary of the Royal Society, took place in late 1667 and 1668 with publication in the *Proceedings of the Society*. Denis had sent a letter to the *Philosophical Transactions*, in London, the official publication of the Royal Society, describing his first transfusion, and this was actually printed, dated July 22, 1667. However, its publication did not take place until September, the editor, Oldenburg, having had what he called an "extraordinary accident" to account for the delay. This was his confinement in the Tower of London on suspicion of treason. Luckily he was declared innocent. Few editors could claim so valid an excuse for delays in publication.

It seems unlikely that Lower profited from Denis' description of the Frenchman's transfusion technique since the English team had carried out blood exchanges between animals beginning in 1665. Yet Lower's human transfusion took place 5 months after Denis'. The best that Oldenburg could contend was that the "English might well have been first if they had not been so tender in hazarding the life of man," a post hoc solicitude with no foundation in fact. The decision regarding priority long remained in doubt and was not really resolved satisfactorily. It finally seemed to be accepted that Lower, of England, deserved the credit for doing and fully describing the first animal transfusions (Chapter Opening Photo), whereas Denis, of France, was credited with the first successful transfusions in humans.

Although the interdiction of transfusion was world wide after 1678, sporadic reports of such treatments are scattered throughout the medical literature of the next 150 years. The usual indications continued to be insanity, manias, or long-lasting unremitting disease, and animals were used as donors. The importance of blood in carrying oxygen from the lungs to the tissues was not appreciated until scientific support was obtained by the researches of

Priestley in 1774 and Lavoisier in 1777 on oxygen and its role in respiration. The danger of acute blood loss could then be understood, making transfusion a logical mode of therapy.

Lifesaving Transfusions: A Physiological Approach

A pioneer in recognizing this fact and an innovator years ahead of his confreres was an English physiologist and obstetrician, James Blundell,[13] of London. Frustrated by his inability to help some of his patients after they suffered massive puerperal hemorrhage, his thoughts turned to means of getting blood into such individuals. Being a scientist as well as a concerned and considerate physician, around 1817–1818 he first experimented on dogs that he exsanguinated. He found that death from hemorrhage could be prevented by transfusion with blood from other dogs. He also observed that it was not necessary to replace all the blood lost, that a smaller transfusion was often adequate. He noted that bubbles of air passing into the recipient's circulation did no harm, even up to 20 ml into a small dog. This refuted the belief that small amounts of air could account for some of the reported fatal transfusion reactions. And, most important, he stated that for transfusion, species lines could not be crossed; therefore, for humans "only human blood should be employed." He also found that venous blood was just as efficacious as arterial blood and that his use of a syringe in making the transfer did not vitiate the value of the blood and did simplify the operation. These important conclusions, based on sound research, should have established transfusion as a lifesaving therapeutic tool and made the procedure easier and practical.

Encouraged by his animal experiments, Blundell proceeded to apply his knowledge and techniques to patients. He devised special instruments, including a warm water–jacketed collection funnel fastened to a chair for the donor, cannulas and syringes, and even three-way stopcocks, so successfully used almost 100 years later. Blundell transfused 10 seriously ill patients: two were already moribund or dead, so rescue proved impossible; of the remaining eight, success was achieved in five, a truly remarkable result considering the obstacles of possible blood group incompatibility and clotting of the blood.

A few other obstetricians, chiefly his associates, followed his lead, and, undoubtedly, some lives were saved thereby. Yet the impact of this pioneer's well-established principles was not as great as it should have been. Throughout the nineteenth century and even into the twentieth, animal blood was used in humans. Blundell's statement that the prime indication for transfusion was blood loss seemed to be ignored since mood change was still often mentioned. His development of a less immediate, less hasty type of transfusion methodology was not pursued for a long time. His ingenuity and his skills might have advanced such therapy further, but unfortunately, following a dispute with Guy's Hospital, where he held the chair of obstetrics, he resigned at age 48 and left London. Having amassed a fortune from a lucrative practice and also inherited much money, he retired to his estate to live the life of a country squire for another 40 years. Nevertheless, his influence and his contributions are well recognized and interestingly reported. He did the first real transfusions after Denis and Lower and deserves to be ranked with the pioneers in the development of blood transfusion therapy[14] (Figure 19-1).

Blundell's successful transfusions stimulated others, not only in Europe but even in the United States. Too often, however, it was a measure of last resort, thereby further handicapping its effectiveness. Reactions continued at a high rate, whether from the use of human or animal blood. Despite the introduction of a syringe method by Blundell and modifications of this by others, as well as the development of greater skill with direct transfusions, the technical difficulties in performing the procedure also hindered its more widespread and more frequent use.

Figure 19-1 Several instruments devised by James Blundell for performing blood transfusion. Upper left: Blundell's "impellor" attached to a chair in which the donor was seated. Lower left: cross section of "impellor" showing syringe and valve mechanism for changing direction of flow. Blood was impelled by "long strokes and sharp movements." Right: additional devices originated by Blundell. (*Courtesy of Dr. Michael E. DeBakey; from Kilduffe RA, DeBakey ME: The Blood Bank and the Technique and Therapeutics of Transfusion. St. Louis, Mosby, 1943, 558 pp, p 27.*)

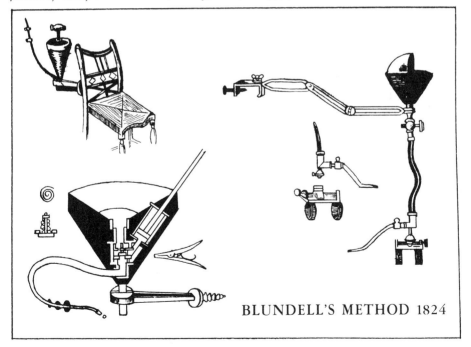

BLUNDELL'S METHOD 1824

In seeking less troublesome substitutes for blood, a short-lived attempt (1873–1880) was made to introduce milk for intravenous therapy. It was first used by Bovell[15] and Hodder in Toronto during a cholera epidemic in 1854, their rationale being an old theory that milk could be converted into white corpuscles of the blood. Two patients given 12 ounces (or more) of cow's milk did well, but two others died. Three more, also so treated, died. This less than encouraging experiment in Canada was nevertheless tried again by Joseph Howe, of New York City, almost 20 years later. In 1873, he injected goat's milk[16] into two patients terminally ill with tuberculosis. One died in 4 hours, the other in 24 hours. Reversing present day procedures, Howe then experimented on dogs. Here, too, milk transfusions resulted in death. He tried one more goat's milk transfusion on a patient with advanced tuberculosis. She survived a 4 ounce injection and seemed to be improved.

A strong advocate of milk transfusions was T.G. Thomas,[17] also of New York City. From 1875 to 1878, he administered these to seven patients. They had severe reactions, with fever, tachycardia, and headache, but recovered. He predicted "a brilliant and useful future for intravenous lacteal injections" since, he claimed, "milk is more allied to chyle, the material of which nature makes blood." There were even some enthusiasts who predicted that milk would supersede blood for transfusions. One final experiment in 1880 by Howe[18] utilized 2 ounces of human milk intravenously for a patient with pulmonary disease. She did badly. After 1880, enthusiasm for milk transfusions quickly faded both here and abroad.[19]

At about this time, intravenous isotonic saline solution[20] was found to be simpler and safer. It was increasingly popular as long as the difficulties attending the transfer of blood made this a measure of last resort. Too often blood transfusion carried the hazards both of immediate and of delayed reactions and complications. Problems occurred in three different areas. First, there was the danger of infection, often local (phlebitis) but sometimes systemic. Then, the clotting of the blood frequently interrupted its free flow, and practical methods of circumventing this had to be developed. Third, and most important, was the long unrecognized problem of immunologic incompatibility between species, and even between humans, the latter risking at least a 35 percent likelihood of agglutination and hemolysis of the red cells.

Control of infection did not begin until after 1867, when the great English surgeon Joseph Lister introduced the use of antiseptics following the demonstration 2 years earlier by Pasteur that bacterial and fungal contamination caused putrefaction. Sterilization of instruments and aseptic methods of operation eventually made the hazard of infection quite negligible.

As had long been known, particularly from the first attempts at transfusion in animals, blood tended to clot within a few minutes after it left the protection of the blood vessels. Successful transfer required as brief outside exposure as possible and speed of flow. The most efficient method in this respect was to connect the blood vessels of the donor and recipient, the animals being placed close to each other so that the connecting quills, tubes, or cannulas would be short as possible. Usually, in the experimental animal transfusions and also in animal-to-human transfusions, a donor's artery was connected to a recipient's vein so as to use the pump action of the heart to give a forceful rapid flow and, thus, avoid stagnation and clotting of the blood. When human donors came increasingly into use during the nineteenth century and vein-to-vein connections were practiced, clotting became a serious handicap to the successful transfer of adequate amounts of blood.

Direct Transfusion: Artery to Vein

Special equipment had to be devised to overcome or delay clot formation. Before reviewing such measures, it is interesting to look at the brief period around the turn of the nineteenth century, when direct transfusion via artery-to-vein anastomoses came into vogue, and skillful surgeons dominated the field. This method, by connecting intima to intima of vessels and avoiding all foreign surfaces, seemed like the solution to the clotting problems of blood transfusion.

Alexis Carrel, a talented and innovative French investigator, who came to the Rockefeller Institute in New York, had been doing organ transplantation experiments on animals.[21] This required delicate suturing of cut blood vessels leading to the organs. His surgical skill resulted in successful transplantations, thereby opening up a new field in reparative medicine. For this he won the Nobel Prize in 1912. A dramatic and attention-attracting application of his skill occurred in 1908, when he was asked to transfuse a 5-day-old infant bleeding uncontrollably from hemorrhagic disease of the newborn. She was the daughter of a prominent surgeon, whose brothers were also well-known physicians. Dr. Carrel, whose previous experience had been limited to animals, was persuaded to try to rescue the dying infant. He was able to transfuse her by anastomosing her popliteal vein to her father's radial artery. This delicate surgery was performed on a kitchen table. The bleeding ceased promptly, the infant recovered, and the story of this lifesaving happening was reported in the daily papers as "a first successful blood transfusion in New York City," which it was not. The publicity, emphasizing that the surgeon had acquired his skill by experiments on animals, helped turn the tide against a strongly supported bill of the antivivisectionists about to be passed by the New York State Legislature.[22]

In the meantime, a well-known Cleveland surgeon, G.W. Crile,[23] had been practicing direct transfusions by artery-to-vein anastomoses beginning in 1898. He called it the "Carrel" technique. To facilitate the difficult vascular suturing, Crile devised a metal tube through which the recipient's vein could

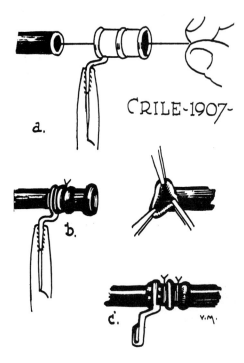

Figure 19-2 Artery-to-vein direct transfusion. *(a)* Pulling vein through cannula. *(b)* Vein cuffed and tied into place in groove near handle of cannula; artery ready to be drawn over vein. *(c)* Completed anastomosis of artery and vein. *(Courtesy of Dr. Michael E. DeBakey; from Kilduffe RA, DeBakey ME: The Blood Bank and the Technique and Therapeutics of Transfusion. St. Louis, Mosby, 1943, 558 pp, p 28.)*

be drawn and cuffed over the end (Figure 19-2). The artery could then be sewn over the cuff more easily. Crile[24] performed 61 transfusions on 55 patients by this method and reported these in 1909 in his book on transfusion, the first of its kind in this country. He did not carry out any blood grouping or crossmatching tests, although Hektoen, of Chicago, had strongly suggested these in 1907. Instead, he recommended, and had performed, when time permitted, an elaborate series of tests for hemolysins by mixing blood samples of donors and recipients and observing them for 24 to 48 hours. The reaction rate of 35 percent or more was about the number to be expected from chance incompatibility of ABO groups.

The direct transfusion method of Crile and the modifications of it by other surgeons, who devised and preferred their own instruments (e.g., Elsberg, Brewer, Janeway, Soresi, Bernheim) introduced several difficulties. The patient and the donor had to lie side by side in an operating room. A team of five or more trained personnel was needed. There was no easy method of judging how much blood was transfused. In some cases several hemoglobin estimates were done, but this required that the transfusion be stopped temporarily. Or, the donor might be weighed before and after the operation and the difference used to estimate the amount of blood withdrawn. Not infrequently, a recipient developed cardiac signs of circulatory overload, or the donor became hypotensive and fainted. And, finally, the donor's radial artery that was usually used had to be tied off, hopefully without jeopardy to the circulation in the hand.

Little wonder the less direct or "mediate" methods of transfusion, dependent on the use of syringes, paraffined tubes, special needles, cannulas, stopcocks, and valves soon became popular.

Keeping the Blood Fluid

As mentioned earlier, the ancients, by astute observation, may have learned that salt—ordinary common salt—kept blood fluid. When transfusion was finally tried in the seventeenth century and clotting often thwarted successful transfer from the donor to the recipient, thoughts about anticoagulants must have occurred to chemists and, particularly, physiologists. An unappreciated lead had been found by William Hewson,[25] the English anatomist and student of John Hunter (Chapter 1). In 1774, he wrote of the anticoagulant effects of various "neutral salts." He stated that Glauber's salt (sodium sulfate) and others prevented shed blood from clotting and kept the color bright rather than dark red. However, he did not see what use this could be in medicine since a high concentration of salts had to be mixed with the blood. Earlier workers, between 1703 and 1743, had also noted the effects of salts on the color and clotting of blood.

Following in Blundell's footsteps, another English obstetrician, J. Braxton-Hicks,[26] in 1868, tried to prevent coagulation by the addition of a solution of "phosphate of soda" to the donor's blood while it was being drawn. He tried this in three transfusions on patients following obstetrical hemorrhage. It kept the blood flowing, but the women all died in shock. Another anticoagulant suggested by Landois in 1892 was hirudin, extracted from leeches. This was actually used by Satterlee and Hooker[27] in 1914, but difficulties in obtaining pure and reliable preparations and the narrow range between effective and toxic doses made this drug dangerous.

The first workers to connect calcium with blood clotting were Swiss physiologists, who found that blood could be kept from coagulating by the addition of small amounts of any soluble salt, such as oxalic acid. A well-known British pathologist, A.E. Wright,[28] wrote an article in 1894 on methods of affecting coagulability of the blood and pointed out that the soluble salts of several acids could postpone clotting indefinitely. However, he seemed to doubt that the nontoxic citrates could bind enough calcium in vivo without producing convulsions. The possible value of citrate for transfusion purposes was, thus, suggested some 21 years before it was used.

An obvious method of obtaining liquid blood was to allow clotting to take place, remove the clot, and use the fluid serum with its (reduced) red cell content. Just when this approach was first put to practical use is not clear, but two French scientists, Prevost and Dumas,[29] published their experiments on animal exsanguination-transfusions in 1821. They showed that defibrinated blood was as effective as untreated blood in resuscitating bled animals. In 1835, Bischoff,[30] of Heidelberg, confirmed this effect by reinfusing into animals that were bled almost to death their own blood after defibrination; recovery resulted. He suggested transfusing human beings with human blood after defibrinating it.

In most instances, the blood was whipped or twirled to defibrinate it. One popular simple method was to collect the blood in an open vessel, beat it with a wire egg beater, lift or strain out the clot, and inject the remaining liquid. Defibrinated blood transfusion, being much the simplest means of avoiding the clotting problem, remained popular all through the latter half of the last century and well into this one. As late as the 1920s, defibrinated blood was used for transfusions in many hospitals in this country. Moss[31] reported on the transfusion practices at the Johns Hopkins Hospital, in Baltimore; the blood was collected in an Erlenmeyer flask containing glass beads and shaken until a firm clot had formed. The remaining liquid portion with the red cells was then poured through a gauze pad into another flask or burette and administered to a recipient via a needle in the antecubital vein connected by rubber tubing to the blood container. Often the blood was warmed in transit by placing coils of the tubing in a basin of warm water. Febrile reactions were not infrequent, probably due to pyrogens in the tubing, needles, glassware, gauze filter, and washing fluid.

Many transfusionists believed the reactions were due to the damaging of red cells by the shaking or whipping of the blood during defibrination. This led to numerous discussions and recommendations in favor of or against the transfusion of defibrinated blood. For example, F. Gesellius,[32] a prominent surgeon in Poland, who devised his own special apparatus for drawing and infusing blood, in 1873 published a monograph on blood transfusion, in which he strongly opposed defibrination. He and a prominent German physician, O. Hasse,[33] once more advocated the use of sheep blood for transfusion. Hasse reported the results of 15 such transfusions in 1874, and, even though reactions were severe, and even fatal, he advocated the use of such blood for various "incurable diseases."

End of Animal-to-Human Transfusions

Important investigations on blood transfusions were carried out by two independent investigators. E. Ponfick,[34] pathologist at Breslau, reported in 1874 and 1875 that heterologous blood transfusions both in animals and in humans produced lysis of red cells, diffuse petechial hemorrhages, bloody urine which was not hematuria but hemoglobinuria, and kidney damage, all of which he demonstrated as resulting from the infused cells. At about the same time, L. Landois,[35] professor of physiology at Greifswald, proved in vitro as well as in vivo that human serum lysed sheep red cells, releasing hemoglobin and leading to oliguria and anuria. Heterologous animal transfusions produced similar pathology. Landois recognized the danger of hyperkalemia from the lysed red cells and the possibility of early death from emboli. In his monograph, Landois published collected statistics on 478 authenticated transfusions up to the end of 1874 beginning with the Denis and Lower cases, of which 129 were from animal donors and 347 from humans. Of the recipients of animal-to-human transfusions, about one-third were said to have been improved, whereas almost half of the human-to-human cases were helped. The studies of the fate of infused blood in heterologous transfusions, especially the thorough experiments and analyses of Landois, should have banished forever the use of animal blood for humans. After a lag of a few years, this occurred almost worldwide. However, as late as 1928, a monograph appeared in France by Cruchet, Ragot, and Caussimon,[36] again advocating transfusion of the blood of animals into humans.

Semidirect or "Mediate" Transfusions

Many transfusionists preferred the transfer of whole blood by a semidirect or "mediate" method with as short a delay as possible to avoid clotting. One which enjoyed some popularity for a time was the use of paraffin-coated vessels.

Curtis and David,[37] in 1911, devised a system of semidirect transfusion which seemed simpler than the direct blood vessel anastomoses of Carrel and of Crile. A Y-shaped glass tube or cannula, paraffin-coated, was tied into the veins of donor and recipient, and a syringe was attached to the neck of the cannula. By alternately compressing and releasing clamps on each vein and filling and emptying the syringe, a measured amount of blood could be transferred in a short time. The advantage of this method was the knowledge of how much blood was given, which by direct transfusion through anastomosed vessels could only be guessed. It also did not require as great surgical skill as vessel-to-vessel suturing. It had considerable vogue between 1911 and 1920, especially in Chicago, the location of its inventors.

In Boston, paraffin was also used in the Kimpton-Brown[38] transfusion apparatus. This consisted of a glass cylinder of 250 ml or greater capacity, the upper end of which was open and the lower end drawn out to a fine hollow cannula which could fit through a slit into a large vein. The glass was paraffin-lined so that clotting was delayed for a considerable time. A pressure bulb could be attached at the top end to hasten the flow of blood into the recipient. Breakage of a tube or blood clotting due to delays in the procedure sometimes led to partial failure (Figure 19-3).*

Several varieties of syringe-needle assemblies were devised and used by transfusion specialists, who spent much of their day giving transfusions in one or more hospitals. Each "transfusionist" usually had his own team of two or more assistants and carried his own special apparatus. There was the Bernheim[39] method of a syringe, two-way stopcock, and U-shaped tube to which needles were attached that could be inserted into the veins of the donor and the patient lying side by side. The Lindeman system[40] was much the same except that a larger cannula-obturator was used in the veins; with the sharp-pointed obturator removed, a freer blood flow was established through the blunt cannula. A well-known transfusionist was Unger.[41] He operated most efficiently with his own system: a large syringe and a four-way stopcock that

---

* The present author served as donor in a Kimpton-Brown transfusion (in 1924), during which a broken cylinder lost 250 ml of his blood. Since the patient was in the operating room with a bleeding brain tumor and urgently needed blood replacement, a third 250-ml tube was drawn, amid much excitement and spilled blood. Fortunately, both recipient and donor recovered.

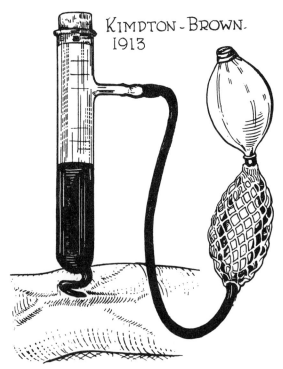

KIMPTON-BROWN.
1913

Figure 19-3 Paraffin-lined glass cylinder of Kimpton-Brown having horizontal side tube for suction or pressure and with the bottom of the tube drawn out in an S-shaped cannula for the donor and the recipient. (*Courtesy of Dr. Michael E. DeBakey; from Kilduffe RA, DeBakey ME: The Blood Bank and the Technique and Therapeutics of Transfusion. St. Louis, Mosby, 1943, 558 pp, p 400.*)

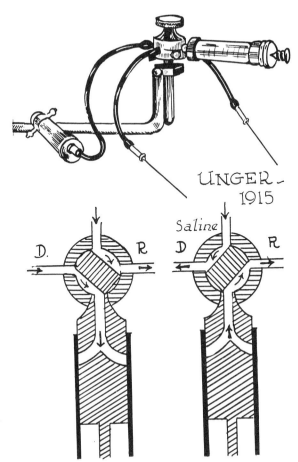

UNGER.
1915

Saline

D.   R   D   R

Figure 19-4 Syringe and stopcock with four outlets to aspirate blood from donor and inject into recipient as well as flush out the system with saline to minimize clot formation. (*Courtesy of Dr. Michael E. DeBakey; from Kilduffe RA, DeBakey ME: The Blood Bank and the Technique and Therapeutics of Transfusion. St. Louis, Mosby, 1943, 558 pp, p 403.*)

permitted him to draw blood through a needle in the donor's vein and, after a turn of the stopcock, to inject it into the recipient (Figure 19-4). The other outlets, connected to a syringe of saline, permitted washing through the system and a flushing out of any small clots that might form and obstruct the flow.

The Discovery of Blood Groups

Around 1900, the most important advance toward safe and effective transfusions took place with the discovery of the human blood groups by Landsteiner. Blood incompatibility between species had been suggested previously by the studies of others, notably by Ponfick[34] in 1874 and Landois[35] in 1873 and 1875. They had each noted hemolysis of the red cells in heterologous blood transfusions, including the commonly used lamb's blood given to humans. Bordet[42] in 1895 showed that hemolysins were produced when he injected red cells of one animal into another of a different species. Ehrlich and Morgenroth[43] in 1900 not only confirmed this but found that there were hemolysins present normally in sera for red cells of other species. The reactions from the use of animal blood in transfusions of humans could now be better understood on the basis of sound in vitro and in vivo experiments.

Stimulated by these studies, Karl Landsteiner,[44] then a young assistant in the Institute of Pathological Anatomy of the University of Vienna, investigated the reactions between red cells and serum of 22 individuals, his associates, and laboratory helpers. He found that certain sera would clump or agglutinate the erythrocytes of certain other persons. This discovery of isoagglutination became the basis of human blood group classification. Originally, Landsteiner was able to separate his blood samples into three types, which he named A, B, and C. The serum of A clumped the cells of B; the serum of B clumped the cells of A; the serum of C clumped the cells of both A and B, but its cells were not clumped by A or B serum. In 1902, Decastello and Sturli,[45] two of Landsteiner's pupils working in Medical Clinic II in Vienna and, therefore, having a more varied and larger number of subjects to study, confirmed Landsteiner's findings in 155 cases. They came upon four individuals (2.5 percent) who had no agglutinins in the serum and whose cells were clumped by the other three sera, the rare group now known as AB. Decastello and Sturli also established the fact that red cell agglutinins had no relationship to disease, being similarly distributed in the 121 patients and in 34 healthy subjects.

Landsteiner recognized the importance of his discovery to human transfusion therapy, although many practitioners failed to appreciate this for a dozen years or more. The significance of the isoagglutinins and their relation to transfusion reactions, and even to possible fatalities, was recognized by Hektoen.[46,47] He emphasized this in two articles in 1907, but they had surprisingly little immediate impact on the practices of transfusionists. Preliminary laboratory testing for blood grouping and cross matching of donor and recipient for transfusions were not carried out routinely and not accepted as mandatory. Some transfusionists, impressed by the studies of Ehrlich and Morgenroth, came to rely on tests for hemolysins. These required the mixing of donor and recipient blood, incubating for several hours or even over night, and then looking for visible hemolysis, obviously a slow and inaccurate process. Other transfusionists relied on a so-called biologic test, which consisted of injecting 5 to 20 ml of donor blood into the recipient and watching for adverse reaction or for hemolysis evidenced by hemoglobinemia. Such results were too crude, reactions usually too long in appearing, and the method even inoperative in a recipient in shock or under anesthesia.

Ottenberg[48] probably performed the first blood transfusions in New York City in 1907 and 1908, using a cannula modification of the direct method developed by Crile and others. Also, and more important, Ottenberg,[49] while still an intern, had his attention directed by Weil, pathologist at the old German Hospital in New York, to the importance of Landsteiner's report on blood types. He put into practice the typing and cross matching of donors and recipients preliminary to transfusions. Despite some opposition, this was eventually accepted as standard procedure. In addition, Ottenberg made other important contributions in this field. In 1908, he first suggested the inheritance of the ABO blood groups. He also showed that group O blood could be given to recipients of the other three groups since the donor's anti-A and anti-B agglutinins would usually be diluted to harmless levels. This initiated the practice of using blood group O people as "universal" donors, especially for urgently needed transfusions. His studies of in vivo and in vitro hemolysis between 1911 and 1913 were of scientific and practical value. He was an unappreciated pioneer in the early days of transfusion therapy.

The discovery of the human blood groups was of fundamental importance to the practice of transfusion. It also proved of inestimable value in several other areas of scientific investigation, such as genetics, anthropology, forensic medicine, immunology, and the pathogenesis of a number of diseases. A more complete story of the discovery of the blood groups and their importance is presented in Chapter 20.

Introduction of Anticoagulants

The use of citrate as an anticoagulant took blood transfusion out of the hands of the surgeon, whose skill in incising blood vessels and anastomosing arteries to veins for direct transfusions was so necessary. Indirect more leisurely transfusion therapy was then possible, although it did not "catch on" as fast as might have been expected. Eventually, however, overcoming the problem of blood clotting led to the free and easy use of transfusion therapy, to storage of blood and, thereby, development of blood banks, to separation of the blood elements and their specific use, and, finally, to fractionation and concentration of plasma components of inestimable value (Chapter 17). In fact, progress in this area is still proceeding.

The citrate story began almost simultaneously in three widely separated countries and involved four different people. As mentioned previously, several investigators had used sodium citrate to render blood fluid for laboratory study purposes. Animal experimentation also was tried using large amounts of anticoagulant salts, but these proved toxic. Two Swiss physiologists, Arthus and Pagés,[50] are credited with first relating calcium and blood clotting, in 1890, and showing that small amounts of the soluble salts of oxalic or citric acid would keep shed blood liquid and could be injected into animals with impunity. The possible practical value of citrate to transfusion problems was overlooked, probably due to the failure of communication. Not until 24 years later was this recognized.

In April 1914, Hustin,[51] of Belgium, reported the use of sodium citrate and glucose as a diluent and anticoagulant solution for a transfusion which he had performed successfully on a patient the previous month. Seven months later, Agote,[52] of Argentina, carried out the first transfusion in which citrate alone was used to keep the blood fluid; he reported this in January 1915. In that same month, Weil,[53] of New York, a pathologist, published in the Journal of the American Medical Association an article on the addition of sodium citrate to blood for purposes of transfusion. He used more salt (1%) than was necessary for 300 ml of blood. This concentration might have been toxic in larger transfusions. However, Weil also noted that citrated blood could be stored in an ice box for several days and then used safely. This was the forerunner of the idea of blood banking. Also, being aware of Landsteiner's work, he advocated cross matching citrated blood samples as an important compatibility test. In the same year, 1915, Lewisohn,[54] a young surgeon in New York, published an article on "a new and greatly simplified method of blood transfusion." He had been studying citrate toxicity in dogs and found that a minimum amount of 0.2% would prevent blood clotting for several hours. He then proved that a massive transfusion of 2500 ml of such citrated blood could be given safely to a patient, even in a brief period. His precise measurement of the minimum amount of citrate needed was an important contribution.

The citrate method of indirect transfusion made the procedure so simple that it might have been expected soon to displace all other methods. But this was still not the case. It was found that as many as 50 percent of patients had pyrexial reactions, whereas some of the transfusionists using direct or "mediate" methods claimed only 10 percent occurrence of such reactions. Lewisohn had to defend what was said to be "citrate toxicity." He was unaware of the 1911 report of Hort and Penfold[55] on the dangers of pyrogens developing in solutions made up with stale distilled water. In 1923, Seibert[56] found that fever-producing substances derived from bacterial growth in standing distilled water accounted for hyperpyrexial reactions; thereafter, double distilling of water to be used in making up citrate and saline solutions diminished this high reaction rate. Finally, Lewisohn and Rosenthal,[57] as they reported in 1933, eliminated all such hyperpyrexias by establishing a well-supervised hospital central supply system to wash all equipment thoroughly and to make up special parenteral fluid solutions for use in transfusions and intravenous therapy.

Acceptance of the Indirect Transfusion Method

The advent of World War I hastened the transition to the indirect method. A Canadian Army medical officer, O.H. Robertson,[58] introduced the use of a citrate-glucose solution of the same volume as the blood being collected. There was some disadvantage in the need to transport such large volumes of fluid to the battlefields and base hospitals, but the blood plus the citrate-glucose solution must have saved many a sufferer from posthemorrhagic shock. Robertson in 1918 also showed that the blood so collected could be stored for as long as 21 days. This had been demonstrated experimentally by Rous and Turner[59] and reported in 1916. These famous investigators at the Rockefeller Institute were seeking a means of preserving rabbit red cells for laboratory test use, as in standard Wasserman reactions and in some culture media. They found that dilute citrate-dextrose solutions would preserve under refrigeration for several weeks the red cells of laboratory animals and, likewise, those of humans. In animal experiments, they proved that after 14 days of such storage, these red cells transfused into animal recipients functioned and survived normally. Their anticoagulant-preservative solution had a volume of 700 ml for each 300 ml of blood. However, they recommended removing the supernatant fluid and administering the sedimented red cells suspended in saline, a proposal strongly advocated 30 to 40 years later for transfusions given to correct severe anemia. The important implications of this to the long-term storage of blood in blood banks were pretty much ignored for 20 years, when World War II restimulated interest in the ready availability and use of whole blood as a lifesaving measure.

Some experience in this direction was gained during the civil war in Spain in 1937–1939, as was reported by Duran-Jorda.[60] In the $2\frac{1}{2}$ years of operation, the blood transfusion service of the Republican Army collected 9000 liters of blood in citrate-dextrose solution, put this up in 300 ml units, and used them efficiently at casualty stations and base hospitals.

The Beginning of Blood Banks

Fantus,[61] at the Cook County Hospital in Chicago, is credited with organizing the first operating hospital blood bank in the United States, as reported by him in 1937. Blood taken in 2% sodium citrate could be refrigerated and used, but only for 7 to 10 days; the wastage of unused blood was therefore high. This made blood storage or banking quite impractical except in large hospitals, where the daily transfusion demands were sufficiently great to make the turnover active and more economical.

With the advent of World War II, the need for blood became acute, and blood procurement organizations were quickly expanded, particularly in Great Britain. There, a "walking-donor service," i.e., volunteer donors of known blood group available on call, had been established for many years. Beginning in 1921 with the London Blood Transfusion Service, assisted by the Red Cross Society, regional centers had been organized around the largest local hospitals and apparatus and methods had been standardized and made reliable and relatively safe. By 1939, when the war started, thousands of "repeat donors" were ready to give blood, and an efficient blood procurement service was operative in numerous regional centers from which the blood could be shipped to wherever it was needed.

In the United States, where distances were much greater and independent blood banks had been established only in large hospitals and in large city centers, a well-organized volunteer donor service had not yet been developed. Paid donors were used much more regularly. When the banked blood became outdated (beyond 7 to 10 days), the cells were discarded, and only the plasma could be saved. Recognition of the value of plasma for treatment of shock led to collection and storage of this more stable product for emergency use, as fully described in Chapter 17. Strumia and McGraw[62] had developed such a plasma collection facility beginning in 1927. In fact, a wave of enthusiasm for using plasma may have led to some unfortunate castastrophes when it was given in place of whole blood for treatment of shock from blood loss.

In June 1940, at a meeting in New York City, it was made known that there was a great need in France and England for plasma to treat shock in battle casualties. A program was then organized to collect large amounts of blood from volunteer donors and to ship the plasma abroad. The American Red Cross, with its countrywide local chapters, joined in this project and helped make it an outstanding success, 13 million units being collected by the end of the war.

As mentioned, late in World War I, Robertson, of the Canadian Army, had shown that blood preserved in citrate-glucose solution, after the method of Rous and Turner (1916), could be safely and effectively used for 2 to 3 weeks after collection. This experience was not exploited in the United States, however, until the advent of World War II. About 1939, DeGowin[63] and his associates developed a somewhat similar formula of citrate-dextrose in 500 ml water and found this satisfactory for as long as 38 days. This, and a modification of it (Alsever's solution), was used in the first whole blood shipments to the European theater of the war beginning in August 1944. In the meantime, in 1943 Loutit and Mollison,[64] of England, had developed an acid-citrate-dextrose (ACD) solution which (in a ratio of 70 ml to 450 ml blood) gave 3 to 4 weeks of preservation and a less dilute therapeutic infusion. It was employed effectively by the United States Navy in the Pacific engagement from December 1944. Incomplete statistics show that after blood shipments were activated in the last year of the war in Europe, about 380,000 units of blood were used in this way. In the Pacific theater, the total was about 180,000 units of blood.[65]

After the end of the war, many physicians and surgeons, who had gained experience with, and had come to rely on, blood in the treatment of injuries and illnesses, returned to find that blood banks were sorely needed to support civilian medical practice. This demand led to the rapid expansion of blood bank facilities in hospitals, in communities, and in regions where the public had become accustomed to making blood donations. With cessation of hostilities, the Red Cross Blood Program ceased, but some local chapters continued to help recruit donors for hospital blood banks. In 1947, the American National

Red Cross formulated a plan for the establishment of regional blood centers to help supply obvious needs for more blood and blood products, both in civilian and military medical practices. From 1948 to 1963, 56 such regional centers were established. By 1962, there were also 4400 hospital blood banks and 123 nonhospital or community or local medical society blood banks. Most of the latter two categories were associated in a national organization, formed in 1948, known as the American Association of Blood Banks.[66] Together, the total blood collections in the United States in 1976 were estimated at about 10 million units.

Originally, blood was collected into rubber-stoppered bottles, using rubber connecting tubes and steel needles, all of which were reused after washing and resterilization. The reutilization of the glass and rubber equipment led to a high incidence of pyrogen reactions due to small amounts of incompletely removed protein matter in the tubing as well as other contaminants remaining in the equipment. Very soon, disposable plastic tubing began to replace the rubber connecting tubes both in the donor and the recipient sets. By 1949, a plastic collecting bag had been developed. After Gibson et al.[67] reported (1952) their exhaustive and convincing trials of this plastic equipment, proving its greater cleanliness, safety, and flexibility for administration of blood and its component parts, glass bottles gradually were replaced worldwide.

After the war, the ACD diluent-preservative of Loutit and Mollison was widely accepted as the standard for 21-day preservation of blood in blood banks. The introduction in 1957 of a citrate-phosphate-dextrose (CPD) preservative, also developed by Gibson et al.,[68] extended the storage period to 28 days with a loss of less than 30 percent of the red cells (the maximum allowed by the NIH) and a normal life expectancy in vivo for the infused cells. Most blood banks in the next decade converted to CPD as the preservative solution, although the dating period by government regulations was maintained at a conservative 21 days. This diluent, being less acid and more protective of the cell, had the added advantage of reducing the collection and storage lesions of the red cell in the bag. Even so, alterations in the stored blood sometimes required considerable readjustment by the recipient's system in order to correct the collection and storage changes. A sick, hypotensive, anoxic, or acidotic individual, especially if given multiple transfusions of older or of poorly collected blood, might be more "helped out" than helped.*

* An anecdote vividly depicts the extent of the storage lesions in banked blood. Dr. Gibson, when he was studying blood preservatives, requested a specimen for his own analysis from a bottle of 21-day-old ACD blood about to be used for transfusion. In error the tube was sent to the hospital laboratory for routine analysis. The report returned was as follows:

This patient, whose red cells show extreme aniso- and poikilocytosis, must be suffering from a bizarre anemia that defies classification. It is obviously hemolytic, the plasma hemoglobin level being 150 mg%; 30 percent of the red cells show markedly increased fragility and hemolysis; he is obviously diabetic, blood sugar being 450 mg%, also probably in renal failure with elevated plasma potassium and inorganic phosphates, as well as high BUN, also in severe acidosis, the pH being 6.65. How long has this patient been dead?

Cadaver Blood, Placental Blood

Another source of blood for transfusion was popularized by Russian scientists in the 1930s. This was from fatally stricken victims of acute cardiac disease or severe trauma brought to a large central emergency hospital in Moscow. Yudin,[69] in 1937, reported on 1000 transfusions with cadaver blood kept for three weeks or more. The results were said to be entirely satisfactory, particularly when postmortem fibrinolysis kept the blood fluid and necessitated no citrate anticoagulant. Large amounts of blood could be made available from this source. Cadaver blood has been exploited in few other countries. An evaluation of its suitability for use in transfusion was also carried out by Vyas et al.[70] in Bombay, India in 1968 with complete hematologic, biochemical, and bacteriologic testing. Only minor chemical changes were found, and the survival value of the red cells did not show any significant fall. Long-term storage was not tried. Cadaver blood had advantages in the large amount available from a single donor and its utility for massive transfusions. It was found, however, that it was distinctly noncompetitive from the point of view of expense. In addition, the idea of obtaining and using cadaver blood has had little appeal in the United States.

An obvious source of possibly useful material, long discarded, has been the human placenta. In fact, in the 1930s and 1940s, it was used by several pharmaceutical firms to manufacture gamma globulin (then called placental extract) for prophylaxis against measles.* During and after World War II, when large stores of plasma were available for production of much wanted albumin, gamma globulin was a by-product available in amounts far beyond its needs. Plasmapheresis made placental extraction uneconomical. In 1938, an obstetrician, J.R. Goodall,[71] and his associates in Montreal published an article entitled, "An Inexhaustible Source of Blood for Transfusion and Its Preservation," claiming that they could collect 100 to 150 ml of blood per placenta. With sterile precautions, and taken into a special citrate preservative, this was said to yield satisfactory blood for transfusion purposes. They stated it could be kept satisfactorily under refrigeration up to 60 days with only minor hemolysis being evident and this "was harmless." No bacterial cultures were taken. "Many" transfusions were given, according to the authors, with no reactions noted. A year later, Boland et al.,[72] of London, reported that in a trial they carried out with 40 specimens of placental blood, long-term cultures yielded 30 positive results. In the use of either sterile placental blood or blood from a vein, they noted four severe reactions, only with the placental source. The "inexhaustible source" of blood from placentae for transfusion purposes seemed to have been overly optimistic.

A giant step forward in the efficient use of blood and all its parts was made

* See Chapter 17.

in the 1940s through the vision and efforts of one man, E.J. Cohn,[73] of Boston, as described in Chapter 17. He was responsible for the fractionation of plasma into useful concentrated albumin and gamma globulin components and foresaw a time when no part or derivative of the blood would be wasted, each derivative being used to treat specific conditions. By the 1970s, 40 years later, his vision had been almost completely fulfilled.

Long-term Storage: Frozen Blood

Attempts to preserve blood for long periods, measured in years, through freezing of red cells achieved considerable success in the 1960s with the use of cryoprotective agents, such as glycerol.[74] Thawing and washing methods were developed that permitted recovery of from 75 to 90 percent of the frozen red cells, some of which had been in storage 10 years.[75] The advantages of using frozen red cells were: (1) long-term storage, permitting stockpiling for an emergency; (2) preservation of rare blood types for later autologous or homologous transfusions; (3) accumulation of quantities of group O Rh-negative cells, safely usable as "universal donor" blood since the plasma was completely removed; (4) complete freedom from leukocytes and plasma, which could cause reactions in sensitized or immunosuppressed donors or transplantation recipients; and (5) possibly low or absent hazard of hepatitis infection. There were certain recognized disadvantages:[76] (1) time and personnel involved in preparation were considerable; (2) much space was needed for preparation and storage; and most important (3) costs were high, not only for needed basic equipment but for expendable supplies, which cost over four times the cost of a unit of banked liquid blood.

For special purposes, for disastrous situations, possibly for wartime use, frozen blood resources promised to fill an important gap. Simplification and economies in methodology are being studied that may solve problems that handicap the freer use of frozen blood.

Modern Blood Transfusion Therapy

Finally, it seems appropriate to mention briefly the present status of the science of blood transfusion. Certainly, there is little cause to feel proud of its slow development over a period of more than 300 years. But it is now one of the major forms of medical therapy, involving as it does the use of whole blood, its separated cellular components, its plasma, and the derivatives of this fluid portion. According to crude statistics, more than 10 million blood transfusions are now given yearly in the United States. Added to this are uncounted thousands of injections of plasma and derivatives, such as albumin, gamma globulin, and clotting factors, needed for specific treatment, for prophylaxis, and for support of many surgical and medical procedures.

Forty years ago, a blood bank was called on to supply only two items, whole blood and plasma from outdated blood. The modern large hospital or community blood bank may have or can make available 17 or more preparations. These are: (1) whole blood in ACD or CPD, 2 to 21 days old, of group- and type-specific varieties; (2) heparinized fresh blood, 1 to 2 days old; (3) sedimented or packed red cell concentrates; (4) red cell concentrates washed free of plasma, platelets, and white cells for multitransfused sensitized patients; (5) reconstituted frozen red cells for highly sensitized recipients or for individuals with rare groups; (6) red cell packs irradiated to destroy all residual lymphocytes for transfusion of immunodeficient and immunosuppressed recipients, who require protection from graft versus host disease; (7) platelet concentrates procured by thrombopheresis; (8) white cell concentrates (on special order) from leukopheresis; (9) plasma, fresh or stored; (10) albumin—20% solution; (11) cryoprecipitate for hemophilia-A patients; (12) factor VIII higher potency concentrate (glycine method); (13) factor IX concentrate for hemophilia-B patients; (14) fibrinogen; (15) gamma globulin derivative from normal plasma; (16) anti-Rh gamma globulin from sensitized Rh-negative donors; (17) gamma globulin concentrates from high antibody level serum against specific diseases, such as measles, mumps, and chicken pox.

Research in progress promises further improvements in blood banking techniques. The use of CPD with additives such as adenine[77] has the possibility of extending refrigerator shelf life to 35 days. Methods for pH adjustments, possibly by means of enclosed bag containers (Gibson and McCue,[78] Bensinger et al.[79]), may extend red cell storage to 42 days or more. These improvements have yet to be made operative.

A further development has been the attempt to find a soluble vehicle as a temporary replacement for the red cell oxygen transport in the circulation. Fluorocarbons in emulsion have been the most promising.[80] When combined with plasma volume expanders and glucose, salt, and water and then injected into rats rendered bloodless, the circulation has been maintained up to three days. Much more information will have to be accumulated before human trials can be considered, but, eventually, some patients with chronic aplastic anemia, kidney failure, or other deficiencies might benefit from such new blood substitutes.

As Bernheim[81] said in 1942:

> If the history of blood transfusion were charted it would present a picture not unlike that of an intermittent fever, with its uneven ups and downs, its periods of quiescence—some longer than others—followed by renewed outbreaks . . . until the gradual drop to the normalcy of ultimate recovery. A basic idea of intense interest and huge potentialities for the human race held the minds of men enthralled throughout the centuries, yet so formidable were the difficulties of execution that despite almost constant even inspired effort, progress was so painfully slow and uncertain as to make some despair of ever reaching the desired goal.

Although victory over our ailments is still far from complete, the proper use of blood and blood products is a great step toward this goal.

Acknowledgments

It is a pleasure to acknowledge my indebtedness to a number of individuals who gave invaluable assistance during preparation of this chapter. Dr. Thomas E. Cone, Jr., supplied references to historical books and papers. Dr. Richard E. Rosenfield, of New York, made available his excellent review of transfusion history at Mt. Sinai Hospital. Dr. Paul J. Schmidt, of Tampa, Florida, generously permitted the use of his illustrations of blood transfusion apparatus, and the American Association of Blood Banks approved reprinting these from *Seminar on Current Technical Topics*, November 1974, as did also Dr. Michael DeBakey and the C.V. Mosby Company, publishers of *The Blood Bank and the Technique and Therapeutics of Transfusions*, 1942. Mrs. Anne Schmid was most helpful in using her editorial skills to make the manuscript correct and more readable. Mrs. Mickie Ochi assisted in finding old as well as new pertinent references and typed and proofread the manuscript most efficiently.

This review was prepared during tenure as a Henry J. Kaiser Senior Fellow at the Center for Advanced Study in the Behavioral Sciences, Stanford, California.

There are a number of reviews of the history of blood transfusion that are invaluable sources of information and references. These are references 82–87.

References

1 Libavius A: 1615, quoted by Maluf NSR: History of blood transfusion. *J Hist Med* 9:59–107, 1954.
2 Folli F: 1680, quoted by Keynes G: *Blood Transfusion*. Bristol, John Wright, 1949, 574 pp, pp 5–6.
3 Dormandy TL: Harvey at 400. *Lancet* i:708, 1978.
4 Webster C: The origins of blood transfusion: a reassessment. *Med Hist* 15:387–392, 1971.
5 Hoff HE, Guilleman R: The first experiments on transfusion in France. *J Hist Med* 18:103–124, 1963.
6 Hollingsworth MW: Blood transfusion by Richard Lower in 1665. *Ann Med Hist* 10:213–225, 1928.
7 Hutchin P: History of blood transfusion. A tercentennial look. *Surgery* 64:685–700, 1968.
8 Keynes G: Tercentenary of blood transfusion. *Br Med J* 4:410–411, 1967.
9 Nicolson MH: *Pepys' Diary and the New Science*. Charlottesville, University Press of Virginia, 1965, 224 pp.
10 Nicolson MH, Rodes DS (eds): *Plays of Shadwell, T.: The Virtuoso*. Lincoln, University of Nebraska Press, 1965, 186 pp.

11 Siewers AB: A case of madness cured by blood transfusion. *Bull Hist Med* 6:1010–1014, 1938.

12 Walton MT: The first blood transfusion: French or English? *Med Hist* 18:360–364, 1974.

13 Blundell J: Observations on transfusion of blood by Dr. Blundell with a description of his gravitator. *Lancet* ii:321–324, 1828.

14 Jones HW, Mackmul G: The influence of James Blundell on the development of blood transfusion. *Ann Med Hist* 10:242–248, 1928.

15 Bovell J: On the transfusion of milk, as practised in cholera, at the cholera sheds. *Can J* 3:188, 1855.

16 Howe JW: Transfusion of goat's milk. *NY State J Med* 21:506–508, 1875.

17 Thomas TG: The intravenous injection of milk as a substitute for the transfusion of blood. *NY State J Med* 27:449–465, 1878.

18 Howe JW: Intravenous injection of human milk. *NY State J Med* 31:383–384, 1880.

19 Oberman HA: Early history of blood substitutes: transfusion of milk. *Transfusion* 9:74–77, 1969.

20 Bull WT: On the intravenous injection of saline solutions as a substitute for transfusion of blood. *Med Rec* 25:6–8, 1884.

21 Carrel A: The surgery of blood vessels. *Johns Hopkins Med J* 18:18–28, 1907.

22 Walker LG: Carrel's direct transfusion of a 5-day old infant. *Surg Gynecol Obstet* 137:494–496, 1973.

23 Crile GW: The technique of direct transfusion of blood. *Ann Surg* 46:329–332, 1907.

24 Crile GW: *Hemorrhage and Transfusion*. New York and London, Appleton, 1909, 560 pp.

25 Hewson W: *Experimental Inquiries*. London, Johnson, 1774, 239 pp, pt 2.

26 Hicks JB: On transfusion and new mode of management. *Br Med J* 2:151, 1868.

27 Satterlee HS, Hooker RS: Transfusion of blood with special reference to the use of anticoagulants. *JAMA* 66:618–624, 1916.

28 Wright AE: Methods of increasing and diminishing the coagulability of the blood, with special reference to their therapeutic employment. *Br Med J* 14:57–61, 1894.

29 Prevost JL, Dumas JB: 1821, quoted by Maluf NSR: History of blood transfusion. *J Hist Med* 9:59–107, 1954.

30 Bischoff THW: Beiträge zur Lehre von dem Blute und der Transfusion desselben. *Arch Anat Physiol Wissensch Med* 347, 1835.

31 Moss WL: A simple method for the indirect transfusion of blood. *Am J Med Sci* 147:698–703, 1914.

32 Gesellius F: *Die Transfusion des Blutes*. Leipzig, Wagner, 1873. (Quoted by Maluf NSR: History of blood transfusion. *J Hist Med* 9:59–107, 1954.)

33 Hasse O: *Die Lammblut-Transfusion beim Menschen*. St. Petersburg, Edward Hoppe, 1874, 78 pp.

34 Ponfick E: Experimentelle Beitrage zur Lehre von der Transfusion. *Virchows Arch* 62:273–335, 1875.

35 Landois L: *Die Transfusion des Blutes*. Leipzig, Vogel, 1875, 358 pp.

36 Cruchet R, Ragot A, Caussimon J: *La Transfusion du Sang de l'Animal a l'Homme*. Paris, 1928. (Quoted by Zimmerman LM, Howell KM: History of blood transfusion. *Ann Med Hist* 4:415–433, 1932.)

37 Curtis AH, David VC: The transfusion of blood. Further notes on a new method. *JAMA* 57:1453–1454, 1911.

38 Kimpton AR, Brown JH: A new and simple method of transfusion. *JAMA* 61:117–118, 1913.

39 Bernheim BM: A simple instrument for the direct transfusion of blood. *JAMA* 65:1278, 1915.

40 Lindeman E: Reactions following blood transfusion by the syringe cannula system. *JAMA* 66:624–626, 1916.

41 Unger LL: A new method of syringe transfusion. *JAMA* 64:582–584, 1915.

42 Bordet J: Les leucocytes et les propriétés due sérum chez les vaccinés, *Ann Inst Pasteur (Paris)* 9:462, 1895; 15:129, 1901.

43 Ehrlich P, Morgenroth J: Ueber Haemolysine. *Berl Klin Wochenschr* 36:6, 481, 1899; 37:452, 681, 1900.

44 Landsteiner K: Über Agglutinationserscheinungen normalen menschlichen Blutes. *Wien Klin Wochenschr* 14:1132–1134, 1901.

45 Decastello A, Sturli A: Über die Iso-agglutinine im Serum gesunder und kranker Menschen. *Münch Med Wochenschr* 49:1090–1095, 1902.

46 Hektoen L: Isoagglutination of human corpuscles. *J Infect Dis* 4:297–303, 1907.

47 Hektoen L: Isoagglutination of human corpuscles with respect to demonstration of opsonic index and to transfusion of blood. *JAMA* 48:1739–1740, 1907.

48 Ottenberg R: Transfusion and arterial anastomosis. *Ann Surg* 47:486–502, 1908.

49 Ottenberg R: Reminiscences of the history of blood transfusion. *Mt Sinai J Med NY* 4:264–271, 1937.

50 Arthus M, Pagés C: Nouvelle théorie chimique de la coagulation du sang. *Physiol Norm Pathol* 2:739–746, 1890.

51 Hustin A: Principe d'une nouvelle méthode de transfusion muqueuse. *J Med Brux* 12:436–439, 1914.

52 Agote L: Nueva procedimento para la transfusion de sangre. *An Inst Modelo Clin Med* 1:25, 1915.

53 Weil R: Sodium citrate in the transfusion of blood. *JAMA* 64:425–426, 1915.

54 Lewisohn R: Blood transfusion by the citrate method. *Surg Gynecol Obstet* 21:37–47, 1915.

55 Hort EC, Penfold WJ: The dangers of saline injections. *Br Med J* 2:1589–91, 1911.

56 Seibert FB: Fever-producing substances found in some distilled water. *Am J Physiol* 67:90–104, 1923–1924.

57 Lewisohn R, Rosenthal N: Prevention of chills following transfusion of citrated blood. *JAMA* 100:466–469, 1933.

58 Robertson OH: Transfusion with preserved red blood cells. *Br Med J* 1:691–695, 1918.

59 Rous P, Turner JR: The preservation of living red blood cells in vitro. I. Methods of preservation. *J Exp Med* 23:219–237, 1916; II. The transfusion of kept cells. 239–248.

60 Duran-Jorda F: The Barcelona blood transfusion service. *Lancet* i:773–775, 1939.

61 Fantus B: The therapy of the Cook County Hospital. *JAMA* 109:128–131, 1937.

62 Strumia MM, McGraw JJ: The development of plasma preparations for transfusions. *Ann Intern Med* 15:80–87, 1941.

63 DeGowin EL, Hardin RC, Alsever JB: *Blood Transfusion*. Philadelphia and London, Saunders, 1949, 475 pp.

64 Loutit JF, Mollison PL: Advantages of a disodium-citrate-glucose mixture as a blood preservative. *Br Med J* 2:744–745, 1943.

65 Kendrick DB: *Blood Program in World War II, Historical Note.* Washington, DC, Office of Surgeon General, Dept. of the Army, U.S. Govt. Printing Office, 1964, 922 pp.

66 Diamond LK: History of blood banking in the United States. *JAMA* 193:40–45, 1965.

67 Gibson JG II, Sack T, Buckley ES Jr: The preservation of whole ACD blood, collected, stored and transfused in plastic equipment. *Surg Gynecol Obstet* 95:113–119, 1952.

68 Gibson JG II, Rees SB, McManus TJ, Scheitlin WA: A citrate-phosphate-dextrose solution for the preservation of human blood. *Am J Clin Pathol* 28:569–578, 1957.

69 Yudin SS: Transfusion of stored cadaver blood. *Lancet* ii:361–366, 1937.

70 Vyas GN, Munver UL, Salgaonkar DS, Purandare NM: Human cadaver blood for transfusion. *Transfusion* 8:250–253, 1968.

71 Goodall JR, Anderson FO, Altemas GT, MacPhail FG: An inexhaustible source of blood for transfusion and its preservation. *Surg Gynecol Obstet* 66:176–178, 1938.

72 Boland CR, Craig NS, Jacobs AL: Collection and transfusion of preserved blood. *Lancet* i:388–391, 1939.

73 Cohn EJ: The separation of blood into fractions of therapeutic value. *Ann Intern Med* 26:341–352, 1947.

74 Huggins CE: Frozen blood. *JAMA* 193:941–944, 1965.

75 Valeri CR: Liquid and freeze preservation of human red blood cells, in Surgenor DM (ed): *The Red Blood Cell,* 2d ed. New York, Academic Press, 1974, vol 1, 612 pp, pp 511–574.

76 Chaplin H, Jr: Frozen blood. *N Engl J Med* 298:679–681, 1978.

77 Beutler E: Experimental blood preservatives for liquid storage, in Greenwalt TJ, Jamieson GA (eds): *The Human Red Cell in Vitro.* New York, Grune and Stratton, 1974, 363 pp, pp 182–216.

78 Gibson JS II, McCue JP: Reversal of the storage lesion of CPD bank blood: A problem in clinical medicine. *Transfusion* 18:524–529, 1978.

79 Bensinger TA, Chillar RK, Beutler E: Prolonged maintenance of 2,3-DPG in liquid blood storage: use of an internal CO_2 trap to stabilize pH. *J Lab Clin Med* 39:498–503, 1977.

80 Editorial: New blood substitutes. *Lancet* i:126, 1974.

81 Bernheim BM: *Adventures in Blood Transfusion.* New York, Smith and Durrell, 1942, 182 pp, p xv.

82 Maluf NSR: History of blood transfusion. *J Hist Med* 9:59–107, 1954.

83 Kilduffe RA, DeBakey M: *The Blood Bank and the Technique and Therapeutics of Transfusions.* St. Louis, Mosby, 1942, 558 pp.

84 Zimmerman LM, Howell KM: History of blood transfusion. *Ann Med Hist* 4:415–433, 1932.

85 Keynes G: *Blood Transfusion.* Bristol, John Wright and Son, 1949, 574 pp.

86 Rosenfield RE: Early 20th century origins of modern blood transfusion therapy. *Mt Sinai J Med NY* 41:626–635, 1974.

87 Schmidt PJ: Transfusion in historical perspective, in *Seminars on Current Technical Topics.* Am Assn of Blood Banks Annual Meeting, 1974. Washington, DC, Am Assn of Blood Banks, 1974, 176 pp.

CHAPTER 20

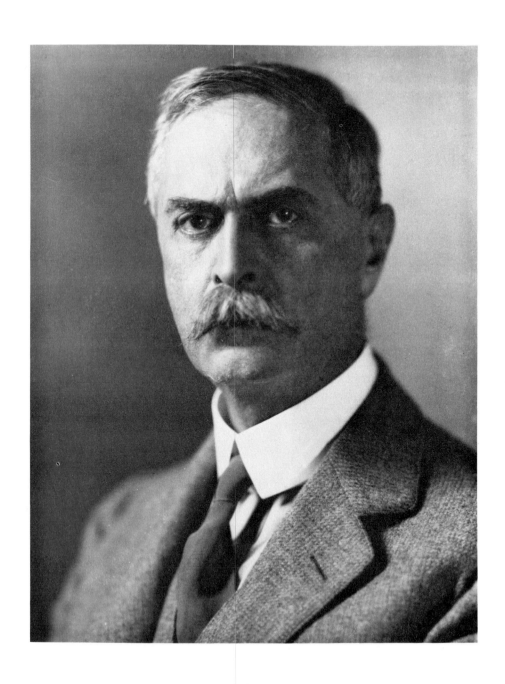

THE STORY OF OUR BLOOD GROUPS

Louis K. Diamond

B lut ist ein ganz besondrer Saft,"* said Goethe in 1808.[1] Just how special, and even individual, human blood is could not be fully appreciated until 1901, when Karl Landsteiner[2] found that red cells could be separated into three different groups. In 1902, a fourth much rarer group was found. From this modest start of four types, the individual characteristics of blood cells have been so greatly expanded that it is now highly improbable that any two people except identical twins would have the same combination of red cell surface markers. In other words, every person on earth is unique in his or her combination of blood groups—a fact recognized only in the past 30 years.

Early in the seventeenth century, there were hints that all bloods were not alike; when blood transfusions were attempted from one animal species to another, and from animals to humans, there were inexplicable reactions. Reasoning from this, James Blundell,[3] an English physiologist-obstetrician and

* "Blood is a very special kind of fluid."

Chapter Opening Photo Karl Landsteiner (1868–1943).

an early advocate of blood transfusion to prevent death from hemorrhage, said in 1828 that only human blood should be used for transfusion of humans, but his advice was ignored for the next half-century. More precise scientific evidence came from the 1875 observations of Landois,[4] of Germany, who found that by mixing the red cells of one animal species with the serum of another, he could produce agglutination similar to the results of mixing bacteria with appropriate immune serum.

An English pathologist, Shattock,[5] actually came close to discovering human blood groups in 1899 and 1900, when he reported seeing in the test tube clumping of normal red cells by serum from patients with acute pneumonia and certain other diseases. He called the phenomenon "irregular rouleaux" formation, although his illustrations suggest agglutination. He found no such occurrence in the serum from a few normal people, however, and, therefore, decided it was caused by the patient's inflammatory disease. It was understandably tempting to ascribe the phenomenon to a pathologic process and, thereby, have a diagnostic test for a disease state, but his failure to control this important observation by using a larger number of normal people caused him to miss the underlying principle of human blood-group differentiation.

Stimulated by these observations and the studies of Landois and of Ehrlich and Morgenroth, Karl Landsteiner (Chapter Opening Photo), then a young assistant in the Institute of Pathological Anatomy of the University of Vienna, investigated the reactions between the red cells and the sera of 22 associates, all normal healthy individuals. He found that certain sera would agglutinate the red cells of certain other people. This discovery of isoagglutination became the basis of human blood-group classification.

Originally, Landsteiner was able to separate his blood samples into three types, which he called A, B, and C. He noted that the serum of A clumped the cells of B, the serum of B clumped the cells of A, and the serum of C clumped the cells of both A and B but were not clumped by A or B serum. According to Philip Levine,[6] his assistant and associate from 1925 through 1932, such careful work was characteristic of Landsteiner, who had previously noted red cell agglutinins and hemolysins in the sera of sick patients but, unsatisfied by a few such observations, had turned to testing a larger number of healthy people. This led him to the basic immunologic principle of human blood-group differentiation. In his characteristically brief but data-filled paper of 1901, Landsteiner further noted and pointed out that the blood isoagglutinins retained their activity after drying and redissolving. Also, he observed agglutination with serum extracted after 14 days from blood dried on a cloth. "The reaction may be suited to establish the identity or more correctly the non-identity of a blood specimen." This predicted the value of Landsteiner's discovery to forensic medicine in the future. The closing statement in his paper was, "Finally, it might be mentioned that the reported observations may assist in the explanation of various consequences of therapeutical blood transfusions." In three pages, Landsteiner compressed knowledge that would fill thousands of pages in the future. Of the 345 publications listed in his bibliography, 240 consisted of articles taking up six pages or fewer, the majority only one or two pages.

As his assistant Philip Levine describes him,[6] he was a tall, stern-looking man, "utterly and completely dedicated to scientific endeavors and had a passion for clear, logical and concise thinking." Underlying his austere appearance was a "warmth, gentleness, and sincerity" and willingness to share his knowledge with younger people, including the present author, who sought an interview and was given not only that but a generous sample of Landsteiner's new anti-Rh serum for his laboratory in Boston.

In 1902, two of Landsteiner's pupils, Decastello and Sturli,[7] working in a large medical clinic in Vienna with a larger and more varied number of subjects, confirmed Landsteiner's findings in 155 cases. They found four people, however, who had no agglutinins in their serum and whose cells were clumped by the other three serums; this was the fourth and rarest group (2.5 percent). They also established the fact that the red cell agglutinins had no relationship to disease and were distributed similarly in 121 patients and 34 healthy subjects.

After Landsteiner had pointed out the importance of his discovery to human transfusion therapy, it is difficult to understand why practitioners failed to appreciate and utilize his findings for almost 10 years. In the United States, this might be blamed on lack of familiarity with the foreign literature; in Europe, it must have been the perennial failure of communication between the clinician and the basic scientist, which then was even greater than now. Even Landsteiner could not have foreseen that eventually humans would be characterized by hundreds of red cell antigens, which would become important to genetics, anthropology, forensic medicine, and some disease states.

Landsteiner was a careful, meticulous worker. In his original paper on the agglutination of normal human blood, he described his method for testing as comprising the mixing of equal amounts of serum and of 5% red cell suspension in 0.6% sodium chloride. This technique, carried out at room temperature or in the cold, favored the agglutinating reaction of anti-A and anti-B antibodies on susceptible red cells but masked the reaction of warm "incomplete" antibodies against the still undiscovered Rh and Kell antigens and numerous others, particularly in a dilute saline suspension. Only chance and the alert mind of Landsteiner's pupil Levine led to the reawakening of interest in blood-group serology 40 years after the original discovery.

ABO Blood Groups

It is not unusual for great discoveries to have little impact at the time they are made. Certainly, the significance of the A and B isoagglutinins and their relation to transfusion reactions went unrecognized for quite a few years and failed to influence the practice of transfusionists. Hektoen, of Chicago, however, realized the practical importance of Landsteiner's discovery and in 1907 published a paper in an infectious disease journal[8] on the isoagglutination of human red cells, repeating such tests on 76 people and confirming the original results. To call attention to the significance of this in transfusion therapy, he also wrote a short summary of his findings for the widely read *Journal of the American Medical Association,*[9] but this, too, had little influence on transfusion practices.

In 1907, Jansky,[10] of Czechoslovakia, worked out the reciprocal relationship (the agglutination reactions) of the four blood groups and numbered them, beginning with the term group I for the most common. His report, however, was published in Bohemian and was little known even on the continent. In 1910, Moss,[11] of Baltimore, quite independently made the same finding, but his classification began with group I as the rarest and group IV as the commonest. This led later to confusion and the necessity of stating whether one was using the nomenclature of Jansky or Moss. It was ultimately resolved in 1927 by the adoption of Landsteiner's notation classifying the groups by letters for each of the agglutinogens, A, B, AB, and O.

It was Epstein and Ottenberg[12] who in 1908 first suggested that the blood groups are hereditary. Two years later, von Dungern and Hirszfeld[13] clearly established the mendelian inheritance of the blood groups, though the exact manner of their inheritance was not detailed until 1924 by Bernstein.[14]

Subgroups of A (A_1 and A_2) were first described in 1911.[15] Further elaboration of subgroups in the ABO system and the sera and methods to detect these were described in ensuing years. This brief review would become encumbered even if it only listed the numerous variants of blood-group factors in the ABO system and other independent systems. For such information, the most authoritative textbook is Race and Sanger's *Blood Groups in Man,*[16] deservedly known as the "bible of bloodgroupers."

A number of years after the ABO groups were discovered, it was found independently by several investigators that the antigens were not limited to the red cells but were present in all tissues except the brain. They could, thus, more correctly be called body or tissue group factors rather than blood-group factors. This is not true of blood groups other than those of the ABO system.

In addition, it was noted by Yamakami[17] that A and B antigens were present in saliva. Hartmann[18] showed that there were two distinct forms of the antigens, a water-soluble form present in most body fluids but not in the red cells or serum and an alcohol-soluble form present in all the tissues and in the red cells but not in the secretions. The ability to secrete the A, B, or O antigens in the saliva was found to be inherited as a mendelian dominant character. This gene, known as Se, is linked to the Lewis blood-group system. About 80 percent of whites are secretors, 20 percent nonsecretors. These figures vary slightly in different countries. The differences are much greater in some ethnic groups. In blacks, nonsecretors number 50 percent, in Amerindians, 1 percent or less.

Blood Groups M, N, and P

No other blood-group systems were recognized until 1927. Landsteiner and Philip Levine had been engaged in seeking additional antigenic differences in human blood by injecting rabbits with different human red cells and absorbing the resulting rabbit immune sera with other red cell samples. They eventually found antibodies that could distinguish between different bloods, independent of the ABO differences. In 1927, they named a new factor,[19] "M" (for immune), and in the same year identified the allele to it, the "N" factor,[20] and a new agglutinogen which they named "P." In 1928, they detailed the inheritance and the frequencies of the M and N factors.[21,22] They showed that two allelic genes, M and N, determine the presence of the corresponding antigens on the red cells, thus resulting in three genotypes, MM, MN, and NN, and three corresponding phenotypes M, MN, and N. This was soon confirmed by family studies in hundreds of cases.

Although some rare alleles were found, no important additions to the MN system were discovered until 1947; then, Walsh and Montgomery[23] uncovered an antibody which, in additional tests by Sanger and Race,[24] subdivided the M and N blood groups by an antigen called S. A few years later, Levine et al.[25] found the predicted serum anti-s and, thereby, identified the allelic antigen, called s. Human bloods were then identified as having the phenotypes MS, Ms, NS, and Ns. Antibodies against these are rarely associated with hemolytic reactions, and the M, N, and P systems can, therefore, be ignored in typing and cross matching for transfusions. They are mentioned here as examples of the complexities of many of the blood-group systems that have been discovered as immunoserology has expanded.

The Rh Blood Groups

Considerable excitement was generated in blood-banking circles in 1939 when Levine and Stetson[26] reported an unusual hemolytic reaction in a group O woman transfused with her husband's blood, also group O. Such an intra-group reaction (group O versus group O) was inexplicable. On testing her serum against her husband's cells, Levine found that agglutination resulted. An unappreciated fact was that this woman had just given birth to a stillborn infant with erythroblastosis fetalis (EF), a fulminant form of hemolytic anemia, the cause of which was then unknown. Levine later reasoned that the infant might have had a red cell agglutinogen inherited from the father but foreign to the mother. In response to transplacental stimulation by this antigen, she had produced an antibody, which, entering the infant's circulation, caused the severe hemolytic anemia. This antibody could also agglutinate her husband's red cells and, thereby, cause her hemolytic transfusion reaction. On testing her serum against 104 ABO compatible blood samples, agglutination resulted in 80. A publication by Levine and associates[27] 2 years later proved conclusively that this new and unusual maternal antibody was the cause of EF, thereafter more accurately called hemolytic disease of the fetus and newborn (HDNB).

In the meantime, Landsteiner and Wiener[28] had found a new antibody resulting from the immunization of rabbits and guinea pigs with the blood of rhesus monkeys. This agglutinated the monkey red cells, and, when tested against the red cells of Caucasians in New York City, clumping ensued in 85 percent of the specimens. They called these individuals "rhesus-positive" and the remaining 15 percent "rhesus-negative." Parallel tests with Levine's serum yielded about the same percentage distribution of positive and negative as the rabbit antirhesus serum; thus, the terms rhesus (Rh) factor and anti-rhesus (anti-Rh) antibody were established. Landsteiner and Wiener,[29] from studies on 60 families, confirmed the presence of the Rh antigen in about 85 percent of white people and showed it to be a dominant character. Meanwhile, Wiener and Peters[30] found that the anti-Rh antibody was, indeed, the cause of intragroup hemolytic transfusion reactions and, therefore, was of real clinical importance. This was confirmed innumerable times thereafter in Rh-negative persons given Rh-positive blood after sensitization by previous transfusion or by pregnancies involving infants who were Rh-positive.

Years later (1961), Levine et al.[31] established that the rabbit antirhesus antibody and the human anti-Rh antibody are not truly the same, and Levine suggested that the rabbit antirhesus antibody be known as anti-LW to honor Landsteiner and Wiener. By then, however, it was impossible to change the term Rh because of the thousands of publications that had accumulated. Had Levine with less modesty given a name to the blood-group system which he and Stetson discovered in 1939, it would have been the heading of this section rather than Rh or rhesus factor of human blood; however, the name may remind us that we are not too far removed from our animal ancestors.

Levine was fortunate in that his first patient's serum also contained the form of antibody detected by the standard tests with dilute suspensions of susceptible red cells in saline. Most antibodies resulting from Rh sensitization yield no agglutination by such tests. For about 4 years, the diagnosis of EF in an infant depended on clinical criteria, supported by finding that the father and the patient were Rh-positive and the mother, Rh-negative; anti-Rh antibodies could not be detected in the maternal serum by standard testing methods. In 1944 and 1945, however, these antibodies were demonstrated to be present on the Rh-positive red cells. Race[32] called them "incomplete" and Wiener,[33] "blocking" antibodies. Each independently showed that the Rh-positive red cell coated with such a serum was "blocked" from reacting with a known anti-Rh serum of the saline-agglutinating type. This "blocking test" proved helpful in diagnosis.

Shortly thereafter, Diamond and Abelson[34] demonstrated that such "incomplete" or "blocking" anti-Rh antibodies produce easily visible agglutination of a thick drop of blood on a slide, especially when warmed. This rapid "slide test" made the diagnosis of EF and of certain transfusion reactions very simple. A further advance occurred when Diamond and Denton,[35] also in 1945, showed that plasma or, still better, human or bovine albumin in place of saline in the test tube would reveal potent, easily titratable anti-Rh antibodies in all cases of EF and of transfusion-sensitized Rh-negative persons. Added sensitivity and accuracy in the detection of "incomplete" antibodies were developed in the same year by Coombs, Mourant, and Race.[36] Theirs was the antiglobulin test, in which the addition of serum from a rabbit sensitized against human globulin produces agglutination of the antibody- (globulin) coated cells. This test could be used not only to detect anti-Rh in the serum but also the anti-Rh coated red cells of the infant with EF and of any other hemolytic anemia due to iso- or autoantibodies, as discussed in Chapter 8. It was most valuable in demonstrating the existence of new blood-group systems, such as the Kell, in 1946, the Kidd, in 1951, and others. The subsequent discovery of new antibodies and detection thereby of new blood factors created a veritable explosion in what had been a quiescent field.

Another refinement in technique for detecting red cell agglutinogens was introduced by Pickles. By enzyme treatment of the cells, she and Morton[37] showed that they were made agglutinable in saline by incomplete antibody. This became the basis for several mechanized agglutination methods and permitted hundreds of tests to be performed in a short time by a small number of technicians.

Shortly after the Rh discovery, as antisera of different specificities were recognized, Rh began to unfold as a complex system with several alleles. Wiener[38] defined six alleles, while Race[39] and his associates had seven. By 1944, the English geneticist Fisher had worked out a logical scheme for the Rh subtypes as three sets of alleles, which he called C and c, D and d, and E and e. The most common Rh factor was called D. He assumed that the three sets of genes were closely linked and that the gene complexes would be inherited as a unit. The Rh gene complex, therefore, could be assembled in eight different ways: CDe, cDE, cde, cDe, cdE, Cde, CDE, and CdE. Fisher's prediction that the until then unknown complex CdE and a new serum, anti-e, would be found was soon borne out, but the "d" factor, if there is such, has never been found.

In the meantime, Wiener had named the common Rh factor Rh_0, the allele (Rh-negative) Hr, the variants Rh-prime (Rh') and Rh-double-prime (Rh''), and their alleles hr' and hr''. As more variants appeared, his nomenclature used a collection of symbols that were difficult to remember, to write, and to speak, such as rh_i, rh^{W1}, rh^x, hr, rh^{W2}, rh^G, and others. The English nomenclature, based on the letters C, D, and E, with lettered superscripts for variants of these, was generally regarded as simpler and more consistent and, thus, became more widely used everywhere. However, no nomenclature for the Rh system in 1945 could have predicted the undiscovered variants in any logical and easily remembered fashion. As Race and Sanger[40] put it, "Neither the CDE nor Dr. Wiener's Rh-Hr notations have found it easy to digest the surfeit of more recent complex antibodies and antigens."

Rosenfield et al.[41] developed a numerical notation in 1962, and elaborated it in 1973,[42] by which time it listed variants up to Rh 35, with probably more yet to be discovered (now up to Rh 37). For common use, the combinations of the letters C, D, and E or the use of Wiener's symbols R_0, R_1, R_2, etc., serve to designate the ordinary Rh subtypes.

In contrast to the ABO blood-group system, in which the antigens are present on all body cells, the Rh antigen has been identified only on the red cell membrane; it is well developed long before birth. Chown[43] proved that a 6-week-old fetus already has the Rh antigens; it could be typed as cDE/cde or Rh_2 heterozygous by the Wiener classification.

The Growing Number of Blood Groups

As already mentioned, Levine's discoveries in 1939 and Landsteiner and Wiener's in 1940–1941 stimulated renewed interest in the blood groups. Serologists, geneticists, and clinicians soon realized that an area of practical as well as theoretic importance had been opened up for exploration. It only required new and more sensitive testing methods to uncover new blood-group systems and new red cell factors within them. And by 1945–1947, these had been developed. Thereafter, the number of blood-group antibodies and the antigens that they detected increased almost exponentially. There were the Lutheran, Kell, Duffy, Kidd, and Diego systems, and many others, often consisting of two or more antigenic determinants. So rapidly did they proliferate from all over the world that there was no time to develop an orderly classification and nomenclature. Accordingly, the names originated in each case from that of the donor or patient whose serum disclosed the new system, usually in investigation of the cause of a case of EF or of an unexplained transfusion reaction. To describe or even name here all the new blood-group systems with the specific red cell antigens and their numerous variants would make as dull reading as the catalogue of ships in Homer's *Iliad*. Table 20-1 lists most of these blood groups with references to the original papers. For full discussions of each the reader may consult Race and Sanger.[16]

It was immediately obvious that the greater number of heritable red cell markers would be important in identifying individuals and ethnic groups. That they might have other values was not apparent. Soon, however, certain blood-group antigens were found to have significant relation to anthropology, pathology, and, also, clinical medicine. Some of these relationships will be briefly pointed out in the succeeding discussions.

Table 20-1 *Blood-group antigens in humans* (adapted from Race and Sanger[16])*

SYSTEM	ANTIGENS	REFERENCE†
ABO	A_1, A_2, A_3, A_x, B, B_x, H	Landsteiner,[2] Decastello[7]
MNSs	M, M_1, M^g, N, S, s, U, Tm, Sj, Hu, and others	Landsteiner,[19,20] Walsh,[23] Levine[25]
P	P, P_1, P^k, Luke, p	Landsteiner[22]
Lewis	Le^a, Le^b, Le^c, Le^d, Le^x	Mourant,[44] Andresen[45]
Ii	I, i	Wiener,[46] Marsh[47]
Rh	D, C, c, E, e (these being Rh 1–5), and variants to total number Rh 35 + LW	Levine,[26] Landsteiner,[28] Wiener,[38] Race[39]
Lutheran	Lu^a, Lu^b, and variants to total number Lu 17	Callender,[48] Cutbush[49]
Kell	K, k, Kp^a, Kp^b, K_u, and variants to total number K 18	Coombs,[50] Allen,[51] Giblett,[52] Levine,[53] Stroup[54]
Duffy	Fy^a, Fy^b, Fy^x, Fy3, Fy4, Fy5	Cutbush,[55] Ikin[56]
Kidd	Jk^a, Jk^b, Jk3	Allen,[57] Plaut[58]
Diego	Di^a, Di^b	Layrisse,[59] Thompson[60]
Xg	Xg^a	Mann[61]
Others	Auberger, Cotton, Dombrock, Scianna, Sid, Yt, and others	Race and Sanger[16]
Common or "public" antigens	13 published and many unpublished examples	Race and Sanger[16]
Rare or "private" antigens	31 published and many unpublished examples	Race and Sanger[16]

*403 red cell antigenic determinants have been recognized to date.
† For brevity, only the first author's name is given. The numbered reference lists other names and the title of the publication.

At this point, it would seem appropriate to give due credit to the three outstanding immunoserologists (or "blood groupers"), whose original contributions expanded this field so remarkably and made its impact on clinical medicine so great. First and foremost is Philip Levine (Figure 20-1). This gifted pupil of Karl Landsteiner began his research activities in the master's laboratory at the Rockefeller Institute in 1925. In the 53 years of his still productive career, he has advanced our knowledge of blood groups and blood-group antibodies to an extent that is unmatched and unmatchable. His instinct or insight for clinical medicine has permitted him to point out the practical applications of his basic scientific discoveries. A few examples of these are: maternal immunization to Rh and other blood-group antigens as the cause of

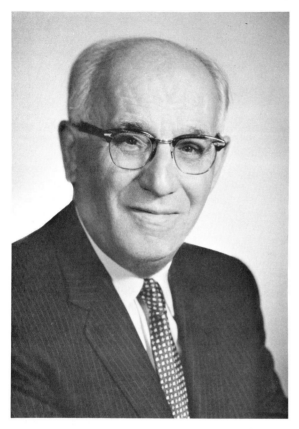

Figure 20-1   Philip Levine (1900–   ).

hemolytic disease of the fetus (EF) and newborn (HDNB) and, as will be described shortly, the protective effect of ABO maternal-fetal incompatibility on Rh sensitization (a basis for anti-Rh immunoglobulin protection of Rh-negative women); the mechanism of some abortions due to development of antibodies[62] (anti-Tj[a] or "p"); and, most recently, the possible relation of antibodies against blood-group factors to cancer.[63] His bibliography is full of such important basic and clinical discoveries. He even contributed to the health and welfare of horses[64] by pointing out that transplacental isoimmunization can occur in the mare after several pregnancies if the foals inherit from the stallion red cell antigens foreign to her. Hemolytic anemia of the newborn then develops in the colt but only after nursing on the mare's colostrum, which is rich in specific antibodies. In utero, the fetus is protected by the ruminant's four-layered placenta, which is impermeable to these antibodies. Well-merited honors have been bestowed on Levine not only for his many specific contributions but for rejuvenating the interest in immunoserology that has led to great advances in so many disciplines.

Alexander S. Wiener (1907–1976) likewise had his start in Landsteiner's laboratory. His interest and work in blood groups and blood transfusions established him as an authority in this field. After Landsteiner and he found the rhesus factor in monkeys, he quickly and initially identified a similar antibody as the cause of numerous previously unexplained intragroup hemolytic transfusion reactions. He discovered several of the subtypes in the Rh system using a nomenclature that he originated. He devoted considerable energy to defending his concept of the mode of inheritance of the Rh variants, publishing numerous papers on it, but since this could not be proved or disproved, it remained unsettled. His symbols R_0, R_1, R_2, and rh still are used universally, and his many contributions in the area of blood grouping and blood transfusion are a lasting memorial to his originality and productivity.

The English arm of the Rh corpus was engrafted by the now famous serologist and geneticist R.R. Race (1907–   ). He wrote his Ph.D. thesis on human blood groups and, with foresight, presented the manuscript on a roll of paper, suggesting a continuum rather than a finite volume of numbered pages. And a continuum it has been, as he and his scientific (as well as marital) partner Ruth Sanger have constantly added to the knowledge of human blood groups. They popularized the C, D, E nomenclature for the Rh system after the original proposals of Sir Ronald Fisher. They unraveled and identified the complicated heredity of dozens of new blood-group factors.

Racial Distribution of Blood Groups

The differences in blood-group distribution due to racial or ethnic origins could not be appreciated at first because the original and most of the subsequent tests were on Europeans. In 1919, Hirszfeld and Hirszfeld[65] published blood typing tests they had done on soldiers fighting on the Macedonian front in World War I. These soldiers were from 16 countries, mostly European but also Asio-African and Middle Eastern and Slavic. The Hirszfelds found that blood-group frequencies differed systematically according to ethnic background. Since then, this has been confirmed by millions of tests. The results from all over the world have been comprehensively reviewed and thoroughly tabulated by Mourant et al.[66] Physical anthropologists were able to augment the data on ethnic background and to trace migrations of aboriginal and ancient peoples. Sometimes, reasonable conclusions could be drawn therefrom; other times, only additional questions were raised. For example, the high incidence of group B in central China (35 percent) showed a slight diminution going south into India and further lowering going west into Europe via the valleys of the major rivers which were the routes of invasion and migration from central Asia (Figure 20-2). Traveling eastward, there was a fall in percentage of group B people in Siberia; they crossed the Bering Straits, once the land bridge to Alaska, and moved on down along the coast of Central and South America.

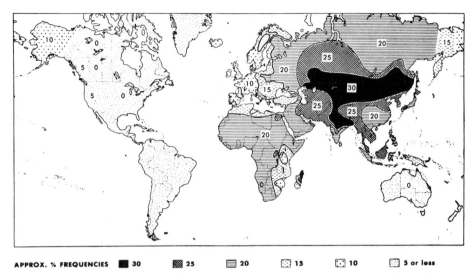

APPROX. % FREQUENCIES   ■ 30   ▨ 25   ☰ 20   ▦ 15   ⊡ 10   ▢ 5 or less

Figure 20-2 An example of blood-group gene frequencies in aboriginal populations resulting from migrations and invasions along trade routes and major river valleys in the Old World and over the prehistoric land bridge between Asia and Alaska in the New World. Environmental factors and genetic drift may have contributed (adapted from Mourant et al.[66]).

The Alaskan and Canadian Eskimos and Amerindians showed 10 percent group B, and the Central and South American Indians 5 percent. The North American Indians showed none.

An interesting discovery was made by W.C. and L.G. Boyd[67,68] in 1934 and 1937. Using serums with known titers of anti-A and anti-B specificities, they were able by absorption experiments to type the dried tissues of ancient Egyptian and American Indian mummies. They decided that the former were group A and the latter group B.

The ethnic distribution of various other blood-group factors, as first demonstrated by the Hirszfelds, has been noted repeatedly as new blood groups have been discovered. Many of these have proved of clinical as well as of anthropological importance. Some deserve mention here.

When the Rh factor was discovered and anti-Rh serums became generally available, it soon became evident that there was considerable variation in Rh negativity and, therefore, in the potential for EF and for transfusion reactions in individuals of certain races. Although whites in Europe and in the United States and Canada were found to be about 15 percent negative for the common Rh_0 or D factor, blacks in New York City were about 5 percent Rh-negative and Orientals 0 to 2 percent negative. Unexpectedly, a larger percentage of Rh-negatives (25 to 35 percent) were uncovered among the Basques of northern Spain and southern France and among the Berbers of Africa (18 to 30 percent) and the Bedouins of the Sinai peninsula. Isolation of an ancestor group plus customary intermarriage may account for this. A rare Rh antigen, V, appeared as diagnostic of Negro blood. Similarly, the antigen Js^a of the Kell system identified the blood of blacks. An unusual phenotype, completely negative for the Duffy antigens, was found only in West African blacks and proved to be of great clinical importance (vide infra). An interesting blood-group system, found by Layrisse et al.[59] in South America and named the Diego factor, was recognized as identifying Indian blood and also was present in Japanese and Chinese up to 10 percent. It therefore indicates Mongolian background. Curiously, though, it has not been found in Eskimos, who have other Mongol features.

Even though he discovered only three types, Landsteiner, in his landmark publication of 1901, predicted the use of blood groups for identification of individuals in medicolegal controversies. He could not foresee that within another six to seven decades there would be several hundred red cell antigens for characterization of each person. If there is a question of identity or of involvement of certain individuals in crimes where blood has been shed, grouping and typing of fresh blood, using the large number of sera now available, can characterize each person beyond reasonable doubt. Even dried blood may serve; its ability to absorb specific typing sera is tested. Significant reduction in titers of each serum identifies a blood factor in the unknown blood cells.

Testing by blood grouping has been accepted in law courts in most states in the United States and in many countries of Europe to settle disputes as to paternity. By the use of seven readily available antisera (ABO, MNS, Rh, Kell, Lutheran, Duffy, and Kidd), an expert laboratory could exonerate about 62 percent of wrongfully accused men. In fact, one laboratory,[69] which has available 37 typing sera for red cell and plasma factors, can exonerate 88 percent of "guiltless" men. Positive proof of paternity is much more difficult, but as Race and Sanger[16] have stated in their book (p. 505), "on rare occasions paternity could be proved beyond all reasonable doubt. If, for example, the accused man and the child were both B, NS, C^{w}D^{u}e/cde, Lu(a+), K+ (a combination of less common factors) and the mother was of common groups, paternity would be proved, provided that the brothers of the accused had alibis. Outside the family of the accused there would not be another such man in ten million."

Kell Blood Groups

This important system was found in 1946 by Coombs et al.[50] through the use of the antiglobulin test on the red cells of an infant thought to have EF but not explainable by Rh incompatibility between mother and child. The antibody that coated the infant's cells was found in the serum of the mother and could sensitize the cells of her husband and her older child. Soon, another example of anti-K was uncovered in a severe transfusion reaction, and this was followed by other examples of this antibody within a short time. The antithetical antibody, anti-k, was found by Levine et al.,[53] and this, too, was confirmed.

The frequency of the Kell antigens is of considerable interest. K^+ constitutes slightly less than 10 percent of the population, 0.2 percent of whom are homozygous (K^+K^+). Despite its rarity, the Kell factor must be a fairly potent antigen. An appreciable number of cases of EF have been caused by it, and transfusion reactions involving anti-K in the common kk individuals also have been noted.

The complexity of the Kell system was revealed in 1957 when Allen and Lewis[51] found the variant Kp^a and its allele Kp^b. A year later, Giblett[52] described a new blood-group system found only in blacks and named it Sutter, or Js; in 1965, Stroup et al.[54] showed that Js^a and Js^b belong to the Kell system.

Eighteen related antigenic determinants in the Kell blood-group system have been identified. One of these was first described by Allen et al.[70] and was called the McLeod phenotype after the family. Later, Giblett et al.[71] noted that a rare sex-linked disease of young boys, chronic granulomatous disease, was often associated with this blood type. In 1977, Marsh[72] showed that boys with this fatal defect lack one of the Kell factors, Kx, on their red cells as well as on their leukocytes. The latter leads to an enzymatic and functional disorder of the white cells with defective bacteriocidal function and resulting chronic infection, chiefly with staphylococci. The red blood cells of these patients, lacking Kx, are prone to destruction; their serum after transfusion may develop antibodies against all Kell factors, making further transfusions difficult.

Duffy Blood Groups

This antibody, discovered in 1950 by Cutbush, Mollison, and Parkin,[55] and more fully described by Cutbush and Mollison,[73] appeared at first to be just another independent agglutinin developed by a hemophiliac, Mr. Duffy, who had had a number of transfusions during the previous 20 years. The antigen, named Fy^a, appears in the red cells of about two-thirds of English people.

Other examples of anti-Fy^a were soon found, and the antithetical antibody anti-Fy^b was discovered.[56] These antibodies have caused serious transfusion reactions, at least two fatalities, and EF has resulted from maternal sensitization.

The unusual feature of the Duffy blood group, discovered in 1955 by Sanger et al.,[74] was that most blacks of West African ancestry were Fy(a-b-), a phenotype not found in whites. In other words, these blacks failed to react to sera of the specificity anti-Fy^a and anti-Fy^b. This system, thereby, became extremely important for genetic discrimination. The Duffy-negative status was symbolized as FyFy, i.e., homozygous for a lacking antigen. Of special interest is that individuals with this phenotype have been found to be resistant to invasion by certain malarial parasites; protected persons have invariably been African blacks. This protection against malaria, furthermore, has proved to be absolute. In contrast, sickle hemoglobin, β-thalassemia, and G6PD deficiency confer only partial protection against malaria (see section on blood groups and disease).

The I ("Big I") and i ("Little i") Blood Groups

This system was uncovered by Wiener et al.[46] in 1956 during investigation of a patient with acquired hemolytic anemia whose serum contained an antibody that agglutinated almost all potential donor cells. After several thousand tests, two compatible donors were found, and the patient was successfully transfused. The antigen was called "I" for "individual." A few years later, a serum was found that identified the rare allele, named "little i." The studies of Marsh,[47] Race and Sanger,[16] and others established that the I antigen was almost universally present on the red cells of almost all people, though in variable strength or amount. The rare person who lacked it or had an extremely weak I could have a natural anti-I in the serum or develop it under certain circumstances. Further studies showed that in fetal blood and in cord blood of newborns, the i antigen was always present, but variable small amounts of "I" might also be found. In the fetus, the I antigen slowly increases with maturation and continues to do so after birth so that by the age of 2 months, the infant has about half the adult level; the full amount is reached by about 18 months.[75]

A further association of the I-i antibodies with clinical conditions remains to be explained. Patients with "primary atypical pneumonia," an infection associated with pleuropneumonia-like organisms (PPLO),[76] may develop high-titer anti-I. This rarely produces a hemolytic anemia since it is usually only a cold agglutinin. Another frequent association has been the appearance of antibodies of i specificity in patients with infectious mononucleosis.[76] One wonders whether the Epstein-Barr virus, the cause of infectious mononucleosis, shares an antigen with i and, thereby, stimulates anti-i production.

An important finding has been that in certain severe anemias[77,78] and malignancies, such as leukemias,[79] increased amounts of i antigen may appear in young red cells. Its concentration may vary from time to time, and, during disease remissions, it may disappear. Marrow stress from repeated phlebotomies or chronic anemia can induce the appearance and elevation of i. Hillman and Giblett[80] concluded that shortened intramarrow transit time and premature release of red cells lead to retention of a property that normally disappears with maturation within the marrow. In some respects, these changes in the i antigen with marrow stress and in certain anemias parallel the appearance and the increase in fetal hemoglobin (hemoglobin F) under some circumstances. The percentage change in each varies widely. The reciprocal relationship of I and i in various conditions has been reviewed recently.[75]

Other Blood Groups

Blood-group systems of lesser importance have been uncovered,[16] most of them still with little clinical or even historical significance. Among them are the Yt, the Au (Auberger), the Do (Dombrock), the Co (Cotton), the Sd (Sid), and the Sc (Scianna) systems. The nomenclature of blood groups is usually derived from the names of the first recognized serum donors; by using two letters of the alphabet, this allows for about 700 combinations as they are discovered. With the increasing number of blood transfusions and the uniqueness of each individual's blood-group profile, the number of possible sensitizations to some factor the recipient lacks would seem infinite—and there is also the pathway of sensitization of a mother by a factor in her fetus. Fortunately, many blood-group agglutinogens are poor or weak antigens, and most individuals seem unable to produce antibodies against them. Also, there are many very common antigens called "public" antigens (present in 99.9 percent of persons), and even more that are very infrequent called "private" antigens (present in one of thousands). Undoubtedly, with continued careful matching of blood for transfusions and transplantations, as well as investigation of antibodies causing hemolytic transfusion reactions and hemolytic disease of the newborn, more blood-group systems will be found. As the old prospectors used to say, "There's still gold in them thar hills." It may require deeper digging in these worked-over mines, but new methods or instruments may uncover valuable material.

Our Blood Groups: Are They Helpful, Harmful, or Neutral?

This question was not even asked in the first 40 years after the discovery of the human blood groups. Except for the possibly harmful results of the "unnatural" procedure of blood transfusion, no influence of blood-group factors on health and well-being was recognized. The blood groups, therefore, were considered to be "neutral" genes. However, prominent geneticists, notably Sir Ronald Fisher and Dr. E.B. Ford, of England, had long held that no gene was neutral, that the blood groups were subject to natural selection, and that different environments and unusual circumstances might favor one gene rather than another. The first convincing proof of a potentially harmful effect of blood groups was Levine's discovery of maternal isoimmunization causing hemolytic disease of the newborn in the Rh system. The evidence of blood-group incompatibility between mother and fetus leading to EF as the result of maternal isoagglutinins, either naturally occurring or following isosensitization by pregnancies or blood injections, was startling. Then, Halbrecht,[81] of

Israel, related severe jaundice of the newborn to the presence of immune anti-A and anti-B in mothers of blood group A or B infants. We now appreciate that hemolytic disease of the newborn on this basis is about $1\frac{1}{2}$ to 2 times as frequent as that due to Rh and other antibodies, but it is generally milder and does not usually require emergency treatment. However, rarely, ABO EF may cause death from anemia or neurologic damage from severe jaundice (kernicterus).

As new blood-group systems were uncovered, the possibility of isoimmunization affecting fertility, gestation, and neonatal mortality became an important question. As early as 1943, Levine[82] had postulated that serologic factors could be a cause of spontaneous abortions. In women with two or more early miscarriages or stillbirths, over 55 percent were incompatible with their husbands according to group A and B factors, compared with 35 percent in random matings. In 1954, he found[62] that a rare isoagglutinin, anti-Tj[a], was a cause of habitual abortion in certain families.

As more and more mass blood typings were done, during the wars for treatment of battle casualties, in blood banks for donors, and in hospitals for possible transfusions, statistical information was accumulated on the blood groups of persons with various diseases. In 1953, convincing evidence of the nonneutrality of the blood-group factors ABO was obtained by Aird, Bentall, and Fraser Roberts,[83] who showed statistically that there was an increased incidence of stomach cancer in group A persons. The following year, Aird[84] noted a greater susceptibility to peptic ulcer in those with blood group O than in persons with other blood groups. The ulcers were more often present in the duodenum.[85] A series collected from a number of centers demonstrated that there was a significant statistical association between pernicious anemia and blood group A.[86] Other such relationships between pathologic conditions and specific blood groups (e.g., diabetes, bronchopneumonia) were less striking. The possible association of ABO factors and infectious diseases worldwide roused considerable controversy favoring or refuting such associations. Experts were lined up on both sides.

Plague, Pestilence, and Population

When Hirszfeld and Hirszfeld[65] published their serologic studies showing that the distribution of the ABO blood groups differed among the races, their report aroused much speculation about the reasons for the considerable variations found in subsequent typings of large populations. Humanlike blood-group antigens have been traced back to primates, so that balanced polymorphisms have had many centuries to become established uniformly. Differences in blood-group genes have been ascribed to propagation within isolated ancestral groups, so-called genetic drift, but this seemed an unlikely explanation on a worldwide basis. A far better explanation was that the blood-group factors had selective evolutionary value, with advantages or disadvantages under different environmental conditions. The possible influence of repeated devastating epidemics of disease seemed a likely factor to help explain the wide fluctuations from one continent to another, or even between countries.

Differences in susceptibility to disease or its severity had a certain logic. If an invading disease organism had an antigen similar to one of the blood-group antigens, a carrier of the latter might not have, or be able to elaborate, an antibody against the invader. The antigenic determinants on many disease-causing organisms were found to have the same specificities as the A, B, or H agglutinogens. According to this concept, pandemics of plague, smallpox, cholera, and influenza could cause almost complete annihilation of people of one or another blood group in a given population. This might explain the distribution of A, B, and O in different races or countries. For example, Vogel, Pettenkofer, and Helmbold[87] claimed that the organism of plague, *Pasteurella pestis,* had an antigen similar to the human H antigen, present on group O red cells. Since group O individuals would then presumably be unable to produce anti-H, they might be most vulnerable. Some of the plague epidemics carried off 80 to 90 percent of the population in scourges of the black death. This might explain the low incidence of group O's in the ancient plague centers of Mongolia, Turkey, and lower Egypt. Similarly, the virus of smallpox has antigenic similarity[87] to group A agglutinogen, thereby suggesting a reason for the great virulence of smallpox epidemics in high group A populations. Another possible association was shown between group O and type A_2 influenza. Still other associations have been claimed between enteric organisms and ABO factors.

All these suggestions have been open to criticism, however, since the organisms cultured on various media may have borne contaminants of blood-group specificities from the media on which they were grown. In addition, there can be no proof that the causative agents of the devastating epidemics of olden times had the same antigenic components as those isolated and cultured now. The pros and cons of blood groups, disease, and natural selection have been well discussed and documented by Muschel,[88] Otten,[89] and Wiener,[90] to mention only a few of the protagonists in this controversy. Accumulating evidence favors the concept that the blood-group genes are not neutral, and again, as Sir Ronald Fisher stated,[91] "*All* genes have selective value in evolution, examples of which are being revealed in startling fashion from time to time."

Blood Groups and Malaria

An elegant and thoroughly convincing proof of the survival value of a blood-group phenotype was assembled by Miller and associates[92] with regard to the Duffy factors. They knew that most West Africans and many American blacks are resistant to infection by *Plasmodium vivax,* although they were susceptible to the other three species of malaria that infect humans. The vivax resistance factor in these West Africans blocks infection completely; the sickle-cell trait, which decreases mortality from *Plasmodium falciparum* (Chapter 11), does not block infection. They hypothesized that the resistance factor, therefore, must interfere with the ability of the parasite to invade the erythrocyte. To test this, they exposed red cells with different antigenic determinants (blood-group factors) to invasion by a simian malaria, *Plasmodium knowlesi*. *P. vivax* does not grow in culture, but this species (*P. knowlesi*) invades the human red cell in culture and can infect humans. Only one type of individual was found to be resistant to invasion; this was a Duffy-negative person (FyFy), lacking both Fy^a and Fy^b antigens. This genotype is present in approximately 90 percent of West Africans but is extremely rare in other racial groups who are susceptible to *P. vivax*. Further proof was obtained by in vitro exposure of erythrocytes from white and black persons, whose Duffy blood groups were known, to *P. knowlesi*–infected rhesus monkey red cells. Only the red cells of the blacks who were Duffy-negative (FyFy) were not invaded by the parasites. Miller and his associates also showed that enzymatic digestion of the red cell surface of Fy^a or Fy^b cells, which removes the Duffy blood-group determinant, rendered the cells resistant to invasion. Moreover, coating Fy^a red cells with potent anti-Fy^a serum, and, thus, covering the Fy^a site, markedly reduced invasion by the parasite. Finally, by video microscopy, it was shown that the plasmodium was unable to penetrate the membrane of the Duffy-negative red cell, a Duffy-positive surface antigen being necessary for this. The evidence was irrefutable.

In a subsequent publication, Miller et al.[93] restudied 17 volunteer subjects of an experiment performed several years earlier to test their resistance to *P. vivax* malaria. It was found that five Duffy-negative (FyFy) blacks were resistant, whereas six blacks and six whites who were Duffy-positive were infected when bitten by mosquitoes with heavily infected salivary glands. Other conclusive experiments on humans and primates also proved that the Fy^a and/or Fy^b determinants on the red cell are necessary for invasion by *P. knowlesi*.

One final word about the Duffy blood group: its genes have now been localized to the number 1 chromosome, as suggested by Donahue[94] in 1968. This was the first blood group to have a definite chromosome assignment in humans. Marsh[95] in 1977 found that the Rh gene was also localized on chromosome 1 near the end of the short arm, whereas the Duffy gene was close to the centromere. Such localizations serve as markers for linkage studies and have potential value diagnostically and prognostically in genetic analyses.

More on Blood Groups and Cancer

A development of considerable interest and great potential importance with reference to malignancies has been the observation that cancer cells may have blood-group antigens which are foreign to the host and to which the host may have specific antibodies,[96] though in low titers. Twenty-five years following a first report, Levine[97] discovered that his original patient, who recovered from her gastric adenocarcinoma, had developed a high-titer serum antibody against the tumor cell blood group. Häkkinen, of Finland,[98] had reported a similar situation in patients with gastric cancer, i.e., the presence of a foreign blood-group factor in the tumor cells of specificity A in persons of group B and O. He called this a "neo-A" antigen. Levine labeled it an *illegitimate* blood-group antigen and pointed out the possibility of immunotherapy.

Another provocative report of human tumor-associated blood-group antigens and levels of antibodies against them was that regarding an MN precursor (T factor) in human breast carcinoma.[99] Numerous other reports have been appearing in cancer journals. They need not be reviewed here.

It is sufficient to say that the evidence is overwhelming that blood groups are not neutral genes. They are often helpful (e.g., the Duffy factors in malaria) but sometimes harmful (e.g., Rh negativity). One hopes that our ingenuity will minimize such adverse effects. A prime example of this latter development merits recording here.

Prevention of Rh Sensitization

After 1946, hemolytic disease of the newborn in the Rh-positive infant of the sensitized Rh-negative woman was successfully treated by exchange transfusion. Prevention of Rh isoimmunization of the woman remained a challenging problem since it potentially involved 13 percent of all pregnancies in whites. Actually, since the father could be heterozygous Rh-positive, and consequently father an Rh-negative infant, the chance was only about 10 percent. This still placed more than a hundred thousand women at risk each year in the United States. Levine,[100] in 1959, noted that there was a protective effect of ABO incompatibility between mother and child that prevented isoimmunization, i.e., a group O Rh-negative woman having a group A Rh-positive baby did not become sensitized, presumably because the fetal Rh-positive cells which leaked into the mother's circulation were destroyed or blocked by her anti-A antibodies and could not stimulate anti-Rh production.

Two groups of investigators 3000 miles apart, each beginning with a different idea, came to a similar solution of the problem at about the same time. In New York City, V.J. Freda, an obstetrician, recalled that the famous Boston bacteriologist Theobald Smith in 1900 had blocked antibody stimulation after injections of diphtheria toxin into rabbits by giving them diphtheria antitoxin simultaneously. This passively present antibody prevented the animal's active response to the toxin. Freda reasoned that an anti-Rh antibody administered to an unsensitized Rh-negative woman might interfere with her reaction to her infant's Rh-positive red cells and prevent her developing anti-Rh antibodies.

In Liverpool, England, Finn and Clarke, knowing of the protective effect of maternal anti-A in the Rh-negative group O woman exposed to group A Rh-positive infant red blood cells wondered about a possible "blocking factor" that might suppress the action of the Rh antigen. Clarke, a knowledgeable geneticist and lepidopterist, recalled that in butterfly breeding, a "suppressor factor" could interfere with the expression of wing color inheritance. Extrapolating from the butterfly to the human was no great step for this nimble scientist. Clarke conceived of the possibility of suppressing the mother's anti-Rh production by giving her anti-Rh serum. Beginning in 1960–1961, Finn and Clarke tested an experimental approach to the problem by using anti-Rh antibody and Rh-positive red cell injections in Rh-negative male volunteers. Their results reported in 1961[101] were most encouraging.

In the meantime, Freda, Gorman, and Pollack, in New York, carried out controlled experiments on Rh-negative male volunteers given Rh-positive red cells and anti-Rh antibodies simultaneously. In order to avoid having to inject large amounts of anti-Rh serum and also risk infection with its possible contaminant of hepatitis virus, they resorted to the use of a gamma globulin concentrate of the serum, thereby circumventing both problems. Their experiments were completely successful.[102] They thereupon embarked on a countrywide trial in more than a dozen obstetric centers. Rh-negative unsensitized women were given 1 ml (later 0.5 ml) of anti-Rh gamma globulin concentrate intramuscularly shortly after delivery of an Rh-positive infant. This was almost completely protective, except in the rare cases when a large "bleed" from baby into mother had occurred. In 1800 women so treated within 72 hours after delivery, only two Rh sensitizations occurred, whereas in controls, there was the expected rate of 16 percent sensitization.[103]

The English investigators likewise turned to the use of gamma globulin concentrate of anti-Rh serum for the protective injection and had similar success.[104] By this means, the Rh sensitization problem could be almost eliminated in one generation. Also, sensitizations by incompatible transfusions given through error were treated by larger injections of anti-Rh gamma globulin.[105] Thousands of persons worldwide were, and continue to be, the beneficiaries of this mode of treatment of blood-group incompatibility problems. Thus, from colors in butterfly wings and diphtheria antitoxin in rabbits came the ideas for prevention of blood-group sensitization and avoidance of hemolytic disease of the newborn and hemolytic transfusion reactions in humans.

Research directed toward antibody detection in the serum of individuals sensitized by pregnancies or transfusions has led to still other important discoveries. In the search for abnormal antibodies in the serum of multiparous women, Payne,[106] in this country, Dausset,[107] in France, and van Loghem[108] and van Rood,[109] in the Netherlands, discovered antibodies against leukocytes, these arising chiefly as a result of maternal sensitization to fetal antigens on white cells. This led to the typing of human lymphocytes and the discovery of human lymphocyte antigens (HLA). These inherited characteristics have now proved crucial to the matching of tissues and organs for transplantation. It has been discovered, furthermore, that certain diseases are associated more commonly with one or more HLA specificities, suggesting that susceptibility to these diseases may be influenced by hereditary antigen patterns. The entire field of immunity has been restimulated and reoriented through the increased understanding of the role of the HLA factors, of which more than 50 had been identified by 1976. It is possible that diagnosis, prognosis and form of treatment may someday be influenced by an individual's HLA status.

In retrospect, it is difficult to believe that so many scientific and therapeutic advances could have resulted from the discovery 40 years ago of an abnormal red cell agglutinin in the serum of the mother of an infant with EF. Alert minds, imaginative theories, and inspired research have advanced medicine phenomenally.

Almost 300 years ago, Charles Morton,[110] a renowned Harvard teacher, published his famous textbook of science *Compendium Physicae*. In it he introduced general principles by many aphorisms, one of which is appropriate here.

> Where New appearance is before the Eyes,
> New Suppositions thereupon arise.

The appearance of a new antibody in a postpartum woman in 1939 led to dozens of "new suppositions," many of which have proved of inestimable value to all humanity.

Acknowledgments

It is a pleasure to acknowledge the generous assistance of several persons in the preparation of this chapter. I am indebted to Dr. Philip Levine for unpublished information about blood-group research; Dr. Girish Vyas, who updated the recent advances in blood-group classification; Mrs. Anne Schmid for her editorial review and helpful suggestions; and Mrs. Mickie Ochi for her proficiency in locating references and in typing and proofreading the paper.

This work was done during tenure as a Henry J. Kaiser Senior Fellow at the Center for Advanced Study in the Behavioral Sciences at Stanford, California.

References

1   Goethe JW: *I, Faust*, 1. 1808.
2   Landsteiner K: Uber Agglutinationserscheinungen normalen menschlichen Blutes. *Wien Klin Wochenschr* 14:1132–1134, 1901.

3 Blundell J: Quoted by Jones HW, Mackmul G: The influence of James Blundell on the development of blood transfusion. *Ann Med Hist* 10:242–248, 1928.

4 Landois L: *Die Transfusion des Blutes.* Leipzig, Vogel, 1875, 358 pp.

5 Shattock SG: Chromacyte clumping in acute pneumonia and certain other diseases and the significance of the buffy coat in shed blood. *J Pathol Bacteriol* 6:303–314, 1900.

6 Levine P: A review of Landsteiner's contributions to human blood groups. *Transfusion* 1:45–52, 1961.

7 Decastello A von, Sturli A: Über die Isoagglutinine in Serum gesunder und kranker Menschen. *Munch Med Wochenschr* 26:1090–1095, 1902.

8 Hektoen L: Isoagglutination of human corpuscles. *J Infect Dis* 4:297–303, 1907.

9 Hektoen L: Isoagglutination of human corpuscles with respect to demonstration of opsonic index and to transfusion of blood. *JAMA* 48:1739–1740, 1907.

10 Jansky J: Haematologické, studie u. psychotikü. *Sb Klin Praze* 8:85–139, 1906–1907. [Études hematologiques, dans les malades mentales, Rês. 131–133, 1907.]

11 Moss WL: Studies of isoagglutinins and isohemolysins. *Johns Hopkins Med J* 21:63–69, 1910.

12 Epstein AA, Ottenberg R: Simple method of performing serum reactions. *Proc NY Pathol Soc* 8:117–123, 1908.

13 Dungern E von, Hirszfeld L: Ueber Vererbung gruppenspezifischer Strukturen des Blutes. *Z Immunitaetsforch* 6:284–292, 1909. (Pohlmann GB [trans]: *Transfusion* 2:70–74, 1962.)

14 Bernstein F: Ergebnisse einer biostatischen zusammenfassenden Betrachtung uber die erblichen Blutstrukturen des Menschen. *Klin Wochenschr* 3:1495–1497, 1924.

15 Dungern E von, Hirszfeld L: Uber gruppenspezifische Strukturen des Blutes III. *Z Immunitaetsforch* 8:526–562, 1911.

16 Race RR, Sanger R: *Blood Groups in Man*, 6th ed. Oxford, Blackwell Scientific, 1975, 659 pp.

17 Yamakami K: The individuality of semen, with reference to its property of inhibiting specifically isohemoagglutination. *J Immunol* 12:185–189, 1926.

18 Hartmann G: *Group Antigens in Human Organs.* Copenhagen, Munksgaard, 1941, 142 pp. (Translation published by the Blood Bank Center, U.S. Army Medical Research Laboratory, Fort Knox, Kentucky.)

19 Landsteiner K, Levine P: A new agglutinable factor differentiating individual human bloods. *Proc Soc Exp Biol Med* 24:600–602, 1927.

20 Landsteiner K, Levine P: Further observations on individual differences of human blood. *Proc Soc Exp Biol Med* 24:941–942, 1927.

21 Landsteiner K, Levine P: On individual differences in human blood. *J Exp Med* 47:757–775, 1928.

22 Landsteiner K, Levine P: On the inheritance of agglutinogens of human blood demonstrable by immune agglutinins. *J Exp Med* 48:731–749, 1928.

23 Walsh RJ, Montgomery C: A new human isoagglutinin subdividing the MN blood groups. *Nature* 160:504–505, 1947.

24 Sanger R, Race RR: Subdivisions of the MN blood groups in man. *Nature* 160:505, 1947.

25 Levine P, Kuhmichel AB, Wigod M, Koch E: A new blood factor, s, allelic to S. *Proc Soc Exp Biol Med* 78:218–220, 1951.

26 Levine P, Stetson RE: An unusual case of intragroup agglutination. *JAMA* 113:126–127, 1939.

27 Levine P, Burnham L, Katzin EM, Vogel P: The role of isoimmunization in the pathogenesis of erythroblastosis fetalis. *Am J Obstet Gynecol* 42:925–937, 1941.

28 Landsteiner K, Wiener AS: An agglutinable factor in human blood recognized by immune sera for rhesus blood. *Proc Soc Exp Biol Med* 43:223, 1940.

29 Landsteiner K, Wiener AS: Studies on an agglutinogen (Rh) in human blood reacting with anti-rhesus sera and with human isoantibodies. *J Exp Med* 74:309–320, 1941.

30 Wiener AS, Peters HR: Hemolytic reactions following transfusions of blood of the homologous group, with three cases in which the same agglutinogen was responsible. *Ann Intern Med* 13:2306–2322, 1940.

31 Levine P, Celano M, Fenichel R, Singher H: A 'D'-like antigen in Rhesus red blood cells and in Rh-positive and Rh-negative red cells. *Science* 133:332–333, 1961.

32 Race RR: An 'incomplete' antibody in human serum. *Nature* 153:771–772, 1944.

33 Wiener AS: A new test (blocking test) for Rh sensitization. *Proc Soc Exp Biol Med* 56:173–176, 1944.

34 Diamond LK, Abelson NM: The demonstration of Rh agglutinins, an accurate and rapid slide test. *J Lab Clin Med* 30:204–212, 1945.

35 Diamond LK, Denton RL: Rh agglutination in various media with particular reference to the value of albumin. *J Lab Clin Med* 30:821–830, 1945.

36 Coombs RRA, Mourant AE, Race RR: A new test for the detection of weak and 'incomplete' Rh agglutinins. *Br J Exp Pathol* 26:255–266, 1945.

37 Morton JA, Pickles MM: Use of trypsin in detection of incomplete anti-Rh antibodies. *Nature* 159:779–780, 1947.

38 Wiener AS: Genetic theory of the Rh blood types. *Proc Soc Exp Biol Med* 54:316–319, 1943.

39 Race RR, Taylor GL, Cappell DF, McFarlane MN: Recognition of further common Rh genotypes in man. *Nature* 153:52–53, 1944.

40 Race RR, Sanger R: *Blood Groups in Man,* 5th ed. Oxford, Blackwell Scientific, 1968, 599 pp, p 176.

41 Rosenfield RE, Allen FH, Swisher SN, Kochwa S: A review of Rh serology and presentation of a new terminology. *Transfusion* 2:287–312, 1962.

42 Rosenfield RE, Allen FH, Rubinstein P: Genetic model for the Rh blood group system. *Proc Natl Acad Sci USA* 70:1303–1307, 1973.

43 Chown B: On a search for rhesus antibodies in very young fetuses. *Arch Dis Child* 30:232–233, 1955.

44 Mourant AE: A "new" human blood group antigen of frequent occurence. *Nature* 158:237, 1946.

45 Andresen PH: The blood group system L. A new blood group L$_2$. A case of epistasy within the blood groups. *Acta Pathol Microbiol Scand* 25:728–731, 1948.

46 Wiener AS, Unger LJ, Cohen L, Feldman J: Type-specific cold auto-antibodies as a cause of acquired hemolytic anemia and hemolytic transfusion reactions: biologic test with bovine red cells. *Ann Intern Med* 44:221–240, 1956.

47 Marsh WL, Jenkins WJ: Anti-i: a new cold antibody. *Nature* 188:753, 1960.

48 Callender ST, Race RR: A serological and genetical study of multiple antibodies formed in response to blood transfusion by a patient with lupus erythematosus diffusus. *Ann Eugenics* 13:102–117, 1946.

49   Cutbush M, Chanarin I: The expected blood-group antibody, anti-Lu[b]. *Nature* 178:855–856, 1956.

50   Coombs RRA, Mourant AE, Race RR: In-vivo isosensitization of red cells in babies with haemolytic disease. *Lancet* i:264–266, 1946.

51   Allen FH, Lewis SJ: Kp[a] (Penny), a new antigen in the Kell blood group system. *Vox Sang* 2:81–87, 1957.

52   Giblett ER: Js, a new blood group antigen found in Negroes. *Nature* 181:1221–1222, 1958.

53   Levine P, Backer M, Wigod M, Ponder R: A new human hereditary blood property (Cellano) present in 99.8% of all bloods. *Science* 109:464–466, 1949.

54   Stroup M, MacIlroy M, Walker R, Aydelotte JV: Evidence that Sutter belongs to the Kell blood group system. *Transfusion* 5:309–314, 1965.

55   Cutbush M, Mollison PL, Parkin DM: A new human blood group. *Nature* 165:188, 1950.

56   Ikin EW, Mourant AE, Pettenkofer HJ, Blumenthal G: Discovery of the expected haemagglutinin, anti-Fy[b]. *Nature* 168:1077, 1951.

57   Allen FH, Diamond LK, Niedziela B: A new blood group antigen. *Nature* 167:482, 1951.

58   Plaut G, Ikin EW, Mourant AE, Sanger R, Race RR: A new blood group antibody, anti-Jk[b]. *Nature* 171:431, 1953.

59   Layrisse M, Arends T: The 'Diego' blood factor distribution: Genetic clinical and anthropological significance, in Hollaender L (ed): *Proc. 6th Cong. Int. Soc. Blood Transfusion.* Basel, Karger, 1958, pp 114–116.

60   Thompson PR, Childers DM, Hatcher DE: Anti-Di[b]: first and second examples. *Vox Sang* 13:314–318, 1967.

61   Mann JD, Cahan A, Gelb AG, Fisher N, Hamper J, Tippett P, Sanger R, Race RR: A sex-linked blood group. *Lancet* i:8–10, 1962.

62   Levine P, Koch EA: The rare human isoagglutinin anti-Tj[a] and habitual abortion. *Science* 120:239–241, 1954.

63   Levine P: Illegitimate blood group antigens P_1, a, and MN(T) in malignancy—a possible therapeutic approach with anti-Tj[a], anti-A, and anti-T. *Ann NY Acad Sci* 277:428–435, 1976.

64   Levine P: Transplacental isoimmunization in horses. *J Hered* 39:285–288, 1948.

65   Hirszfeld L, Hirszfeld H: Serological differences between the blood of different races. The result of researches on the Macedonian front. *Lancet* ii:675–679, 1919.

66   Mourant AE, Kopeć AC, Domaniewska-Sobczak K: *The Distribution of Human Blood Groups and Other Polymorphisms,* 2d ed. London, Oxford University Press, 1976, 1055 pp.

67   Boyd WC, Boyd LG: An attempt to determine the blood groups of mummies. *Proc Soc Exp Biol Med* 31:671–672, 1934.

68   Boyd WC, Boyd LG: Blood grouping tests on 300 mummies. *J Immunol* 32:307–319, 1937.

69   Umansky I: Personal communication, 1978.

70   Allen FH, Krabbe SMR, Corcoran PA: A new phenotype (McLeod) in the Kell blood group system. *Vox Sang* 6:555–560, 1961.

71   Giblett ER, Klebanoff SJ, Pincus SH, Swanson J, Park BH, McCullough J: Kell phenotypes in chronic granulomatous disease: a potential transfusion hazard. *Lancet* i:1235–1236, 1971.

72 Marsh WL: The Kell blood group, Kx antigen, and chronic granulomatous disease. *Mayo Clin Proc* 52:150–152, 1977.

73 Cutbush M, Mollison PL: The Duffy blood group. *Heredity (Lond)* 4:383–389, 1950.

74 Sanger R, Race RR, Jack J: The Duffy blood groups of New York negroes: the phenotype Fy(a-b-). *Br J Haematol* 1:370–374, 1955.

75 Marsh WL: Anti-i: a cold antibody defining the Ii relationship in human red cells. *Br J Haematol* 7:200–209, 1961.

76 Mollison PL: *Blood Transfusion in Clinical Medicine*, 5th ed. Oxford, Blackwell Scientific, 1972, 833 pp.

77 Giblett ER, Crookston MC: Agglutinability of red cells by anti-i in patients with thalassaemia major and other haematological disorders. *Nature* 201:1138–1139, 1964.

78 Crookston JH, Dacie JW, Rossi V: Differences in the agglutinability of human red cells by the high-titre cold antibodies of acquired haemolytic anemia. *Br J Haematol* 2:321–331, 1956.

79 Jenkins WJ, Marsh WL, Gold ER: Reciprocal relationship of antigens 'I' and 'i' in health and disease. *Nature* 205:813, 1965.

80 Hillman RS, Giblett ER: Red cell membrane alteration associated with 'marrow stress.' *J Clin Invest* 44:1730–1736, 1965.

81 Halbrecht I: Role of hemagglutinins anti-A and anti-B in pathogenesis of jaundice of the newborn (icterus neonatorum precox). *Am J Dis Child* 68:248–249, 1944.

82 Levine P: Serological factors as possible causes in spontaneous abortions. *J Hered* 34:71–82, 1943.

83 Aird I, Bentall HH, Roberts JAF: Relation between cancer of the stomach and the ABO blood groups. *Br Med J* 1:799–801, 1953.

84 Aird I, Bentall HH, Mehigan JA, Roberts JAF: The blood groups in relation to peptic ulceration. *Br Med J* 2:315–321, 1954.

85 Clarke CA, Edwards JW, Haddock DRW, Howel-Evans AW, McConnell RB, Sheppard PM: ABO blood groups and secretor character in duodenal ulcer. *Br Med J* 2:725–731, 1956.

86 Aird I, Bentall HH, Bingham J, et al (21 coauthors): An association between blood group A and pernicious anemia. A collective series from a number of centres. *Br Med J* 2:723–724, 1956.

87 Vogel FH, Pettenkofer J, Helmbold W: Uber die Populations-genetik der ABO-Blutruppen, 2. Mitteilung Gehautigkeit und epidemische Erkrankungen, *Acta Genet Statistica Med* 10:267–294, 1960. (Quoted by Otten CM: *Curr Anthropol* 8:209–226, 1967.)

88 Muschel LH: Blood groups, disease and selection. *Bacteriol Rev* 30:427–441, 1966.

89 Otten CM: On pestilence, diet, natural selection, and the distribution of microbial and human blood group antigens and antibodies. *Curr Anthropol* 8:209–226, 1967.

90 Wiener AS: Blood groups and disease. *Am J Hum Genet* 22:476–483, 1970.

91 Fisher RA: Personal communication, 1946.

92 Miller LH, Mason SJ, Dvorak JA, McGinniss MH, Rothman IK: Erythrocyte receptors for (*Plasmodium knowlesi*) malaria. Duffy blood group determinants. *Science* 189:561–563, 1975.

93 Miller LH, Mason SJ, Clyde DF, McGinniss MH: The resistance factor to *Plasmodium vivax* in Blacks. The Duffy blood group genotype, FyFy. *N Engl J Med* 295:302–304, 1976.

94   Donahue RP, Bias WB, Renwick JH, McKusick VA: Probable assignment of the Duffy blood group locus to chromosome 1 in man. *Proc Natl Acad Sci USA* 61:949–955, 1968.

95   Marsh WL: Mapping assignment of the Rh and Duffy blood group genes to chromosome 1. *Mayo Clin Proc* 52:145–148, 1977.

96   Levine P: Blood group and tissue genetic markers in familial adenocarcinoma: potential specific immunotherapy. *Semin Oncol* 5:25–34, 1978.

97   Levine P, Bobbitt OB, Waller RK, Kuhmichel A: Isoimmunization by a new blood factor in tumor cells. *Proc Soc Exp Biol Med* 77:403–405, 1951.

98   Häkkinen I: A-like blood group antigen in gastric cancer cells of patients in blood groups O or B. *J Natl Cancer Inst* 44:1183–1188, 1970.

99   Springer GF, Desai PM, Scanlon EF: Blood group MN precursors (T) as human breast carcinoma–associated antigens and "naturally" occurring human cytotoxins against them. *Cancer* 37:169–176, 1976.

100 Levine P: The protective action of ABO incompatibility on Rh isoimmunization and Rh hemolytic disease—theoretical and clinical implications. *Am J Hum Genet* 11:418, 1959.

101 Finn R, Clarke CA, Donohoe WTA, McConnell RB, Sheppard PM, Lehane D, Kulke W: Experimental studies on the prevention of Rh haemolytic disease. *Br Med J* 1486–1490, 1961.

102 Freda VJ, Gorman JG, Pollack W: Successful prevention of sensitization with an experimental anti-Rh gamma globulin. *Transfusion* 4:26–32, 1964.

103 Freda VJ, Gorman JG, Pollack W, Robertson JG, Jennings ER, Sullivan JF: Prevention of Rh isoimmunization. *JAMA* 199:390–394, 1967.

104 Clarke CA: Prevention of Rh hemolytic disease. *Br Med J* 4:7–12, 1967.

105 Diamond LK: Unpublished. Personal experiences.

106 Payne R: Leukocyte agglutinins in human sera. *Arch Intern Med* 99:587–606, 1957.

107 Dausset J: Leuco-agglutinins. *Vox Sang* 6:190–198, 1954.

108 Loghem JJ van, van der Hart M, Hijmans W, Schuit HRE: The incidence and significance of complete and incomplete white cell antibodies with special reference to the use of the Coombs consumption test. *Vox Sang* 3:203–223, 1958.

109 Rood JJ van, Eernisse JG, Leeuwen A van: Leucocyte antibodies in sera from pregnant women. *Nature* 181:1735–1736, 1958.

110 Morton C: *Compendium Physicae.* Boston, Publications of The Colonial Society of Massachusetts, 1940, vol 33, 237 pp, p 4.

CHAPTER 21

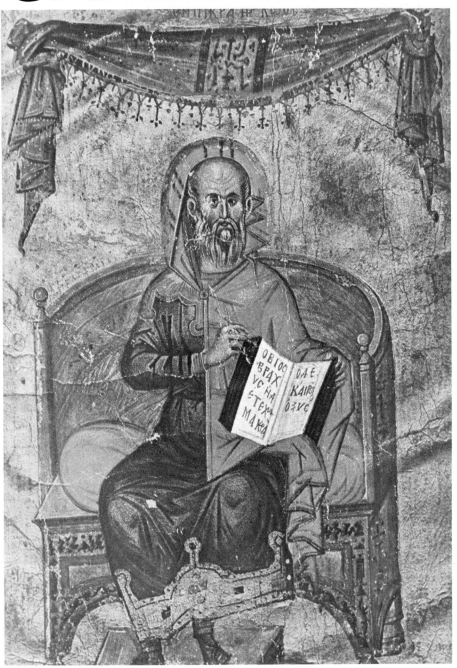

THE LESSONS OF HISTORY
Maxwell M. Wintrobe

E veryone who has read the preceding stories of discovery in what has come to be called the field of hematology—the early gropings in the midst of profound ignorance and the difficulties that confronted the investigators—must be impressed with their patience and their persistence, as well as the astounding consequences of their efforts. One marvels at the present-day outcome of the inquisitiveness of the early microscopists, the ramifications of Metchnikov's observations on the response of a starfish larva to the thorn of a rose (Chapter 13), and the fundamentally important outcome of the examination and description of a Jamaican student by an observant

Chapter Opening Photo   Hippocrates, as envisioned by a Byzantine artist in the fourteenth century. Hippocrates was born and taught on the island of Cos in the fifth century B.C. Until his time, medicine was based on magical arts and supernatural deities. In contrast, the teachings of the hippocratic school stressed facts and reasoning, systematic and thoroughgoing examination of patients, critical evaluation of results, and the utility of experience based on observation. Thus, for the first time a foundation for scientific medicine was established. *(Reproduced from Lyons AS, Petrucelli RJ II: Medicine, an Illustrated History. New York, Harry N. Abrams, 1978, by permission of Bibliotheque Nationale, Paris.)*

physician in Chicago, as described by Dr. Conley in Chapter 11. We have gained an understanding of biology that could hardly have been dreamed of only a short time ago, let alone at the time of the first tentative forays into the unknown. Moreover, understanding has been crowned by tangible benefits for humanity.

It is worthwhile to consider how such great progress comes about and why. How is knowledge achieved? This question has been disputed by historians of science[1] and by philosophers alike and has been the subject of much discussion.[2]

A simple answer is the concept of logical empiricism, which holds that the acquisition of knowledge is a strictly logical process. Theory leads to experiment, and experiment then confirms the concept, or results in its modification, each step or discovery naturally leading to the next. Writers of textbooks tend to present the past in this manner because pedagogically this is the easiest and most efficient way to present the current dogma.

Yet the first lesson to be learned of history is that the path of progress is anything but straight. It is rough and rocky and often seems to wander endlessly and in all directions; it has many blind alleys and is strewn with the debris of false hopes, of failures, and discouragement. The course of research has been likened to the flow of a stream that ultimately becomes a rushing torrent. A trickle here, a meandering flow of water there, go in one direction and another, seemingly without purpose. Finally a small stream is formed, and this is joined by other streams of equally unpretentious nature to form a river of ever-growing size that ultimately becomes an imposing waterway whose importance is obvious. This certainly has been the history of research in hematology.

It does not follow that, because a concept is plausible and is in accord with the understanding of the time, it is necessarily correct. The preceding pages provide many examples of misinterpretations resulting from such an assumption. Furthermore, because they have been plausible, such views often have endured and have stood in the way of acceptance of observations and interpretations that proved to be the correct ones.

Another lesson of history is that what was held to be the truth yesterday may not be so regarded today, and tomorrow the story may again be somewhat different.

Discovery begins with an observation or the posing of a question. But observation is not as simple as it sounds.

A third lesson of history is that many look, but few see. It is the exceptional person who recognizes the unusual event or manifestation. Still fewer pursue it to new understanding. Many may ask questions but few have the imagination, the energy, and the overpowering drive to persist in the search for an answer, especially when this must be done in the face of difficulties and failures and even in spite of scorn from their peers.

The unveiling of the truth is accomplished by the pursuit of ideas. The stuff of scientists, therefore, must include imagination and creativity. Coupled with these are intuition and confidence in their own insights and hypotheses. They cannot allow themselves to be easily dissuaded. As the preceding chapters have illustrated, it has been the individuals who have been endowed with these attributes and who were dogged in their quest who forged the paths and laid the milestones marking the history of hematology. To do this they not only collected facts and accurately recorded their observations but they persistently, stubbornly, and critically sought to comprehend.

The arrival on the scene of an individual with an inquisitive and imaginative mind, one who was determined in his inquiry, has been the key element in the advancement of knowledge about the blood. Such a person sought to decipher and interpret nature rather than to parrot the "Ancients." This person was the kind who, to quote Dwight Ingle,[3] rises "above that sizeable group of scientists who argue themselves out of venturesome thoughts and research and are limited to cut-and-dried projects of the sort which follow the pioneering of a bolder mind." Such a person treads new paths, undaunted by the opinions of others. As we have seen, Paul Ehrlich was one of these.

Imagination and industry alone, however, have not sufficed. Means have had to be devised to explore the questions that were posed. When these were provided, it is impressive to see what the introduction of a new technique made possible for an area of inquiry. Repeatedly, such an advance was like the planting of a seed, the acorn that ultimately becomes a giant oak, dispersing additional acorns into farther fields. Illustrating this point, as far as hematology is concerned, are the invention of the compound microscope, the introduction of the aniline dyes, the discovery of electrophoresis, chromatography and the "fingerprinting" of proteins, and, still more recently, the development of cell culture techniques and advances in cytochemistry and in microscopy.

Nevertheless, improvements in methods alone are not enough. The seed cannot grow unless properly nurtured. A suitable soil is essential. Leeuwenhoek with his microscope saw the red corpuscles of the blood, but his observations remained meaningless curiosities until the importance of oxidation in life processes was demonstrated and until hemoglobin, with its special properties, was discovered. The essential soil is science; technology is but the handmaiden of science.

Furthermore, the limitations of a technique must be recognized. As Dr. Tavassoli has shown so well in his chapter on the bone marrow, when scientists have exploited a methodology and have reached the boundaries of the potential of their method, they must be careful not to overstep "the circle of permissible conclusions." Unless at this stage new methods are developed, disagreement and confusion are likely to ensue.

Progress has depended, naturally, on the contributions of many. All investigators stand on the shoulders of their predecessors. Moreover, every scientific discipline has benefited from developments in other fields, progress in one field spurring another, and vice versa. The history of discovery is replete with examples. At first, the philosopher, the scientist, and even the physician were one and the same individual. In time, as knowledge grew, it became impossible for a single human being to encompass the whole, and the discovery and growth of understanding have become more and more dependent on interchange among scientific disciplines. Unfortunately, many times there has been a long delay between the development of insight in one field and its application in another. This is still true but much less so than it once was. The interdependence of the sciences has made it obvious that a broad cultivation of science is essential if advances are to be made. It follows that, in supporting scientific effort, one field must not be stressed to the exclusion or neglect of another. Many examples of these truisms are found in the preceding chapters.

We must recognize, also, that sometimes, especially in earlier days, humanity was the beneficiary of people who, uninhibited by the discipline of formal education and not influenced by the observations of others, simply allowed their curiosity free rein. Leeuwenhoek was that kind of person.

Likewise of importance has been the spirit of the times—the "climate of opinion."[4] This can exert a negative effect and discourage imagination, investigation, and innovation. It was pointed out in Chapter 1 that Galen's reputation was such that his views held sway for more than 14 centuries. His authority was rarely questioned. This can be explained in part by the importance of his anatomical contributions, the astuteness of his observations, and the wisdom of his teachings. But to a greater degree it is attributable to the prevailing acceptance of authority; as might be expected, many of Galen's concepts were erroneous and not free from contradictions. However, as Temkin points out, from childhood, medieval man was brought up to accept authority. This was no less true in his attitude toward events of the day and to the established social order, which he believed was divinely established, than in his acceptance of religious doctrine. Physicians also did not question authority. Truth was assumed to have been revealed in the past rather than being something that might be achieved in the future. As a consequence, for centuries Galen's teachings were blindly accepted. His erroneous ideas were given equal weight with his correct observations; no new authorities rivaled his teachings.

On the positive side, it is noteworthy how often it was during the most memorable periods of great intellectual ferment that many of the persons of whom we have written lived and worked. Thus, Hippocrates made his mark during the Golden Age of Greece, the period of its greatest philosophers, statesmen, historians, sculptors, dramatists, and poets. That was, incidentally, only shortly after Confucius and Zoroaster made their contributions of mind and spirit to the other side of the world. Similarly, in the mid-nineteenth century, when some independence of thought in medicine was evident, the political climate in Europe was one which encouraged people to challenge authority and to question traditional ideas. There, especially in the country in which a number of small states had just been united and was led by a man of Bismarck's stamp, the spirit was one of achievement. Both the political and the scientific environments were stimulating. Scholarship and research were greatly encouraged and esteemed, and facilities were provided for such endeavors.

Ehrlich turned out to be the outstanding medical scientist of them all, but there were at that time in Germany and also in France, England, and elsewhere others of considerable achievement. In a similar fashion, in the United States after World War I, a golden age of clinical investigation began for a determined few with the support of the Rockefeller Institute and the help of various other private foundations. After World War II, with the establishment of the research grants and of related programs of the National Institutes of Health, one could even say to young people contemplating careers in research that if they were imaginative and dedicated and were willing to work hard, they could count on long-term reasonable support for their investigations and for themselves and their families. The atmosphere became one that encouraged men and women who were dedicated to inquiry. The results of their efforts conducted in such circumstances have spoken for themselves. Such golden periods in the history of humanity, however, do not last forever. Expectations were exaggerated, the difficulties inherent in groping into the unknown have not been appreciated, patience has been taxed. Consequently, these and various social, economic, and political factors have taken their toll.

The preceding pages illustrate over and over again the fact that research for research's sake is a good investment and that basic science, even fundamental research that may seem abstruse and without hope of ultimate practical value, provides the essential foundation for advances that ultimately lead to better understanding, treatment, and even prevention of disease.

What role has serendipity, the lucky chance, played in the advancement of understanding? The anomalous behavior of the hemoglobin of the sickle-cell anemia red cell upon deoxygenation was clearly shown by Hahn and Gillespie in 1927[5]—but its significance was not appreciated at a molecular level until 1950.[6] Even so, it was only by chance that Pauling learned about the interesting but unexplained fact that sickled red cells appear birefringent in polarized light.[7] The story of the remarkable developments that followed, not only in regard to sickle-cell disease and other abnormal hemoglobin disorders but also in our understanding of another widely prevalent genetic disorder, thalassemia, as well as of human genetics and molecular biology is told in Chapters 11 and 12.

There are many other instances of capitalization on accidental occurrences or observations by keen observers and imaginative investigators. The way in which the feeding of spoiled sweet clover hay to cattle, resorted to by an impoverished farmer, led to the discovery of vitamin K, as recounted by Dr. Ratnoff (Chapter 18), is such an example.

But chance alone has played only a limited role. It is commonly stated that Alexander Fleming's discovery of penicillin was due to the accident of a spore of *Penicillium* floating onto his culture plates. However, the story of the discovery of penicillin which is usually presented misses the point. The chance observation in itself does not suffice—equally important is the prepared mind. The intruding spore was a stimulus to a prepared mind, not just a mischance, for the intrusion would have been unnoticed or disregarded by some other investigator. Alexander Fleming had been looking all his life for antibacterial substances, and consequently, "when by accident penicillin with its properties obtruded itself upon his attention, he was perfectly well attuned to recognize its potentialities."[8] Similarly, a brilliant physical chemist, when he learned about the birefringence of sickled red cells when deoxygenated, was led to explore the suggestion made to him by Castle that this might be due to some type of molecular alignment or orientation; he then went on to deeper insights.

Still another aspect of the progress of understanding is worth noting. It is not generally appreciated how often curiosity concerning an observation made at the bedside by clinicians has led to far-reaching investigations which ultimately enriched many diverse branches of science. The fact that the concept of molecular disease arose out of curiosity about the sickling of the blood of patients with sickle-cell anemia has been mentioned already. Curiosity concerning the cause of certain changes in the blood of several individuals of Italian extraction stimulated the study of mild and asymptomatic forms of what turned out to be the heterozygous inheritance of the thalassemia trait.[9] This observation played an important role in the explosion of knowledge about human genetics that began in the 1940s.[10]

There are many more examples of the part played by searching bedside observations and investigation. The way in which George Minot's concern for the victims of pernicious anemia and the studies initiated by his young assistant, Bill Castle, led to a revolutionary new approach in the field of hematology is described in Chapters 1 and 10. How clinical laboratory investigators applied the great advances made in the biological and physical sciences to the problems of increased red cell destruction and the anemias caused thereby is recounted by John Dacie in Chapter 8. The way in which the discovery and investigation of "experiments of nature"—abnormalities in individuals resulting from unique failures of normal biologic processes—have revealed new and until then unimagined vistas of the wondrous workings of nature is described in Chapters 5, 6, and 18, among others. As Diamond has pointed out in Chapter 20, it is astounding how many scientific and therapeutic advances resulted from the discovery of an abnormal red cell agglutinin in the serum of a mother of an infant with erythroblastosis fetalis.

It also is interesting to observe how often a search with one objective has led to totally unexpected results in another direction. Planners and "directors," in particular, need to be aware of this fact. An imaginative scientist cannot and should not be bridled. The history of science is replete with examples. As is described in Chapter 6, the discovery of G6PD deficiency and the subsequent illumination of red cell metabolism, as well as of various ill effects resulting from enzyme deficiencies of the red cell, were the result of scientific investigations that sought to learn why black troops were unusually sensitive to an antimalarial compound. Again, as mentioned in Chapter 1, the study for military reasons of a war gas, nitrogen mustard, was the key that opened the door to modern antitumor therapy. That the research eventuated so favorably was not just good luck. It is testimony to the quality of human observation, to the breadth of human imagination, and to the persistence of human curiosity.

The road builders, being human, have not always been farseeing and logical, moving steadily and directly to their goal, nor did they fail to make mistakes. Indeed, incorrect theories often have hampered the advance of knowledge, especially when these theories were widely disseminated and were pronounced by eminent authorities. Hewson's observations and ideas were truly remarkable; yet his concept that lymphocytes are transformed into red corpuscles in the spleen dominated thinking and created great confusion for more than a hundred years. Progress has been delayed by the worship of authority and by the failure to recognize or accept truth. As described in Chapter 3, even when Ernst Neumann and Giulio Bizzozero described the production of red blood cells in the bone marrow in 1868, for a number of years thereafter their observations were not accepted. The dominating influence of authority is not new to us, but, fortunately, mistaken concepts today no longer remain unchallenged quite so long.

It should be noted also that concepts that ultimately proved to be incorrect have on occasion initiated experimental advances which turned out to be of great significance.[11] It was mentioned earlier that the assumption which led to the use of liver in the treatment of pernicious anemia was wrong. The immediate result, fortunately, was the saving of many lives. It took another 20 years to discover vitamin B_{12}. In the delightful essay by Dwight Ingle entitled "Fallacies and Errors in the Wonderlands of Biology, Medicine and Lewis Carroll,"[3] the author points out that it is commonly assumed that a fallacy always leads to error. This is itself a fallacy.

It follows that authorities must be humble and novices skeptical.

References

1   Kuhn S: The structure of scientific revolutions, in *International Encyclopedia of Unified Science*, 2d ed. Chicago, University of Chicago Press, 1970, vol II, no 2, 210 pp.
2   Wade N: Thomas S. Kuhn: revolutionary theorist of science. *Science* 197:143–145, 1977.

3   Ingle DJ: Fallacies and errors in the wonderlands of biology, medicine, and Lewis Carroll. *Perspect Biol Med* 15:254–281, 1972.
4   Temkin O: Scientific medicine and historical research. *Perspect Biol Med* 3:70–85, 1959.
5   Hahn EV, Gillespie EB: Sickle cell anemia. A report of a case improved by a splenectomy. Experimental study of sickle cell formation. *Arch Intern Med* 39:233–254, 1927.
6   Harris JW: Molecular orientation in sickle cell hemoglobin solutions. *Proc Soc Exp Biol Med* 75:197–201, 1950.
7   Wintrobe MM: Anemia, serendipity, and science. *JAMA,* 210:318–321, 1969.
8   Medowar P: Scientific method in science and medicine. *Perspect Biol Med* 18:345–352, 1975.
9   Wintrobe MM, Matthews E, Pollack R, Dobyns BM: A familial hemopoietic disorder in Italian adolescents and adults. *JAMA* 114:1530–1538, 1940.
10 Neel JV: Human genetics, in Bowers JZ, Purcell EF (eds): *Advances in American Medicine, Essays at the Bicentennial.* New York, Josiah Macy Jr Foundation, 1976, vol I, 457 pp, p 62.
11 Robb-Smith AHT: The advantages of false assumptions. *Oxford Med Sch Gaz* 1:2, 1–50, 1949–1950.

EXPOSITION AND GLOSSARY

Insofar as possible, technical terms employed in the preceding chapters have been explained as they have been used. Nevertheless the reader may find it helpful to have readily available definitions of some of the words that are used frequently in the text. In addition, the following explanation of the hematopoietic system may be found helpful.

The terms commonly used to denote blood production derive from the Greek stems "hemo" (or "hemato"), meaning blood, "cyte" or ("cyto"), meaning cell, and "poiesis," meaning production. Thus, the term *hemopoiesis* is a contraction of hemo-cyto-poiesis, denoting blood cell production; *erythropoiesis* denotes red blood cell production; *thrombocytopoiesis*, platelet (thrombocyte) production; and *leukopoiesis*, white blood cell production.

Hemopoiesis involves both cell multiplication (often denoted *proliferation*) by cell division or *mitosis* and the progressive *maturation* (also denoted *differentiation*) of cells as they acquire the physical, chemical, and functional features of mature, functional cells. Cells that are not fully differentiated (mature) are called precursor cells; some of these are capable of division; each of the various stages of maturation, recognizable microscopically, is denoted by a certain term.

The term *blast cell* denotes the earliest form of immature precursor; if the blast cell has certain microscopic stigmata, it may be subclassified as an *erythroblast,* a *myeloblast,* or a *lymphoblast,* the earliest identifiable stages of the red cell series, the granular leukocyte series, and the lymphocyte series, respectively. The term *stem cell* is used to designate those immature cells that are the sources of the various hemic elements; that is to say, stem cells not only produce blood elements which circulate as mature cells after several successive divisions and maturational steps, but they maintain their capability of replenishing blood cells indefinitely. Some stem cells are believed to be restricted to providing only one or very few of the various mature cell lineages; others have been shown to be capable of providing all of the various cell lineages. The latter are denoted *pluripotent* or *pluripotential* stem cells.

This complex system of hemopoiesis daily provides billions of differentiated functional blood cells essential to life. The process has to be closely controlled. There are chemical signal or control systems ("feedback loops") from various parts of the body, both positive (stimulatory) and negative (inhibitory), that help to regulate the rate of production of various cell types. Those chemical stimuli that signal the blood-forming tissue to increase cell production (-poiesis) are denoted as *poietins.* Thus, *erythropoietin* has been shown to be the hormonal stimulus calling for increased erythropoiesis (Chapter 9). *Thrombocytopoietin* and several *granulocytopoietins* and *monocyto-poietins* have been postulated and, to some extent, demonstrated.

The hematologist uses certain general terms to denote abnormalities in blood cell number (or concentration). *Erythrocytosis* (and/or polycythemia), *thrombocytosis,* and *leukocytosis* (subdivided into neutrophilic, eosinophilic, basophilic, monocytic, lymphocytic) denote, respectively, increased numbers of circulating red blood cells, platelets, or various white blood cells. *Anemia, thrombocytopenia,* and *leukopenia* (again with various subcategories) denote, respectively, decreased numbers of circulating red blood cells, platelets, or various white blood cells.

Terms referring to white blood cells and their precursors are the following: *myeloblast, promyelocyte, myelocyte* (these cells are capable of cell division), *metamyelocyte (juvenile), banded cell* (or *stab* form, referring to the cell nucleus, which is elongated and indented but not segmented), *segmented* or *polymorphonuclear* granulocytes (nucleus divided into segments joined by filamentous strands). The last of these is the mature form of this cell, which circulates and enters various body tissues. *Granulocytes* are so denoted because of their content of granules that contain various enzymes and other substances necessary to their function. These granules are denoted as *lysosomes* (see Chapter 13). The granulocytes are subdivided into *neutrophils, eosinophils,* and *basophils,* according to whether they stain neutral, pink, or blue with stains containing certain dyes. *Mast cells* are tissue-fixed cells that resemble basophils.

Both granulocytes and monocytes are capable of engulfing foreign material by a process of *phagocytosis*, whereby the engulfed material is enclosed within a vacuole lined by a portion of the cell's membrane. This process is imperative in the body's defense against living bacteria, fungi, or viruses, which may invade the body to cause infection, and precedes the killing of the microbe within the phagocytic cell (*microbicidal* action). *Monocytes*, which are believed to derive normally from the same stem cell as granulocytes, mature into various types of *macrophages*, cells so named because of their capacity to engulf and store large particles of foreign material. Macrophages engulfing body cells are denoted *histiocytes*; if the engulfed cells are erythrocytes, the process is called *erythrophagocytosis*. The bodywide tissue capable of phagocytosis and immune expression is known as the *reticuloendothelial or monocyte-phagocyte system.*

Macrophages are aided in their antimicrobial action by soluble protein molecules present in blood plasma that are known as *antibodies*. Antibodies are produced by *plasma cells (plasmacytes)*, which are morphologically distinctive derivatives of certain lymphocytes (B lymphocytes). The antibodies are produced by the encounter of these cells with foreign material containing chemical characteristics recognized by the body's immune apparatus as "foreign," a characteristic of an *antigen*. The production and secretion of antibody by plasma cells reacting to antigen often requires interaction with macrophages which have digested the foreign material, a process often denoted *antigen processing*. The effect of the antibody on the foreign material is often to render it more susceptible to phagocytosis; the term often used for such antibody effect on antigenic material is *opsonin* (from the Greek *opsonein*, "to buy victuals"). Phagocytic granulocytes and monocytes or macrophages have the capacity of purposeful movement (-taxis) by extension and retraction of pseudopods in response to chemical stimuli, a process known as *chemotaxis*. Their movement through the endothelial lining of small blood vessels is called *diapedesis*. Phagocytic cells are also influenced in their migration and function by secretions derived from other lymphocytes (T lymphocytes, see below) responding to foreign antigens. These other secretions are grouped under the general heading of *lymphokines* and include *transfer factor, migration inhibition factor* (MIF), *eosinophil chemotactic factor,* and other poorly defined substances. Phagocytic cell function is importantly influenced by the activation of a complex system of soluble proteins in blood plasma known collectively as *complement* (complementary to cellular defense). The complement system is activated by events such as microbial invasion.

Lymphocytes play a central role in the body's defensive reactions; that is, in immune responses. All lymphocytes ultimately arise from precursors in the bone marrow, but according to their subsequent pathway of differentiation lymphocytes can be classified as B lymphocytes and T lymphocytes. *B lymphocytes* are stimulated by antigen (usually with the help of T lymphocytes) to give rise to antibody-secreting plasma cells. They are able to react to antigen because they display antibody molecules as receptors on their surface membrane. The letter *B* denotes their origin in birds in a special lymphatic organ near the anal end of the gut, termed the *bursa of Fabricius*. In many respects this resembles the thymus.

T lymphocytes are cells which have been processed or "educated" in the thymus by the influence of thymus epithelial cells on incoming migrants from the bone marrow. (The *thymus* is a mass of lymphopoietic tissue located in the upper chest or neck of mammals.) After being dispersed from the thymus to the spleen and to lymph nodes and other sites these T cells can react to antigen and divide and differentiate further to give rise to clones of sensitized T cells. (A *clone* of cells is produced by repeated division of a single cell. All the members of a clone are generally identical.) Sensitized T lymphocytes do not secrete antibody but can implement immune reactions by a radically different mechanism called *cell-mediated immunity*. This demands the physical contact of sensitized T cells and antigen (for example, in the skin) and is one reason for the remarkable widespread migration of lymphocytes between the blood and many tissues. One demonstration of cell-mediated immunity is the inflammation following the injection of tuberculin into an immune subject (*delayed hypersensitivity*).

Lymphocytes and their precursors are distributed from the marrow and thymus to the blood whence they enter most tissues of the body. The proliferation of B and T lymphocytes usually takes place in the spleen and in lymph nodes. The latter are found in many parts of the body. Their architecture is designed to facilitate the access of large numbers of T and B lymphocytes to antigen-laden macrophages.

An essential feature of the immune system is that an antigen alters the body's capacity to respond to a second encounter with the same antigen without affecting other immune capacities. Generally, a faster and more vigorous response ensues (*immunological memory*), but under certain circumstances, particularly in embryonic life, antigen can induce a state of unresponsiveness confined to that specific immune response (*immunological tolerance*).

Terms referring to red cells are *normoblast*, the nucleated stage found normally in the bone marrow and not in the blood; *reticulocyte*, a later stage in red cell development in which the nucleus has been lost, although the cell still contains some reticular remnants of the nucleus; and *red blood corpuscle*, the nonnucleated form that is the normal constituent of the blood. The red corpuscle is composed chiefly of *hemoglobin*, the pigment which has the unique property of binding oxygen, thereby to transport it throughout the body.

Red blood cells normally are of uniform size and shape but in disease may vary in size (*anisocytosis*) or shape (*poikilocytosis*) or may manifest a slightly varied and bluish tint (*polychromatophilia*) when stained with Wright's or Giemsa's stain. In disease, red cells may be spherical (*spherocyte*) or be of other shapes (elliptical, etc.). The large, immature nucleated red cell characteristically seen in the bone marrow in pernicious anemia is known as a *megaloblast.*

Platelets, the tiny nonnucleated structures found in the blood that are involved in the process of blood coagulation and in maintaining the integrity of the blood vessels are formed in the bone marrow from the cytoplasm of very large, usually multinucleated cells known as *megakaryocytes.*

The clotting of blood, *coagulation,* is the ultimate consequence of the interaction of a number of factors, most of which now are designated by Roman numerals and, in most instances, have been given names as well, e.g., factor I, fibrinogen. These are discussed in Chapter 18.

adoptive transfer: The transfer of a certain immune capacity by injecting living lymphocytes from one animal into another.

adrenal cortical hormones: Hormones secreted by the cortex of the adrenal gland.

agglutination: A phenomenon consisting of the collection into clumps of the cells distributed in a fluid, caused by specific substances called agglutinins, the molecules of which become attached to the cells.

agglutinin: An antibody present in plasma which produces agglutination or clumping of red cells containing a susceptible agglutinogen or antigen (e.g., an anti-Rh agglutinin acting on Rh positive red cells).

allele: One of a pair, or of a series, of variants of a gene having the same locus on homologous (i.e., corresponding in structure or function) chromosomes.

anephric: Without a kidney.

anisocytosis: Inequality in the size of erythrocytes.

antibody: One of a class of substances, natural or induced by exposure to an antigen, which have the capacity to react as agglutinins, lysins, or precipitins with the specific or related antigens. In the serum, they are intimately associated with certain globulin fractions.

antigen: Any substance eliciting an immunologic response, such as the production of antibody specific for that substance.

autoagglutinin: An agglutinin contained in the serum of an individual which causes an agglutination of his own erythrocytes.

basophil: A cell showing an affinity for basic dyes.

basophilic stippling: Bluish or bluish black granules in red cells stained by Wright's or similar stains.

blood film or blood smear: Preparation of blood for microscopic study, made by spreading it on a glass slide or cover slip.

chemotaxis: The response of organisms to chemical stimuli; attraction toward a substance is positive and repulsion is negative chemotaxis.

chromatin: The chromosomal material in a nucleus that readily stains with nuclear stains.

chromatography: The procedure by which a mixture of substances is separated by fractional extraction or adsorption or ion exchange on a porous solid (such as a column of aluminum oxide or filter paper) by means of one or more flowing liquid or gaseous solvents, especially by the process of partition chromatography. The principal types of chromatography are: column, gas, paper, and thin-layer.

chromosome: Any one of the separate, deeply staining bodies, commonly rod-, J- (or L-), or V-shaped, which arise from the nuclear network during mitosis and meiosis. They carry the hereditary factors (genes) and are present in constant number in each species. In humans, there are 46 in each cell except in the mature ovum and sperm, where the number is halved. A complete set of 23 is inherited from each parent.

clone: A group of cells derived from a single cell by repeated mitoses.

complement: Any one of a group of at least nine factors, designated C'1, C'2, etc., that occur in the serum of normal animals, enter into various immunologic reactions, are generally absorbed by combinations of antigen and antibody, and, with the appropriate antibody, may lyse (break down) erythrocytes, kill or lyse bacteria, enhance phagocytosis and immune adherence, and exert other effects. Complement activity is destroyed by heating the serum at 56°C for 30 minutes.

cryoprecipitate: A precipitate (e.g., of a protein) produced by a low temperature process.

cupping: A method of bloodletting by means of the application of cupping glasses to the surface of the body.

cytolytic: Adjective form of cytolysis—the disintegration or dissolution of cells.

cytoplasm: The protoplasm of a cell other than the nucleus.

dendritic: Branching in treelike or rootlike fashion.

diapedesis: The passage of blood cells through unruptured vessel walls into the tissues.

DNA (deoxyribonucleic acid): Any of the high molecular weight polymers of deoxyribonucleotides, found principally in the chromosomes of the nucleus; varies in composition with the source; able to reproduce in the presence of the appropriate enzyme and substrates; bears coded genetic information.

electrolyte: A substance which in solution is capable of conducting an electric current, and is decomposed by it.

electrophoresis: The migration of charged colloidal particles through the medium in which they are dispersed when placed under the influence of an applied electric potential.

embolism: The occlusion of a blood vessel by an embolus, such as a blood clot, causing various syndromes depending on the size of the vessel occluded, the part supplied, and the character of the embolus.

endothelium: The cell layer lining the inside of blood vessels and lymphatics.

enzyme: A catalytic substance, protein in nature, formed by living cells and having a specific action in promoting a chemical change.

eosinophil: A type of granulocytic cell of the peripheral blood or bone marrow whose granules stain red with eosin or other acid dyes.

epithelium: A tissue composed of contiguous cells with a minimum of intercellular substance. It forms the outer layer of the skin and lines hollow organs and all passages of the respiratory, digestive, and genitourinary systems.

erythroblastosis fetalis: A condition which becomes manifest late in fetal life or soon after birth with excessive destruction of red blood cells and extensive compensatory overdevelopment of erythropoietic tissue. It may occur as a result of transplacental passage of an anti-Rh agglutinin produced in an Rh-negative mother who has been immunized by the Rh-positive red cells of the fetus or by a transfusion of Rh-positive blood.

erythrophagocytosis: The ingestion of an erythrocyte by a phagocytic cell, such as a blood monocyte or a tissue macrophage.

erythropoiesis (erythrocytopoiesis): The formation or development of erythrocytes.

erythropoietin: A humoral substance concerned in the regulation of erythrocyte production, found in a variety of animals including humans, and characterized as a glycoprotein migrating in blood plasma with α_2-globulins.

etiology: The study of the causation of diseases.

eukaryotic: Pertaining to an organism with a true nucleus, in contrast to bacteria and viruses.

fibrinogen: A protein of the globulin class present in blood plasma and serous transudations; the soluble precursor of fibrin.

gene: A hereditary factor; the unit of transmission of hereditary characteristics, capable of self-reproduction, which usually occupies a definite locus on a chromosome. Genes, in general, are constituted of DNA, although in some viruses they consist of RNA.

genotype: The hereditary constitution of an organism resulting from its particular combination of genes.

granulocyte: A mature granular leukocyte; especially, a polymorphonuclear leukocyte, either eosinophilic, basophilic, or neutrophilic.

granulopoiesis (granulocytopoiesis): The process of development of the granular leukocytes, occurring normally in the bone marrow.

hematocrit: The special tube in which blood cells are separated by centrifugation.

hematuria: The discharge of urine containing blood.

hemic: Pertaining to or developed by the blood.

hemoglobin: The respiratory pigment of erythrocytes, that has the reversible property of taking up oxygen (oxyhemoglobin, HbO_2) or of releasing it (reduced hemoglobin, Hb), depending primarily on the oxygen tension of the medium surrounding it.

hemoglobinemia: The presence in the blood plasma of hemoglobin.

hemoglobinuria: The presence of hemoglobin in the urine.

hemolysin: An antibody which liberates hemoglobin from red blood corpuscles.

hemolysis: The destruction of red blood cells and the resultant escape of hemoglobin.

hemosiderin: An iron-containing glycoprotein pigment found in liver and in most tissues, representing colloidal iron in the form of granules much larger than ferritin molecules. It is insoluble in water and differs from ferritin in electrophoretic mobility. Pathologic accumulations are known to occur in a number of disease states.

heterozygote: A heterozygous individual (heterozygous = having the two members of one or more pairs of genes dissimilar).

histology: The branch of biology that deals with the minute structure of tissues.

homozygote: A homozygous individual (homozygous = having both members of a given pair of genes alike).

hyperkalemia: An elevation above normal of potassium in the blood.

icterus: The term for jaundice. When the amount of bilirubin, a conversion product of hemoglobin, is increased in the blood and deposits in the skin and in the mucous membranes, a yellowish discoloration results.

immunoglobulin: A generic name for antibody molecules regardless of the particular antigen for which they show specificity; abbreviated Ig.

isoagglutinin: An agglutinin which acts upon the red blood cells of members of the same species.

karyotype: The total of characteristics, including number, form, and size, of chromosomes and their grouping in a cell nucleus; it is characteristic of an individual, race, species, genus, or larger grouping.

leukocyte: One of the colorless, more or less amoeboid cells of the blood, having a nucleus and cytoplasm. Those found in normal blood are usually divided according to their staining reaction into granular leukocytes, consisting of neutrophils, eosinophils, and basophils, and nongranular leukocytes, consisting of lymphocytes and monocytes. Those found in abnormal blood consist of myeloblasts, promyelocytes, neutrophilic myelocytes, eosinophilic myelocytes, basophilic myelocytes, lymphoblasts, and plasma cells. Synonyms: white blood cell, white corpuscle.

leukocytosis: An increase in the leukocyte count above the upper limits of normal.

leukopenia: A decrease below the normal number of leukocytes in the peripheral blood.

leukopheresis: The removal from a donor of a quantity of leukocytes, followed by return to him or her of the remaining portions of the withdrawn blood.

lymph: The fluid in the lymph vessels.

lymph node: Masses of lymphatic tissue 1 to 25 mm long, often bean-shaped, intercalated in the course of lymph vessels, more or less well organized by a connective tissue capsule and trabeculae into cortical nodules and medullary cords, which form lymphocytes, and into lymph sinuses, through which lymph filters, permitting phagocytic activity of reticular cells and macrophages.

lymphatic: A vessel conveying lymph.

lymphopoiesis: The genesis of lymphocytes.

macrocyte: An erythrocyte having either a diameter or a mean corpuscular volume (MCV), or both, exceeding by more than two standard deviations that of the mean normal, as determined by the same method on the blood of healthy persons.

macrophage: A phagocytic cell belonging to the reticuloendothelial system. It has the capacity for accumulating certain aniline dyes, as trypan blue or lithium carmine, in its cytoplasm in the form of granules.

megakaryocyte: A giant cell of bone marrow, 30 to 70 μm, containing a large, irregularly lobulated nucleus; the progenitor of blood platelets. The cytoplasm contains fine azurophil granules.

mesenchyme: The portion of the mesoderm that produces all the connective tissues of the body, the blood vessels and the blood, the entire lymphatic system proper, and the heart; the nonepithelial portions of the mesoderm.

mesoderm: The third germ layer, lying between the ectoderm and entoderm. It gives rise to the connective tissues, muscles, urogenital system, vascular system, and the epithelial lining of the coelom.

mesothelium: The simple squamous epithelium lining the pleural, pericardial, peritoneal, and scrotal cavities.

molecule: A minute mass of matter; the smallest quantity into which a substance can be divided and retain its characteristic properties.

monocyte: A large mononuclear leukocyte with a more or less deeply indented nucleus, slate-gray cytoplasm, and fine, usually azurophilic granulation; the same as, or related to, the large mononuclear cell, transitional cell, resting wandering cell, clasmatocyte, endothelial leukocyte, or histiocyte of other classifications.

monophyletic: Pertaining to, or derived from, a single original ancestral type.

morbidity: The quality or state of being diseased.

neoplasm: An aberrant new growth of abnormal cells or tissues; a tumor.

nephrectomy: Excision of a kidney.

neutropenia: A decrease below normal in the number of neutrophils per unit volume of blood.

neutrophil: Neutrophil leukocyte.

nucleic acid: One of a group of protein-combining compounds found in nuclei and cytoplasm which on complete hydrolysis yields pyrimidine and purine bases, a pentose sugar, and phosphoric acid.

nucleolus: A small spherical body within the cell nucleus.

nucleoprotein: A protein constituent of cell nuclei consisting of nucleic acid and a basic protein.

nucleus: The differentiated central protoplasm of a cell; its trophic center.

oliguria: A diminution in the quantity of urine excreted.

parabiosis: The experimental fusing together of two individuals or embryos so that the effects of one partner upon the other may be studied.

pathogenesis: The origin and course of development of disease.

pathology: The branch of biological science which deals with the nature of disease, through study of its causes, its process, and its effects, together with the associated alterations of structure and function.

phagocyte: A cell having the property of engulfing and digesting foreign or other particles or cells harmful to the body. Fixed phagocytes include the cells of the reticulo-endothelial system and fixed macrophages (histiocytes). Free phagocytes include the leukocytes and free macrophages.

phenotype: (1) The sum total of visible traits which characterize the members of a group. (2) The visible expression of genotype.

phlebotomy: The opening of a vein for the purpose of letting blood.

phytohemagglutin: A protein extracted from beans that agglutinates red cells and, by an independent action, stimulates small T lymphocytes to enlarge and divide.

plasma: The fluid portion of blood or lymph, composed of a mixture of many proteins in a crystalloid solution and corresponding closely to the interstitial fluid of the body.

plasma cell (plasmacyte): A fairly large, generally ovoid cell. The nucleus is small and eccentric in position. The chromatin material is adherent to the nuclear membrane and arranged in clumps in a cartwheel fashion. The cytoplasm is agranular and deeply basophilic everywhere except for a clear area adjacent to the nucleus in the area of the cytocentrum.

plasmapheresis: The removal of blood, separation of plasma by centrifugation, and reinjection of the packed cells suspended in citrate-saline or other suitable medium. It is used as a means of obtaining plasma without waste of erythrocytes. It may also be helpful in treatment of certain pathological conditions.

pluripotent: Characterizing a cell or embryonic tissue capable of producing more than one type of cell or tissue.

poikilocytosis: Abnormality in shape of circulating erythrocytes.

polychromatophilia: The presence in the blood of polychromatophilic (susceptible to staining with more than one dye) cells.

polycythemia: A condition characterized by an increased number of erythrocytes.

polymorphonuclear: Having a nucleus which is lobated, the lobes being connected by more or less thin strands of nuclear substance; for example, the nucleus of a neutrophil leukocyte.

polyphyletic: Pertaining to origin from many lines of descent.

puerperal: Pertaining to, caused by, or following childbirth.

reticulocyte: An immature erythrocyte. Retention of portions of the nucleus accounts for the reticulated appearance when stained supravitally with cresyl blue or when viewed by phase microscopy. It is larger than a normal erythrocyte and usually constitutes less than 1 percent (range: 0.5 to 2.5 percent) of the total. There is an increase during active erythrocytopoiesis. In Wright- or Giemsa-stained blood films, these cells appear as polychromatophilic erythrocytes.

reticulocytosis: An excess of reticulocytes in the peripheral blood.

ribosome: A submicroscopic ribonucleoprotein particle attached to the endoplasmic reticulum of cells that is the site of protein synthesis in cytoplasm.

RNA (ribonucleic acid): Nucleic acid occurring in cell cytoplasm and the nucleolus, first isolated from plants but later found also in animal cells; contains phosphoric acid, D-ribose, adenine, guanine, cytosine, and uracil.

serum: The cell- and fibrinogen-free amber-colored fluid after blood or plasma clots.

sickle cell: A crescent-shaped erythrocyte found in a form of anemia occurring almost exclusively in blacks.

somatic cells: All the cells of the body except the germ cells.

somatic mutation: A mutation during the course of development in a somatic cell, resulting in a mosaic condition.

spherocyte: An erythrocyte which is spherical in form rather than biconcave.

testosterone: A male sex hormone; the principal androgen secreted by human testes.

thrombosis: The formation of a thrombus (thrombus = a clot of blood formed during life within the heart or blood vessels).

thymus: A structure composed mainly of lymphatic tissue, present in the upper part of the chest, which after growing until the second year of life remains stationary until about 14 years of age and then undergoes atrophy.

tritiated thymidine: A radioactive substance that is selectively incorporated into DNA during a certain phase of the cell-generation cycle; thus it labels only actively proliferating populations of cells and can be used to estimate the life-span of cells.

vital staining: In contrast to the usual method of staining of blood cells, as by Wright's or Giemsa stain, which requires their fixation and death, in vital staining the cell takes up the dye while still vital and is not injured by this.

NAME INDEX

Page numbers in *italic* indicate illustrations or tables; page numbers in **boldface** indicate main discussions.

737

SUBJECT INDEX

Page numbers in *italic* indicate illustrations or tables.

753

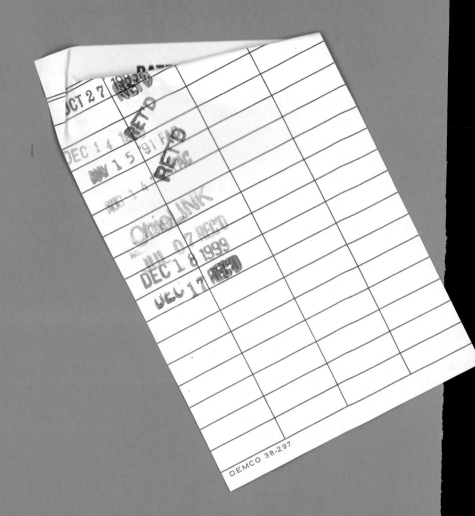